P9-AQE-911

research methods in health

foundations for evidence-based practice

DEDICATION

For my daughters,
Zoe Sanipreeya Rice and Emma Inturatana Rice

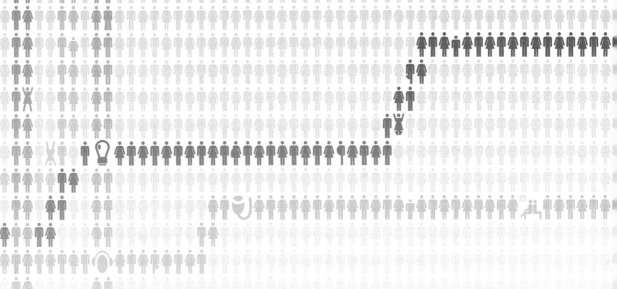

research methods in health
foundations for evidence-based practice

Edited by Pranee Liamputtong

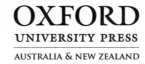

OXFORD
UNIVERSITY PRESS
AUSTRALIA & NEW ZEALAND

OXFORD
UNIVERSITY PRESS

Oxford University Press is a department of the University of Oxford.
It furthers the University's objective of excellence in research,
scholarship, and education by publishing worldwide. Oxford is a registered
trademark of Oxford University Press in the UK and in certain other
countries.

Published in Australia by
Oxford University Press
253 Normanby Road, South Melbourne, Victoria 3205, Australia

© Pranee Liamputtong 2010

The moral rights of the author have been asserted

First published 2010
Reprinted 2010, 2011

All rights reserved. No part of this publication may be reproduced, stored in a retrieval system,
or transmitted, in any form or by any means, without the prior permission in writing of Oxford
University Press, or as expressly permitted by law, by licence, or under terms agreed with the
appropriate reprographics rights organisation. Enquiries concerning reproduction outside the scope
of the above should be sent to the Rights Department, Oxford University Press, at the address above.

You must not circulate this work in any other form and you must impose this same condition on
any acquirer.

National Library of Australia Cataloguing-in-Publication data

Liamputtong, Pranee, 1955–
Research methods in health : foundation for evidence-based
practice / Pranee Liamputtong.
ISBN 978 0 19 556817 2 (pbk)
Bibliography.
Health—Research—Methodology.
Medical sciences—Research—Methodology.
Evidence-based medicine.
Research—Methodology.

610.7

Reproduction and communication for educational purposes
The Australian *Copyright Act 1968* (the Act) allows a maximum of one chapter
or 10% of the pages of this work, whichever is the greater, to be reproduced
and/or communicated by any educational institution for its educational purposes
provided that the educational institution (or the body that administers it) has
given a remuneration notice to Copyright Agency Limited (CAL) under the Act.

For details of the CAL licence for educational institutions contact:

Copyright Agency Limited
Level 15, 233 Castlereagh Street
Sydney NSW 2000
Telephone: (02) 9394 7600
Facsimile: (02) 9394 7601
Email: info@copyright.com.au

Edited by Venetia Somerset
Cover concept design by Luke Foley, Studio Overture
Text design by Ziegler Design
Typeset by Cannon Typesetting
Proofread by Liz Filleul
Indexed by Russell Brooks
Printed in Hong Kong by Sheck Wah Tong Printing Press Ltd

*Links to third party websites are provided by Oxford in good faith and for information only.
Oxford disclaims any responsibility for the materials contained in any third party website
referenced in this work.*

Brief Contents

Expanded Contents

PART I METHODS AND PRINCIPLES   1

1 THE SCIENCE OF WORDS AND THE SCIENCE OF NUMBERS: RESEARCH METHODS AS FOUNDATIONS FOR EVIDENCE-BASED PRACTICE IN HEALTH

Pranee Liamputtong

2 WHAT IS ETHICAL RESEARCH?

Paul Ramcharan

7   Using Grounded Theory in Health Research

Jemma Skeat

8   Phenomenology and Rehabilitation Research

Christine Carpenter

9   USING CLINICAL DATA-MINING AS PRACTICE-BASED EVIDENCE

Martin Ryan and David Nilsson

10   'CLEAR AT A DISTANCE, JUMBLED UP CLOSE': OBSERVATION, IMMERSION AND REFLECTION IN THE PROCESS THAT IS CREATIVE RESEARCH

Mark Furlong

PART III QUANTITATIVE APPROACHES AND PRACTICES   171

11 MEASURE TWICE, CUT ONCE: UNDERSTANDING THE RELIABILITY AND VALIDITY OF THE CLINICAL MEASUREMENT TOOLS USED IN HEALTH RESEARCH

Christine Imms and Susan Greaves

14   How Do We Know What We Know? Epidemiology in Health Research

Melissa Graham

15   CLINICAL TRIALS: THE GOOD, THE BAD AND THE UGLY

Karl B. Landorf

PART IV   EVIDENCE-BASED PRACTICE AND SYSTEMATIC REVIEW

16   EVIDENCE-BASED HEALTH CARE

Deirdre Fetherstonhaugh, Rhonda Nay and Margaret Winbolt

PART V   MIXED METHODOLOGY AND COLLABORATIVE PRACTICES   315

19   INTEGRATED METHODS IN HEALTH RESEARCH

Carol Grbich

20   THE USE OF MIXED METHODS IN HEALTH RESEARCH

Ann Taket

24 DATA ANALYSIS IN QUANTITATIVE RESEARCH

Jane Pierson

25 HOW TO READ AND MAKE SENSE OF STATISTICAL DATA

Paul O'Halloran

Figures and Tables

Preface

Globally, evidence-based practice (EBP) has become a major preoccupation of researchers and practitioners in health care. EBP lends itself neatly to the practice of some health practitioners, particularly those who rely on interventions in their practice. No doubt it is very useful for certain health researchers and practitioners, but the practice overemphasises certain kinds of research and undervalues or ignores other kinds that can contribute greatly to health practices. Politically, this has prompted many researchers to suggest that EBP is developed to privilege certain health researchers, practitioners and health practices. The main debate is the question of what type of evidence we need in health care practice. Of course not all evidence can be gathered from the approach advocated by EBP, and this is when we need to carry out our research to find appropriate evidence that will be suitable for our practice and our clients. This is the precise reason for writing this book.

In this book I bring together contributors who write about research methods that readers can adopt to find their evidence. I include both qualitative and quantitative approaches as we need to select the method that is appropriate for the questions we ask. I also include chapters on the mixed-methods research design so that readers can see that there are times when we need to consider both approaches in finding evidence we need. The volume also introduces ways in which we can make sense of the research data we have collected and instructions on how to write up the data in a more meaningful way.

In any piece of research, ethical issues are crucial. How do we carry out our research without harming our research participants? In our preoccupation with finding evidence, we may forget that there is another party that we must acknowledge, and we must design our research carefully so that they will not be harmed. Chapter 2 deals with this important matter. Also, researchers and practitioners have to find appropriate methods or approaches when dealing with disadvantaged groups, such as indigenous populations. How to work with marginalised people in our research endeavour is dealt with in Chapter 21.

In most textbooks on qualitative and quantitative research, the quantitative approach is treated first. To me this implies that qualitative research takes second place and confirms the common perception that it is a 'soft' science. By putting qualitative research first I am arguing that this approach is as legitimate as the quantitative one in the academic and practical worlds.

As in any good textbook, a Glossary is included at the end of this book. It should be noted that many of the entries in this Glossary are contested in the literature in terms of definition and use. Readers may find that some of the definitions that I use in this book are different from others, but they represent what writers refer to in their chapters. The margin notes are an abbreviated version of the relevant Glossary entry.

This book is intended as a foundation for evidence-based practice in health. It is written mainly for undergraduate students. Each chapter is provided with concrete or real examples.

Each chapter also contains 'Tutorial exercises' at the end, and most contain 'Try it yourself' boxes throughout, which will give students practice in using research to generate evidence. And each chapter provides further reading lists and websites that will also allow students to delve deeper into the methods and issues. Although the book is intended for undergraduates, it will also be useful for postgraduate students and novice researchers who need to make themselves more familiar with different types of research and the processes involved.

I wish to express my gratitude to many people who helped to make this book possible. First, I would like to express my thanks to the contributors, many of whom worked hard to deliver their chapters within the short time-frame that I set. I would like to thank the two reviewers who provided useful comments. I thank Debra James of Oxford University Press in Melbourne who believed in this book and helped to bring it to birth; I greatly appreciate her assistance. I wish to thank Jane Pierson who read one of the chapters that I wrote in this volume. My thanks also go to Tanya Serry, my PhD student and a colleague at La Trobe University, who assisted me with a few chapters that we wrote together. Her enthusiasm about working with me is greatly appreciated. Last, I thank my two children, Zoe Sanipreeya Rice and Emma Inturatana Rice, who understand the busy life of an academic mother.

Two chapters in this book reproduce sections that have been published in journals.

In Chapter 17, Table 17.1 is reproduced from Iles & Davidson (2006), Evidence based practice: A survey of physiotherapists' current practice, in *Physiotherapy Research International*, with permission from Wiley-Blackwell. In Chapter 26, an example from the journal *Sexual Health* (see Rawson & Liamputtong 2009) is used with permission from CSIRO Publishing. The link to this issue of *Sexual Health* is <www.publish.csiro.au/nid/166/issue/5048.htm>. An example from *Archives of Physical Medicine and Rehabilitation* (see Shields, Taylor & Dodd 2008) is used here with permission from Elsevier Science.

Pranee Liamputtong
Melbourne, June 2009

About this Book

This book contains twenty-six chapters and is divided into six parts. Part I contains two introductory chapters. The first, by Pranee Liamputtong, introduces issues relevant to evidence and evidence-based practice. It suggests that evidence can be obtained from different sources. It argues that the hierarchical system used in the EBP model privileges certain research methods and that not all evidence can be found in EBP. It follows with discussion on several salient points in carrying out research in the health sciences. These include the selection of the method appropriate to the questions for which researchers wish to find evidence. When asking qualitative and/or quantitative questions, researchers need to ensure that the method is selected appropriately. Each approach will provide different types of evidence and we should not assume that one approach can provide the best or all the evidence we need. Different ontological and epistemological positions adopted by qualitative and quantitative approaches are introduced in this chapter. Issues of rigour, validity and reliability within both approaches are crucial for good research and are included in this chapter. The last section is dedicated to sampling issues.

In Chapter 2, Paul Ramcharan outlines the emergence of the largely unregulated social research ethical frameworks and, by contrast, those associated with health and medical research that arose from the Helsinki Declaration. The convergence of the two discourses in the past decade is described and explained. This is supplemented by a consideration of the Australian NHMRC National Statement on Ethical Conduct in Human Research and the position of both the National Office for Research Ethics Committees and the Research Ethics Framework of the Economic and Social Research Council in the UK. The nature and principles of contemporary ethical frameworks are described and case studies are provided to highlight issues around anonymity/confidentiality, privacy, informed consent, dependence and vulnerability, data storage and potential conflicts of interest. Readers are given additional examples through which they might work using ethical principles and the seminal concepts of beneficence, non-maleficence, discomfort and justice. In these case studies, students are asked to work as researchers or together as a Human Research Ethics Committee (HREC) to come to a decision about the balance of risk and benefit in each case study. Remaining issues around ethical regulation are described and include the extent to which regulation is paternalistic; difficulties in maintaining independence of decision-making from conflicts of interest; contradictions between the need for clearly established protocols for decision-making versus research with emergent designs; issues around vulnerable groups; and the importance of ethics as process.

Part II commences with Chapter 3 on the in-depth interviewing method in health, by Tanya Serry and Pranee Liamputtong. They argue that among qualitative research methods, the in-depth interviewing method is the most commonly employed by qualitative researchers. Conversation, it is argued, is a fundamental means of interaction between individuals in society. Through conversation, people have an opportunity to know others, learn about their feelings, their experiences, and the world in which they live. The authors suggest that interviewing is a way of collecting empirical data about the social world of individuals by inviting them to talk about their lives in depth. In an interview conversation, the researcher asks questions and then listens to what people say about their dreams, fears and hopes. The researcher will then hear about their perspectives in their own words, and learn about their family and social life and work. Most people, including researchers, will say they know about in-depth interview method, or they have heard about it and it is not difficult to ask questions and talk to people. But as the authors suggest in this chapter, undertaking a good in-depth interview requires a lot more than knowing how to ask questions and talk to people. There are many things to consider and there are techniques that can be used to elicit detailed and accurate information from the research participants. The authors provide practical steps in doing in-depth interviews and case studies from their research in speech pathology and public health.

Chapter 4 is about the focus group method in health and nursing. Patricia Davidson, Elizabeth Halcomb and Leila Gholizadeh argue that focus groups are a useful strategy for obtaining the collective perspective of a group of individuals with common characteristics; they are also useful for studying issues and concerns about a topic that is not well known. Focus groups are particularly valuable in obtaining the views and perspectives of underrepresented and marginalised individuals and can be tailored to address contextual factors and concerns. Commonly, focus groups consist of 5–15 people who share their opinions and experiences about a particular issue with the guidance of a moderator. Focus groups can also promote interaction and encourage deliberation of crucial issues by stimulating group discussion. In health research, this method can be informative in exploring issues as well as providing an evaluation technique. This chapter discusses pragmatic issues in conducting focus groups and proposes strategies to ensure methodological rigour.

In Chapter 5, Linsey Howie writes about narrative enquiry in occupational therapy. She contends that the numerous methodologies comprising qualitative research can be confusing to the uninitiated health professional. Narrative enquiry is a research method used more recently in health science research to examine clients' thoughts and experiences of illness, interventions, rehabilitation and recovery, and service provision. In illuminating experience from a consumer's perspective, narrative enquiry enlarges our understanding of phenomena and engages participants in the research process. However, the potential for narrative research to inform health practice through the retrospective telling of events or experiences relevant to specific professions is not fully appreciated. The aim of this chapter is to provide a detailed account of narrative enquiry and the processes involved in the design and conduct of narrative studies that seek to establish the meaning of human experiences conveyed through stories. This chapter gives an outline of the method, its origins and uses in other disciplines, and an overview of the place of narrative within qualitative research. A clear account of sampling procedures, participant recruitment and engagement, data collection and analysis, with reference to key authors in this area of research, is presented using a step-by-step approach to demystify poorly understood aspects of this method.

Jon Willis and Karen Anderson discuss the use of ethnography in health research in Chapter 6. They suggest that ethnography focuses on describing and understanding the practices and beliefs of groups of people within the context of the shared cultures that structure and give meaning to their actions and interactions. From the health perspective, ethnography provides unique insights into the ways that patients understand illness and the struggle for health; the social contexts in which health practitioners are trained; the ways in which we organise and validate health-related actions, whether as consumers or practitioners; and how societies privilege particular models of health and illness, while dismissing others. In this chapter, the authors explore the origins of ethnography in early 20th-century anthropological practice, and chart its development as a methodological paradigm. Using examples, they demonstrate the array of tools and approaches that ethnographic methodology now encompasses in a range of social and health science disciplines. They explore in particular the influence of the Chicago School and the symbolic interactionists on the application of ecological principles in the ethnography of urban societies, as well as the impact of postmodernism, and the insights offered by cultural theory to our understanding of the circulation of health-related information, meanings and rationalities within complex social networks. Finally, they examine recent examples of ethnography in the area of health, including focused ethnography, institutional ethnography and ethno-nursing.

Chapter 7, by Jemma Skeat, is about using grounded theory in health research. Jemma points out that qualitative methods have been used in health professions such as speech pathology for many years to describe, interpret and better understand the perspectives of clients, families and clinicians. Grounded theory is a qualitative method that allows researchers to explore and explain social processes, structures and interactions. The focus for grounded theory research is on discovering the main concern of people in the situation, the processes that are at work for these people, and how these processes are maintained or limited. For example, health professionals could explore the goal-setting process from the client's perspective, in order to understand better how to negotiate this process with clients and provide client-centred care. There are several approaches to grounded theory, but each includes a core set of methods that researchers apply in order to develop an explanatory framework for the situation. The aim of this chapter is to introduce the grounded theory method, including the main techniques that distinguish it from other methods. The chapter begins with a brief description of the history of grounded theory, and a consideration of different modes or approaches. It then describes the steps to be taken in a grounded theory study—including theoretical sampling, constant comparison for analysis, and development of theory. An example of some of these steps is given using the authors' research. Potential uses of the method for understanding social processes and interactions in speech pathology, including examples of published research in the field, are also provided. As an example of its application, Jemma explores the potential uses of the method for understanding social processes and interactions in speech pathology, including examples of published research in the field.

Christine Carpenter, in Chapter 8, discusses phenomenology as a methodological approach to rehabilitation research. She contends that the aim of phenomenological research is to understand the lived experience of a phenomenon, for example spinal cord injury or physiotherapy services in the home, from the individual's perspective, and to examine the meanings they give to that experience. The choice of a particular method reflects the type of question being asked, and the method in turn contributes to a coherent and rigorous qualitative study design that includes data collection methods, participant recruitment, data analysis, and the role of the researcher. These design features are discussed and illustrated by drawing on research examples relevant to rehabilitation practice and physical therapy. In order to listen actively and genuinely to research participants' perspectives, researchers are required to reflect upon, and make explicit, their own understandings and beliefs about the phenomenon being studied, and this is examined in this chapter. Christine suggests that health care practitioners are required to be accountable in terms of the evidence supporting the clinical decisions they make on behalf of patients or clients. Evidence-based practice, as originally conceived, privileged a hierarchy of evidence derived primarily from experimental research. Practitioners recognised that this narrow definition of 'best' evidence did not reflect the complex issues involved in living with a chronic condition or disability, or of the model of patient-focused or client-centred and interdisciplinary approaches characteristic of rehabilitation practice. Qualitative research can make a significant contribution to the generation of evidence to support clinical reasoning and practice. This contribution is also discussed using examples of phenomenological research relevant to rehabilitation.

Chapter 9, by Martin Ryan and David Nilsson, presents the use of clinical data-mining as practice-based evidence for social workers. They argue that clinical data-mining involves the use and analysis of available clinical information research purposes. It is a form of practice-based research that is carried out by practitioners and is designed to inform and address practice issues. It is essentially a specific form of a secondary data analysis. It has been used by social work practitioners and other health professionals in a range of research studies. This chapter begins by defining this method, provides a context for its use, compares it to other research methods, and outlines its advantages and drawbacks for social work practitioners. The process involved in clinical data-mining is then outlined, followed by a case study using David's study of psychosocial problems faced by 'frequent flyers' in a paediatric diabetes unit in a children's hospital. As well as outlining the methodology and findings of the study, they provide a reflexive account of David's experience of using clinical data-mining in this example.

In Chapter 10, Mark Furlong argues that clinical and field-based observation has played a key role in developing much of the knowledge that is fundamental to good practice in the health and human service settings. Despite this contribution, the status of observation has receded as standardised models of data collection and results analysis—'hands off' research methods based on the idealisation of experimental distance—have become prevalent. Against this background, this chapter outlines a positive position for observation as a component of a mixed-model approach to research, outlines the decision points that require attention in the design and implementation of observational protocols and discusses the process of immersion that tends to occur when we engage intensively with the experience of observing.

Part III is dedicated to quantitative research methods and comprises five chapters. In Chapter 11, Christine Imms and Susan Greaves argue that health clinicians use tools frequently in clinical practice and during research. We use the data obtained to support practice, to understand the condition of the client, to determine intervention choices and measure change. We must know how and for what purpose these tools were developed so we can choose the right measure for our intended use. Understanding the psychometric properties of the tools we use is critical to knowing how much trust we can place in the findings. Christine and Susan point out that research studies that do this, that is, investigate the properties of clinical measurement tools, seek to evaluate aspects of validity and reliability. Validity studies aim to demonstrate that a measurement tool actually measures what it intended. Reliability studies evaluate the ability of the tool to measure consistently. Often, preliminary validity and reliability studies are conducted during development of a measurement tool, but as validity and reliability are not 'all or none' constructs, evidence about a tool's reliability and validity must be built over time. This places a requirement on the clinician to have the knowledge to be a critical consumer of validity and reliability studies. This chapter provides a basic framework to enable clinicians to become critical consumers of measurement studies. Readers are introduced to two theories of measurement development—classical test theory and item response theory—and are helped to understand the range of research studies required to develop a valid and reliable measure. They learn to critically appraise the research methods used to validate a clinical measurement tool and interpret reliability statistics. Reading this research critically will enable the clinician to determine the relative validity and reliability of the measurement tools they require in daily practice and as a result assist their selection of optimum tools for use with clients.

Miranda Rose's Chapter 12 is about single-subject experimental designs in the health sciences. This chapter covers salient issues relevant to single-subject experimental designs (SSEDs). It defines SSEDs, describes their history and the need for them, and contextualises them within the broader research design schema to highlight the phases and stages of research activity they are best suited to. The chapter describes the types of SSEDs commonly used in health science research. It discusses the statistical and visual analysis techniques commonly used in SSEDs, outlines their limitations, highlights current controversies in their implementation and analysis, and suggests possible future directions for their development. A practical case study and reflective account regarding the use of the method is provided. It also describes the use of a published SSED in the investigation of treatment efficacy for aphasic word retrieval impairments. The strengths and limitations of the design and analysis methods are also discussed. Last, alternative designs and the decision-making process in selecting a SSED are described.

Chapter 13, by Margot Schofield and Christine Knauss, introduces surveys and questionnaires in health research. Surveys are a very common descriptive research method.

They are particularly useful for collecting data about research phenomena that are not directly observable. This chapter provides an overview of the types of surveys used in health research, such as cross-sectional and longitudinal surveys, and describes how these relate to study aims and design. A variety of methods of administering surveys is described, including paper and pencil surveys, online surveys, and interviewer-administered surveys (face-to-face, telephone and internet formats). The relative advantages and disadvantages of the different methods are explored such as cost, time, facilities and the personnel required. The chapter also outlines key issues in survey design such as determining the topics to be covered by the survey, use of standardised scales (advantages and disadvantages), how to design questions and response options for surveys, how to sequence questions, use of screening questions, design of questions on sensitive topics, avoiding bias, and consideration of closed versus open-ended responses. Issues about validity and reliability of surveys responses are addressed and methods for checking validity and reliability outlined. Examples of both cross-sectional and longitudinal survey design are also provided.

In Chapter 14, Melissa Graham writes about epidemiology in health research. She argues that epidemiology is concerned with the study of the distribution and determinants of health states in populations. Epidemiology can help us to determine the extent of ill health or disease in the community; identify the cause of ill health and the risk factors for disease; understand the natural history and prognosis of ill-health; investigate disease outbreaks or epidemics; evaluate existing and new preventive and therapeutic programs and services; and provide the foundation for developing public policy and regulation. Essentially, this means that epidemiology can provide the answers to questions asked in the health sector, such as: how much disease is there?; who gets it?; where are most people affected?; when did they have it?; what happens over time? More important is how we as health professionals apply this to prevent and control health problems. This chapter aims to introduce readers to the underlying principles of observational descriptive and analytical epidemiology, drawing on examples from contemporary practice. It also introduces readers to sources of existing epidemiological data and discusses practical applications to help answer questions of person, place and time. A case study drawing on existing data is presented.

Chapter 15, by Karl B. Landorf, introduces clinical trials in health. Karl suggests that clinical trials that evaluate the effectiveness of interventions or treatments are abundant in the health sciences. It is essential that such evaluations ensure that the effects detected are directly attributable to the intervention being investigated and not to other extraneous causes. However, not all clinical trials provide the framework to achieve this. If poorly executed, they may provide invalid results, due to inherent bias or poor methodology. Often such trials—non-randomised or uncontrolled trials ('the bad' or 'the ugly')—overestimate the effectiveness of an intervention. Fortunately, there are methods to overcome this. For some time now, the randomised controlled trial has been considered the 'gold standard' when evaluating the efficacy or effectiveness of an intervention. There are two key features to a randomised controlled trial, which in its simplest form includes (1) comparison of a group that receives an intervention with one that does not, and (2) random allocation into those groups. The main aim of using randomised trials is to ensure as much as possible that the characteristics of the participants (people who receive the interventions) at the beginning of the trial are similar across groups. Nevertheless, some randomised trials fail to adhere to good design principles. As a consequence, if appropriate randomisation is not carried out adequately, bias, or systematic unwanted effects, will be present. This bias will ultimately affect the accuracy of the results of the trial, generally leading to an overestimation of the effectiveness of the intervention being evaluated. Accordingly, all trials are not created equal. Certain clinical trial designs provide more accurate results than others. Randomised controlled trials are considered the gold standard when evaluating the efficacy or effectiveness of interventions. However, if there is not enough attention to detail, results from such trials can also be biased or contain errors. To minimise such errors appropriate methods (e.g. allocation concealment and blinding) and planning (e.g. prospective sample size calculations and statistical analysis) are essential. Clinical trials should also be registered before commencement with a recognised trial register and the results reported on using the recommendations outlined in the CONSORT statement. By being aware of such matters, clinicians and researchers will assist in the process of improving the quality of clinical trials, thus encouraging a higher standard.

Part IV is about evidence-based practice and systematic review. It has three chapters. First, in Chapter 16, Deirdre Fetherstonhaugh, Rhonda Nay and Margaret Winbolt discuss evidence-based health care. They point out that basing practice on the best available evidence is now an expectation in health care. Nevertheless, finding and translating the evidence into practice poses significant challenges for health professionals. This chapter introduces readers to evidence-based concepts in health care, provides a potted history of its development and outlines methods used to locate and appraise the evidence. As most practitioners will be more involved in using the evidence than in primary research or research appraisal, the main focus of the chapter is on translating evidence into everyday practice. There are numerous known barriers to changing practice and these are outlined along with strategies that can be used to overcome them. A case study reporting the trials, failures and successes of translating evidence into practice with relevant activities assist readers to learn by doing. The chapter adopts a person-centred and interdisciplinary care approach.

Megan Davidson and Ross Iles, in Chapter 17, introduce evidence-based practice (EBP) in therapeutic health care. They point out that EBP is defined as the use of best research evidence, along with clinical expertise, available resources and patient's preferences to determine the optimal assessment, treatment or management option in a specific situation. The skills to be acquired for the evidence-based practitioner centre on the use of 'best research evidence'. The five-step EBP approach of Sackett is a widely used framework. Step 1 is to recognise a knowledge gap and formulate an answerable clinical question. The type of question—whether it relates to therapy effectiveness, prognosis, diagnosis or human experiences—dictates the type of research design that is best able to answer the question. In Step 2 the evidence-based practitioner searches for the available research that is best able to answer the clinical question. Important resources for this step include sources of 'pre-appraised' evidence such as clinical practice guidelines and systematic reviews. Databases such as the Cochrane Library, Clinical Evidence and PEDro (the Physiotherapy Evidence Database) are of most value, followed by abstracting databases such as Medline and Cinahl. In Step 3 the practitioner critically evaluates the research evidence against accepted quality criteria in order to determine how much influence the research evidence will have when considering Step 4. Step 4 is the integration of the research evidence with the other aspects of evidence-based practice (expertise, resources, patient preferences) that results in a practical clinical outcome. The final step, Step 5, is to reflect on Steps 1–4, seeking to improve one's effectiveness and efficiency as an evidence-based practitioner. In this chapter, Megan and Ross demonstrate, by an example of a therapy question and a diagnosis question, how the evidence-based physiotherapy practitioner might undertake the five-step process. They also present published surveys of physiotherapy practice that demonstrate that many practitioners do not have sufficient skills to undertake the five steps, and the implications this has for patients and clients of physiotherapists.

In Chapter 18 Nora Shields discusses how to conduct the systematic reviews often used in evidence-based practice. A systematic review is a comprehensive identification and synthesis of all relevant studies on a review question. It is conducted according to an explicit and reproducible method to minimise the risk of reviewer bias. Systematic reviews help health professionals cope with large volumes of literature by summarising it and providing more reliable evidence, which can aid clinical decision-making. They are also used by researchers to identify gaps and strengths of the current literature, assisting research design. Nora argues that the method of conducting a systematic review should be transparent, easily replicated and scientifically rigorous. This chapter offers sets out a six-step process for completing a systematic review, including how to set an answerable clinical question, search for relevant information, decide what should be included and excluded, assess the quality of the included studies, extract relevant data, synthesise the findings of your review and consider the relevance of your review to your clinical practice. The PICO method is recommended to assist with Steps 1–3. Throughout the chapter emphasis is placed on practical advice for students regarding decision-making and where to look for further information. Nora also suggests that despite the advantages systematic reviews offer, this method is not infallible. Areas where potential problems can arise such as sensitivity and specificity of the search strategy, validity of the quality assessment procedure, publication bias and data pooling and interpretation are discussed, so that care can be taken by the review to avoid some of the pitfalls inherent in this research method.

In Part V, chapters relevant to mixed-methods research are included. Chapter 19 presents the writing of Carol Grbich on integrated methods in health research. Carol contends that the nature of allied health with its multidisciplinary focus provides the best environment for a mix of methodological approaches in research. These enable the practitioner to give a wider overview of the setting or situation before going deeper into the reasons why, the experience of and the explanation of particular behaviours. This chapter attempts to clarify the range of mixes in methodological approaches that the health professional may find useful. In particular, parallel methods and the sequencing of methods are discussed together with indications of how these might be used within a range of methodological approaches such as ethnography, narratives, case studies and grounded theory. Multiple data sets can then be put together in order in a variety of ways to enhance the impact of such approaches.

In Chapter 20, Ann Taket introduces the use of mixed methods in health research. She suggests that the term 'mixed methods' can be understood in different ways. First of all, it can refer to different kinds of methods being used within a single study—often it is used to refer to mixing qualitative and quantitative methods—but it can also refer to mixing different kinds of qualitative method within a study. Second, it may refer to mixing that occurs at different stages in the research process, for example in data collection, in data analysis or indeed in both these stages. Third, we need to consider different modes or ways of mixing methods within a single study. Sometimes a research study is divided into a number of stages, carried out sequentially, so we may have a qualitative stage followed by a quantitative stage or vice versa; for example, a qualitative component, focus groups, may be used to help define and pilot a structured survey instrument. Sometimes the mixing is parallel—a qualitative component in a study runs alongside a quantitative one, without interaction, answering different research questions. Or the mixing may be a 'blend'—two (or more) interacting strands, answering the same research question(s). Ann then considers the different potential reasons for mixing different types of qualitative method: promoting choice and empowerment for research participants; enabling participation; accessing different research participants; and triangulation. She also discusses some of the issues involved in using mixed methods in health research, illustrated with examples taken from her own research. The chapter ends with a discussion of some of the challenges (or fears) expressed about mixed methods.

Collaborative participatory research with disadvantaged communities is presented by Priscilla Pyett, Peter Waples-Crowe and Anke van der Sterren in Chapter 21. In recent years the overwhelming evidence of the links between social factors and health inequalities has led to increasing calls for collaborative and partnership approaches to health research with disadvantaged and marginalised groups. Participatory action research (PAR) has a long tradition in developing countries and has been used in health research with many disadvantaged communities. In PAR, community members participate in research to bring about changes that will improve their circumstances. PAR involves a cycle of observe, reflect, plan, act, observe and so on. It is often used by consumer and advocacy groups or by practitioners carrying out evaluation of their programs. Academic research, on the other hand, because of the way it is funded, rarely includes sufficient time or financial resources to carry out the actions required of a PAR project. Collaborative participatory research (CPR) is a term used to describe a more practical approach to partnerships between academics or practitioners and the community groups they are researching. In CPR, participation by community members may vary from cooperating with and supporting the research team, through various levels of collaboration to full engagement as co-researchers. There is no doubt that CPR is more time-consuming than more conventional research methods. But it is also well established that CPR can increase the validity and improve the relevance of the research to the communities involved. This in turn increases the uptake of findings and the likelihood of results being of benefit to the communities. This chapter describes collaborative and participatory research methods for health research, focusing on research with Indigenous communities. It also discusses the ethical, methodological and practical challenges associated with CPR. The case study describes a collaborative project conducted with an urban Indigenous community organisation. The project was carried out in three phases: research, resource development, and training and dissemination.

Part VI is concerned with how to make sense of data and how to present it. In Chapter 22, Pranee Liamputtong and Tanya Serry discuss how to make sense of qualitative data. Once data have been collected, researchers need to organise the data in a more meaningful way. This is what qualitative researchers refer to as data analysis. Qualitative research has several ways of making sense of the data. The simplest and most common are content analysis and thematic analysis. The procedures for these data analysis methods are given in this chapter.

Chapter 23, by Tanya Serry and Pranee Liamputtong, introduces computer-assisted qualitative data analysis (CAQDAS). They argue that in this postmodern world, computers have extensively impacted on our lives, and not surprisingly, this is the case when we do research. For qualitative research, as in other fields of research, the use of computers has gained increasing prominence in both data collection and data analysis. Computer-assisted qualitative data analysis software or CAQDAS refers to a specifically designed program that can take over a substantial amount of the manual labour involved with analysing data. In this chapter, Tanya and Pranee briefly discuss some of the key functions available via CAQDAS. They also describe how they have adopted CAQDAS in their own research along with times when they have decided not to use it. However, they do not present a step-by-step approach to using CAQDAS, nor do they promote any one CAQDAS program over another. There is 'no industry leader' with regards to CAQDAS options. At the end of the chapter, they provide a list of alternative CAQDAS options for readers to explore.

In Chapter 24, Jane Pierson writes about data analysis in quantitative research. This chapter covers essential matters in analysing quantitative data: the place and purpose of quantitative data analysis in health research; selection of data analysis procedures; procedures for examining association and relationships between two or more variables (chi-square, bivariate correlation, and multiple regression); and procedures for examining differences between two or more measures of central tendency (t tests and non-parametric equivalents, ANOVAs and non-parametric equivalents, factorial ANOVAS, and post-hoc tests).

Paul O'Halloran, in Chapter 25, tells us about how to read and make sense of statistical data. He contends that reading and interpreting statistical data, whether it is original data from a computer package or data from a journal article, can be a considerable challenge to students and practitioners alike. Many people become overwhelmed by a mass of figures and are unclear about what specific pieces of information will aid their interpretation of the data. This can be a problem because with the adoption of evidence-based practice, the ability to interpret statistical data is an important skill for all health care professionals. The aim of this chapter is to give readers the background information and tools that will enable them to pinpoint the critical figures and issues when reading and interpreting statistical data. This is conducted by examining core issues related to interpreting statistical data within a health context. That is, a practical case study involving data that are pertinent to health professionals is used to illustrate key issues. Issues examined in the chapter include key issues when interpreting descriptive statistics (e.g. strengths and limitations of descriptive statistics and how to interpret means, standard deviations and confidence intervals); key issues when interpreting inferential statistics (e.g. how to interpret findings that are statistically significant and how to interpret findings that are *not* statistically significant); statistical versus clinical significance (e.g. amount of change, complete elimination of symptoms, and similarity with normative samples at the end of an intervention); and common errors when interpreting statistical data (e.g. overinterpretation of data).

The last chapter, Chapter 26, is about how to present our end product in qualitative and quantitative data. Pranee Liamputtong and Nora Shields point out that once researchers have conducted a piece of research, it is essential to put the information down on paper; we need to write about it. We need to write in order to disseminate our research findings so that other people can read and make use of them, whether for improving current health and welfare practices or using them as the basis for developing new research projects. In many cases, this not only completes the project but is also the best way to disseminate the findings to wider audiences. In this chapter, Pranee and Nora discuss some of the characteristics of qualitative and quantitative writing. They outline the styles of research report commonly used to disseminate findings drawn from both qualitative and quantitative research projects. There are a number of techniques to observe when writing good qualitative and quantitative research papers, and these are included in this chapter.

About the Editor

Pranee Liamputtong holds a Personal Chair in Public Health at the School of Public Health, La Trobe University, Melbourne, Australia. Pranee has previously taught in the School of Sociology and Anthropology and worked as a public health research fellow at the Centre for the Study of Mothers' and Children's Health (now Mothers and Child Health Research), La Trobe University. Pranee's particular interests include issues related to cultural and social influences on childbearing, childrearing, and women's reproductive and sexual health.

Pranee has published several books and a large number of papers in these areas. These include: *Maternity and Reproductive Health in Asian Societies* (with Lenore Manderson, Harwood Academic Press, 1996); *Asian Mothers, Western Birth* (Ausmed Publications, 1999); *Living in a New Country: Understanding Migrants' Health* (Ausmed Publications, 1999); *Hmong Women and Reproduction* (Bergin & Garvey, 2000); *Coming of Age in South and Southeast Asia: Youth, Courtship and Sexuality* (with Lenore Manderson, Curzon Press, 2002); *Health, Social Change and Communities* (with Heather Gardner, Oxford University Press, 2003). Her more recent books include *Reproduction, Childbearing and Motherhood: A Cross-Cultural Perspective* (Nova Science Publishers, 2007); *Childrearing and Infant Care Issues: A Cross-Cultural Perspective* (Nova Science Publishers, 2007); *The Journey of Becoming a Mother amongst Thai Women in Northern Thailand* (Lexington Books, 2007); *Population, Community, and Health Promotion* (with Sansnee Jirojwong, Oxford University Press, 2008); and *Infant Feeding Practices: A Cross-Cultural Perspective* (Springer, New York, 2010).

Pranee has published several research method books. Her first research method book is titled *Qualitative Research Methods: A Health Focus* (with Douglas Ezzy, Oxford University Press, 1999, reprinted in 2000, 2001, 2003, 2004); the second edition of this book is titled *Qualitative Research Methods* (2005, reprinted in 2006, 2007, 2008); and the third edition is authored solely by herself (*Qualitative Research Methods, 3rd edition*, 2009). Pranee has also published a book on doing qualitative research online: *Health Research in Cyberspace: Methodological, Practical and Personal Issues* (Nova Science Publishers, 2006). Her new books include *Researching the Vulnerable: A Guide to Sensitive Research Methods* (Sage, London, 2007); *Undertaking Sensitive Research: Managing Boundaries, Emotions and Risk* (with Virginia Dickson-Swift and Erica James, Cambridge University Press, 2008); *Knowing Differently: Arts-Based and Collaborative Research Methods* (with Jean Rumbold, Nova Science Publishers, 2008); *Doing Cross-Cultural Research: Ethical and Methodological Issues* (Springer, 2008); and *Performing Qualitative Cross-Cultural Research* (Cambridge University Press, 2010). She is completing *Focus Group Methodology: Principles and Practices* for Sage, London, which will be published in late 2010.

About the Contributors

Karen Anderson is a lecturer in Public Health at La Trobe University. She has recently completed a major ethnographic study of the way health promotion principles are deployed in the training and practice of Australian nurses.

Christine Carpenter was educated as a physical therapist in Liverpool, England, and attained her graduate degrees in Educational Studies at the University of British Columbia, Canada. Before becoming an educator and researcher, she worked as a physical therapist for over twenty years in rehabilitation settings, primarily with people who had sustained spinal cord injury. Her current research initiatives are focused on the long-term experience and quality of life issues involved with living with a disability or chronic condition. She has co-written three books on qualitative research and evidence-based practice for occupational and physical therapists.

Megan Davidson is an associate professor and Head of the School of Physiotherapy at La Trobe University. She has eight years' experience in curriculum design and teaching in evidence-based practice for physiotherapy students. Her education research interests are in the areas of interprofessional education, the assessment of clinical performance, and evidence-based practice. Megan has published eighteen papers in peer-reviewed journals, six books chapters and numerous conference papers.

Patricia Davidson is professor and Director of the Cardiovascular and Chronic Care Centre in the School of Nursing and Midwifery at Curtin University of Technology based at Curtin House in Sydney. Patricia is the President of the International Council on Women's Health Issues and Secretary of the International Network for Doctoral Education in Nursing. Her current research activities include models of delivering chronic care; development and evaluation of guidelines for palliative care of patients with heart failure; indigenous health; novel models of care in heart failure management; perspectives of cultural diversity in heart disease; prevention and management and women. She is particularly interested in methods of research that engage vulnerable and marginalised communities.

Deirdre Fetherstonhaugh is the Deputy Director of the Australian Centre for Evidence Based Aged Care (ACEBAC) at La Trobe University. Her research focuses on the translation and implementation of research evidence into practice; the ethical implications of clinical practice; and the conceptualisation and operationalisation of person-centred care.

Mark Furlong is a senior lecturer in the School of Social Work and Social Policy, La Trobe University, where he has worked since mid 1995. Before commencing at La Trobe, Mark undertook direct practice roles for almost twenty years with a particular emphasis on work with families in mental health, disability and child protection. In addition to discipline specific and multidisciplinary teaching and training, Mark has had extensive experience providing secondary consultation. Mark's academic interests are diverse and include researching 'the relationship between casework and counselling', 'case management', 'agency-based practice', 'confidentiality', 'working with men' and 'blame'. He has published in social work, psychiatric, family studies, family therapy, psychotherapeutic, primary health and left-leaning journals.

Leila Gholizadeh is a lecturer at the University of Technology, Sydney and Tabriz University of Medical Sciences. She completed her Master's degree at Tabriz University of Medical Sciences in 1999 and her PhD at the University of Western Sydney in 2009. She is interested in mixed method research and has used this methodology in her PhD project to study the relationship between perceived and estimated absolute risk of cardiovascular disease in Middle Eastern women.

Melissa Graham is a senior lecturer in epidemiology and health research methods at Deakin University. Her area of interest is women's reproductive health, specifically the role of reproductive health on social exclusion, the impact of hysterectomy on health and well-being, the determinants of reproductive health, and the experience of and impact of childlessness on health.

Carol Grbich is a professor in the School of Medicine at Flinders University. She is author of several texts on qualitative research approaches including *Qualitative Research in Health: An introduction*, Prentice Hall 2004; *New Approaches to Social Research*, Sage 2004; and *Qualitative Data Analysis*, Sage 2007. She is also the foundation editor of the *International Journal of Multiple Research Approaches*.

Susan Greaves is Senior Occupational Therapist (Neurodevelopment) at the Royal Children's Hospital and is currently a PhD student at La Trobe University. Her PhD project is the development of a bimanual outcome measure for young infants with hemiplegic cerebral palsy.

Elizabeth Halcomb is a senior lecturer at the University of Western Sydney who completed her PhD in 2006. For her doctoral thesis, Elizabeth conducted a mixed methods project that explored the role of the general practice nurse in chronic heart failure management. She has published 38 papers in peer-reviewed journals since 2001 and has co-authored a book chapter entitled 'Mixed methods Research'. She is co-editor of *Mixed Methods Research for Nursing and the Health Sciences*, published by Wiley-Blackwell in 2009.

Linsey Howie is Head of the School of Occupational Therapy and Deputy Dean of the Faculty of Health Sciences at La Trobe University. She has a keen interest in qualitative research methods and has used narrative inquiry in her own research and that of Honours and postgraduate students she supervises. Linsey strongly believes in the need to support beginning researchers to fully appreciate the methodological principles associated with qualitative research.

Ross Iles is a lecturer and fourth-year coordinator at the School of Physiotherapy at La Trobe University. His interest in physiotherapists' use of evidence-based practice formed the basis of his Honours thesis and he now teaches evidence-based practice to fourth-year physiotherapy students. He is currently undertaking a PhD examining the impact of recovery expectation in recovery from low back pain. He has published three papers in peer-reviewed journals.

Christine Imms' research encompasses intervention effectiveness and outcome measurement for children. She is a lecturer in the School of Occupational Therapy at La Trobe University, and Senior Occupational Therapist (Research) at the Royal Children's Hospital, Melbourne.

Christine Knauss is a research fellow in the Department of Counselling and Psychological Health, School of Public Health, La Trobe University. She completed her PhD in the area of body dissatisfaction in adolescent boys and girls in the Department of Developmental Psychology, the University of Bern, Switzerland. Christine has worked in several research projects in Switzerland and Australia, ranging from eating disorders, evaluation of psychotherapy and school suspension.

Karl B. Landorf is a senior lecturer and research coordinator within the Podiatry Department at La Trobe University. He is also Group Leader of the Foot and Ankle Research Group within the Musculoskeletal Research Centre at La Trobe and Deputy Editor of the free-access, online *Journal of Foot and Ankle Research*.

Rhonda Nay is Professor of Interdisciplinary Aged Care, Director of the Australian Centre for Evidence Based Aged Care; Director of the Victorian and Tasmanian Dementia Training Studies Centre; and Director of the La Trobe University Institute for Social Participation. Her research is focused on dementia and translating research into practice.

David Nilsson is a lecturer in the School of Social Work and Social Policy at La Trobe University's Bundoora campus. His practice experience has largely been in the hospital social work field and he has conducted a number of research studies on health social work.

Paul O'Halloran is a health psychologist and a senior lecturer, who has been lecturing in research methods at La Trobe University at undergraduate and postgraduate level for ten years. As well, Paul is an active researcher in areas such as chronic illness conditions and mood and physical activity.

Jane Pierson is a lecturer in the School of Public Health at La Trobe University. Jane has a substantial history of involvement, in health research and evaluation, in Australia and in the UK. The bulk of this has been in neuropsychology and gerontology, and has provided extensive experience in the analysis of quantitative data and data from mixed-method studies. Jane also has extensive experience, in Australia and in the UK, in educating undergraduate and postgraduate students, and health professionals, in quantitative research methods and related data analysis procedures.

Priscilla Pyett is a sociologist with over 20 years' experience as a health researcher working with collaborative methodologies. She is Associate Professor in Indigenous Health Research at Department of Rural and Indigenous Health, Monash University, and an honorary researcher at the Victorian Aboriginal Community Controlled Health Organisation.

Paul Ramcharan is Senior Lecturer in Disability Studies, RMIT University in Melbourne. Paul has nearly 20 years' experience and between 2001 and 2006 was coordinator of a national research initiative designed to support the implementation of Valuing People (2001), an English national policy around people with intellectual disabilities.

Miranda Rose is a senior lecturer in the School of Human Communication Sciences at La Trobe University. Her doctoral studies used single-subject experimental designs to investigate the efficacy of speech pathology treatments for aphasia. Miranda coordinates the research stream in the Graduate-Entry Master of Speech Pathology and has a special interest in evidence-based practice. She has written several books and a large number of papers within her own discipline. Her recent book, with D. Best, is *Transforming Practice through Clinical Education, Professional Supervision and Mentoring*, published by Elsevier in 2005.

Martin Ryan is a counsellor/community educator at Support After Suicide, a suicide bereavement counselling program run by Jesuit Social Services in Melbourne. Until the end of 2008 he was an associate professor in the School of Social Work and Social Policy at La Trobe University's Bundoora campus. He taught research methods for many years and his most recent research has focused on social work expertise, particularly in mental health social work

Margot Schofield is Professor of Counselling and Psychotherapy in the School of Public Health at La Trobe University, and Director of Research for the Psychotherapy and Counselling Federation of Australia. She has extensive experience in the design of both cross-sectional and longitudinal surveys, and has been a founding investigator on the Australian Longitudinal Study of Women's Health.

Tanya Serry is a speech pathologist, lecturer and researcher at La Trobe University. She has a strong interest in qualitative research and she is currently engaged in PhD work that is aiming to develop an integrated understanding across various stakeholders, about premises and practices for supporting young schoolchildren who have reading difficulty. Tanya has published a number of scholarly articles and a book chapter and has assisted with editing *Australian Communication Quarterly* for a number of years.

Nora Shields is a senior lecturer in the School of Physiotherapy at La Trobe University. She teaches the process of how to conduct a systematic review to both undergraduate and postgraduate students and among her publications has published six high-quality systematic reviews.

Jemma Skeat completed her speech pathology degree at La Trobe University and has worked as a clinical speech pathologist in various paediatric settings. Her PhD used grounded theory to explore speech pathologists' views about implementing outcome measures in the clinical setting. Her current research uses quantitative and qualitative methods to explore various aspects of service delivery for children with speech and language difficulties.

Anke van der Sterren is in the final year of her PhD on Indigenous models of public health. She has twelve years' experience working in Indigenous health research and is currently a research fellow at the Centre for Excellence in Indigenous Tobacco Control.

Ann Taket is Head of the School of Health and Social Development and Professor of Health and Social Exclusion at Deakin University. She has over 20 years' experience in public health-related research. She has particular interests in participatory methods, the use of mixed methods, research with marginalised or disadvantaged groups and the prevention of violence and abuse.

Peter Waples-Crowe is an Aboriginal man with over 15 years' experience working in Indigenous health and is currently a Team Leader at the Victorian Aboriginal Community Controlled Health Organisation.

Jon Willis is an anthropologist and social epidemiologist who has conducted ethnographic research in Singapore, South Africa and in a range of Indigenous communities in Australia. He is best known for his work on the sexual and health cultures of the Pitjantjatjara people of Australia's Western Desert. Jon is a senior lecturer in the School of Public Health at La Trobe University, and a senior research fellow at the Australian Research Centre in Sex, Health and Society.

Margaret Winbolt is a research fellow in the Australian Centre for Evidence Based Aged Care, La Trobe University. She is a registered nurse with many years' experience in the care of older people. She has a strong interest in exploring the transfer of research evidence into everyday practice and her PhD explored changing gerontic nursing practice from task orientation to evidence-based practice.

Abbreviations

ACCHO	Aboriginal community controlled health organisation
ACL	Anterior Cruciate Ligament
AHW	Aboriginal health worker
AMS	Aboriginal Medical Service
ANOVA	analysis of variance
CAQDAS	computer-assisted qualitative data analysis software
CDM	clinical data-mining
CEBM	Centre for Evidence Based Medicine
CONSORT	Consolidated Standards of Reporting Trial
CPG	clinical practice guideline
CPR	collaborative participatory research
CTT	classical test theory
EBP	evidence-based practice
GP	general practitioner
HREC	Human Research Ethics Committee
ICC	intraclass correlation coefficients
IEC	institutional ethics committee
IRT	item response theory
MANOVA	multivariate analysis of variance
MOU	memorandum of understanding
NHMRC	National Health and Medical Research Council
PAR	Participatory action research
PBR	Practise-based research
PEDro	Physiotherapy Evidence Database
PICO	Population, Intervention or indicator, Comparator or control, Outcome
PRR	prevalence rate ratio
RBP	research-based practice
RCT	randomised controlled trial
SDD	smallest detectable difference
SDT	Self Discovery Tapestry
SEM	standard error of measurement
SPSS	Statistical Package for the Social Sciences
SSED	single-subject experimental design
STI	sexually transmitted illness

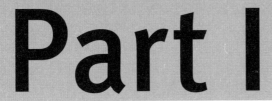

Part I

Methods and Principles

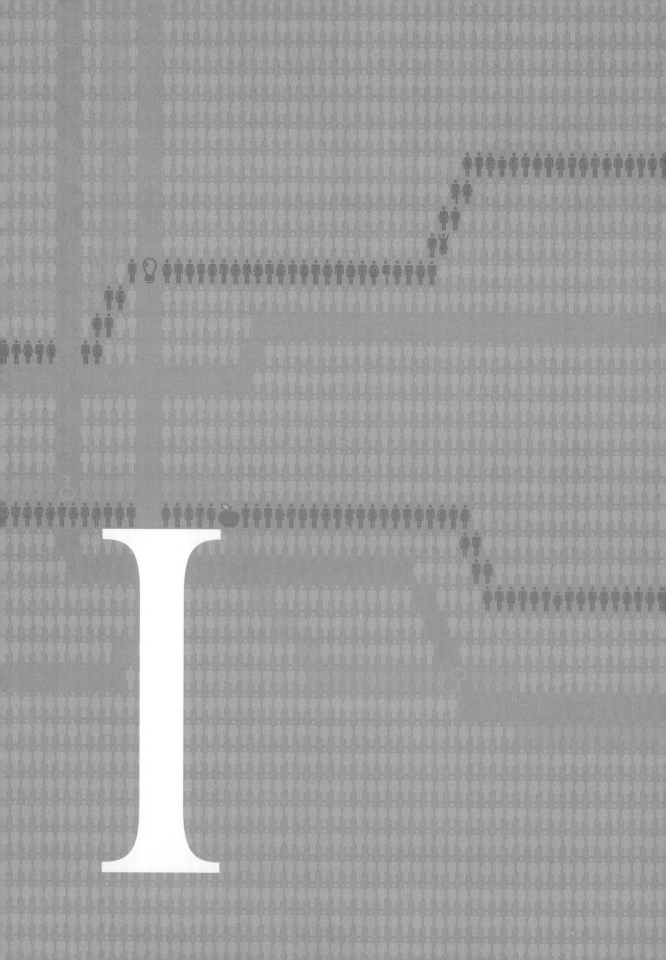

1

The Science of Words and the Science of Numbers: Research Methods as Foundations for Evidence-based Practice in Health

Pranee Liamputtong

CHAPTER OBJECTIVES

In this chapter you will learn:

☐ about evidence and evidence-based practice

☐ about different research designs in health

☐ the nature of qualitative and quantitative approaches

☐ the usefulness of mixed methods

☐ about rigour, and reliability and validity in research

☐ about sampling issues

KEY TERMS

Convenience sampling

Constructivism

Data saturation

Epistemology

Ethnography

Evidence

Evidence-based practice

Knowledge

Knowledge acquisition

Mixed methods

Non-probability sampling

Ontology

Positivism

Pragmatism

Probability sampling method

Purposive sampling

Qualitative research

Quantitative research

Randomised controlled trial

Reliability

Research designs

Rigour

Sample size

Sampling strategies

Validity

INTRODUCTION

Knowledge is essential to human survival. Over the course of history, there have been
many ways of knowing, from divine revelation to tradition and the authority of elders.
By the beginning of the seventeenth century, people began to rely on a different way
of knowing—the research method. (Grinnell et al. 2008, p. 27)

According to Grinnell and associates (2008, p. 9), **knowledge** is 'an accepted body of facts or
ideas which is acquired through the use of senses or reason'. In the old days, we used to believe
that the earth was flat and our belief came about through those who were in 'authority', who
told us so, or because people in our society had always believed that the
world was flat. Now we know that the earth is spherical because scientists
have travelled into space to observe it from this perspective. However,
Grinnell and colleagues argue that the most efficient way of 'knowing
something' (**knowledge acquisition**) is through research findings, which
have been gathered through the use of research methods.

Knowledge: An accepted
body of facts or ideas
acquired through the use
of the senses or reason, or
through research methods.

Knowledge acquisition:
The most efficient way of
'knowing something' is
through research findings,
which have been gathered
through the use of research
methods.

What has knowledge got to do with evidence and evidence-based
practice? I contend that it is through our knowledge that evidence can
be generated. This evidence can then be used for our practice. Without
knowledge, there will not be evidence that we can use. But how can we
find knowledge? The answer is through research and research methods.
According to Grinnell and associates (2008, p. 16), 'the research method of
knowing' comprises two 'complementary research approaches': the qualitative approach and
the quantitative approach. Qualitative research relies on 'qualitative and descriptive methods
of data collection'. Data are presented in the form of words, and sometimes as diagrams,
or drawings, but not as numbers. The quantitative approach, on the other hand, 'relies on
quantification in collecting and analysing data and uses descriptive and inferential statistical
analyses'. Data obtained in a quantitative study are presented in the form of numbers, not in
the form of words, as is the case for the qualitative approach. These two approaches will be
discussed later in this chapter.

EVIDENCE AND EVIDENCE-BASED PRACTICE

It is our belief that you must know the basics of research methodology to even
begin to use the concept of evidence-based practice effectively. (Grinnell &
Unrau 2008, p. v)

This quotation expresses the main reason why this book has been written. Thus it is intended
to provide the foundations for evidence-based practice (EBP) in health. As I have suggested,
evidence can be derived from knowledge and knowledge can be obtained through research.

Evidence, according to Manuel and colleagues (2008, p. 482), is 'information' that can be used to support and guide practices, programs and policies in health and social care in order to enhance the health and well-being of individuals, families and communities. For example, you might be interested in depression among young people and the most effective way to assess their risk for suicide and to prevent it. Types of evidence that you may be interested in may include:

> **Evidence:** 'Information' which can be used to support and guide practices, programs and policies in health and social care in order to enhance the health and well-being of individuals, families and communities.

- ☐ perceptions and experiences of depression and suicide among young people
- ☐ factors that are related to the onset of depression in young people
- ☐ risk factors and protective factors that are relevant to depression and suicide among young people
- ☐ evidence-based methods that can be used to carry out an appropriate assessment of suicide risk
- ☐ strategies or interventions that can be used in practice
- ☐ prevention programs and policies that can have a positive impact on these health and social problems.

As you can see, there are several types of evidence that you can use to find answers to the questions about the health issue in which you are interested. Now it has to be asked which type is the 'best' evidence that you can use and how do you obtain this evidence? This depends on the questions you ask. It has been debated among researchers and practitioners that there is no universal way to judge which evidence is the best. Researchers and practitioners come from different disciplines and surely will have different perspectives on the types of evidence they see as useful or not useful for their research purposes and professional practices (Manuel et al. 2008). What is seen as the best evidence for some researchers and practitioners may not be seen as such by others. It is at this point that I wish to bring up the issue of evidence-based practice.

Fundamentally, **evidence-based practice** in the area of health care refers to 'the process that includes finding empirical evidence regarding the effectiveness and/or efficacy of various treatment options and then determining the relevance of those options to specific client(s). This information is then considered critically, when developing the final treatment plan for the client or clients' (Mullen et al. 2008, pp. 509–10; see also CHAPTERS 15, 16, 17). One approach for evaluating evidence within the model of EBP is through a hierarchical ranking system (Manuel et al. 2008, p. 490; see CHAPTER 17). Within this system, evidence is evaluated according to the research design that was used to generate it. For instance, when evaluating a health care intervention, a well-designed experiment, specifically a randomised controlled trial (RCT),

> **Evidence-based practice:** A process that requires the practitioner to find empirical evidence about the effectiveness or efficacy of different treatment options and then determine the relevance of the evidence to a particular client's situation.

or better, the systematic review of a number of RCTs, is perceived as the 'gold standard' (Hawker et al. 2002; Evans 2003; Aoun & Kristjanson 2005; see CHAPTERS 12, 14, 17, 18).

However, the hierarchical ranking system may ignore some of the limitations of RCTs, and neglect observational studies (Concato 2004; Aoun & Kristjanson 2005; Manuel et al. 2008; see also CHAPTER 12). For instance, confidence in the RCT is based on knowing that the research was correctly undertaken (see CHAPTER 15), but more often than not, published research using RCTs presents conflicting findings (see CHAPTER 12). Some researchers argue that a hierarchical approach is based solely on seeing whether the intervention works as intended, or on the measurement of the efficacy of intervention 'with little attention to the appropriateness and feasibility of the interventions in the real practice world' (Manuel et al. 2008, p. 490; see also Evans 2003; Aoun & Kristjanson 2005).

More importantly, within this hierarchical system, qualitative evidence is often placed at the bottom of the hierarchy and grouped with expert opinion (Grypdonck 2006; Savage 2006). Within this model, the contribution to evidence-based practice of findings from qualitative research is undervalued, and at worst is discounted (Hawker et al. 2002; Gibson & Martin 2003; Aoun & Kristjanson 2005; Grypdonck 2006; Denzin 2009). Qualitative research, despite its increasing contributions to the evidence base of health and social care, is still underrepresented in some health care areas that place a high value on evidence from the hierarchical system (Johnson & Waterfield 2004). This is in part, as Gibson and Martin (2003, p. 353) suggest, due to 'mistaken attempts to evaluate qualitative studies according to the evidence-based hierarchy, where the status of qualitative research is not acknowledged'. Many qualitative researchers argue that this is flawed, as qualitative studies also employ rigorous methods of data collection and analysis (Johnson & Waterfield 2004; Annells 2005; Hammersley 2005; Denzin 2009). Savage (2006, p. 383), for example, argues that **ethnography**, one of the qualitative research methods, 'is particularly valuable because of the attention that it gives to context and its synthesis of findings from different methods'. More importantly, ethnography provides 'a holistic way of exploring the relationship between the different kinds of evidence that underpin clinical practice' (see CHAPTER 6).

Ethnography: A research method that focuses on the scientific study of the lived culture of groups of people, used to discover and describe individual social and cultural groups.

It is argued that the hierarchical model of evidence is only one way of organising different types of evidence. It is important for health researchers and practitioners to know this, so that they can evaluate the quality of evidence that can be found with respect to a specific health issue. And no doubt it can be very useful for some health practices, for example in therapeutic science (see CHAPTERS 15, 17 for example). However, Manuel and colleagues (2008, p. 490) believe that 'the decision on what evidence to use should be placed in context with your research and practice needs'. Researchers and practitioners need to consider the relevance and feasibility of evidence and whether the evidence accords with the values and preferences of the clients. And this is what I advocate in this chapter—that we need to consider different types of evidence and that this evidence can be derived from the findings of different types of research. This book will give readers an understanding of the different methods that researchers and practitioners can use or draw on in producing evidence: qualitative methods (see PART II), quantitative methods (see PART III), mixed-methods (see CHAPTERS 19, 20) and collaborative approaches (see CHAPTER 21).

It is worth noting that EBP has emerged from the long-standing commitment among health practitioners to social research and science. But there has been a significant change in how research and practice are related. According to Mullen and colleagues (2008, p. 521), in the past, research and practice were seen as separate activities and/or as the roles of two different professions. Research was undertaken by researchers to add to the knowledge base, which was eventually drawn upon by practitioners to provide evidence on which to base their practice. Now, these differences are blurred and research and practice are often combined. In EBP, many of the practice questions largely resemble the essential parts of research questions: 'We search for evidence—especially research evidence—to answer our practice questions using established research criteria when the evidence comes from research studies, and we collect data on the processes and outcomes of our interventions' (p. 521).

In evidence-based practice, practitioners need to be clear about what is known and not known about any health problem or health practice that will be 'best' for their clients (Mullen et al. 2008). But all too often we know little about particular health problems of some population groups, or about treatment options that are not empirically based. Although there is research evidence that practitioners may find in existing literature, Mullen and colleagues (2008, p. 523) argue that there are still many health issues that remain unknown to us. Currently, EBP does not apply to many of the health issues of certain population groups, for example certain ethnic minorities and indigenous groups, recent immigrants and refugees, gays and lesbians, rural communities, and people with uncommon or particularly challenging health problems. It is clear that there is a need for more research as part of the EBP process. Also much of the EBP focus, in terms of both research and application, has been centred on only a subset of health issues. Research is needed in other fields, in both health issues and practices.

More importantly, depending on the research or practice question, practitioners may need evidence other than that which relates to the efficacy of interventions, to inform their practice (Aoun & Kristjanson 2005; Manuel et al. 2008). Evidence that we use in evidence-based practice cannot and should not be based solely on the findings of RCTs. Rather, it should be derived from many sources (Hawker et al. 2002). Some health topics or issues are not appropriate for an RCT (see e.g. Aoun & Kristjanson 2005), and there are many ethical concerns regarding RCTs (see CHAPTER 2). For instance, you may be interested in knowing about the meaning and interpretation of body weight because there have been higher rates of diabetes or anorexia nervosa in your city, or you may need to know about the understanding of homelessness among poor families and how they deal with it, because you have noticed that there are increasing numbers of homeless young people in poorer areas of your city. The 'best' evidence for these issues will not be generated by RCTs but by qualitative research (see CHAPTERS 8, 16, 21). These scenarios illustrate situations where you need to look for other types of evidence.

Therefore evidence can be obtained by gaining knowledge through your own research, if there is no available evidence that you can find from systematic reviews or from other sources (e.g. literature). In this book, I contend that evidence can be generated by both qualitative and quantitative research. No doubt, most health care providers will trust the so-called 'hard' evidence obtained through quantitative approaches such as surveys with closed-ended questions, clinical measurements, and RCTs (see chapters in PART III). As I have pointed out, the quantitative approach is seen as being empirical science and as being more systematic than qualitative research, so the findings of this approach are regarded as more reliable. But I argue that evidence derived from the qualitative approach can help you to understand the issue and to use the findings in your practice. Qualitative research provides evidence that you may not be able to obtain from quantitative research or from a **systematic review** of

Systematic review: A comprehensive identification and synthesis of the available literature on a specified topic. In a systematic review, literature is treated like data.

quantitative research. Seeley and colleagues (2008), for example, point out that the quantitative part of their research, which involved more than 2000 participants, failed to provide a good understanding of some of their findings regarding the impact of HIV and AIDS on families. It was only through the life histories of 24 families that they were able to explain these findings in a more meaningful way. Their study clearly points to the importance of qualitative evidence in health care and practice. Indeed, many researchers have argued that 'qualitative research findings have much to offer evidence-based practice' (Hawker et al. 2002, p. 1285; see also Green & Britten 1998; Popay et al. 1998; Grypdonck 2006; Daly et al. 2007; CHAPTER 8). As Sandelowski (2004, p. 1382) puts it, 'Qualitative research is the best thing to be happening to evidence-based practice'.

Within the emergence of evidence-based practice in health care, Grypdonck (2006, p. 1379) contends that qualitative research contributes greatly to the appropriateness of care. She argues that health practitioners need to have a good understanding of

> what it means to be ill, to live with an illness, to be subject to physical limitations, to see one's intellectual capacities gradually diminish, or to be healed again, to rise from [near] death after a bone marrow transplant, leaving one's sick life behind, to meet people who take care of you in a way that makes you feel really understood and really cared for.

Practitioners cannot obtain knowledge from existing literature in order to address these crucial health and illness issues. Such knowledge can only be gained through the integration of research into their daily work (see CHAPTER 8, for example). Surely, by gaining a better understanding of the lived experience of patients and clients, health practitioners will be able to provide more sensitive and appropriate care.

I argue here that qualitative enquiry is an essential means for eliciting evidence from diverse individuals, population groups and contexts (see also Grypdonck 2006; Creswell 2007; Daly 2007; Liamputtong 2007; Munhall 2007; Carpenter & Suto 2008; Padgett 2008). However, there is still a sense of distrust of qualitative research (Johnson & Waterfield 2004; Baum 2008). This is mainly due to a perception that qualitative enquiry is unable to produce useful and valid findings (Hammersley 2008; Torrance 2008), a perception that stems largely from insufficient understanding of the philosophical framework for qualitative work, which has its focus on meaning and experience, the social construction of reality, and the relationship between the researched and the researcher (Creswell 2007; Daly 2007; Bryman 2008; Denzin & Lincoln 2008).

Research designs: which one?

Before selecting a research design, you must think carefully about your research questions. What are the questions or health issues to which you need or wish to find answers? Researchers need to consider carefully whether qualitative or quantitative research is best suited to addressing the research problem. Once you have thought this through, you will be able to select a research design that will be appropriate for the questions you ask. For example, if you wish to understand why some young women smoke and you want to learn from them about their perceptions of smoking, gender issues and societal pressure, their needs and concerns about smoking and their body, or if you want to really understand why many working-class men will not stop smoking, can you find your answers by conducting a randomised controlled trial, or a case-control study? Will these methods allow you to find useful answers? On the other hand, if you wish to find out how many young women smoke, or what the prevalence of diabetes is among young children in your local area, can these questions be addressed by the use of a qualitative approach? Before you can answer these questions, you will need to understand what each approach can offer you and what it cannot (its limitations). Hence a good understanding of research methods is essential.

Often we hear students and novice researchers make comment like, 'I want to do a qualitative research study because I am not very good with numbers', or 'I want to use quantitative research because I am not interested in qualitative research', or, worse, 'I do not want to use qualitative research because I don't like it—too many flowery words and not objective enough'. I would suggest that this is not a good way of going about selecting your approach. You need to find out which approach is the best way for you to find answers to your research questions (or to find evidence for practice), and this can be either a qualitative or a quantitative approach. If you cannot find your complete answers (or evidence) using either of these approaches alone, you may need to go further and use a mixed methods design.

The choice of research design, according to Bryman (2008, p. 26), must be 'dovetailed with the specific research question being investigated'. If researchers are interested in how individuals within a specific social group perceive health and illness, a qualitative approach, which allows us to examine how individuals interpret their social world, will be the most appropriate research strategy to use. Also, if researchers are interested in a topic that we know little about, a more exploratory position is preferable. This is when a qualitative approach will serve our needs better, because such approaches are typically associated with the generation of new findings rather than the testing of existing theory (see chapters in PART II). On the other hand, if researchers are interested in finding the causes of a health problem, or its prevalence, for example the rate of diabetes in Australia, it is the case that a quantitative approach will provide more appropriate answers (see CHAPTERS 13, 14).

Another salient matter relevant to the choice of research designs is the nature of the topic and the characteristics of the individuals or groups being researched. For instance, if the researchers need to talk with hard-to-reach individuals or groups such as those engaged in illicit activities, such as violence, drug use and dealing, or those living with stigmatised illnesses such as mental health problems and HIV/AIDS, or with Indigenous people, it is unlikely that a quantitative approach would allow them to gain the necessary rapport or the confidence of the participants. These are some of the reasons that most researchers in these areas have adopted a qualitative approach as their research strategy (see Liamputtong 2007, 2009; CHAPTER 21).

DOING RESEARCH

A practical consideration in the choice of research approach

Zoe is a podiatrist and owns her practice. She has treated many competitive athletes who come to her with foot injuries. This is particularly so around the time of major competitive events like the Commonwealth and Olympic Games. She does not know the real prevalence of the injuries in her city, so she cannot say exactly what the rate of injuries would be; she only knows that she has treated many athletes. She would like to know about the rate of injury as she needs to prepare her practice in terms of how many podiatrists she should employ and the purchase of essential equipment. Zoe also notices that some athletes do not follow her advice about how to avoid or prevent foot injuries, or adhere to her treatments, despite the fact that she has followed the recommendations from a systematic review, which has shown that the advice she has given and the treatments she has adopted are the best options. This has really puzzled her. She wants to know the reasons for this non-compliance. This is the beginning of her research endeavour.

From reading literature on sports injuries, Zoe realises that there are different ways in which she can find her answers. If she wants to ascertain the prevalence of foot injuries among competitive athletes, she would need to use a quantitative approach, which would allow her to determine the number of such injuries in her city. But if she wants to understand why the athletes do not follow her advice or adhere to her treatment plans, she must talk to them and allow them to tell their stories, because this will give her in-depth understanding of their concerns and may help her to develop treatment plans that cater better for their needs. So Zoe has choices as to how she can obtain evidence that can inform her work.

If you were Zoe, how would you go about doing your research in order to find the evidence you need?

ONTOLOGY AND EPISTEMOLOGY

In any research undertaking, it is crucial that researchers examine the ontological and epistemological positions that underlie the way in which research is undertaken. **Ontology** refers to the question of whether or not there is a single objective reality (Denzin & Lincoln 2005). Here 'reality' refers to the existence of what is real in the natural or social worlds. If we adopt the ontological standpoint of objective reality, we must take a position of objective detachment and ensure that the research process is free from any bias. Researchers who adopt this position would argue that reality can be accurately captured (Grbich 2007). These researchers will adopt a quantitative approach for their research.

> **Ontology** refers to the question of whether or not there is a single objective reality.

Other researchers would reject the position of objective reality. Rather, they would argue that it is impossible to carry out research in a detached way. These researchers would argue that if we wish to understand the realities and experiences of other people, we must acknowledge our own subjectivities, which include our own beliefs, values and emotions, in the process of carrying out research. It is important that we acknowledge our personal impact on the research process (Bryman 2008; Dickson-Swift et al. 2008). These researchers will make use of a qualitative approach for their research.

Epistemology is concerned with the nature of knowledge and how knowledge is obtained (Broom & Willis 2007; Grbich 2007; Bryman 2008; Guba & Lincoln 2008). It begs 'the question of what is (or should be) regarded as acceptable knowledge in a discipline'. A central concern is 'the question of whether the social world can and should be studied according to the same principle, procedures, and ethos as the natural sciences' (Bryman 2008, p. 13). There are five major epistemological paradigms, which can be used to explain the nature of knowledge (Guba & Lincoln 1994, 2008). These paradigms give different understandings of what reality is in the natural and social worlds, and how we come to know that reality (Broom & Willis 2007; Willis 2007). In this chapter I shall focus on the two paradigms on which qualitative and quantitative approaches are respectively based: constructivism and positivism. A more detailed discussion of research paradigms can be found in Denzin and Lincoln (2005), Willis (2007) and Dickson-Swift et al. (2008). See also CHAPTERS 6, 8, 10, 19, 20.

> **Epistemology** is concerned with the nature of knowledge and how knowledge is obtained.

Constructivism suggests that 'reality' is socially constructed. It is also referred to as interpretivism (Bryman 2008). Constructivist researchers reject the ideal of a single truth. Instead, they believe that there are multiple truths, which are individually constructed (Guba & Lincoln 1994, 2008; Grbich 2007; Willis 2007; Dickson-Swift et al. 2008). Reality is seen as being shaped by social factors such as class, gender, race, ethnicity, culture and age (Grbich 2007). To constructivist researchers, reality is not firmly rooted in nature, but is a product of our own making. One of the central beliefs of researchers working within this paradigm is that research is a very subjective process, due to the active involvement of the researcher in the construction and conduct of the research (Grbich 2007). Constructivist researchers also argue that 'reality is defined by the research participants' interpretations of their own realities' (Williams et al. 2008, p. 84). Research situated within this paradigm, as Grbich (2007, p. 8) points out, focuses on 'exploration of the way people interpret and make sense of their experiences in the worlds in which they live, and how the contexts of events and situations and the placement of these within wider social environments have impacted on constructed understanding'.

> **Constructivism:** An epistemology that suggests that 'reality' is socially constructed. Constructivist researchers believe there are multiple truths, individually constructed, and that reality is a product of our own making.

According to Bryman (2008, p. 15) constructivist researchers hold 'a view that the subject matter of the social sciences—people and their institutions—is fundamentally different from that of the natural sciences'. When the social world is studied, it 'requires a different logic of research procedure, one that reflects the distinctiveness of humans as against the natural order'. Within this constructivist paradigm, it requires the researchers to 'grasp the subjective meaning of social action' (p. 16). This necessitates the use of research methods that would allow people to articulate the meanings of their social realities, and this requires the use of a qualitative approach.

On the other hand, **positivism** is underpinned by the ontological belief that there is an objective reality that can be accessed (Guba & Lincoln 1994; Denzin & Lincoln 2005; Broom & Willis 2007; Grbich 2007; Willis 2007; Dickson-Swift et al. 2008). This is often referred to as 'naïve realism' (Dickson-Swift et al. 2008). Positivism is also known as naturalism, logical empiricism, and behaviouralism. It views reality as being independent of our experiences of it, and being accessible through careful thinking, and observing and recording of our experiences (Moses & Knutsen 2007; Bryman 2008). The aim of positivistic enquiry is to explain, predict or control that reality. One of the central ideas of research approaches based on a positivist paradigm is the generation and testing of hypotheses through scientific means (Bryman 2008).

> **Positivism** views reality as being independent of our experiences of it, and being accessible through careful thinking, and observing and recording of our experiences.

According to Unrau and colleagues (2008, p. 64), positivism 'strives toward measurability, objectivity, the reducing of uncertainty, duplication, and the use of standardized procedures'. Knowledge generated through this paradigm is based on 'objective measurements' of the real world, and not on the 'opinions, beliefs, or past experiences' of individuals. Positivism argues that research must be as 'objective' as possible; the things that are being studied must not be affected by the researcher. Positivist researchers attempt to undertake research in such a way that their studies can be duplicated by others. Further, 'a true-to-the-bone positivist researcher' will only use well-accepted standardised procedures. Research is only regarded as credible when others accept its findings, and before they accept them they must be satisfied that the study is 'conducted according to accepted scientific standardised procedures' (p. 65).

Differences in ontology and epistemology lead to different data collection methods (Williams et al. 2008). Objective reality can be explored through the data collection method of standardised observation, which is the practice commonly used in research that uses a quantitative approach. However, it is not possible to establish subjective reality through standardised measurement and observation. The only way to find out about the subjective reality of our research participants is to ask them about it, and the answer will come back in words, not in numbers. This is the hallmark of the qualitative approach. Williams and colleagues (2008, p. 85) state that 'in a nutshell, qualitative research methods produce qualitative data in the form of text. Quantitative research methods produce quantitative data in the form of numbers.'

In summary, constructivism influences qualitative research whereas positivism dominates quantitative research (Willis 2007). If researchers wish to examine the subjective nature of phenomena, and the multiple realities of those involved in the research, a constructivist paradigm is essential, and of course, this necessitates the use of a qualitative approach. If researchers want to investigate the objective nature of phenomena, a positivistic paradigm is crucial, and hence a quantitative approach is indicated (Williams et al. 2008, p. 84).

I wish to point out here that traditional research methods and designs are heavily influenced by scientific positivism, since it is seen as 'the crowning achievement of Western civilization' (Denzin & Lincoln 2005, p. 8). But many constructivist researchers reject the use of positivist assumptions and methods. Positivist methods, for some researchers, are just one way of 'telling stories about societies or social worlds'. These methods may not be better or worse than any other methods, but they 'tell different kinds of stories'. Other constructivist researchers, however, believe that the criteria used in positivist science are 'irrelevant to their work'. They argue that 'such criteria reproduce only a certain kind of science, a science that silences too many voices' (Denzin & Lincoln 2005, p. 12).

In this chapter, I wish to introduce a third paradigm: **pragmatism**. This paradigm has become increasingly popular among health researchers from a variety of disciplines. Pragmatism has been promoted as an attractive philosophical paradigm within 'methodological pluralism' (Greene 2007). Pragmatists argue that reality does not exist only as natural and physical realities, but also as psychological and social realities, which include subjective experience and thought, language and culture. Knowledge, according to pragmatists, is both constructed and based on the reality of the world in which we live and which we experience. As such, pragmatists advocate that researchers should employ a combination of methods that work best for answering their research questions.

> **Pragmatism** argues that reality exists not only as natural and physical realities, but also as psychological and social realities, which include subjective experience and thought, language and culture.

Pranee Liamputtong

Moses and Knutsen (2007) contend that this paradigm offers a 'fully fledged metaphysical position', which combines the most attractive characteristics of constructivism and positivism. See also CHAPTER 19.

The major push for the methodological pluralism that underlies pragmatism is the belief that knowledge can be generated from diverse theories and sources, and in many ways through different research methods. Hence we must embrace methodological diversity in our research. Methodological pluralism encourages objectives-driven research instead of methods-driven research. As I have indicated above, the reason for this is that certain methods, regardless of their ontological and epistemological positions, may be more suitable for some questions than others. In order to understand complex social phenomena, methodological pluralism is crucial (Moses & Knutsen 2007).

QUALITATIVE AND QUANTITATIVE APPROACHES: A COMPARISON

Qualitative research is recognised as 'the word science' (Denzin 2008, p. 321). It relies heavily on words or stories that people tell us, as researchers. Qualitative research is research that has its focus on the social world instead of the world of nature. Fundamentally, researching social life differs from researching natural phenomena. In the social world, we deal with the subjective experiences of human beings, and our 'understanding of reality can change over time and in different social contexts' (Dew 2007, p. 434). This sets qualitative enquiry apart from researching the natural world, which can be treated as 'objects or things'. **Quantitative research**, on the other hand, is known as the science of numbers, and it is also referred to as positivist science. For quantitative researchers, the need to be objective and structured is crucial, as quantitative research attempts to measure things and avoid any bias that could influence the findings.

Qualitative research:
Research strategies that emphasise words rather than numbers in data collection and analysis. The focus of qualitative research is on the generation of theories.

Quantitative research:
Research strategies that emphasise numbers in data collection and analysis. The focus of quantitative research is on the testing of theories.

Qualitative research is more flexible and fluid in its approach than quantitative research. This has led some researchers to see qualitative research as less worthwhile because it is not governed by clear rules. Quantitative researchers have argued that the interpretive nature of qualitative research makes it 'soft' science, lacking in reliability and validity, and of little value in contributing to scientific knowledge (Guba & Lincoln 1994; Hammersley 2007; Baum 2008; Denzin 2008; Torrance 2008). But the interpretive and flexible approach is necessary because the focus of qualitative research is on meaning and interpretation (Liamputtong 2007, 2009). For most qualitative researchers, it is accepted that in order to understand people's behaviour we must attempt to understand the meanings and interpretations that people give to their behaviour. Essentially, qualitative research aims to 'capture lived experiences of the social world and the meanings people give these experiences from their own perspective' (Corti & Thompson 2004, p. 326).

Because of its flexibility and fluidity, qualitative research is more suited to understanding the meanings, interpretations and subjective experiences of individuals than is the quantitative approach (Liamputtong 2007, 2009; Carpenter & Suto 2008; Denzin & Lincoln 2008; Dickson-Swift et al. 2008). Qualitative enquiry allows the researchers to hear the voices of those who are marginalised in society. The in-depth nature of qualitative methods allows the participants to express their feelings and experiences in their own words (Creswell 2007; Daly 2007; Liamputtong 2007, 2009; Barbour 2008; Bryman 2008; Padgett 2008).

While quantitative research has always been the dominant research approach in the health sciences, in the past decade or so qualitative research has been gradually accepted as a crucial component for increasing our understanding of health (see Johnson & Waterfield 2004; Holloway 2005; Finlay & Ballinger 2006; Saks & Allsop 2007; Carpenter & Suto 2008; Seeley et al. 2008; Green & Thorogood 2009; Liamputtong 2009). In many areas of health, researchers have argued about the value of interpretive data. In public health in particular, the 'new public health' recognises the need to 'describe' and 'understand' people. For example, Baum (2008, p. 180) argues for the need for qualitative methods, since they 'offer considerable strength in understanding and interpreting complexities' of human behaviour and health issues. Qualitative research is crucial 'for coping with complexity and naturalistic settings'. This is reflected in the chapters in PART II of this book.

Bryman (2008, pp. 393–5) provides some contrasts between qualitative and quantitative research approaches, which are presented in Table 1.1.

Table 1.1: Comparison of qualitative and quantitative approaches

Qualitative approach	Quantitative approach
Words	Numbers
Participants' points of view	Researcher's point of view
Meaning	Behaviour
Contextual understanding	Generalisation
Rich, deep data	Hard, reliable data
Unstructured	Structured
Process	Static
Micro	Macro
Natural settings	Artificial settings
Theory emergent	Theory testing
Researcher close	Researcher distant

MIXED METHODS

In some ways, the differences between quantitative and qualitative methods involve trade-offs between breadth and depth...Qualitative methods typically produce a wealth of detailed data about a much smaller number of people and cases. (Patton 2002, p. 227)

How then do we combine the depth and the breadth? **Mixed methods** approaches offer a way of doing this. In some situations we find that neither a qualitative nor a quantitative approach alone can provide sufficient information for us to use, so a combination of the two is required. This is referred to as a mixed methods research design (see Johnson et al. 2007; CHAPTERS 19, 20).

Mixed methods: A research design that combines research methods from qualitative and quantitative research approaches within a single research study.

According to Bryman (2008, p. 23), although qualitative and quantitative approaches have different ontologies, epistemologies and research strategies, 'the distinction is not a hard-and-fast one: studies that have the broad characteristics of one research strategy may also have a characteristic of the other'. Thus within one research project the two can be combined, and this is what has been referred to as a mixed methods design. Bryman (2008, p. 603) suggests that this strategy 'would allow the various strengths to be capitalized upon and the weaknesses offset somewhat'.

The term 'mixed methods research' should not be confused with the combination of research methods that come from just one research approach (Bryman, 2008). For example, the combined use of in-depth interview and focus groups is not mixed methods research, because both these methods belong to the qualitative approach. Similarly, the use of both a questionnaire (with closed-ended questions) and a randomised control trial is not mixed methods research because both methods come from the quantitative approach. Only research that employs both qualitative and quantitative methods such as using focus groups and a questionnaire is classed as mixed methods research. Some researchers, however, may use the term to refer to the combination of different methods from one approach (see CHAPTER 20, for example).

There are different ways in which researchers can combine the methods. Hammersley (1996) proposes three approaches: triangulation, facilitation and complementarity. *Triangulation* refers to the use of qualitative research to confirm the findings from quantitative research or vice versa. In *facilitation*, one research approach is used in order to facilitate research using the other approach. When the two approaches are used so that different aspects of an investigation can be articulated, this is referred to as *complementarity*. You may like to read Bryman (2008, pp. 610–23), who provides useful ways of combining qualitative and quantitative research in a mixed methods design. More information on the use of mixed methods research is given in CHAPTERS 19 and 20.

RESEARCH RIGOUR: TRUSTWORTHINESS AND RELIABILITY/VALIDITY

Both qualitative and quantitative research approaches have criteria that can be used to evaluate the **rigour** (authenticity/credibility/strength) of the research. Within the qualitative approach, we use the term 'trustworthiness', which refers to the quality of qualitative enquiry (see also CHAPTERS 4, 8). In health research and practice, for example, trustworthiness means that 'the findings must

Rigour: Rigorous research is trustworthy and can be relied on by other researchers.

be authentic enough to allow practitioners to act upon them with confidence' (Raines 2008, p. 455). In quantitative research, the concepts of reliability and validity are used. Reliability refers to 'the stability of findings' and validity represents 'the truthfulness of findings' (Carpenter & Suto 2008, p. 148). **Reliability** refers to 'the consistency and trustworthiness of research findings; it is often considered in relation to the issue of whether a finding is reproducible, at other times, and by other researchers' (Kvale 2007, p. 22; see also Bryman 2008). **Validity** bears upon measurement and is 'concerned with the integrity of the conclusions that are generated from a piece of research' (Bryman 2008, p. 32). The most commonly used validity concepts are internal and external validity. Internal validity is related to 'the issue of whether a method investigates what it purports to investigate' (Kvale 2007, p. 22), while external validity relates to 'whether the results of a study can be generalised beyond the specific research context' (Bryman 2008, p. 33).

Reliability: The extent to which a measurement instrument is dependable, stable and consistent when repeated under identical conditions.

Validity: The degree to which a scale measures what it is supposed to measure.

The attainment of validity in quantitative research is based on strict observance of the rules and standards of the approach. Thus it follows that attempting to apply those rules to qualitative research becomes problematic (Raines 2008). Angen (2000, p. 379) contends that when qualitative research is judged by the validity criteria used in the quantitative approach, it may be seen as 'being too subjective, lacking in rigour, and/or being unscientific'. As a consequence, qualitative research may be denied legitimacy.

The concepts of validity and reliability are seen as incompatible with the ontological and epistemological foundations of qualitative research (Carpenter & Suto 2008, p. 148; see also Arminio & Hultgren 2002; Tobin & Begley 2004; Raines 2008). As I have suggested earlier, qualitative research is descriptive and unique to a specific historical, social and cultural context (Johnson & Waterfield 2004). It therefore cannot be repeated in order to establish reliability. Qualitative research holds the view that reality is socially constructed by an individual, and while this socially constructed reality cannot be measured, it can be interpreted. For qualitative research, understanding cannot be separated from context. Hence qualitative data cannot be 'tested for validity' using the same rules and standards, which are based on 'assumptions of objective reality and positivist neutrality' (Johnson & Waterfield 2004, pp. 122–3; see also Angen 2000).

Qualitative researchers have, however, developed some criteria that can be used to judge the trustworthiness of qualitative research. Here I refer to the work of Lincoln and Guba (1989), who propose criteria that qualitative researchers can adopt. They remain the 'gold standard' that many qualitative researchers have followed. The four criteria that Lincoln and Guba (1985, 1989) have developed can be used 'as a translation of the more traditional terms associated with quantitative research' (Carpenter & Suto 2008, p. 149). Hence credibility equates to internal validity, and transferability to external validity, dependability to reliability, and confirmability to objectivity (see also Creswell 2007; Bryman 2008; Padgett 2008; Raines 2008; Liamputtong 2009).

Credibility relates to the question: 'Can these findings be regarded as truthful?' (Raines 2008, p. 455), or 'How believable are the findings?' (Bryman 2008, p. 34). It scrutinises the matter of 'fit' between what the participants say and the representation of these viewpoints by the researchers (Padgett 2008). Credibility asks whether 'the explanation fits the description and whether the description is credible' (Tobin & Begley 2004, p. 391).

Transferability (or applicability) relates to the question: 'To what degree can the study findings be generalised or applied to other individuals or groups, contexts, or settings?', or 'Do the findings apply to other contexts?' (Bryman 2008, p. 34). It attempts to establish the 'generalisability of inquiry' (Tobin & Begley 2004, p. 392; Padgett 2008). Transferability pertains to 'the degree to which qualitative findings inform and facilitate insights within contexts other than that in which the research was conducted' (Carpenter & Suto 2008, pp. 149–50; see also Padgett 2008).

Dependability raises questions about whether the research findings 'fit' the data that have been collected (Carpenter & Suto 2008), or 'are the findings likely to apply at other times' (Bryman 2008, p. 34). Dependability 'addresses the consistency or congruency of the results' (Raines 2008, p. 456). It is gained through an auditing process, which requires the researchers to ensure that 'the process of research is logical, traceable and clearly documented' (Tobin & Begley 2004, p. 392).

Confirmability asks if the researcher has 'allowed his or her values to intrude to a high degree?' (Bryman 2008, p. 34). It attempts to show that the findings and the interpretations of the findings do not derive from the imagination of the researchers, but are clearly linked with the data (Tobin & Begley 2004; Padgett 2008). Confirmability, according to Lincoln and Guba (1985, p. 290), is seen as 'the degree to which findings are determined by the respondents and conditions of the inquiry and not by the biases, motivations, interests or perspectives of the inquirer'.

Table 1.2 compares rigour criteria employed in qualitative research with those used in quantitative research.

Table 1.2: Rigour criteria employed in qualitative and quantitative research

Qualitative research	Quantitative research
Credibility	Internal validity
Transferability	External validity
Dependability	Reliability
Confirmability	Objectivity

Source: Carpenter & Suto 2008, p. 149

As you can see, both qualitative and quantitative approaches do have criteria that allow researchers to evaluate the usefulness and the strength of each enquiry. Due to space limitations in this chapter, I refer readers to other works for further information. See Carpenter and Suto

(2008), Raines (2008) and Liamputtong (2009), who give detailed discussions of rigour and strategies to ensure it is inherent in qualitative research. Issues relevant to reliability and validity in quantitative research are discussed in CHAPTERS 11, 12, 15.

SAMPLING ISSUES

Here I discuss two salient issues in relation to sampling: sampling methods and sample size.

Sampling methods

Sampling issues in the context of sampling methods centre around whether the sample is based on a probability or a non-probability sampling method. **Probability sampling** methods 'are those in which the probability of an element being selected is known in advance' (Schutt 2008, p. 143). In research involving people, an element equates to a **research participant**. Within these methods, elements are randomly selected and hence there should be no systematic bias as 'nothing but chance determines which elements are included in the sample' (Schutt 2008, p. 143). Because of this characteristic, probability sample methods are important in quantitative research where, in most cases, the intent is to generalise the findings for the sample to the population from which the sample was taken (see also CHAPTERS 11–15, 24, 25). The four most common methods for drawing random samples include simple random sampling, systematic random sampling, stratified random sampling, and cluster random sampling (Schutt 2008; see CHAPTER 15).

Probability sampling: The probability of an element being selected is known in advance. The intent is to generalise the findings for the sample to the population from which it was taken.

For **non-probability sampling** methods, on the other hand, the likelihood of a potential research participant being selected is not known in advance (Schutt 2008). Additionally, random selection procedures commonly employed in probability sampling are not used in non-probability sampling methods. The latter do not provide 'representative samples' for the populations from which they are drawn, so the findings cannot be generalised to a larger group of people. However, these methods are useful for research questions that do not need to involve large populations, and particularly for qualitative research projects (Johnson & Waterfield 2004; Schutt 2008).

Research participant: A person who agrees to take part in the study on equal terms.

Non-probability sampling: The probability of a potential research participant being selected is not known in advance. The findings cannot be generalised to a larger group of people.

Qualitative researchers therefore usually rely on non-probability sampling methods. Since qualitative research is concerned with in-depth understanding of the issue or issues under examination, it relies heavily on individuals who are able to provide information-rich accounts of their experiences. It usually involves a small numbers of individuals. Morse (2007, p. 530, original emphasis) contends that 'qualitative researchers sample for *meaning*, rather than frequency. We are not interested in how much, or how many, but in *what*'. Qualitative research aims to examine a 'process' or the 'meanings' that people give to their own social situations. It does not require a generalisation of the findings as in positivist science (Hesse-Biber & Leavy 2005, p. 70). Qualitative research also relies heavily on **purposive sampling** strategies (Patton 2002; Hesse-Biber & Leavy 2005; Morse 2007; Teddlie & Yu 2007). Purposive sampling refers to a deliberate selection of specific individuals, events or settings because of the crucial information they can provide, which cannot be obtained as adequately through other channels (Carpenter & Suto 2008). For example, purposive sampling, in research that is concerned with how cancer patients cope with pain, will require the researcher to find participants who have pain, instead of randomly selecting any cancer patients from an oncologist's patient list (Padgett 2008). The powers of purposive sampling techniques, Patton (2002, p. 230, original emphasis) suggests, 'lie in selecting *information-rich cases* for study in depth'. Information-rich

Purposive sampling looks for cases that will be able to provide rich or in-depth information about the issue being examined, not a representative sample as in quantitative research.

Convenience sampling allows researchers to find individuals who are conveniently available and willing to participate in a study.

cases are individuals or events or settings from which researchers can learn extensively about issues they wish to examine. Such cases offer in-depth understanding and insights into the findings, instead of empirical generalisations. See also CHAPTERS 5, 7.

Another sampling method commonly adopted in qualitative research is **convenience sampling**. This method allows researchers to find individuals who are conveniently available and willing to participate in a study. Convenience sampling is crucial when it is difficult to find individuals who meet some specified criteria such as age, gender, ethnicity, or social class. This may happen more often in research that requires the conduct of fieldwork, such as ethnography. Researchers need to find key informants who are able to provide in-depth information on the research issues and site. Often researchers make decisions on the basis of 'who is available, who has some specialized knowledge of the setting, and who is willing to serve in that role' (Hesse-Biber & Leavy 2005, p. 71; see also Bryman 2008).

Sample size

The issue of sample size is considered differently in qualitative and quantitative approaches. A crucial point in qualitative research is to select the research participants meaningfully and strategically, instead of attempting to make statistical comparisons or to 'create a representative sample' (Carpenter & Suto 2008, p. 80; see also Patton 2002). Hence the important question to ask, when deciding about the sample size in qualitative research, is whether the sample provides data to allow the research questions or aims to be thoroughly addressed (Mason 2002; see also CHAPTER 7). The focus of decisions about sample size in qualitative research is on 'flexibility and depth'. A fundamental concern of qualitative research is on quality, not quantity. Qualitative researchers do not intend to maximise the breadth of their research (Padgett 2008).

In qualitative research, no set formula is rigidly used to determine the sample size, as is the case for quantitative research (Morse 1998; Patton 2002). The sampling process is flexible and, at the commencement of the research, the number of participants to be recruited is not definitely known. However, **data saturation**, a concept associated with grounded theory, is used by qualitative researchers as a way of justifying the number of research participants, and this is established during the data collection process. Saturation is considered to occur when little or no new data is being generated (Padgett 2008). The sample is adequate when 'the emerging themes have been efficiently and effectively saturated with optimal quality data' (Carpenter & Suto 2008, p. 152), and that 'sufficient data to account for all aspects of the phenomenon have been obtained' (Morse et al. 2002, p. 12). See also CHAPTER 7.

> **Data saturation** occurs when little or no new data is being generated and new data fits into the categories already developed.

In quantitative research, sample sizes tend to be larger than those of qualitative research. Researchers have more confidence about generalising their results if they have larger samples. Often, during the planning stage of their research, quantitative researchers attempt to determine how large a sample they must have in order to achieve their purposes. As Schutt (2008, p. 154) points out, quantitative researchers must 'consider the degree of confidence desired, the homogeneity of the population, the complexity of the analysis they plan, and the expected strength of the relationships they will measure'. Generally, quantitative researchers can use the following criteria when considering their sample size (Schutt 2008):

☐ The larger the sample size, the less the sampling error.

☐ Samples of more diverse populations need to be larger than samples of more homogeneous populations.

☐ If only a few variables are to be examined, a smaller sample is needed, but if a more complex analysis involving sample subgroups is required, then a larger sample will be needed.

☐ If the researchers wish to test hypotheses, and expect very strong effects, they will need a smaller sample size to find these effects, but if they expect smaller effects, a larger sample is required.

Sample size can be estimated by using existing tables (Peat 2001), or calculated using relevant formulae (Friedman et al. 1998). Ideally, more precise estimation of the necessary sample size should be carried out by the use of the statistical power analysis method (Kraemer & Thiemann 1987). This analysis allows 'a good advance estimate of the strength of the hypothesized relationship in the population' (Schutt 2008, p. 155). However, it is a complicated analysis and it may require researchers to work with a statistician to determine the size of their research sample. See also CHAPTERS 15, 19.

DOING RESEARCH

Obtaining evidence from women living with HIV/AIDS in Thailand

Before ending this chapter, I would like to give readers a reflective practice example from my own research that I conducted collaboratively with colleagues from two universities in Thailand (see Liamputtong et al. 2009).

Pranee Liamputtong

Thai women are now experiencing a high prevalence of HIV and AIDS. Therefore there is an urgent need for health care providers to understand their experiences so that more sensitive health care can be made available to these women. In this study, we examined the women's perspectives on community attitudes towards women currently living with HIV/AIDS. We also looked at strategies employed by women in order to deal with any stigma and discrimination they might feel or experience in their communities. Last, we examined the reasons that women had for participating in drug/vaccine trials.

A qualitative approach was adopted in this study. The qualitative approach is appropriate because qualitative researchers accept that in order to understand people's behaviour we must attempt to understand the meanings and interpretations that people give to their behaviour. Using a qualitative method enables the researcher to examine the interpretations and meanings of HIV/AIDS within the women's perspectives. The strength of using qualitative methodology is that it has a holistic focus, which allows for flexibility and also allows the participants to raise issues and topics that may not have been included by the researcher, so adding to the quality of the data collected. This approach is particularly appropriate when the researcher has little knowledge of the researched participants and their views.

A purposive sampling technique was adopted for this research; that is, only Thai women who had HIV/AIDS and who were participating, or had participated, in HIV clinical trials, and female drug users who had been participating in vaccine trials, were approached to participate in the study. The participants were recruited through advertisements on bulletin boards at hospitals and personal contacts made by the Thai co-researchers, who have carried out a number of HIV and AIDS research projects with Thai women. In conducting research related to HIV/AIDS, the recruitment process needs to be highly sensitive to the needs of the participants. The sensitivity of this research guided our discussion of how we would approach the women and invite them to take part. We directly contacted potential participants ourselves only after they were introduced by our network or our gatekeepers. Because of the sensitive nature of this study, we also relied on snowball sampling techniques; that is, our participants suggested others who were interested in participating. We also enlisted the assistance of leaders of two HIV and AIDS support groups to access the women in this study.

In-depth interviews and some participant observations were conducted with 26 Thai women. The number of participants was determined by the theoretical sampling technique, which dictates that recruiting stops when little new data emerges. We interviewed the women in places that they selected. Most often, the interviews were done in a café or in a shopping mall. Since the women wished to preserve their confidentiality and identities as HIV persons, they did not wish us to interview them in their own homes.

Interviews were conducted in the Thai language to maintain as much as possible of the subtlety and any hidden meanings of the participant's statements. Before the study began, ethical approval was obtained from the Faculty of Health Sciences Human Ethics Committee, La Trobe University, Australia, and from the Ethics Committee at Chulalongkorn University, Thailand. Before making an appointment for interviews, each participant's consent to participate in the study was sought. After a full explanation of the study had been given, and the length of interviewing time and the scope of questions had been explained, the participants were asked to sign a consent form. Each interview took between one and two hours. Each participant was paid 200 Thai baht as compensation for their time spent in taking part in the study. This incentive is necessary for sensitive research such as this, as it is a way to show research participants that their time and knowledge are respected.

With permission from the participants, interviews were tape-recorded. The tapes were then transcribed in Thai, for data analysis. The in-depth data were analysed using a thematic analysis. All transcripts were coded, and emerging themes were subsequently identified. The emerging themes were presented in the results section of the report on the research. In presenting women's verbatim responses, we used fictitious names in order to preserve confidentiality and avoid disclosure of the women's identity.

As you can see, there are many issues we need to consider in carrying out a piece of research, not only which approach and which method to use, but who will be our research participants, how we will find them and how many we need for our project. Also, ethical issues requiring consideration need to be identified, and we need to consider how we will make sense of the data we have collected, and how we will present this data and its analysis. All these matters are covered in this book. I encourage all readers to consult most of the chapters in the book, to make themselves familiar with the way that we can use research methods to gather evidence that we can use in practice. In the case of the example that I present in this box, it is the evidence that we gather from women living with HIV/AIDS that can be used to develop sensitive health care practice for vulnerable and marginalised women in Thailand.

SUMMARY

> Neither quantitative nor qualitative methodology is in any ultimate sense superior to the other. The two approaches exist along a continuum on which neither pole is more 'scientific' or more suited to…knowledge development. (Williams et al. 2008, p. 100)

In this chapter, I have introduced the concept of evidence and evidence-based practice in health. I have argued that in many situations and for many health issues, researchers and practitioners need to find the 'best' evidence, and this may require us to carry out a research study to find our answers. I have provided readers with firm foundations for carrying out research in health. I have suggested that researchers should not favour one method over another based on their own preferences. Rather, we need to consider carefully the research questions to which we wish to find answers.

Qualitative and quantitative research approaches, as Williams and colleagues (2008, p. 100) contend, 'have existed side by side since the beginning of contemporary social science. They both attempt to describe and explain social reality. The main difference between them lies in the way that they do it. Despite their differences, however, both approaches are planful, systematic, and empirical. They are equally valid approaches to…knowledge generation.' Each research approach, be it qualitative or quantitative, has its special uses. Rather than asking which approach is best, it would be more appropriate for us to ask 'under what conditions each approach is better than the other in order to answer a particular research question' (Williams et al. 2008, p. 99). This is what I have advocated in this chapter.

Taking a step further from the debate about using either a qualitative or quantitative approach, I have also suggested that perhaps we need to consider the use of a mixed methods design in our research. This will allow us to make the best use of evidence from both research approaches, and the information we generate from using this design may be the best evidence for our practice.

In summary, I argue that knowledge is essential in the era of evidence-based practice in health care. Without knowledge, evidence cannot be generated. Without 'appropriate' evidence, our practice may not be applicable or suitable to those who health care providers/practitioners need to serve.

TUTORIAL EXERCISES

1   You have been asked by your superior to find the 'best' evidence that can be used to develop culturally sensitive maternal and child health services for Indigenous Australians. How would you find this 'best' evidence? Discuss various types of evidence that you could obtain.

2   There has been a good deal of discussion in your local area about young people, who are seen to be likely to engage in risky health-related behaviour, such as smoking heavily, driving very fast, and not paying attention to their dietary make-up. You want to understand why young people tend to take such health risks. Which research approach (qualitative or quantitative) is likely to provide you with the greater in-depth understanding of their life, the meaning they attach to risk-taking behaviour and their lived experiences of risk? Discuss.

3   You want to ascertain the prevalence of risk-taking behaviour among young people in your city. What approach will provide you with an estimate of this prevalence and how will you go about doing this? Discuss.

4   As you need to design a research study that will provide the best answers that you can find, what important issues do you need to consider? Please write up a short account of your proposed research, taking into account salient issues that have been discussed in this chapter.

FURTHER READING

Aoun, S.M. & Kristjanson, L.J. (2005). Evidence in palliative care research: How should it be gathered? *Medical Journal of Australia*, 183(5), 264–6.

Creswell, J. & Plano Clark, V.L. (2007). *Designing and conducting mixed methods research*. Thousand Oaks, CA: Sage Publications.

Denzin, N.K. (2009). The elephant in the living room: Or extending the conversation about the politics of evidence. *Qualitative Research*, 9(2), 139–60.

Gibson, B.E. & Martin, D.K. (2003). Qualitative research and evidence-based physiotherapy practice. *Physiotherapy*, 89, 350–58.

Grypdonck, M.H.F. (2006). Qualitative health research in the era of evidence-based practice. *Qualitative Health Research*, 16(10), 1371–85.

Hammell, K.W. & Carpenter, C. (2004). *Qualitative research in evidence-based rehabilitation*. Edinburgh: Churchill Livingstone.

Hawker, S., Payne, S., Kerr, C., Hardey, M. & Powell, J. (2002). Appraising the evidence: Reviewing disparate data systematically. *Qualitative Health Research*, 12(9), 1284–99.

Johnson, R. & Waterfield, J. (2004). Making words count: The value of qualitative research. *Physiotherapy Research International*, 9(3), 121–31.

Liamputtong, P. (2009). *Qualitative research methods*, 3rd edn. Melbourne: Oxford University Press.

Mullen, E.J., Bellamy, J.L. & Bledsoe, S.E. (2008). Evidence-based practice. In R.M. Grinnell & Y.A. Unrau (eds), *Social work research and evaluation: Foundations of evidence-based practice*, 8th edn. New York: Oxford University Press, 508–24.

WEBSITES

www.womenandhealthcarereform.ca/en/work_evidence.html

This website provides useful discussions on evidence and women's health care. It argues that 'because women are not all the same, changes to the health care system may variously affect the health, well-being and work of particular groups of women. This means that when evidence is used by decision-makers in the development and implementation of health care reforms, women need to question what is being counted as evidence, whose perspective and experience is being counted, if the differing contexts of women's lives are being considered, and which women's needs are being included and excluded.'

http://en.wikipedia.org/wiki/Evidence-based_medicine

This website provides good discussion on EBP and its limitations.

www.gla.ac.uk/media/media_48396_en.pdf

This website contains a set of slides on the contribution of the qualitative approach to EBP, which will be useful for the many readers who are sceptical about the value of qualitative research.

www.conted.ox.ac.uk/courses/details.php?id=48

This is the website of Oxford University's MSc in Evidence-Based Health Care program. It is part of the Oxford International Programme in Evidence-Based Health Care. It is offered as a part-time course consisting of six taught modules and a dissertation. The course provides extensive coverage of the role of research methods, including both qualitative and quantitative approaches, in providing the information needed for EBP.

www.nationalschool.gov.uk/policyhub/evaluating_policy/how_res_eval_evid.asp

This website provides discussions of the ways in which evidence contributes to policy-making. It suggests that evidence-based policy involves a balance between professional judgment and expertise and the use of valid, reliable and relevant research evidence.

2

What is Ethical Research?

Paul Ramcharan

CHAPTER OBJECTIVES

In this chapter you will learn:

☐ basic principles of research ethics as they relate to health and social care research

☐ about developments and changes to ethical regulation since Helsinki (1964)

☐ how contemporary Human Research Ethics Committees operate

☐ how to critically appraise ethical regulation and key topics of continuing debate

☐ how to support readers to apply their learning in their review of other studies and in constructing their own research ethically

KEY TERMS

Anonymity

Confidentiality

Deontological ethics

Ethical principles

Etics

Human research ethics committee

Informed consent

Regulation

Research ethics

Research participant

Research subject

Risk and harm

Sensitive topics

Utilitarian

Virtue ethics

Vulnerable people

INTRODUCTION

All human interaction produces a relationship between the people involved. These relationships can be passing or long term; they can be affective or businesslike; they can be warm or distanced; they can be pleasurable or not, as the case might be. Like all forms of human interaction, research undertaken on human research subjects or in which human subjects are participants raises issues about what motivates a person to enter into an interaction, how a person should comport themselves, and how a person's interaction affects the other(s) involved. Researchers in health and social care research rely on members of the public who choose to continue to accept invitations to be involved in research. As such, it is in the interests of researchers to carry out their research in a way that supports this outcome. But how do researchers accomplish this? What are the rules of conduct for such relationships? And how can we be sure that researchers are acting in a moral or ethical way? This area of research is often referred to as **research ethics**, the subject matter of this chapter.

Research ethics is understood as finding the balance between the risks associated with a research project and its benefits.

TRY IT YOURSELF

Consider why you see the following as questionable. What does this tell you about your own values?

- ☐ Living prisoners are given by the King to a medical practitioner for research using vivisection, i.e. surgery while alive (reported of Herophilus, 335–280BC).
- ☐ In 1796 a doctor, Edward Jenner, injects a young boy with the material in cowpox blisters from a sufferer of the disease in order to examine the effects and later continues to do so on many more research subjects.

These and other examples are reported on the following website: ‹http://en.wikipedia.org/wiki/Human_experimentation#History›

There are more recent examples. Under Nazi experimentation 400 000 people were subjected to varying means of sterilisation as a means of ensuring that feeble genes would not damage the national gene pool; experiments were conducted on 1500 pairs of twins, of which only 200 survived; thousands were subjected to freezing experiments to establish how best to protect Nazi troops on the front line. Between 1932 and 1972, a total of 399 poor African Americans were denied treatment for syphilis despite penicillin having been found to be a cure in 1947. The Tuskegee Syphilis study, as it was called, resulted in the death of some study patients, passing on their syphilis to others as well as suffering discomfort unnecessarily (see also Liamputtong 2009, 2010).

The power relationships in these examples are worth noting: researchers gained power by royal decree and, in Jenner's case, by government plaudit and public funding. In situations of sanctioned coercion or in working with vulnerable or ill-informed subjects, it is easier for researchers to exert their will over the research 'subject'—a term that has long been rejected in favour of 'participant'. In contrast, '**research participant**' refers to a person who agrees to take part in the study on equal terms. Equality of power in the research relationship therefore requires the freedom, that is, *autonomy and will*, to choose to take part in a study whose nature is well understood by the prospective participants.

> **Research participant:** A person who agrees to take part in the study on equal terms.

Given the experiences of the Second World War, in 1948 principles of medical research were established at Nuremberg, and in 1964 the World Medical Association extended and formalised the Nuremberg principles in their Helsinki Declaration, a declaration considered to be the seminal work on which ethical regulation to the present day is based.

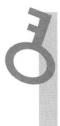

TRY IT YOURSELF

☐ Is it enough to have *principles* for doing research ethically that researchers follow by choice? Or should there be *regulation* where what researchers do or intend to do is scrutinised, granted permission, and where sanctions can be applied?

☐ If you think there should be regulation, then who should have the power to say whether a piece of research is ethical and can go ahead?

The Helsinki Declaration, part of which will be considered later, was written originally for medical research, and much social research did not come under its regulatory aegis until fairly recently. Consider the following two case studies.

DOING RESEARCH

A researcher acted as a 'Watch Queen', warning men participating in homosexual acts in public lavatories if a member of the public was approaching. The researcher undertook 50 interviews there and then. However, where this was not possible, the researcher copied the men's car registration numbers and traced their home addresses. He later disguised himself and undertook a 'health survey' with 50 more participants, part of which covered homosexuality (Humphreys 1975).

DOING RESEARCH

A researcher recruited research participants and paid them a small sum to take part in an experiment which they were told was about memory and learning in different conditions. The participant was introduced to a 'learner' (an actor) and an 'experimenter' (the

Paul Ramcharan

researcher). The experimenter told the participant that the learner would have to memorise word pairs and that when they got one wrong a shock would be administered by the participant (no shock was actually administered, but the participant did not know this). The participant was given a small shock to indicate the 'learner's' experience. The participant was told they would have to raise the shock intensity 15 volts for each incorrect answer. The 'learner' cried out each time a 'shock' was administered, more loudly as the voltage increased. If the participant wanted to stop taking part the researcher used successive prompts: Please continue; the experiment requires that you continue; it is absolutely essential that you continue; you have no other choice; you must go on (Milgram 1974).

TRY IT YOURSELF

☐ In small groups consider the case studies. Have the researchers done anything wrong? Why? Report your group's view and discuss whether there are any differences in your opinions.

☐ Have your views on whether to regulate research or not changed through your discussions?

CONVERGING PRINCIPLES IN MEDICAL, HEALTH AND SOCIAL CARE RESEARCH?

There remained within social research considerable debate around the probity of covert or disguised research up to the 1980s (see e.g. Erikson 1967; Douglas 1976; Denzin 1982). Bulmer (1982) contends that the covert research debate lays bare some of the key principles on which contemporary research ethics are based, and to the end of this section, therefore, key ethical principles will be italicised (or bolded). For example, some would argue that Humphreys' (1975) covert study of homosexuality did not allow **informed consent**, that is, that people from whom data was collected understood the research and agreed to participate on the basis of this understanding; the research approach used both *disguise* and *deception*; it also involved an invasion of *privacy* with records linking car registration and home addresses.

Informed consent: Before data collection, participants are informed of the aims and methods of the research and asked for their consent.

Anonymity refers to a person being unknown to the researcher and hence to anyone else.

Confidentiality conceals the true identity of participants to protect them from any negative consequences, particularly those marginalised and stigmatised in society.

Humphreys points out that although he used deception and invaded people's privacy, at no time was the **anonymity** of the person breached. The term 'anonymity' refers to a person being unknown to the researcher and hence to anyone else. Furthermore, where the person took part in the public health survey their **confidentiality** was maintained. Confidentiality differs from anonymity in that the researcher knows the person's identity and further things about them but does not divulge this identity or acts, circumstances or places that might lead to identification in any way at any time. Humphreys argues that his study *benefited* a population that was deeply misunderstood and one that was persecuted for its sexuality and most certainly for its public expression. In short, Humphreys' argument was that the *risks* of the research were outweighed by the research *benefits*. This central issue is one that will be revisited shortly.

Milgram's experiment has similar issues around deception and confidentiality (of people 'willing to administer shocks' to strangers!). Three further principles emerge from this study. The first is that if a person is paid to become involved in a piece of research, they are more likely to do what they are told or to give answers or views they expect will be those the researcher wishes to hear. This is methodologically as well as ethically unsound. Such payment could be seen as an *inducement* if it covers more than expenses or token appreciation (Grady 2001). Second, the researcher exerted undue pressure for compliance so that the participant did not actively consent and did not have *equal power* to that of the researcher. Third, many of the participants showed signs of stress and distress at what they were doing; they showed *discomfort* and may well have been harmed by their experience.

Unifying concepts for these principles have been widely attributed to the work of Beauchamp and Childress (2001) in their *Principles of Biomedical Ethics*, first published in 1979. The authors argue for four key **ethical principles**: *respecting autonomy*—the person making an informed decision about being involved; *beneficence*—the obligation to provide benefits not to the participant necessarily, but certainly to the 'public good'; *non-maleficence*—avoiding bad intention or the causing of harm or discomfort disproportionate to the benefits of the research; and *justice*—the concept that benefits, risks and costs are equitably distributed. These ideas appear widely in contemporary regulatory research ethics frameworks.

Ethical principles: There are four principles that researchers must adhere to in their research: respecting autonomy, beneficence, non-maleficence, and justice.

UNDERSTANDING AND APPLYING THE PRINCIPLES OF ETHICAL RESEARCH

Even where the principles of research ethics have been shared (Lacey 1998), the organisational response has varied across countries and in relation to health as opposed to social or behaviourally focused research. For example, in the USA, Institutional Review Boards (set up after the Belmont Report 1979) have gradually extended from medical and behavioural studies to cover social and social care research. In contrast, in the UK the regulation of social care research remains a hot topic for debate (Dominelli & Holloway 2008), with a new Social Care Research Ethics Committee housed at the Social Care Institute of Excellence, a quasi-government organisation, only being announced in 2008.

In Australia, the Medical Council *Statement on human experimentation* was issued in 1966 in direct response to Helsinki, followed by a subcommittee recommendation in 1976 in Supplementary Note 1 to make it a requirement for all proposed research involving human subjects to be examined by an institutional ethics committee (IEC). By 1985, no human research without permission from the appropriate committee could be accorded public funding. Before that, research in social sciences such as psychology, sociology and anthropology were guided by statements by their Australian Associations. The National Health and Medical Research Council (NHMRC), established in 1992, issued its *National statement on ethical conduct in research involving humans* (NHMRC 1999b), and more recently this has been updated in the *National statement on ethical conduct in human research* (2007). In what follows, the regulatory framework is considered in relation to some of the key ethical principles outlined above.

The membership of the **human research ethics committee** (HREC) can be a decisive factor in that it needs to carry knowledge and expertise of the merit and standards that apply across research paradigms and groups to make fair and just decisions and to do so with 'due process' (De Vries et al. 2004; Edwards et al. 2004). The NHMRC guidelines (2007) recommend an ethics committee makeup that includes researchers, health and social care professionals, a lawyer, lay members, and someone with a pastoral role in the community. They also indicate the need to have a balance of men and women as well as people who are regularly present or are co-opted for specialist expertise.

Human research ethics committee: A group of people that includes researchers, health and social care professionals, a lawyer, lay members, and a balance of men and women.

Below is a summary of key requirements for research ethics committees and the key issues around their decision-making.

Generic requirements

When submitting an application to an HREC, the researcher will be required to submit a research proposal. In this regard the 2008 Helsinki Declaration says:

> Article 12 'Medical research involving human subjects must conform to generally accepted scientific principles.'

> Article 14 'The design and performance of each research study involving human subjects must be clearly described in a research protocol. The protocol should contain a statement of the ethical considerations involved.'

The reason for this is that 'a poorly designed study is by definition unethical' (Lynoe et al. 1999, p. 152) since it cannot produce the benefits claimed. Any risk would be too great when set against a study that has no benefit. The protocol is likely to require some review of literature, a statement of the study's aims, the numbers in the sample and means of recruitment, the approach to analysis, and research tools such as questionnaires being used alongside consideration of the ethical issues. However, there are some issues around Lynoe's dictum.

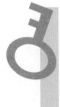

TRY IT YOURSELF

Is there anything ethically questionable about the following research? A new drug for cancer is being tested. The researchers have proposed a double-blind randomised controlled trial (see CHAPTER 15). This means that before analysis of results neither the researcher nor the subjects know which of the sample are given the new drug and which a placebo.

In this example, a sacrifice of methodological rigour is important because it would be wrong to ask people to forgo a life-saving treatment and 'intolerable' if they did not know whether they were in the experimental or placebo group (Kent 1996). Not all well-designed projects are, by being well designed, ethical.

A second criticism is that qualitative studies and their research relationships can be complex (de Laine 2000; Guillemin & Gillam 2004). Moreover, an emergent research design means that the researcher is initially less clear on samples and sample size and has to alter the approach to data collection to test emergent theories. Action research, which is being used increasingly in the health and social care fields, requires reorientation of the research as it proceeds (Khanlou & Peter 2004; see Chapter 1). There are also issues around 'proportionality'. The latter argument is that, judged against the invasiveness and potential threats to the physical integrity of the body in much medical research, health and social research produces far less risk. It is far more efficient to use a 'lighter touch' than subject all research to the same level of scrutiny to satisfy the surveillance needs of an 'audit culture' (Strathern 2000). Moreover, that a committee has the right to judge whether a person can themselves respond suggests a degree of paternalism that infringes autonomy and the individual's own right to choose.

In stating the four principles listed above, the most recent NHMRC guidelines (2007) implicitly recognise a broad base of research approaches. Further, the guidelines on qualitative research adapt the Helsinki emphasis on 'generally accepted scientific principles' and 'scientific protocols' to, *inter alia*, emphasis on the applicability of findings and not capacity for generalisation (para 3.1.4), and rigour not being judged on sample size (para 3.1.6) or validity and reliability as in quantitative approaches (para 3.18) but on 'quality and credibility of data collection and analysis' (para 3.18). See also Chapter 1.

Beneficence/non-maleficence

The UK has for a long time had an electronic ethics application form, and in Australia the National Ethics Application Form has been introduced at the time of writing (early 2009). So what in addition to the proposal will the health researcher need to do to complete these forms? Earlier, it was argued that at all times the benefits of research must outweigh its risks, and this is a central equation on which ethics committee members seek to form their judgment.

TRY IT YOURSELF

Write a list of what risks and what benefits you think might arise in health and social care research.

Lists of risks are provided in Table 2.1. These are not exhaustive, and in their deliberations ethics committee members will also consider the seriousness of the risk, its probability of occurrence, and the strategies to minimise the risk and to address any risk that remains (see NHMRC 2007, *passim* 15–18).

Paul Ramcharan

Table 2.1: Thinking about potential ethical risks in a research project

Potential risks	
Health	Injury to body (e.g. through invasive medical procedure); using healthy volunteers for experiment (e.g. sleep deprivation and mechanical manipulation study); side effects (e.g. of a new drug); discomfort or inconvenience (e.g. of procedure from lengthy sessions, interviews or focus groups); placebo and delay of treatment; indirect risk (e.g. on public transport as a result of a procedure).
Psychological	Stress (e.g. of procedure or of memories and thoughts); emotional (memories, procedure or effect on relationships); identity (e.g. a person's self-ascription of deviance, vulnerability, powerlessness); distress (e.g. as a result of the approach taken to data collection or its inconvenience); worry over effects of participating (e.g. of a service provider who knows a person who has taken part); arrangements for withdrawal from the study.
To the community	Disproportionate impacts on marginalised groups or in sensitive areas; economic, political, social effects of working with some groups (e.g. from minority ethnic or religious communities, indigenous groups, those seeking asylum, those socio-economically disadvantaged, those who are disenfranchised and those without a voice).

As well as the actual process of carrying out research, harm can be produced by the way in which data is collected, stored and then published. Data collection for web surveys, for example, should be undertaken using methods in which identities cannot be accessed; transcript data should de-identify the participants and be stored in locked filing cabinets and on password-protected computers. In publication, major problems can emerge around the identity of participants even where names are not used. For example, giving the participant's gender and the city location of a facility (the only one in that city) that provides a service for very few clients may, given additional information on the participant's history, inadvertently give away their identity. There needs to be sensitivity towards maintaining confidentiality and anonymity, for example by using pseudonyms, making sure quotations are not attributed, or using 'composite stories' combining the views of several participants to describe a recurrent **theme** or theory (see also Dickson-Swift et al. 2008; Liamputtong 2009).

Theme: A grouping of data emerging from the research and to which the researcher gives a name.

So if there are substantial risks, what are the benefits against which these should be offset? Table 2.2 lists some of the benefits against which risks can be offset.

Table 2.2: Some potential benefits accruing from a research study

Benefits	
To knowledge	Knowledge may have direct application (utility) or it may be for 'enlightenment'; it may be personal in terms of increase in skills, insight or understanding.
To the participant	Taking part, hope, a chance to reconsider life, identity and relationships may benefit; public service (i.e. giving back by contributing); the direct change to services, life outcome; identity (e.g. chance to reformulate their identity by taking part); new technology and interventions; learning resources.
To the public good	Knowledge of the public about an issue; Practitioner resources and knowledge; contributing to the community's ability to address problems of health or disadvantage, to deliver economic benefits, challenge injustice and promote equality.

Given the complexity of research, there are a number of other key issues that are considered below with a focus on completing the ethics committee application forms.

AUTONOMY

TRY IT YOURSELF

Discuss the ethics of the following scenarios:

1   A part-time doctoral student also runs a counselling service in which she has developed a new method of working with clients. The student has submitted an application to the HREC to evaluate this new method of counselling. Participants are receiving treatment free as long as they agree to complete a questionnaire and a battery of health measures every two weeks and undergo an interview at the end. The cost of the eight sessions would ordinarily be $720.

2   In a study of quality of life and health outcomes among people with intellectual disabilities, a participant is unable to answer some questions about the health professionals with whom he has had contact. With the participant's permission, a member of staff has joined in the discussion but remains seated for the rest of the interview in which the participant is evaluating the service she receives.

In the first scenario, there is a potential conflict of interest as it is in the interests of the student to produce results that promote their own counselling approach. The payment at *the end* of the therapy sessions may mean that participants carry on with sessions even where these create discomfort and, especially where it is the researcher who administers the questionnaires or conducts the final interview, the participants may not feel free to give their real views.

In the second scenario, the professional service received by the client might not be honestly reported because of the presence of one of the providers.

Another aspect of autonomy is the prospective participant's understanding of the research in making a decision about whether to participate. In this regard, as well as the research proposal, the applicant is also required to produce a plain language statement that outlines the details of the study in language understandable to participants. This should inform the potential participant about the project's title and aim; the investigators involved; the funding source; rights as a participant (including the right to withdraw, to have identifiable data withdrawn, to have questions answered); what is expected; the risks and relevant safeguards; the benefits of the research; and to whom complaints or questions should be directed. Similar information should be included in a letter or frontispiece to postal questionnaires or as a series of boxes that have to be clicked before completion of web-based surveys. This approach assumes that return of a questionnaire or submission via the web implies consent to participate.

The plain language statement above is submitted with the HREC application along with a consent form that is signed by the participant (and in some circumstances by their guardian or advocate) and witnessed by the researcher. These should be kept in a locked filing cabinet. Consent forms usually have statements or tick boxes in which the participant says they have read the plain language statement, understand confidentiality and anonymity issues for the study, recognise that they have the rights to withdraw from the study at any time without consequence, and understand that the researcher commits to keeping the data secure.

Issues around consent and autonomy

ARE THERE EXCEPTIONS?

TRY IT YOURSELF

Discuss whether consent is necessary in the following case studies.

1   A study was undertaken to assess the impact of HIV status on outcomes of intensive care treatment and to assess whether HIV patients should be prioritised for non-HIV intensive care treatment. The participants were not told they were being tested for HIV and no staff were informed about the person's HIV status (see Bhagwanjee et al. 1997a).

2   Although questions later arose around his 'interviews' and methods (Fleck & Muller 1997), a Nazi concentration camp inmate collects data that, when he is released, later forms the basis of a book on the psychology of living in extreme conditions (Bettelheim 1943).

In defence of their HIV study, Bhagwanjee and associates (1997b) point out that the ethics committee had given consent for their study, they could not have gained consent on admission, and no staff were informed of any person's HIV status. The study was undertaken in Natal, South Africa where they report that: 'By the end of 1992 over 300 000 people were infected... If the worst case scenario materialises, by 2010 it is estimated that 28–52% of all deaths will be related to HIV infection' (p. 1082). The ethics committee held that the study was of national importance and sufficiently in the *public interest* to waive the right to consent in this case, though this position was by no means universally accepted (e.g. Kale 1997).

Had Bettelheim made known his data collection and study intentions, it is probable that he would not have survived the concentration camp. In such situations is the study's benefit great enough to warrant disguise and deception? As recently pointed out by Liamputtong (2007, p. 138), 'Sensitive researchers need to think carefully about what method will be best for them to use to work with vulnerable individuals and groups and the moral and ethical issues that go with the method.' This raises wider issues in relation to working with sensitive topics and with vulnerable groups as discussed below.

SENSITIVE TOPICS AND VULNERABLE GROUPS

Lee and Renzetti (1993) delineate **sensitive topics** as among those that may touch deep emotions (e.g. death or dying, eating disorders, sexual abuse), areas that may be culturally taboo for research (e.g. religion or homosexuality in some cultures), areas in which the research threatens powerful interests (e.g. the arms trade or large corporations) or areas of deviance (e.g. drug-taking cultures or places in which there is or may be illegal activity). Awareness of the likely effects of participation is important in this respect alongside the methodology being adopted and the strategy for withdrawal. For example, interviews may be one-off or they may require more time and more visits. If the interview takes place on one occasion the researcher needs to have a view on whether the sensitivity of the interview may lead to an emotional reaction at a later date (see also Liamputtong 2007; Dickson-Swift et al. 2008).

> **Sensitive topics** arise in research that may cause emotional upset or pose some physical and emotional risks to the research participants.

Where the interview is held over several meetings, other ethical issues arise because of the different level of rapport and emotional involvement involved (Minichiello et al. 2008). A number of further ethical issues arise in these circumstances. A one-off consent sheet hardly suffices and it is important to establish 'consent as a process' (Cutcliffe & Ramcharan 2002; Royal College of Nursing Research Society 2005; Wiles et al. 2005). The closeness of the relationship may lead to a 'delusion of alliance' (Stacey 1988) or to new issues about gauging how much trust exists within the research relationship (McDonald et al. 2008). Researchers need to be careful not to exert subtle pressure and to ensure the relationship does not become too intrusive (Stalker 1998). And, given the relationship that develops, the researcher needs to manage an exit strategy that does the least harm (Booth 1999).

In considering such issues, ethics committee members tend to perceive such issues of 'vulnerability' in terms of the 'level of risk'. This is a third area of contention in much ethics committee decision-making, as outlined below.

Paul Ramcharan

RISK AND VULNERABILITY

Some **vulnerable people** may find it difficult to understand the language and concepts of research and therefore informed consent sheets or plain language statements will be beyond them (Liamputtong 2007, 2010). The irony for much health and social care research is that social justice, that is, that all people are treated fairly and equally, means a disproportionate interest in such groups. It is also inconceivable that such research should be suspended, for it would be unethical to stop potentially useful research on the grounds of difficulty in understanding. There have been a number of responses to this issue.

Vulnerable people:
Individuals who are marginalised or discriminated against because of their class, ethnicity, gender, age, illness, disability or sexual preference.

In the past some organisations have sought to organise in-house ethics procedures for the 'best interests' of 'their' clients, meaning that researchers have to submit ethics applications to more than one ethics committee. Iacono (2006) also reports that one HREC in Australia empowered the Office of the Public Advocate to assess the capacity of potential participants to consent to 'subjecting vulnerable people to a substantial number of probing questions, thus multiplying the effects any research might subsequently have had' (Ramcharan 2006, p. 183). Thankfully, the present Australian NHMRC guidelines propose a responsibility to 'adopt a review process that eliminates unnecessary duplication of ethical review' (NHMRC 2007, Section 5.3.1, p. 87), but the institution still has a responsibility to 'identify any local circumstances…and provide for their management' (Section 5.3.3a, p. 87).

In the UK the latter point has been formalised into a research governance framework (Department of Health 2005). This has meant that researchers have had to apply to the institutions in which the research is taking place, which again involves committees. As well as the resulting delays, there are issues about the independence of local services to make such decisions. The Helsinki Declaration understandably specified that decision-making should remain independent of the researcher and sponsor to ensure no conflicts of interest, and it is conceivable that some organisations might use this power to prevent challenging or unwanted research and to claim, for example, that their clients are overresearched or would be unable to participate meaningfully.

A second approach is that ethics committees identify levels of risk for each application. One of the criteria around risk relates to 'vulnerable groups', for example children, indigenous populations and people with intellectual disability, mental illness or cognitive impairment (see also CHAPTER 21). The present Australian guidelines carry a significant list in these respects (NHMRC 2007, Section 5). However, the danger is that to identify whole groups as 'higher risk' or 'unable to consent' can be seen as a labelling issue that infringes the rights of at least some individuals in these groups to decide for themselves whether to take part (Ramcharan 2006, p. 184). It is then difficult to establish a balance between protection of the potentially vulnerable and paternalism and stereotyping.

Such surveillance might be construed by some as a sinister attempt by powerful interests to control the free-minded. It also indicates a loss of trust: here '**virtue ethics**', where judgments are made about a person (*qua* researcher) by their demonstrated moral character, and '**deontological ethics**', in which a person acts in accord with (researcher) obligations and duties, have no place. Instead the dominant model is '**utilitarian**', based on the assumption that it is possible to predict the likely consequences of an action (in this case research) and the likely benefit it will have for the greatest number of people.

Having established many of the ethical principles and pointed to the ways in which they are made operational, it is important to recognise that the decision-making by research ethics committees is a form of peer review. It is not a scientific process with an easily calculated answer. In this respect, the decisions made by committees are made on the information provided and the case made will ultimately be subject to both the frailties and the benefits of human decision-making processes.

Virtue ethics: A situation where judgments are made about a person (*qua* researcher) by their demonstrated moral character.

Deontological ethics: Ethics in which a person acts in accord with (researcher) obligations and duties.

Utilitarian: A model based on the assumption that it is possible to predict the likely consequences of research and the likely benefit it will have for the greatest number of people.

SUMMARY

The framework for ethical regulation has come a long way since the Helsinki Declaration and there is now certainly a system in place to which medical, health, behavioural and social care researchers are required to submit their research proposals for scrutiny. But there are a number of remaining issues, some fundamental and others of a more practical and evidential kind. First and foremost is the fundamental issue about the extent to which regulation is necessary at all. At one level, there are arguments here about the extent to which surveillance by regulatory bodies is itself infringing freedoms: the freedom of some participants to make their own decision rather than having a formal body with the power to take away that right; as well as the freedom of thought so necessary for researchers to break new ground and create knowledge.

But even if the utilitarian model is used, there are some really thorny problems. First, since the decision is taken by an ethics committee before the research begins, it is conceivable that the researcher might comport him or herself in an unpalatable way during the research, particularly for research among those who are most vulnerable and who have least voice and power. Second, no research evidence-base drawing on previous research (again, particularly with vulnerable groups) has been used to demonstrate the ethical dilemmas that have actually been encountered. The problem here is that the regulatory system tends to operate from a worst case scenario. The surveillance approach may therefore be highly inefficient, and unnecessary. Additionally, there is an issue around proportionality in the ethical regulation process. How dangerous is an

Paul Ramcharan

interview or participant observation compared to physically invasive research? Is the same level of regulation really necessary?

Since research and its associated methods change and adapt, so too do the principles that guide the ethical regulation of research. For example, participatory and emancipatory research paradigms will involve the collection and use of data by the beneficiaries of the research. What new relationships are created when the researched become researchers, when they are privy to information and when they seek to publish their findings (see CHAPTER 21)? As the world contracts by transport and through new media, how can we rethink regulation across national boundaries and fend off the cultural imperialism of frameworks imposed on other cultures and nations? If the majority of the population gain through technology access to information on which they base their everyday decisions, what responsibility do researchers have to record their reservations around such information given their alternative perspectives and evidence? In a world of e-technology, artificial intelligence, robotics and cloning, what will be the implications for ethical regulation and who will be in a position to police these areas?

TUTORIAL EXERCISES

1   In a group, a few students choose a recent empirical study from a doctoral thesis that is available in your library or from your tutor. Identify the ethical issues in this study. The other students should listen to the students relating the ethical issues that arise in this study and question them about how they will resolve these issues.

2   As a group, write a *wiki* that outlines the key contemporary issues and debates on research ethics in health and related research.

3   Most health research is not invasive or ethically challenging. Ethics committees are therefore a waste of time and money. Debate.

4   Your tutor will provide you with one or more research proposals. You are to form into ethics committees (with different roles) and make a decision about the research using the learning from this chapter. After you have made your decision in relation to the proposal(s), discuss how you feel about how the process operates and the difficulties HREC members may encounter in their role.

FURTHER READING

Beauchamp, T.L. & Childress, J.F. (2001). *Principles of biomedical ethics*, 5th edn. Oxford: Oxford University Press.

Bulmer, M. (2001). The ethics of social research. In N. Gilbert (ed.) *Researching social life*. London: Sage Publications.

Dickson-Swift, V., James, E. & Liamputtong, P. (2008). *Undertaking sensitive research in the health and social sciences: Managing boundaries, emotions and risks*. Cambridge: Cambridge University Press.

Liamputtong, P. (2007). *Researching the vulnerable: A guide to sensitive research methods*. London: Sage Publications.

Malone, S. (2003). Ethics at home: Informed consent in your own backyard. *Qualitative Studies in Education*, 16(6), 797–815.

Mann, C. & Stewart, F. (2000). *Internet communication and qualitative research: A handbook for researching online*. London: Sage Publications.

Mauthner, M., Birch, M., Jessop, J. & Miller, T. (2002). *Ethics in qualitative research*. London: Sage Publications.

Punch, M. (1986). *The politics and ethics of fieldwork*. Beverley Hills, CA: Sage Publications.

Shaw, I.F. (2003). Ethics in qualitative research and evaluation, *Journal of Social Work*, 3(1), 9–29.

WEBSITES

www.nhmrc.gov.au/health_ethics/research/index.htm#

The NHMRC hosts this useful website.

www.nres.npsa.nhs.uk

UK National Research Ethics Service.

www.esrc.ac.uk/ESRCInfoCentre/Images/ESRC_Re_Ethics_Frame_tcm6-11291.pdf

Economic and Social Research Council (UK, Research Ethics Framework).

http://en.wikipedia.org/wiki/Human_experimentation#History

This page contains some history around unethical human research.

www.wma.net/e/policy/b3.htm

The World Medical Association has the latest version of the Declaration of Helsinki and other resources.

www.esteve.org/FEsteve/content/publicaciones/docInteres/1074785709.67/1093864680.57/endoc.pdf

You will find the Belmont Report at this address.

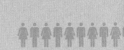

Part II

Qualitative Approaches and Practices

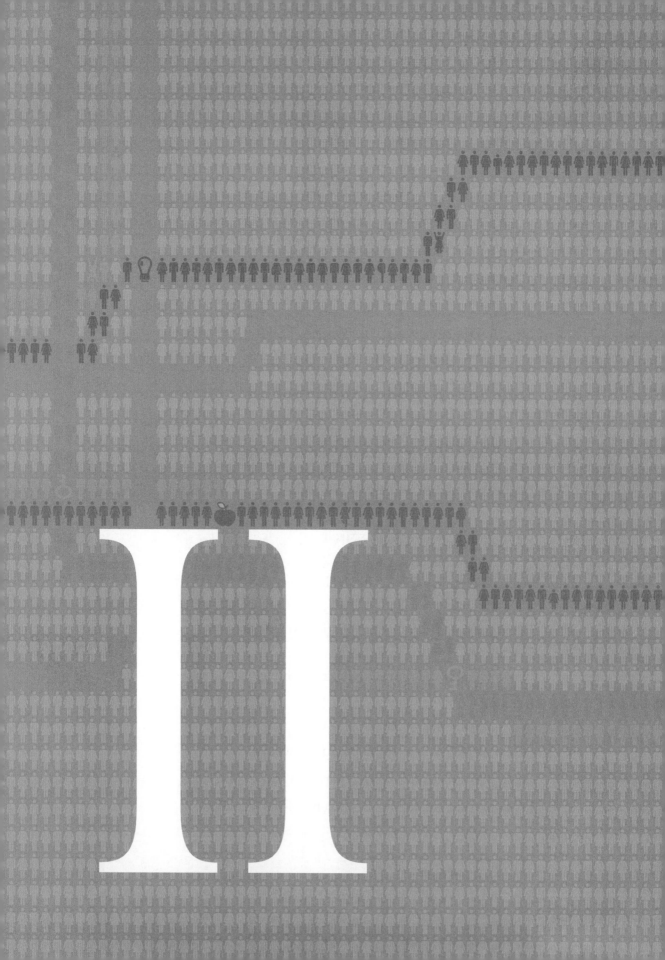

II

3

The In-depth Interviewing Method in Health

Tanya Serry and Pranee Liamputtong

CHAPTER OBJECTIVES

In this chapter you will learn:

- [ ] about the essence of the in-depth interviewing method
- [ ] how to prepare the interview structure and sequence
- [ ] how to ask questions to elicit maximal information
- [ ] about some practical considerations

KEY TERMS

In-depth interviewing

Interview transcript

Semi-structured interview

INTRODUCTION

> Interviewing is rather like marriage: Everybody knows what it is, an awful lot of people do it, and yet behind each closed front door there is a world of secrets.
> (Oakley 2009, p. 93)

In-depth interviewing:
A method of qualitative data collection. The interview does not use fixed questions, but aims to engage interviewees in conversation to elicit their understandings and interpretations.

Among qualitative research methods, **in-depth interviewing** is the most commonly known and is widely employed (Patton 2002; Holstein & Gubrium 2003; Kvale 2007; Bryman 2008; Minichiello et al. 2008; Liamputtong 2009). Conversation itself is a fundamental means of interaction among individuals in society. Through conversation, Kvale (2007) contends, individuals have an opportunity to know others, to learn about their feelings, their experiences, and the world in which they live. So if we wish to learn how people see their world, we need to talk with people (see also CHAPTER 8).

Interviews in social research are seen as 'special conversations'. Holstein and Gubrium (2003) suggest that interviewing is a way of collecting empirical data about the social world of individuals by inviting them to talk about their lives in great depth. In an interview conversation, the researcher asks questions and then listens to what individuals say about their lived experiences, such as their dreams, fears and hopes. The researcher will then hear about the interviewees' perspectives in their own words, and learn about their family and social life and work (Kvale 2007).

Most people, including researchers, will claim that they know about in-depth interviews, and that it is not difficult to ask questions and talk to people. But conducting a quality in-depth interview requires a lot more skill than just asking questions and talking to people. There are many salient matters and techniques that researchers must consider to enable the eliciting of rich, detailed and accurate information from their participants.

WHAT IS AN IN-DEPTH INTERVIEW?

An in-depth interview is in many ways similar to conversation (Liamputtong 2009) because it involves two participants who mutually observe and abide by rules of verbal interchange. Yet, as Cheek and colleagues (2004, p. 148) indicate, 'simply interviewing someone is not qualitative research'. Ritchie and Lewis (2005) point out that there is a specific purpose to the in-depth interview. Furthermore, the interviewee typically contributes more to the conversation, while the interviewer is actively engaged in listening and facilitating the flow of conversation.

Accordingly, the in-depth interview aims to elicit fruitful information from the interviewee's perspective on a selected topic. Through a partnership, researchers can delve into the 'hidden perceptions' of their research participants (Marvasti 2004, p. 21). For example, if researchers wish to examine people's attitudes towards the death penalty, in-depth interviews will allow people to adopt 'it depends' expressions. Instead of making people indicate whether they agree or disagree with capital punishment, they may say something like, 'It depends on who the victim was and how I felt about him or her' (p. 22).

An in-depth interview usually means a one-on-one, face-to-face interaction between researcher and participant. In-depth interviewing requires a greater depth of self-expression by the participant than do other interviewing methods such as focus groups (see CHAPTER 4).

'The aim of the in-depth interview is to explore the "insider perspective", to capture, in the participants' own words, their thoughts, perceptions, feelings and experiences' (Taylor 2005, p. 39).

FRAMEWORK OPTIONS FOR THE IN-DEPTH INTERVIEW

Patton (2002) describes three levels of structure in interviewing. The choice typically depends on the type of qualitative research undertaken. These options are: the informal conversational interview, the interview guide or semi-structured interview, and the standardised open-ended interview. The informal conversational interview allows for vast flexibility but is best suited to ethnographically oriented qualitative research by virtue of its informality and spontaneity (see CHAPTER 6). The standardised open-ended interview is carefully worded and ensures that all participants are asked similar questions, but it affords far less opportunity to explore themes and issues as they arise. The **semi-structured interview** provides a balance between the two more extreme approaches. Figure 3.1 depicts the options for structure in an in-depth interview along a continuum.

Semi-structured interview: An interview where the researchers elicit information from prepared questions, but at the same time allow the participants to elaborate on their responses.

Figure 3.1: Options for structure in an in-depth interview: A continuum

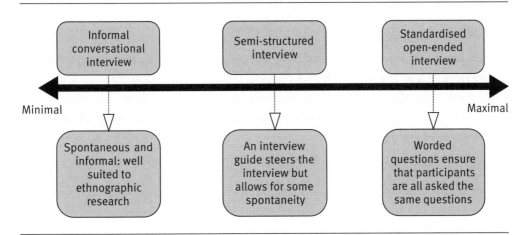

We have chosen to focus primarily on the semi-structured interview in this chapter for two reasons. First, in our experience the semi-structured format is commonly used in the health and social sciences. Second, since the semi-structured interview option takes the middle ground, it serves as a useful framework on which researchers can adapt their in-depth interview format depending on their specific research needs.

QUESTIONS AND IN-DEPTH INTERVIEWS

In order to create a comfortable and non-judgmental environment, the language and specific jargon need to be used with care if sufficient accurate and rich information is to be elicited (Fontana & Prokos 2007). Having said this, in our experience attentive researchers will intuitively use many of the attributes we outline below when formulating their questions. Our suggestions can facilitate your interaction style with participants for optimal information-gathering

Open-ended questions

Questions should be dominated by an open-ended style rather than a closed format or where forced options are given by the interviewer. Open-ended questions can allow for 'unexpected turns or digressions that follow the informants' interest or knowledge' (Johnson 2002, p. 111). In making the question open-ended, you must speak as little as possible. This will allow the participants to talk about their lived experiences in their own terms (Low 2007).

Active listening

This is a critical aspect and involves listening not only to what is said but to how it is said. Non-verbal features such as hesitations, pauses and volume changes will optimise your capacity to be actively engaged with your participant. Bryman (2008) says that researchers must also listen carefully to what the participant is not saying. This will allow you to follow up with further prompts and explore unexpected territory.

Monitoring linguistic choices

Your linguistic style should vary with different participants. Liamputtong (2009) suggests that the interviewer should monitor their own vocabulary to meet the needs of the interviewee while also ensuring that questions are grammatically clear and concise. To accommodate the diverse socio-cultural and linguistic needs of individual participants, she recommends avoiding the use of a fixed wording format.

Monitoring the use of jargon

The use of jargon should also be carefully monitored as over- or underuse can rapidly derail an interview. You will need to make astute judgments based on participants' personal or professional background and how the person presents at the interview.

The assumption of 'not knowing'

Questions presented with the implied assumption on the researcher's behalf of 'not knowing' are useful to provide an environment for the participant to talk freely and without assuming that the researcher is an expert in the field. When we explored the experiences of parents whose children have reading difficulty, we came to each interview with an intimate theoretical knowledge about the mechanisms underlying reading difficulty. Yet when asking parents how or why they think their child might have reading difficulty, we asked questions such as: 'Do you have any thoughts on how your child might have run into difficulty with reading?' This format allows parents to respond in any number of ways. For example, some parents may talk about a premature birth while others may talk about their own struggles with reading. Others may lay blame or worry that they sent their child to school too early. A poorly worded question that presents the interviewer as 'knowing' runs the risk of limiting such options.

Attention to participant's silences

Silence is important when conducting an in-depth interview. You need to be aware of the ramifications of silences in interviews. Charmaz (2002, p. 303) suggests that 'not all experiences are stories, nor are all experiences stored for ready recall. Silences have meaning too. Silences signify an absence—of words and/or perceivable emotions…[and] may…reflect active signals—of meaning, boundaries, and rules.'

Silences, as Low (2007, p. 78) suggests, may also tell you that the participant is tired. Sometimes their illness or disability prevents them from speaking, or causes pain. Silence may also mean that you have said something that makes the participant fall silent or not wish to respond to the question (Charmaz 2002). Silences should also be recorded and used in the analysis of data.

Avoid appearing to 'test' the interviewee

A question such as 'Have you thought about XYZ as a possible issue?' may appear to put the participant on trial by highlighting a fact that they may not have considered. Such questions may be perceived by your participant as disrespectful and lacking in sensitivity. Furthermore, you run the risk of introducing bias to the interview data by presenting an idea not generated by the participant.

Avoid leading questions

Similarly, asking leading questions that can influence responses should also be avoided. Leading questions are those that force the participants to respond with specific answers; inevitably, they do not allow the participants to say what they really think. A question such as 'Don't you think the system is just too underresourced?' is one such example. A more appropriate version would be 'What is your view on the resources available for people in your situation?'

Avoid dichotomies

It is crucial to limit the number of questions that can easily be answered with a simple 'yes' or 'no' or a forced choice. These questions are referred to as 'dichotomous questions' since there are only two possible answers to them. They do not encourage the participants to continue their stories, and this will shorten the interview or it will not allow the researcher to elicit in-depth information.

The question 'Why?'

Researchers must be cautious about asking the question 'Why?'. Often participants may not know *why* they behave or think in a certain manner. As a result, they may feel defensive or perhaps confronted when asked to explain the reasons for their behaviour. This does not mean that the question should not be asked in an interview, but it should be put in a different way. For example, instead of asking, 'Why do you find it hard to settle your baby?' you might ask, 'Can you tell me what you worry about when you try to settle your baby?' Occasionally, simply saying 'How come?' rather than 'Why?' can reduce the sense of confrontation potentially felt by the participant.

Non-questioning responses

An in-depth interview, as in a regular conversation, is not solely a question-and-answer exercise. Researchers also will need to engage in a variety of responses other than questions to ensure that active listening and participant engagement is maintained. Strategies may include:

- verbal or non-verbal expressions encouraging the participant to continue.
- retelling the interviewee's narrative as a tool to ensure that the researcher has understood the information correctly. For example:
  - 'So just to clarify, first you approached the classroom teacher and then you felt you really had to take it further. Is that correct?'
- acknowledging difficult questions or topics. Recently, we were interested in asking our participants about sensitive terminology. We approached the topic by framing the question as follows:
  - 'It's a bit of an "elephant in the room" but I was just wondering what your views are on ...'
- validating a participant's response, often as a springboard to further probing. For example:
  - 'You make a very interesting point about the program. Can you tell me...'
  - 'I hear that very strongly...'

Researchers must be cautious about asking the question 'Why?'. Often participants may not know why they behave or think in a certain manner.

DOING RESEARCH

Questioning examples

Below are some questions that could be asked to parents of children with reading difficulty. Would you word anything a bit differently? If not, why not? If so, please attempt to do so.

- ☐ I wonder what you think it was about the intervention program that just clicked with him.
- ☐ Were there particular things that you thought were really helpful for him?
- ☐ Do you know why your daughter had such difficulty when she started school?
- ☐ What else do you think could have made it easier for you?
- ☐ How did you get over that hurdle?
- ☐ Do you think children should be 5 or 6 when they start school?
- ☐ What would be helpful for parents who are just interested and who just want to know the latest research?

TYPES OF QUESTIONS

Researchers can use different types of questions for different purposes. The following question types combine suggestions made by Kvale (2007, pp. 60–62) and Bryman (2008, pp. 445–7). Table 3.1 describes a variety of question types and provides examples.

Table 3.1: Question types available for the in-depth interview

Question	Useful for:	Example:
Introductory or opening question	☐ allows the participant to talk at great length, typically offering spontaneous and rich descriptions ☐ participants can provide what *they* see as the main issues or phenomena under investigation	☐ In your own words, please tell me about your recent illness. ☐ How would you describe your experience of becoming a single mother?
Follow-up question	☐ to encourage participants to say more about the answer they have just given ☐ participants' responses can be further elaborated ☐ usually asked as a direct question	☐ Do you mean you had a negative experience with your doctor? ☐ You said earlier that you'd prefer not to have a child. Could you tell me more about this?'
Probing question	☐ researcher probes for further discussion so that they have a clear understanding of the matter being examined	☐ Can you give me some more examples of this issue? ☐ Can you say more about what you have just told me? ☐ What happened? When did it happen? How did it happen?

Table 3.1: (*cont.*)

Question	Useful for:	Example:
Specifying question	☐ similar to follow-up questions; asking more specific questions so that a more explicit response can be obtained	☐ How did you react when the teacher told you about his difficulty in the classroom?
Direct question	☐ used to clarify the issues or some ambiguity during the interview ☐ should be left until later in the interview, when participants have given offered their own explanations ☐ researcher is sure that the topic of the direct question is of key importance	☐ Have you ever experienced discrimination from others in your community? ☐ What stops you from looking after your baby as you would like to do?
Indirect question	☐ several indirect questioning techniques such as 'projective' and 'contextualising' questions can be used. Although the participant will typically talk 'outside him/herself' in response, their own attitudes may be revealed to some extent ☐ further careful questioning is essential in order to accurately interpret participants' responses to indirect questioning	☐ How do you think other men would react to domestic violence? ☐ What do other parents say about the resources available for children with learning difficulty? ☐ What do you think may make your experience different from others'?
Structuring question	☐ this type of question assists the participant to move on to the next line of questioning ☐ researchers should indicate to the participants when a topic of the previous question has been dealt with ☐ useful also when the participant gives a long discussion of matters that may not be directly relevant to the research	☐ The researcher may summarise their understanding of the answer given by the participants and then say, 'I would now like to introduce another topic…' (Kvale 2007, p. 61). ☐ When the participant pauses momentarily, the researcher may introduce the next line of questions as a way of bringing the participant back to topic.
Interpreting question	☐ questions that assist researcher to interpret or clarify what the participants have suggested ☐ may simply be rephrasing the participant's response	☐ Is it correct that you feel that you feel he is being discriminated against at school?

The nature of questions used in the in-depth interviewing also warrants careful consideration before commencement. Researchers can use different types of questions for different purposes.

DOING RESEARCH

We have often used a 'funnelling technique' as described by Smith (1995) for our in-depth semi-structured interviews. To do so, we start with an introductory question such as 'Could you start by telling me about your role in the school with regard to children with reading difficulty?' Such an open question aims to put the interviewee at ease but, importantly, also helps to ensure neutrality in the researcher (Liamputtong 2009). We maintain that a funnelling technique minimises the potential bias that might arise if we had set the structure and themes for the interview by probing specific points at the outset.

Typically, we find that interviewees tend to respond to our introductory question with rich, detailed and lengthy responses. We are then able to 'funnel' questions to probe specific issues that were raised. The funnelled questions may be of any format (direct, prompting, indirect, etc.) and allow us to pick up on key issues raised by the participant in tandem with following up on points pertinent to the research. Our sense of this technique based on reading our transcripts is that it is a rather 'gentle' and respectful way to seek in-depth information.

Examples of questions

Here are examples of some questions Pranee used in research with women living with HIV/ AIDS in Thailand. You will see that most are open-ended, but occasionally there are some direct questions about their feelings. Pranee had some introductory questions and these were followed by some probing, specifying, direct and indirect questions:

- Can you please tell me about your thoughts about HIV/AIDS?
    - In your view, how do people get HIV?
    - Is there any way people can prevent it?
    - In your view, what can people do to prevent it?
    - Some people may say that it is difficult for them to prevent HIV. What do you think about this?
- I would like to ask you about health care or treatment of HIV/AIDS that people might have.
    - Have you ever received any health care or treatment of HIV/AIDS?
    - If yes, what type of treament have you received?
    - Can you please tell me more about this?
    - Where did you seek health care?
    - How did health care providers treat you?
- As a woman and a mother, can you please tell me about your experience of living with HIV/AIDS?
- Is there anything we have not discussed that you would like to tell me more about?
- Is there any advice you would like to give to other women who are in the same situation as you?

Doing an in-depth interview: the sequence

Below is a typical sequence for conducting your in-depth interview from meeting your participant until the time you leave. In doing so, we have considered some strategies such as how to facilitate a flowing interaction, managing and containing the verbose participant, and how to provide closure at the end of the interview.

On arrival and introduction

☐ Engage in 'small talk' and make the participant feel comfortable with having you in their home.

☐ Feel free to accept or acknowledge the hospitality of the participant as a way of developing rapport.

☐ Introduce the research and explain the purpose of the study and their involvement.

☐ Reassure confidentiality, and ask for consent. Request permission to record, even if this has been mentioned in a written consent form.

☐ You are now ready to commence the interview.

Beginning the interview

☐ Using your interview guide, start with an opening question (see previous section). Encourage the participant to keep talking by using probes and tactics as suggested above.

☐ Be mindful of your body language and verbal cues. These can act as subtly powerful cues for your participant to continue talking, showing that you are interested in hearing their stories.

☐ You may wish to take brief notes as a way of following up or clarifying issues. If you plan to do this, inform your participant beforehand to avoid uncertainty about what you are doing.

☐ Let the interview flow as naturally as possible. Although some responses may seem irrelevant to the questions, it is essential that you allow the participant to finish their story.

☐ As Barbour (2008) notes, often participants want to tell their stories and the researchers should acknowledge this need.

Ending the interview: some options

☐ You may choose to summarise some of the main points the participant has given.

☐ You may indicate that you have no further questions and then ask if the participant would like to add anything further. For example: 'I have no further questions. Is there anything else you would like to bring up, or ask about, before we finish the interview?' (Kvale 2007, p. 56).

☐ Barbour (2008) suggests ending on a positive note and often asking participants to share advice for others in the same situation.

☐ These options may give closure to the interview. Yet further valuable data may arise when you initiate the end.

After the interview

☐ You may need to debrief with the participant. Make sure the participant is left with good feelings.

☐ It is important not to underestimate how moving and powerful it may be for participants to disclose information about their world.

☐ It is likely that some participants will experience great distress during or at the end of an interview. It is important not to rush off. Occasionally, you may need to refer someone for appropriate support.

☐ You may also ask the participant about their experience of the interview. Often we have found that the participant initiates such a reflection.

☐ Take time to thank the participants and reconfirm how their contribution will help your research (Daly 2007).

Practical issues in doing an interview

Preparing an interview guide

An interview guide will help you cover the issues you wish to examine. It will contain these issues and the general wording of your questions. However, you are unlikely to follow the guide strictly. Depending on the answers of the participants, you will probably ask additional questions based on the progression of each interview (Taylor 2005; Kvale 2007). You may need to rephrase questions and change their order. We present some key suggestions that can help you plan an interview guide:

☐ Construct the guide to help you address what puzzles you or what you have identified as crucial to your research (Daly 2007).

☐ Prepare an individual interview guide for each participant. In this way you can also use the interview guide page to record a person's socio-demographic details and other relevant information.

DOING RESEARCH

Recently, we studied perspectives of both parents and teachers of children with reading difficulty. Here is a subsection of the interview guide from our interviews with parents:

☐ reaction and response to confirmation of child's reading difficulty
☐ impact of child's reading difficulty on parent (home, work, social etc.)
☐ expectations of support intervention provided at school.

What might you include in an interview guide for the teachers that support young children with reading difficulty?

Location of the interview

The interview location is extremely important. As a practical measure, Bryman (2008) recommends selecting a quiet setting so that recording quality is not marred. To protect the confidentiality of the participants, the setting should also be private so that others cannot overhear the conversation.

As far as possible, we ask participants where they would feel most comfortable being interviewed. Participants tend to request their own home as the most comfortable and practical location for the interview. Sometimes they may prefer to be interviewed away from home for reasons such as privacy, shame and suspicion from others. Researchers have conducted interviews in cafés, libraries, health care centres, parks, playgrounds and supermarkets, wherever participants suggest.

DOING RESEARCH

As a novice researcher, one of Tanya's projects necessitated interviewing school staff. It was usually possible to find a quiet space. On one occasion, an interview had to be conducted in the staff room because of limited room availability. This became a problem. With the experience of hindsight, I would set about finding an alternative, even if it meant sitting on a park bench down the road. I became aware of a number of limitations with the interview.

First and foremost, there was the matter of privacy. Although it was teaching time, various staff members did come in and out of the staff room. People typically attended to their task at hand. Nevertheless, the presence of one particular person appeared to constrain my participant's dialogue. As subtly as I could, I asked her if she in fact did feel some discomfort with certain people in earshot of our conversation. She indicated that was all right even though her body language did not seem to convey this. I used my observation as data, although I do believe I may have missed out on some valuable data. Second, there was the simple fact that it became somewhat distracting for both of us when people walked in and out. And finally, the photocopier in the background made listening to my recording rather a challenge. Although interviews in cafés and other public places can be noisy and distracting, the effect was greatly exacerbated in my staff room experience when the distractions were from peers and colleagues.

Recording interviews

It is highly desirable that you record an in-depth interview, preferably using a digital recorder. Since you need to pay close attention and respond accordingly to what participants say, it is difficult to try to write down the conversation at the same time. Kvale (2007, p. 94) says that 'taking extensive notes during an interview may be distracting, interrupting the free flow of the conversation'. He points out that 'the words and their tone, pauses and the like are recorded in a permanent form that it is possible to return to again and again for re-listening' (p. 93). We present some key issues to be mindful of when recording interviews.

RECORDING EQUIPMENT

In the past, researchers had to rely on cassette tape-recorders. Nowadays digital audio recorders give excellent sound quality and can record for many hours without interruption (Gibbs 2007; Kvale 2007). Digital recorders also allow you to transfer audio files directly to a computer. Software is also available that can assist with transcribing interviews from digital recordings. We use an easily downloadable program called Express-Scribe (<www.nch.com.au/scribe/>) to transcribe audiofiles. Features such as key-pad controls for rewinding and slowing down the speed of the recording make Express-Scribe a very useful tool.

AUDIBILITY

Poor audibility of recorded interviews has been a problem for many researchers. If indoors, ensure that the interview room does not have too much background noise. In an open space or a café, noise can obscure or distort the conversation. Be mindful of how you set up seating and positioning for such an interview. Fortunately, many digital recorders are able to cope well with background noise.

CONSENT TO RECORD: ISSUES AND CONSIDERATIONS

Consent must be sought before recording a participant. Most often participants will agree to have the conversations recorded. Nevertheless, some participants will refuse for various reasons and this must be respected. For example, women from some ethnic groups may suggest that their religion forbids their voices being recorded, to be heard by anyone other than their husbands.

Sometimes researchers may feel it is unethical to record the interview as it is too intrusive for the participants. Additionally, it may not always be practical to tape-record interviews. In his ethnographic research into the manufacture of authentic blues music in Chicago blues clubs, Grazian (2003) started out using a cassette recorder to record interviews with musicians and members of the audiences, but he soon gave it up because the background chatter and music made the recordings useless.

NON-RECORDED DATA

To end our discussion of recording, we wish to highlight a situation that can easily occur whereby the interview ends, the tape is turned off, but the participant adds additional information that is 'off the record' (Bryman 2008, p. 457). It may be that people forget to talk about an issue during the interview, or they feel more able to speak freely when the tape is not running. Daly (2007, p. 149) calls this the 'door handle disclosure' and it presents the researchers with a 'difficult dilemma'. However, by asking participants for consent to include the unrecorded content in their research, this ethical dilemma can be solved.

Interview transcript: The written record of an interview that has been transcribed from the verbal conversation. It is used for in-depth data analysis in qualitative research.

Transcribing interviews

Interview data must be transcribed into the written form to enable data analysis. This written form of data is called an **interview transcript**.

Transcribing interviews is in fact your initial data analysis (Gibbs 2007; Rapley 2007; Bailey 2008). Transcribing interview material is time-consuming, tiring and even stressful (Kvale 2007). An hour interview may take an experienced transcriber up to six hours to transcribe (Daly 2007; Gibbs 2007).

WHO SHOULD TRANSCRIBE THE INTERVIEW?

We recommend that the researcher or the interviewers should transcribe their own interviews, as they 'will learn much about their interviewing style; to some extent they will have the social and emotional aspects of the interview situation present or reawakened during transcription, and will already have started the analysis of the meaning of what was said' (Kvale 2007, p. 95).

Some researchers may prefer to have a research assistant or pay for a transcription service. This is not a preferred option, but if done, you must ensure that interviews are transcribed verbatim (Rapley 2007) with regard to verbal and non-verbal features (see paragraph below).

HOW SHOULD INTERVIEWS BE TRANSCRIBED?

We suggest that each interview is transcribed verbatim, word by word, keeping all the informal conversation style and emotional expressions, such as pauses, emphases, laughter, sighing, and sounds like 'hmm', 'oh', 'ah'. Importantly, both questions and answers should be transcribed for contextual clarity. What questions, how the researchers ask the questions and how the participants answer are all important (Esterberg 2002).

DOING RESEARCH

When participants review their transcripts

In a recent study, we routinely offered participants the opportunity to view their written transcript before conducting our analysis. Additionally, participants were informed that they were welcome to delete, add or modify any of their content. Our primary motive was to ensure that participants knew they could delete content that they now felt was too sensitive—because of the topic of discussion, sensitive information was often discussed.

The outcomes

A substantial number of participants took up the offer to review an electronic version of their written transcript, but very few requested changes. More often than not, people were shocked at how their spoken output appeared as a written transcript. These were the types of comments I received from people—usually in jest.

People use far more informal language in spoken output than they would in written form. It is only when people (including myself as interviewer) are confronted with their spoken words on paper that they realise that they may use 'um', filler phrases like 'you know' and so forth habitually. It may be useful in some cases to gently alert people that their written transcript is unlikely to be perfectly grammatical and fluent.

SUMMARY

As we have articulated in this chapter, in-depth interviewing is the method most commonly employed in qualitative research. A skilful performance from the researcher is required to obtain sufficient, detailed and quality information. We conclude by presenting a list of key attributes that we believe are essential foundations for conducting in-depth interviews.

- Be well informed and well organised when approaching an interview.
- To optimise the interview process, bring strong investigative skills and a well-developed capacity to draw people out (Miles & Huberman 1994).
- Be actively engaged in listening and responding to the interviewee in a supportive and non-judgmental manner.
- Facilitate the flow of conversation and be attentive to verbal and non-verbal cues from the interviewee.
- Ensure the interviewee has sufficient time and opportunity to respond to questions.
- Bring 'empathic neutrality' (Patton 2002) to the interview whereby the researcher can validate the interviewee while remaining neutral to the content of what is being said.

TUTORIAL EXERCISES

You are planning to investigate how people who have had a chronic illness learn to live with their physical and/or cognitive disability. You want to explore your participants' experiences of their changed abilities and you have chosen to use in-depth interviews to gather data.

- What interview framework will you choose? Think about the rationale for your choice.
- What questions will you use to elicit information from the participants? Make a list of some potential questions. Identify what types of questions they are.
- How will you ensure that you will obtain in-depth information? Think of some strategies that you may use.

Write down your plans and your question guide, which will help you to have more focus on your research.

FURTHER READING

Bird, C.M. (2005). How I stopped dreading and learned to love transcription. *Qualitative Inquiry*, 11(2), 226–48.

Davies, P. (2000). Doing interviews with female offenders. In V. Jupp, P. Davies and P. Frances (eds), *Doing criminological research*. London: Sage Publications, 82–96.

Tanya Serry and Pranee Liamputtong

Fontana, A. & Prokos, A. H. (2007). *The interview: From formal to postmodern.* Walnut Creek, CA: Left Coast Press.

Kvale, S. & Brinkmann, S. (2008). *InterViews: Learning the craft of qualitative research interviewing.* London: Sage Publications.

Minichiello, V., Aroni, R. & Hays, T. (2008). *In-depth interviewing,* 3rd edn. Sydney: Pearson Prentice Hall.

Pooley, J., Breen, L., Pike, L.T., Cohen, L. & Drew, N.M. (2008). Critiquing the school community: A qualitative study of children's conceptualizations of their school. *International Journal of Qualitative Studies in Education,* 21(2), 87–98.

WEBSITES

www.pathfind.org/site/DocServer/m_e_tool_series_indepth_interviews.pdf?docID=6301

This website links to Pathfinder International Tool Series and includes a report on the use of an in-depth interviewing method.

http://elt.britcoun.org.pl/elt/forum/howint.htm

This page provides an article on how to conduct a successful in-depth interview.

www.blc.lsbu.ac.uk/aa/aa/Multimedia/In-Depth%20Interviewing%20Techniques/player.html

This page provides a set of slides with sound track given by Professor Yvonne Guerrier to her students about why and how to use an in-depth interviewing method.

www.nch.com.au/scribe

A program called Express-Scribe used to transcribe audiofiles.

4

Focus Groups in Health Research

Patricia Davidson, Elizabeth Halcomb and Leila Gholizadeh

CHAPTER OBJECTIVES

In this chapter you will learn:

☐ the value of the focus group method in nursing and health research

☐ about the advantages of obtaining a group perspective in health research

☐ factors to consider when choosing the focus group method

☐ the importance of preparation and promoting methodological rigour

☐ about professional development strategies to assist you in undertaking focus groups

KEY TERMS

Data analysis

Focus groups

Moderator

Qualitative approach

Thematic analysis

Theme

INTRODUCTION

Obtaining the views and perspectives of stakeholders is crucial not only in assessing needs and documenting health issues, but also in developing and evaluating interventions. Originating in the realm of market research, **focus groups** have evolved to fill an important niche in health research and nursing for both exploration and evaluation (Morgan 1998; Halcomb et al. 2007; Krueger & Casey 2009). The rapid growth of the popularity of this method demonstrates the utility of focus groups to elicit a range of views and opinions in a moderated setting. Some innovative approaches of the focus group method are being adopted with the online moderation of focus groups (see Liamputtong in press). In contrast to other methods, such as interviews and surveys (see CHAPTERS 3, 13), focus groups generate data to provide a collective perspective (Liamputtong 2010, in press). Not only does this method generate a collective perspective, but it can also illustrate the polarity and diversity of opinions. Although debate continues on the value and merit of focus groups, like most approaches to research, high-quality focus groups are dependent on planning and adhering to methodological rigour (Morgan 1998; Wilkinson 1998; Willis et al. 2009). In focus groups, planning that encompasses the logistics of recruitment, organising venues and managing group dynamics is just as important as the development of your proposal, data analysis, report writing and manuscript preparation. In this chapter we will outline the rationale for choosing focus groups as a method of data collection, the advantages and disadvantages of this approach and the sequential steps involved in planning and undertaking a focus group in nursing and health research.

Focus groups: A data collection method based on group discussion. The participants express their views by interacting in a group discussion of the issues.

WHY CHOOSE FOCUS GROUPS AS A METHOD OF ENQUIRY?

Qualitative approach: Research strategies that emphasise words rather than numbers in data collection and analysis. The focus of qualitative research is on the generation of theories.

All research focuses on establishing new knowledge and is a prospective, systematic form of enquiry. Since **qualitative research** is an inductive approach, the intent is exploration and the questions are open-ended (see CHAPTER 1). The focus group method sits neatly within this framework. Focus groups can be used in many ways. The box below summarises the purposes of focus groups.

Purposes of focus groups

- □ assessing needs
- □ describing contexts
- □ eliciting knowledge, attitudes and beliefs on a group basis

☐   evaluating health care interventions
☐   exploring knowledge, attitudes, and beliefs
☐   generating hypotheses
☐   elucidating quantitative study findings

When planning and conducting research, it is important to consider the feasibility of selecting an appropriate methodology. The collective perspective and the capacity to capture multiple participants' views in a single interview setting make focus groups a prudent use of limited research resources (Gibbs 1997; Madriz 2000; Vogt et al. 2004). Ideally, focus groups consist of 5–15 participants. This size is recommended to allow all participants to contribute and achieve cohesion within the group. However, the size of a focus group can vary depending on the research topic and social context of the participants (Hennink 2007; Liamputtong 2009, in press).

According to Gibbs (1997), the interaction among participants is the novelty of the focus group method. Hence focus groups are useful in obtaining information on perceptions, insights, attitudes, experiences and beliefs (Davidson et al. 2003; Liamputtong in press). Focus groups are also useful in obtaining unique subjective perspectives, particularly as they pertain to collectives or groups. This collective perspective is achieved by creating an opportunity for group members to stimulate each other to comment and question. For example, an investigation was undertaken of how nurses working in cardiology and respiratory clinical areas viewed end-of-life and palliative care in the acute care setting. As nursing care is a collaborative activity this group perspective was important. Advantages of focus groups are that the group dynamic can yield useful information that individual data collection does not provide, particularly when exploring collective views. As in the example given above, health care delivery is dependent on the attitudes of professional groups and therefore this collective viewpoint is as important to obtain as an individual one (Davidson et al. 2003; Willis et al. 2009).

The focus group method also allows access to research participants who may find individual interviews intimidating (see CHAPTER 3), or where it may not be culturally appropriate to interview individuals alone (Madriz 2000; Liamputtong 2010). Focus groups can also be useful in gaining insight into a topic that may be more difficult to gather through other data collection methods. For example, in individuals who have limited literacy or language, focus groups can provide an excellent vehicle for accessing marginalised and vulnerable groups (Liamputtong 2007). Focus groups are particularly suggested in studying underrepresented and marginalised populations such as women and those who are not part of the mainstream culture, and are particularly suited for research investigating cultural perspectives (Halcomb et al. 2007; Liamputtong 2007, 2010). The method can be tailored to meet situational factors and the needs of the target population (Wilkinson 1998; Halcomb et al. 2007). For example, focus groups can be conducted in community settings and at times convenient to participants. The use of

Patricia Davidson, Elizabeth Halcomb and Leila Gholizadeh

community leaders and cultural brokering can also assist in recruiting participants and ensuring that structure and process are commensurate to their needs.

Risks associated with the focus group method are that they can be susceptible to moderator bias and that there is the potential for the discussion to be dominated by a minority. Yet these risks can be minimised with effective planning, such as the critical analysis of audiotapes to assess the moderator's role and other forms of ensuring the integrity of qualitative data (Morgan 1998). The focus group method does not allow for in-depth information at the individual level, and therefore if this is the intention of the research other methods should be employed. The strongly contextual aspect of focus groups means that the information is not representative of other groups and therefore the ability to generalise findings is limited (Morgan 1998). In spite of these limitations, an expanding literature illustrates the potential of this method to evoke crucial perspectives to inform health care delivery. The focus group method can be a primary form of enquiry where the data generated is the sole source, or a part of a mixed method enquiry where focus groups are complementary to quantitative data collection to further elucidate findings (Phillips & Davidson 2009; Liamputtong in press). Considering potential risks to rigour in the planning stages of your research can maximise the data yield from focus groups.

In spite of these limitations, an important advantage of the focus group method is that it is suited to investigating cultural perspectives and diverse views (Halcomb et al. 2007; Hennink 2007; Liamputtong 2010). Facilitating social interaction and maximising group dynamics can encourage and stimulate the participants to share their beliefs and ideas with those of similar socio-economic or cultural backgrounds (Gibbs 1997; Wilkinson 1998; Madriz 2000; Hennink 2007). It is often the assumption of commonality and acceptance that increases the utility of focus groups in investigating cultural perspectives. Leila Gholizadeh (2009) undertook a systematic enquiry of Middle Eastern women's perception of the risk of cardiovascular disease. As Gholizadeh is a Middle Eastern woman, this facilitated her access to participants as well as her capacity to interpret study data. Middle Eastern women are potentially among the most marginalised and underrepresented populations in Australia, and social, political and economic factors have fuelled this marginalisation (Albrechtsen 2006). These factors contribute to the limited knowledge available to health professionals concerning the health beliefs and behaviours of immigrant Middle Eastern women and underscore the importance of assessing needs and implementing and evaluating effective health care interventions and public health messages. Vogt and colleagues (2004) argue that when researchers use quantitative methods they often explore, and therefore interpret, the experiences of participants from other cultures from the viewpoint of their own cultural beliefs and values. This can lead to making inaccurate assumptions regarding knowledge, practices and experiences. The use of qualitative methods is an important strategy to provide a voice for underrepresented participants (see CHAPTER 1).

The advantages and disadvantages of the focus group method are summarised in Table 4.1.

Table 4.1: Advantages and disadvantages of the focus group method

Advantages	Disadvantages
☐ Can provide a collective perspective of the topic of interest. ☐ Allows access to groups that may not always access traditional data collection methods such as surveys because of language issues. ☐ Facilitates cultural brokering and culturally appropriate strategies. ☐ Group perspective provides clarification and synthesis of views and opinions. ☐ Facilitates access to a large number of participants with similar resources to individual interviews.	☐ It is more difficult <u>to control</u> for confidentiality issues and <u>to manage</u> issues that are distressing to individual participants. ☐ Conflicts may arise in the group through discussion. ☐ Group dynamics may influence participants' level of participation. ☐ The success of the focus group is dependent on the skill of the moderator. ☐ The monitoring of verbal and non-verbal responses is challenging because of the number of participants.

PLANNING THE FOCUS GROUPS

The research questions underpinning the project plan should inform the organisation of the focus group. These questions will inform the question route for the group and determine the number and characteristics of participants and the interview setting.

There are two aspects of data collection that must be considered. First, it is often useful initially to obtain basic demographics of participants, such as age and gender. The depth of socio-demographic data collection will depend on the study questions and may require the completion of a brief questionnaire (see CHAPTER 13). Subsequently, developing the focus group guide is an important step that leads researchers through the different parts of the discussion. Table 4.2 provides a guide for planning the question route and includes the framework of introductory and transitional questions. It is also important to consider the need for questions that probe points raised by participants and search for explanation and meaning. If questions and discussion are superficial, the data emerging from the study will lack depth and fail to address the study questions. See also CHAPTER 3 for questions used in interviews.

Table 4.2: Examples of a focus group question route

Introductory question	Can you please tell us about your experience of having a heart attack?
Transition question	Can you tell us briefly about what helped your recovery from a heart attack?
Transition question	Do you know of any help or support services that are available for people who have had a heart attack?
Focus questions (these should be based on research questions)	What are the greatest needs faced by people after a heart attack? What can health professionals do to help people recover from a heart attack?
Summarising question	As you know, we are going to be implementing a program to assist those who have recently experienced a heart attack. Think back on your experiences and our discussions today and tell us what we can do to improve the care people receive.
Concluding question	Is there anything else that anyone feels we should have talked about but didn't?

Source: Halcomb et al. 2007

Patricia Davidson, Elizabeth Halcomb and Leila Gholizadeh

During the planning process, the recruitment of research participants needs to be considered. In many instances, engaging key stakeholders, such as community leaders or clinical champions, can be crucial in recruiting participants. Getting together a group of participants who meet the inclusion criteria involves careful planning and can often be a lengthy procedure. It is also important to carefully explore the ethical implications of the research and take the time to consider matters that may impact on the welfare of participants. Please refer to CHAPTER 2 to help you in working through ethical issues pertaining to planning research.

UNDERTAKING THE FOCUS GROUPS

The questions and the manner in which the focus group is facilitated are dependent on the participants and study setting. Further, the level of structure and direction depends on the purpose of the focus groups (Beaudin & Pelletier 1996). For example, consideration of cultural expectations and customs is important when undertaking focus groups with culturally and linguistically diverse groups (Hennink 2007; Liamputtong 2010); in some cultural groups it may be inappropriate to have a male moderator conduct focus groups with female participants.

Moderator: A key person in focus groups, who may or may not be the researcher. A moderator leads and controls group discussions.

The role of the **moderator** is crucial in generating data from the focus group and skilfully navigating the discussion to derive rich and meaningful information (Krueger 1998). In essence, the moderator becomes a tool not only to facilitate the group discussion, but also to generate the first level of analysis by providing their initial perceptions of participants' views.

Ideally, the moderator should be someone with whom the participants feel comfortable and can potentially relate to and with whom they are likely to feel that they can openly disclose information.

'Doing research' below describes how an occupational therapist and social worker used the focus group method to evaluate the use of an open group mutual aid model in a secondary prevention cardiac rehabilitation program. As they were really interested in participants' views, the focus groups were conducted and moderated by experienced health professionals who were not actively involved in the delivery of the mutual aid groups.

DOING RESEARCH

Evaluating program delivery is a critical element of health service delivery. The use of a single method of evaluation, such as a survey (see CHAPTER 13), can be limited primarily because of floor and ceiling effects of instruments—that is, when instruments capture extreme ranges of scores. Focus groups are often useful for health service evaluation as they provide both an individual and a collective picture. In a cardiac rehabilitation program in metropolitan Sydney, a mixed methods study design (see CHAPTERS 19, 20), using questionnaire and focus group data, was used to evaluate a co-facilitated mutual aid, open-group model of providing information and support by a social worker and occupational therapist (Arndt et al. 2009). These focus groups were conducted by health professionals not involved in the program delivery and the data was analysed collaboratively. If the clinicians providing the course undertook the evaluation, participants may have felt less forthcoming in providing opinions. Analysis of the focus group data generated the following themes: (1) the need for provision of hope; (2) a desire for structure and support; (3) appreciation of support of fellow group participants; and (4) the need for patients to review process and interpret their illness trajectory. Participants also supplied information to the investigators to improve service delivery, such as providing name badges and leaving discussion of sensitive matters such as sexual activity to a time when there was more group cohesion.

The moderator should not only be skilled in facilitating group dynamics, but should have a genuine sense of reciprocity and respect for the target group. The moderator should also be familiar with the issues being explored in the focus groups. In some instances, focus groups can be dual-moderated and this will require careful planning and a cohesive and respectful relationship between the moderators. The question route provides the prompts for the moderator. The box 'Guidelines for moderators' provides some guiding principles for the moderator. Summarising the critical points at the end of each focus group and asking the participants to confirm their accuracy is an important strategy for maintaining the accuracy of findings. The notetaker also plays an important role in accurately representing discussions. It is useful for the moderator and notetaker to critically analyse the audiotapes of the focus group to appraise their performance and to modify their technique and question route where appropriate. Questions to ask oneself upon preliminary analysis include: Is the moderator dominating the conversation and not allowing participants to discuss and debate? Is the moderator successful in probing and clarifying positions espoused by participants? Is the conversation focused on addressing the study questions?

Guidelines for moderators

Introduce yourself and your role and thank participants for agreeing to come. Explain the reason they were chosen and the main purpose of focus groups. Explain group guidelines, emphasising respect for others' opinions and confidentiality of issues disclosed, and tell participants how long the focus group will last. The following provides a checklist of points to raise during the introduction of the focus group.

- ☐ We have the discussion scheduled for approximately one hour today. During the group we want to obtain your views on [Briefly describe the content area].
- ☐ My role is to facilitate the session today. You won't offend me, whatever opinions you give. We are interested in hearing *your* point of view even if it disagrees with others' opinions.

Patricia Davidson, Elizabeth Halcomb and Leila Gholizadeh

☐ It is my role to keep the discussion focused on the topic we are here to discuss, so I may need to move the conversation along so we can cover all of the items and to make sure that we get to hear from everyone here today.

☐ It is important that we maintain confidentiality and respect others' beliefs and opinions.

☐ We will be audiotaping the discussion, with your permission, because we don't want to miss any comments. It is important for you to realise that no names will be attached to the report or any publications. You may be assured of complete confidentiality in the report and publications.

☐ I would like to introduce you to my colleagues [notetakers and co-moderators].

☐ I would also like you to introduce yourselves. [Level of introduction and affiliations depends on the purpose and context of the focus group.]

☐ Before we start the group I would like to emphasise the need for respect and confidentiality and the importance of hearing everyone's views.

After briefing participants on the purpose of the focus group and allowing the group time to become acquainted, the moderator will pose the questions to the group and allow time for participants to respond to each other's comments. Some flexibility is required to allow views to be expressed and to explore issues that may not have been anticipated by the researchers. It is also important to ensure that voices of all participants are heard and that certain members do not dominate the conversation and prevent the group view from emerging. Strategies should be implemented to ensure that offensive comments are not made and that people's views and opinions are respected. It is the moderator's role to address inappropriate comments and maintain mutual respect within the group. Undertaking role-plays as part of preparation for focus groups can be useful in preparing the research team to deal with the challenges of group dynamics.

In addition to the moderator, it is important to have an observer or a notetaker during the session. The box 'Example of focus group data collection template' gives a template that may be useful for notetaking based on the question route provided in Table 4.2. Assigning a research team member to take responsibility for audiotaping and also observation is important, as assembling the same participants and repeating the interview is not usually feasible. Practical considerations such as ensuring that recording material is working effectively and is optimally placed is fundamental to ensuring that effective data is obtained (see also CHAPTER 3). In some instances, videotaping is also undertaken and this requires additional planning and explicit consent of participants. Taking the time at the end of each focus group to reflect and comment on the outcomes of the session is crucial. This is particularly important because transcription can be challenging when multiple participants are talking at once. Therefore not only is this initial debriefing the first step in data analysis, but it also contributes to the planning for subsequent focus groups where it may be necessary to probe emerging issues or add questions to elicit information. It is also a risk mitigation process in case of recording failure or transcription challenges.

Example of focus group data collection template

Date: ....

Start Time: ....

Stop Time: ....

Moderator: ....

Notetaker: ....

Observer (s): ....

Venue: ....

Participants: ....

Focus question	Responses	Key issues
What were the greatest needs or most important issues faced by people suffering from a heart attack?		
What are the barriers and facilitators to recovery from a heart attack?		
What can health professionals do to promote recovery from a heart attack?		
Summary and reflections		

It is important that after each focus group the research team takes the time to reflect on the group and assess the efficacy of the question route as well as the dynamics for eliciting information. Scheduling adequate time between focus groups to allow preliminary data analysis is generally recommended (Krueger 1998). The number of focus groups is determined by the depth of data required and whether the focus group is a primary, adjunctive or secondary data source. As in other forms of qualitative data, determining when data saturation has been achieved is important and underscores the importance of an iterative and reflective process. Generally, data saturation is said to occur when no or little new data emerges (Liamputtong 2009; see also CHAPTER 1). Although there is no rigid rule, it is generally useful to conduct another one or two focus groups, following the perception of data saturation, to ensure that saturation has indeed occurred. Optimally, you should conduct at least two focus groups with each type of participant.

DATA ANALYSIS

The method of data analysis should be driven by the study questions, and more information is available in CHAPTER 22. When beginning the review of focus group data, **data analysis** is at first mechanistic, looking for recurrent patterns and themes. In the next phase, the analysis is interpretive, searching for meaning and conclusions. As in all forms of qualitative data analysis, the process of the researcher immersing themselves in the data is crucial to true understanding of participants' perspectives. When using qualitative approaches, the researcher acts as a research instrument and is pivotal to data analysis and interpretation. As a consequence, declaring the values, perspectives and experiences that the researcher brings to the research process is important. Researchers should consider their assumptions, biases and experiences that may shape the research process and the level of acceptance by study participants and influence data analysis and interpretation (Morse et al. 2002). Although qualitative methods are challenged in providing subjective, biased and unreliable findings, the openness and closedness of a qualitative researcher to the study participants' experience is more likely to derive a better understanding of the subject under investigation (Rossman & Rallis 2003).

Data analysis: The way that researchers make sense of their data. In qualitative research it means looking for patterns or themes, whereas in quantitative research numerical data are analysed and statistics are used.

Data collection and analysis should be concurrent and simultaneous activities (Liamputtong 2009; see CHAPTER 22). Krueger (1998) recommends that if analysis is delayed the sense of the group, its mood and meanings may be lost among the data collected from other subsequent focus groups. It is also important to include as many members of the research team as possible in this fundamental stage of analysis. Data sources available for interpretation include the verbatim transcriptions of the data, handwritten field notes, and the researchers' thoughts following each group, which should be recorded as a personal file. The personal file should include the individual researcher's reflections and perceptions as well as commentary on interactions and emerging issues (Krueger 1998). Transcriptions should be reviewed repeatedly to allow immersion in the data. Methods of data management vary from paper notes through to qualitative data analysis software such as NVivo (see CHAPTER 23). It is important to note that regardless of the method of data management, the researcher remains the tool through which the views of participants are filtered and synthesised.

Generally, **thematic analysis** is used to analyse focus group data (Krueger 1998). This process classifies words and observations into categories based on their conceptual significance. In the initial phases of analysis, ideas, observations and concepts are coded and subsequently similar incidents, reflections and comments are grouped together. It is important to continually return to audiotapes, transcripts and field notes to verify reflections and observations. Gomm (2004) advocates that the names of codes should emerge from the data and that the use of predetermined codes loses the nuances of the qualitative method. Once data is organised into categories based on groups of words with similar meanings, this may lead to the emergence of common issues

Thematic analysis: The identification of themes through a careful reading and rereading of the data.

and meanings described as **themes**. The search for commonality should not lead to disregarding the range and diversity of experiences and perceptions (Krueger 1998). As focus groups and data collection progress, initial themes should be validated and explored in subsequent groups. Emerging themes and the degree of relevance to the study questions should be considered within the context of field notes, personal notes and discussions within the research team. See more detail in CHAPTER 22.

> **Theme:** A grouping of data that emerges from the research and to which the researcher gives a name.

A reflective and iterative process should be used to maximise the validity of data interpretation and minimise external bias (Krueger 1998). The need to ensure rigour as a measure of reliability and validity in qualitative research has been well recognised (Guba & Lincoln 1981; Davies & Dodd 2002; Golafshani 2003; Liamputtong 2009). Some qualitative researchers argue that the reliability of qualitative research should not be judged according to quantitative criteria and suggest an alternative terminology to describe different concepts of qualitative studies, such as trustworthiness, whereby researchers attempt to show that their research process is auditable so that the reader would be able to track and verify the research process (Davies & Dodd 2002; Rolfe 2006; Liamputtong 2009). The research is trustworthy if the results reflect the experiences of the participants as much as possible (Clayton & Thorne 2000). Trustworthiness includes credibility, which reflects the accuracy of presenting the data and specifically participants' views (Clayton & Thorne 2000). Dependability relates to reliability and transferability of the data. A study is said to be trustworthy when the data has been presented accurately and truthfully (Clayton & Thorne 2000). Member checking, where participants are asked to review and comment on study findings, is one way of assessing for credibility (see Liamputtong 2009). The process of member checking may not, however, be feasible in the context of multiple focus groups. See also, CHAPTER 1.

Summary of steps to achieve rigour in focus groups

1 Developing a protocol involving a comprehensive and critical literature review

2 Outlining the roles and responsibilities of the research team

3 Generating research questions that address the study aims

4 Engaging key stakeholders' support and submission for ethical approval

5 Anticipating ethical issues and implementing appropriate strategies such as access to counselling if necessary

6 Considering unique issues relating to culture, gender and socio-economic circumstances

7 Declaring researchers' stance in relation to the target population and the study project

8 Planning for participant recruitment, participation and identification of appropriate and accessible venues

Patricia Davidson, Elizabeth Halcomb and Leila Gholizadeh

9 Audio/video-recording focus groups and documenting observations of interactions, in particular non-verbal communication and group dynamics

10 Note-taking by observers and the use of field notes and summary templates in the data analysis plan

11 Summarising critical points at the end of each focus group and asking participants to confirm their accuracy

12 Undertaking a debriefing session between the moderator(s) and observer(s) immediately after each focus group to capture initial impressions and highlight similarities and differences with preceding focus groups

13 Planning for a systematic process of data analysis to ensure credible representation of participants' views

14 Undertaking careful documentation of study processes including planning, data collection, analysis and dissemination of findings.

DOING RESEARCH

A practical case study and reflective account of the use of focus groups

In this case study, we would like to describe the experience of Leila Gholizadeh (2009) in using focus groups as part of her PhD. Leila is a female nurse and was born in Azerbaijan, a province in the northwest of Iran, which adjoins Turkey and Azerbaijan. After completing her Bachelors and Masters degrees in Iran, Leila worked as a cardiovascular nurse and nurse educator in Madani Heart Hospital, Azerbaijan for 7 years. During this period she encountered patients and carers who had limited knowledge of risk factors for heart disease and inaccurate perceptions about their personal risk factors and who made inaccurate casual attributions about their heart disease. For example, one patient was re-hospitalised for another heart attack after being discharged from hospital just two weeks before. He had resumed high-intensity manual work on his farm, contradicting health care recommendations. In another instance, Leila was explaining to another patient about his heart attack and the importance of reducing risk factors. During this encounter, a relative of the patient pulled Leila aside and told her that she was not supposed to tell the patient about his diagnosis, as his doctor would not approve. In contrast, health professionals were struck by some patients' low adherence to prescribed medical regimens. This stance of non-disclosure challenged many of her assumptions of what is considered as best practice in cardiovascular care, where there is a large emphasis on providing information and empowerment.

In embarking on her PhD program in Australia, Leila investigated factors impacting on the perception of cardiovascular disease of Middle Eastern women. As part of this data collection process, focus groups were used to describe the views of immigrant Turkish, Persian and Arabic women regarding their perceptions of the risk of heart disease, their causal attributions, and risk-reducing behaviours. Using the focus group method, Leila was able to reach out to women through community-based groups and interact with women who do not commonly interact with the health care system. She moderated the focus groups with the assistance of bilingual health care workers and health care interpreters. Themes emerging from the focus group discussions were: (1) Middle Eastern women underestimate the risk of cardiovascular disease; (2) stress is a pervasive factor in the lives of Middle Eastern women; and (3) Middle Eastern women face many barriers to reducing their risk of cardiovascular disease. Overwhelmingly, participants underestimated their risk of cardiovascular disease. This is in contrast to the fact that cardiovascular disease is the predominant cause of death and disability in women globally. In this study, women attributed the risk of cardiovascular disease to psychological status rather than lifestyle factors.

To ensure the validity of the findings, a debriefing session between the moderator (Leila), observer, health care workers and health care interpreters was conducted immediately after each focus group. This enabled capturing the first impressions and highlighting similarities and diversities in the participants' views and perceptions. Finally, the researcher's principal supervisor and an experienced research assistant read the raw data and gave their comments on the themes that emerged. This technique is widely used in qualitative studies (Pilote & Hlatky 1995; Edmonds 2005).

In this study, the use of the focus group method allowed exploration of issues from the perspective of participants and elucidated views and comments previously unexpected. Findings of this study have implications for health care services to develop culturally and linguistically competent programs for Middle Eastern women while taking into account cultural differences in beliefs and traditions.

DEVELOPING PROFICIENCY IN UNDERTAKING FOCUS GROUPS

As in most scenarios, practice makes perfect. As well as reading about focus groups, if you intend to use focus groups as a method of data collection, it is important that you take the time to dissect the anatomy of focus groups, identifying the elements that make them successful (Morgan 1998). The important considerations in perfecting the focus group technique are preparing the research questions, taking the time to understand the dynamics and nuances of the target group, preparing the setting and data collection methods, and undertaking a process of self-reflection to ensure that the moderator becomes the voice of the target group and ensures the well-being of participants. Preparation and planning for focus groups includes not only organisational aspects but also considering factors such as group dynamics and anticipating needs and perspectives of participants (Willis et al. 2009). Implementation and dynamics of focus groups may be related to perspectives of authority, gender, class and culture (Halcomb et al. 2007). For example, do not be dismayed if some focus group participants decline to have interviews audio- or videotaped (see Liamputtong 2007, 2010). In some cultural groups this can be perceived as authoritative, with potentially punitive consequences. Denying participants a voice and access to potentially valuable data through rigid protocol adherence can be a limited view.

Devising strategies to understand the target group means that many of the challenges of focus groups can be anticipated and included in the study protocol. Being receptive to participants' needs, as well as maintaining methodological rigour (see CHAPTER 1), is part of the art as well as the science of conducting effective focus group interviews. Participating in role-plays and critical analyses of individual performances is crucial if the data yield is to be maximised. This requires critical self-reflection in order to improve quality. Critical analysis of audiotapes and calculating the ratio of participant versus moderator dialogue is one example of implementing strategies to elicit high-quality data. It is also important to consider non-verbal factors of communication and strategies for achieving group perceptions and how these will be included in the process of analysis and interpretation. Other strategies, such as preparing standard phrases—'It is important that everyone has the opportunity to express their ideas, regardless of your individual perspective', or 'Thank you for sharing that opinion, but it is important that we consider everyone's view'—can ensure that respect and reciprocity are prevailing themes of the focus groups.

It is also important that the moderator be prepared to deal with disagreements in the group and also be astute in targeting participants who appear distressed and may need follow-up. Providing participants with contact details for counselling services if they are distressed or require support or more information is part of the researchers' responsibility and ethical requirements. Therefore taking the time to understand the group you are targeting is important and allows you to anticipate potential challenges. Developing templates and effective forms of data management as outlined in this chapter are important considerations in preparing for focus groups and can make your experience of focus groups less stressful and more productive in the data yield.

SUMMARY

In this chapter, we have suggested that focus groups are a useful strategy for obtaining the collective perspective of a group of individuals with common characteristics. After reading this chapter, it is likely that you are impressed by the fact that undertaking a focus group is a team activity and therefore roles and responsibilities of the research team need to be emphasised. The box 'Summary of steps to achieve rigour in focus groups' summarises important factors for you to consider when preparing to conduct focus groups. This method is particularly valuable in obtaining the views and perspectives of underrepresented and marginalised individuals where issues such as low literacy prevent participation in many other forms of research, such as surveys. This chapter has also shown that the focus group method can be tailored to address a number of practice settings. Within health research, it can be informative in exploring issues as well as being useful as an evaluation technique. This chapter has also emphasised the importance of planning and effective data management to promote methodological rigour and strategies to ensure the well-being of participants.

TUTORIAL EXERCISES

1   A successful focus group is contingent on planning and coordination. Another crucial factor is the proficiency of the moderator. In your tutorial group, identify what are the ideal characteristics of a moderator. Discuss how you may be able to identify the facilitation of the moderator by listening to audiotapes and reviewing transcripts.

2   Describe the strategies you would use to facilitate engagement of all participants in focus group discussions. What are some statements that you could use to maximise participation?

3   Discuss the process of data management in focus groups. Identify strategies for data recording, transcription and analysis. What are the strategies that you would employ to achieve methodological rigour?

FURTHER READING

Hennink, M.M. (2007). *International focus group research: A handbook for the health and social sciences*. Cambridge: Cambridge University Press.

Krueger, R.A. & Casey, M.A. (2009). *Focus groups: A practical guide for applied research*, 4th edn. Thousand Oaks, CA: Sage Publications.

Liamputtong, P. (in press) *Focus group methodology: Principles and practices*. London: Sage Publications.

Morgan, D.L. (1998). *Focus group kit* vol. 1: *Focus group guidebook*. Thousand Oaks, CA: Sage Publications.

Phillips, J.L. & Davidson, P.M. (2009). Focus group methodology: Being guided along a pathway from novice to expert. In V. Minichello & J. Kottler (eds), *Qualitative journeys: Student and mentoring experiences with research*. Thousand Oaks, CA: Sage Publications, 255–76.

St John, W. (2004). Focus group interviews. In V. Minichiello, G. Sullivan, K. Greenwood & R. Axford (eds), *Handbook of research methods for nursing and health science*, 2nd edn. Sydney: Pearson Education Australia, 448–61.

Willis, K., Green, J., Daly, J., Williamson, L. & Bandyopadhyay, M. (2009). Perils and possibilities: Achieving best evidence from focus groups in public health research. *Australian & New Zealand Journal of Public Health*, 33(2), 131–6.

WEBSITES

www2.fhs.usyd.edu.au/arow/o/m01/rlewis.htm

Action and Research OpenWeb. Focus Groups. *This site provides an overview of the origins of the focus group method as well as some examples of the use of the focus group method.*

www.scu.edu.au/schools/gcm/ar/arp/focus.html

Resource papers in action research. Structured focus groups. *This site provides information regarding structuring focus groups and preparation for conducting focus groups.*

www.agpn.com.au/site/index.cfm?display=24910

Australian General Practice Network. Focus Groups. *This site provides information regarding the potential and application of the focus group method. It also provides access to examples of focus group research conducted in community-based settings and access to additional references.*

www.eowa.gov.au/Developing_a_Workplace_Program/Six_Steps_to_a_Workplace_
Program/Step_2/Consultation_Tools/Consultation_Moving_Forward/Focus_Groups.asp

Australian Government. Equal Opportunity forWomen in theWorkplace. Moving Forward: Focus groups. *This site provides examples of using focus groups as an adjunct to survey data.*

5

Narrative Enquiry and Health Research

Linsey Howie

CHAPTER OBJECTIVES

In this chapter you will learn:

☐ about the nature of narrative enquiry

☐ how to use narrative enquiry in qualitative research

☐ about the narrative enquiry method: sampling, participants, data collection and analysis

☐ what steps to take in narrative analysis and analysis of narratives

KEY TERMS

Analysis of narratives

Data analysis

Discourse

Metaphor

Narrative analysis

Narrative enquiry

Plot

Purposive sampling

Snowball sampling

INTRODUCTION

It is fitting in a chapter on narrative enquiry to begin with a brief story about my background in occupational therapy, and subsequent engagement in higher degrees in sociology. I was drawn to investigate qualitative research methods anticipating they would reflect my interest in understanding people's lived experience, and the link between occupation and states of health and ill health. Exploring the range of qualitative methods available to me, I realised the potential of **narrative enquiry** to answer a range of questions relevant to people receiving occupational therapy and other health services. More than that, however, I have come to appreciate the value that narrative enquiry places on people's lives, their individual experiences and responses to

Narrative enquiry:
A research method that focuses on the structure and nature of the narratives, or stories, produced.

specific events, circumstances, relationships and environments. Hearing an individual story, my curiosity about people in similar circumstances is aroused and I enter the world of human experience, which further develops my critical appraisal of professional practice with particular populations.

With its focus on enabling storytelling to reveal people's experience, narrative enquiry is a method that foregrounds what people bring to matters of importance to them. In addition, it offers the opportunity for research participants to describe in detail the wider context shaping their experience of the phenomenon in question. Narrative enquiry, as Pinnegar and Daynes (2007, p. 5) observe, 'begins in experience as expressed in lived and told stories'. The narrative researcher studies particular stories elicited through a range of methods to facilitate the in-depth telling of pertinent experience (Liamputtong 2009).

My reading of the works of leading authors in the area of narrative enquiry (especially Goodfellow 1997; Polkinghorne 1998; Mishler 1999; Clandinin 2007; Riessman 2008) has informed this chapter. My own experience of using a narrative framework while conducting research and supervising higher degree students is included in the form of exemplars, tutorial exercises and reflections on past studies in occupational therapy (see Howie et al. 2004; Kelly & Howie 2007; Feldman & Howie 2009).

WHAT IS NARRATIVE ENQUIRY?

The field of narrative enquiry can be confusing to the beginning researcher, or the seasoned researcher coming to qualitative research methods for the first time. While the study of narrative can be traced to origins in hermeneutics and phenomenology (Josselson 2006), it has been widely adopted in history, anthropology and sociology, and across a variety of professions such as law and education, medicine, psychology, nursing, social work and occupational therapy (Riessman 2008; Liamputtong 2009). Some of the confusion associated with what constitutes narrative enquiry is understandable given the variety of ways researchers have approached this field of study. Writing about a special issue in *Narrative Inquiry* devoted to understanding contemporary uses of the method, Smith (2007, p. 392) notes how narrative enquiry can 'mean different things to different people'. He adds: 'Narrative enquiry might therefore be best considered an umbrella term for a mosaic of research efforts, with diverse theoretical musings, methods, empirical groundings, and/or significance all revolving around an interest in narrative.'

This is useful to keep in mind. There are many ways to conduct a narrative enquiry, and while the literature is extensive, it is characterised by disparate views as well as corresponding ideas (see Liamputtong 2009). The pages that follow provide one way of understanding narrative enquiry; other authors will have different perspectives or make different emphases. This does not give researchers free rein to do whatever they like. Rather, it invites you to read widely and think carefully about how to construct a narrative study.

Schwandt's definition (1997, p. 98) draws attention to the centrality of story to this method: 'Narrative inquiry is concerned with the means of generating data in the form of stories, means of interpreting that data, and means of representing it in narrative or storied form.' Josselson (2006, p. 4) reminds us that narrative research 'strives to preserve the complexity of what it means to be human and to locate these observations of people and phenomena in society, history and time'. Polkinghorne (1995, p. 5) describes it as a 'subset of qualitative research designs in which stories are used to describe human action'. However, to distinguish narrative enquiry as a research *method* from the word 'narrative' commonly used in qualitative research, he emphasises that narrative in narrative enquiry 'refers to a discourse form in which events and happenings are configured into a temporal unity by means of a plot'. Goodfellow (1997, p. 61), on the other hand, describes narrative in this context in terms of 'a form of natural **discourse** in which the narrator conveys the nature of what has been experienced through the sequential telling of that experience'.

Three further elements of narrative enquiry are important to grasp at this point: the significance of *meaning-making* in people's use of stories, and the relevance of *plot* and *metaphor* to this process. Kielhofner (2002, p. 125) says that as humans we 'draw meaning from life by locating ourselves in unfolding narratives that integrate our past, present, and future selves'. **Plot**, he maintains with reference to Gergen and Gergen (1988), is a 'forestructure of narrative' indicating how people think in recounting stories and revealing the meaning and significance of various story elements. Plot also indicates how people extract understanding from past events to make sense of present circumstances. The use of **metaphor** in narratives also enhances the meaning of stories by suggesting an analogy with something familiar, or emphasising the meaning of experience that might be difficult to understand or convey in any other way.

The literature proposes many uses for narrative enquiry. Reissman (2008, pp. 8–9) reflects on narratives and people's everyday use of stories to 'remember, argue, justify, persuade, engage, entertain and even mislead

Discourse: In this chapter it means 'communication of thought by words; talk; conversation' rather than its specific meaning in the social sciences.

Plot: The narrative structure of a story, indicating how people extract understanding from past events to make sense of present circumstances.

Metaphor is used in narrative enquiry to enhance the meaning of stories by suggesting an analogy with something familiar.

Linsey Howie

an audience'. She emphasises that recalling past experiences supports individuals to make sense of painful or fragmented memories. This, she argues, is achieved through therapeutic processes or through writing, reading, or dramatic or other cultural or political events. Narratives, she maintains, are 'strategic, functional and purposeful' and they can 'mobilise others into action for progressive and social change'. Gergen and Gergen (2006) note the uses of narrative practices in therapy and in organisational transformation and conflict reduction. They maintain that understanding narratives as embedded in social interaction in various contexts reveals the potential for stories to enhance relationships and produce personal and social change. Smith (2007, pp. 391–2) too observes that narratives are 'effective in social and individual transformation' as well as 'constructing selves and identities'. These examples illuminate the uses of narrative enquiry beyond the individual memoir or reflection on a particular experience and invite discussion about how narrative research can be used to bring about social change or action.

Narrative researchers have varying views on what a narrative enquiry entails, but the literature appears to concur that stories, freely told, reveal human activity in all its complexity and these stories have the potential to enhance understanding of people in their environments. There is no absolute 'right way' to implement a narrative enquiry, but researchers are encouraged to record, discuss and debate their practices to expand knowledge of the potential for this research method to answer contemporary questions of individual or social importance. Stories are foregrounded in every aspect of a narrative enquiry: in data collection, in analysis and in the findings. Last, the unpredictable nature of storytelling and the different perspectives that humans put on a story, depending on the audience or the moment of telling or the environment in which stories are communicated, are instructive ideas for all researchers undertaking a narrative enquiry. While certainty is not guaranteed, establishing procedures to guide the conduct of a narrative study can be very beneficial.

Narrative enquiry method

So how do qualitative researchers set about designing and conducting a narrative enquiry? A reading of contemporary narrative studies confirms there are many ways to proceed. Smith (2007) notes the tendency of studies reviewed in the special issue of *Narrative Inquiry* (2006) and published as a book (Bamberg 2007) to distinguish between those that are more formulaic in structure and those that tend to be playful or more creative in method. I find this distinction helpful but consider it more useful in this context to describe a systematic approach to doing narrative research, and to present information gleaned from my reading and research experience over recent years.

Sampling procedures and participants

In line with most qualitative studies, the sampling method used in narrative enquiry will necessarily include participants who are information-rich and able to express their experiences or recall events in depth (see also CHAPTER 1). There are a number of sampling strategies assembled under the umbrella term 'purposive sampling' to guide researchers engaging participants in narrative studies. **Purposive sampling** is widely used to select small numbers of people who share perceptions, behaviours, experience or contexts relevant to the study aims. It allows the establishment of inclusion and exclusion criteria to ensure participants have the desired qualities or abilities. In narrative enquiry, it is usual to select participants without cognitive limitations, people who are able to recollect significant events and relationships, and people who are able to range freely around the research question. People with a good command of the language in which the study is undertaken are also valuable in this type of research.

> **Purposive sampling** looks for cases that will be able to provide rich or in-depth information about the issue being examined, not a representative sample as in quantitative research.

Selecting the right sampling method for a study largely involves common sense and a willingness to review the various types of sampling in order to select people who meet the objectives of the study. Purposive sampling includes criterion sampling, extreme case sampling, homogeneous sampling and **snowball sampling** (Liamputtong 2009; see also CHAPTER 8). The last begins by selecting one or a few participants with pertinent knowledge or experience and asking them to identify others with similar experience. We used this form of sampling in a study of psychiatric nurses to determine the influence of training in Gestalt psychotherapy on their nursing practice (Kelly & Howie 2007). In another study (Feldman & Howie 2009), we used criterion sampling to select a particular group of older people who assessed themselves as in good health, were actively engaged in leisure occupations, and were able to reflect on their histories of occupational participation.

> **Snowball sampling:** Sampling that relies on existing participants to identify acquaintances who fit the inclusion criteria of a study in order to increase the size of the sample.

Data collection

During data collection in narrative enquiry, the researcher engages in thoughtful conversations with participants, in an attempt to enter their world and understand the story or stories at the heart of the study. Data collection may use various methods. In-depth interviews (see CHAPTER 3), journal and diary entries are common, but researchers might like to use graphic techniques, or electronic methods such as email, or narratives recorded by the participants. In a recent narrative study, my colleague Susan Feldman and I used the Self Discovery Tapestry (SDT) (Meltzer et al. 2002), a life history review tool during individual face-to-face interviews, to assist 11 participants, aged 81 to 99 years, to evoke past events and reflect on their long lives and consider how they were adapting to changing capacities and environments. The SDT, unlike autobiographical methods, uses a matrix and coloured pens to denote significant events or periods in a lifetime and provides an orderly framework and immediate graphic representation to facilitate recollection.

DOING RESEARCH

When researchers question how they collect data

Having collected data for a study of older people using the SDT to guide the research interviews in which a number of researchers were involved, Susan and I questioned what was inherent in the instrument that did not support the participants to share their experiences in the way we had anticipated.

Our concerns

In a recent publication we reflected on our data collection procedures (Feldman & Howie 2009). First, it was apparent that 'reflecting on a long life and recalling significant events and relationships was not necessarily an easy experience for the participants'. Second, 'despite modifying the SDT to accommodate older participants in this specific study, it remained difficult for them to complete without considerable assistance. For instance, choosing a coloured pen to resonate with an experience, and an inability to "stay within the lines" of the matrix caused frustration and concern to some participants and most participants asked the researcher to fill in the matrix for them'. Third, 'some participants were also concerned to "get the facts right". The longevity of the participants meant that for some it was difficult to recall exact dates and sequence of events. Even recalling major events such as weddings, births, the death of a spouse required extra effort and many could not indicate times of turmoil or confusion or when they were happy or unhappy' as the SDT asked them to do.

What can we learn from this?

We have learnt that greater participation of the older people themselves in trialling the matrix, in the early stages of this study, would have been valuable in confirming the use of the instrument with this age group. It was not sufficient to rely on the literature or our experience with a younger population. We considered that 'conducting focus group research with older people would establish the value and appropriateness of the tool in exploring changes across the life course'. We also learnt that 'a matrix-based instrument which allows for more spontaneous recall of events, memories and dispositions identified by participants rather than insisting on linear recall could be more encouraging and less threatening to this age group'.

In an earlier study (Howie et al. 2004), we used traditional in-depth interview techniques to focus older participants' lifelong participation in a craft such as painting, woodwork or knitting. In this and other studies I have used an interview schedule to guide data collection to support researchers to engage fully with participants and their story and track their progress through the interview. In the narrative study of psychiatric nurses who did further training in

Gestalt psychotherapy (Kelly & Howie 2007), we wanted participants to freely develop their own account of the research topic, so we designed a minimalist guide to focus on the narrative as the participant was telling it, and to seek the rich, complex and varied elements of each story.

Table 5.1: Interview schedule—'Working with Stories in Nursing Research'

Before Gestalt therapy training	Prompt the participant to recount their story of beginning Gestalt therapy training in the context of their psychiatric nursing practice.
During Gestalt therapy training	Prompt the participant to recount their story of doing Gestalt therapy training in the context of their psychiatric nursing practice.
After Gestalt therapy training	Prompt the participant to recount their story of what their professional experience is like having completed training in Gestalt therapy. Prompt the participant to identify a word or metaphor to describe the influence of Gestalt therapy training on their psychiatric nursing practice.

Note: Gestalt therapy refers to an approach to psychotherapy concerned with people's experiences in the here and now. It is an existential and experiential psychotherapy with training programs and practitioners located globally but particularly in Australia and New Zealand, North America and Europe, including the UK.

You will notice that the schedule is not comprised of multiple questions. Rather, it contains a series of prompts so that the interviewer can track the development of the participant's narrative according to specific periods in their professional lives. Notice too the final prompt, which asks for a metaphor or word to describe the influence of Gestalt training on their current practice. This is a useful technique to elicit a spontaneous idea, or ideas. This technique often generates further details to enhance understandings of the research question.

DOING RESEARCH

Designing an interview schedule

Consider for a moment a research topic that is of interest to you. How would you know if it is suitable to be designed as a narrative enquiry? I suggest you ask yourself, does the topic lend itself to a story format with a beginning, middle and an end? If so, imagine you are now ready to construct the interview schedule.

An example I encountered with an Honours student, Emily Stapleton (2008), was how to construct an interview schedule for a study of older parents caring for an adult child with a long history of mental illness. We were interested in caring as an occupation. Emily designed a schedule that had three sections: caring then, caring now, caring in the future. To begin with she asked for some preliminary information about their role as carers and then she asked about significant milestones in their lives (education, work, children, family, leisure interests etc.). Next, she invited the participant to look back to the time of their son or daughter's diagnosis and the impact this had on their lives (caring then).

Linsey Howie

Then she asked them about their current experience, what caring involves now and how the demands of caring impact on their work, leisure and social relationships. Finally, Emily asked about their thoughts and plans for caring for their child in the future.

TRY IT YOURSELF

Remembering that questions you ask must have direct relevance to the overall research question, write a brief interview schedule on the topic you identified.

1   Outline your research topic to a friend or colleague and ask them for feedback on this schedule.

2   Trial the schedule on someone who shares your interest in the topic or someone who is familiar with the issues, even if that person does not have direct experience of the topic.

3   Reflect on the feedback you have received and highlight what are important changes to make to your original schedule.

4   Rewrite the schedule.

Notice that you have just completed a process of drafting, trialling, reflecting and rewriting an interview schedule—an important process in conducting a qualitative study. A well-developed interview guide supports the quality of the data we collect.

Data analysis

Following data collection, transcription of data and preparation of a master transcript, (including de-identifying data, listening to the interview and editing the transcript to ensure accuracy, line numbering, and page set-up according to standard qualitative research procedures), data analysis in narrative enquiry is ready to commence (see also CHAPTERS 3, 22). I prefer each line of the transcript left-adjusted, with 70 characters to a line (approximately), allowing room on the right-hand side to record your analytic response to the data.

Data analysis: The way researchers make sense of their data. In qualitative research it means looking for patterns or themes; in quantitative research numerical data are analysed and statistics are used.

Many beginning researchers become apprehensive in approaching **data analysis**, wondering how to assume responsibility for interpreting other people's stories (see CHAPTER 22). However, as Josselson (2006, pp. 4–5) reminds us, every aspect of narrative research is an interpretive act. She observes that from the initial choice of research question and participants, 'deciding what to ask them, with what phrasing, transcribing from spoken language to text, understanding the verbal locutions, making sense of meanings thus encoded, to deciding what to attend to and to highlight—the work is interpretive at every point'. This is helpful as it reminds us that having reached the data analysis stage of a study we have already engaged in interpretive practices.

Data analysis, like data collection procedures, searches for the story inherent in the individual telling of experience. When you have the experience of transcribing an interview, you will observe that people do not usually recount experience in an orderly, chronological fashion, and it can be daunting to sit with pages and pages of narrative data and not have a clear sense of how to begin or proceed with analysis (Liamputtong 2009). I propose a sequence of steps to guide data analysis. This may appear overly formulaic, but in my experience it is useful for researchers new to narrative enquiry. The steps I propose are drawn from the work of Goodfellow (1997) and Polkinghorne (1995) and include my experience of imposing order on narrative data, first by creating a storied account of the data (**narrative analysis**) and second by deriving themes across the stories to demonstrate commonalities and dissimilar experiences (**analysis of narratives**).

Narrative analysis:
A method of creating a story by imposing order on narrative data.

Analysis of narratives:
The type of data analysis where themes are derived across the stories to demonstrate commonalities and dissimilar experiences.

Table 5.2: Data analysis—Step 1, narrative analysis (story creation)

Steps	Researcher actions
1 Transcript review	☐ Read, and if necessary reread, the final or master transcript to get a sense of the whole interview.
	☐ Pay particular attention to what is being said that extends your understanding of the research question—what is familiar, or what offers a novel appreciation of the topic.
	☐ Notice how things are said, what the participant emphasises (the strength of words, use of metaphors or figures of speech).
	☐ Reflect on what is avoided or minimised.
	☐ Make file notes and record line numbers at particular points of interest. These notes support the deeply intellectual work associated with data analysis and will develop your central argument about the phenomenon in question.
2 Story preparation	☐ Create headings that permit a chronological or logical sequencing of the data into a story with a beginning, middle and end.
	☐ Ensure these headings will reflect data collected from all participants and will incorporate the central concepts, behaviours or events relevant to the research question.
	☐ Colour-code the transcripts to indicate the heading to which the data are best assigned. Note that some data may not be relevant to the research and will not be included.
	☐ Transpose the data to a separate document for each participant according to the matching headings.

Table 5.2: (*cont.*)

Steps	Researcher actions
3 Story creation	☐ Write a story for each participant using the headings identified in Step 2.
	☐ Write the story in the third person past tense. For example in Emily Stapleton's thesis (2008) on caring for an adult child with a mental illness, she began Maggie's story under the heading 'Early Days' as follows: 'Maggie recalled that Emma (daughter) 'loved primary school' but on entering high school she revealed, 'it was shocking. She was bullied from the day she went'… Reflecting on that time, Maggie was saddened that she 'couldn't protect her' from the other children and regretted having not done something about it at the time. 'I should have put my foot down' she said, 'it ruined everything' (p. 22).
	☐ Continue in a similar vein until you have written a short and lucid account of the participant's experience, inserting direct references to the transcript where appropriate.
	☐ Edit the story carefully and ensure that references to the transcript are accurate.
	☐ Send a copy of the story, neatly printed and soft-bound, to the participant.
	☐ Request feedback from the participant if ethics approval has been granted to do so.

Note: the results of a narrative enquiry are presented in the form of individual stories created according to the steps outlined above.

Following this creative act of writing a story derived from the original transcript, the second step in analysis involves a shift in focus to analysing the individual story in conjunction with all the stories comprising the study to arrive at deeper understanding of the stated research question.

Table 5.3: Data analysis—Step 2, analysis of narratives

Steps	Researcher actions
1 Transcript and narrative review	☐ Revisit each transcript *and* story to appreciate fully the participants' experiences in preparation for analysis of each story and the development of themes relevant to all the stories.
2 Story preparation for analysis	Create a new document for each story, allowing 70 characters per line and two columns to the right of equal width to facilitate the next step in analysis
3 Analysing the stories: First response to the story	In the column closest to the story, enter your initial response to the details contained in each sentence.
	☐ Ask the question, 'What is this sentence about?'
	☐ Insert your interpretation in a few words or a phrase.
	☐ Repeat this process for the whole story.
	☐ Observe that the central column now has a distilled version of the story in your own words.
	☐ Repeat for all stories in the study.

4 Analysing the stories: Developing provisional categories and creating a thematic schema

In the right-hand column, create a *provisional category* against each sentence in the story that best reflects the content of the sentence in question.

☐ In a separate Word file provide a definition for this category to assist you to assert with confidence that this category is sound for each sentence in the story bearing this category.
☐ Repeat this process for the whole story.
☐ Notice that you now have a number of categories that convey the central issues relevant to this participant's story.
☐ Repeat this process for all the participants' stories.

Discuss this process with a supervisor or co-researcher to confirm the attribution of categories (and their definitions) to each story. Once you have verified these categories to your satisfaction, map out a categorising system to represent the relationship within and between each category. You will most likely develop a hierarchical categorising system to reflect these relationships.

You are now positioned to convert your categorising system into a *thematic* system or schema that provides you with the themes and their subthemes relevant to the study findings.

☐ For example—Emily Stapleton developed three themes in her thesis on older caregivers of an adult child with a mental illness. They included: a) *Caring—A Productive Occupation*; b) *Caring & Growing Older*; and c) *Influences on Occupations in Later Life*. Three of the five subthemes relating to the first theme were identified as 1) Providing a home; 2) Managing and monitoring the Illness; and 3) Providing links to the community (Stapleton 2008, p. 43).
☐ Write the discussion according to the themes derived from the stories and outlined above. The discussion follows a logical progression according to the themes and subthemes identified in this process.

THE BENEFITS OF NARRATIVE ENQUIRY

The literature proposes a number of advantages in conducting narrative enquiry, some of which have been touched on earlier. Goodfellow (1997) observes the value of giving voice to participants and researchers, and the importance of narratives *resonating* to the extent that stories can be 'readily understood' (p. 72). Resonance in this context, she states, refers to the 'dynamic process of making connections between the complex relations which may exist within and between images, experience and human relations' (p. 72). The capacity of stories to hold an overall or holistic account of phenomena, as opposed to fragmented parts of the whole picture, is offered as another benefit of narrative enquiry (Goodfellow 1997).

In my experience, another benefit is that most participants welcome the return of created stories in an attractively presented document and few request changes to researchers' interpretation of their story. This seems to me to be an important acknowledgment of the participant's commitment to the research project and a worthwhile aspect of the study when participants value a record of their experience, skills or knowledge in a particular domain.

Linsey Howie

On the other hand, Josselson (2006) has argued that small studies that produce 'highly individualised' accounts of phenomena in different locations, with different researchers, raise questions about how to 'build a knowledge base that can amalgamate the insight and understandings across researchers' (p. 3). This is an important issue and one that warrants serious consideration in health sciences research. There are clear arguments for narrative studies in the health sciences to develop beyond individual accounts of experience if we are 'to understand', as Josselson states, 'the patterns that cohere among individuals and the aspects of lived experience that differentiate' them (p. 5). Josselson's article sets out a number of ideas that might contribute to this 'amalgamation of narrative knowledge' (p. 8) and invites researchers to enter conversations about how to enable this to happen. By extension, the challenge to expand the benefits and uses of narrative enquiry in the health sciences is worth taking up. In this historical moment, there are any number of health professionals engaging in narrative research supported by a proliferation of journals and texts on the subject. Bringing together a community of researchers to envisage integrating knowledge derived from multiple studies is both timely and essential. The effort of narrative health sciences researchers to deliver best practice and fully understand the range of human experiences and behaviours is worth pursuing.

SUMMARY

This chapter has introduced health science researchers to the main components in conducting a narrative enquiry. The method offers a creative means of studying a phenomenon while drawing on the strengths of individuals to recount their experience of events, and the researchers' skill in entering a dialogue in order to elicit the richness of individual experience. The chapter has provided a background to narrative enquiry, its origins and practical application, and has outlined specific procedures to support the conduct of research when research questions lend themselves to exploration of experience through the story form.

The inventive and interpretive steps associated with this method can be disquieting to researchers steeped in positivist approaches to research. This chapter set out to describe rigorous data collection and analysis procedures, and transparent reporting mechanisms to illuminate aspects of the method and guide the further development of narrative enquiry in the health sciences.

TUTORIAL EXERCISES

1   You are preparing to conduct a narrative enquiry and want some experience of analysing data to create a story. In the *first person*, past tense write 2–4 pages on an everyday, recent experience that you can readily recall, such as preparing a meal for friends or family, taking a trip to the zoo or going to the beach for a swim. Without

too much thought, begin to write (word-process) your account of the experience beginning at a point in time that seems right to you. Continue to write in as much detail as you can remember about the experience: what you did, where it happened, who was present, and include your thoughts and feelings about the experience (to the extent you are prepared to commit them to paper) until you reach a conclusion to your story. You now have a *transcript* with which to practise writing a story.

2   Follow steps 1–3 outlined in Table 5.2 until you have written a short and lucid account of the your experience in the *third person*, inserting direct references to your transcript where appropriate and adding interpretive details if they seem relevant, given a second or third reading of your story.

3   Let us assume your name is Mary and you chose to write about going to the beach for a swim. Your created story will be different from the transcript, but it will reflect the facts, situation, elements or mood in your original account and may provide insights not evident in your original telling of events. It might begin as follows:

> *Mary remembered that the night before she arranged to go to the beach with friends, the weather forecast had been for a hot summer day. She was not looking forward to the day. She recalled she had moved unexpectedly from interstate and she did not want to 'disappoint her new friends'.*

4   This small excerpt raises questions about collecting and analysing data in narrative studies. You will be aware that there are many factors influencing an individual's experience and telling of events and they are open to various interpretations, depending on a multitude of prior experiences, memories, cultural and societal values and other factors. In this passage, some researchers might be surprised that Mary did not eagerly anticipate a day at the beach on a hot day. Others might question the relevance of her recent and unexpected move from interstate. The questions we choose to ask in research interviews and what we bring to interpreting data are relevant to narrative enquiry and qualitative research.

   (a) Are you familiar with the literature on reflexivity and ethical aspects of the research relationship in qualitative research?

   (b) Are you aware of the standpoint in narrative studies, that researcher self-knowledge is of prime importance in all aspects of the enquiry?

   (c) If you would like to know more about this issue, see Carpenter and Hammell (2000, pp. 107–19), Fossey et al. (2002) and Josselson (2007, pp 537–66).

   (d) What areas of research are of the most interest to you, what specific population, age group or gender, and why? How did you develop this interest? Why is this important to establish?

Linsey Howie

5 Reread your created story carefully and observe the impact on you of reading your story when written in the third person. In a few words, or a sentence or two, write about the impact on you, beginning with an 'I' statement and using the present tense. 'I am...' What have you learnt in completing this exercise?

(a) as a researcher

(b) as a potential participant in a narrative study.

FURTHER READING

Dollard, J. (1949). *Criteria for the life history*, 2nd edn. New York: Peter Smith.

Emden, C. (1998a). Conducting narrative analysis. *Collegian*, 5(3), 34–9.

Emden, C. (1998b). Theoretical perspectives on narrative inquiry. *Collegian*, 5(2), 30–35.

Feldman, S. & Howie, L. (2009). Looking back, looking forward: Reflections on using a life history review tool with older people. *Journal of Applied Gerontology*, 28(5), 621–37.

Josselson, R. (2007). The ethical attitude in narrative research: Principles and practicalities. In J.D. Clandinin (ed.), *Handbook of narrative inquiry: Mapping the methodology*. Thousand Oaks, CA: Sage Publications, 537–66.

Reissman, C.K. (2008). *Narrative methods for the human sciences*. Los Angeles: Sage Publications.

WEBSITES

www.clarku.edu/faculty/mbamberg/narrativeINQ

Narrative Inquiry *is the continuation of the* Journal of Narrative and Life History *1990–97 and its focus on theoretical approaches and analysis of narratives is very useful for researchers in health sciences, nursing and social work.*

http://qix.sagepub.com

This website is a link to Sage publications and the journals Qualitative Inquiry *and* Qualitative Health Research. *They offer you a free sample of an issue that can be printed but not saved to your computer.*

6

Ethnography as Health Research

Jon Willis and Karen Anderson

CHAPTER OBJECTIVES

In this chapter you will learn:

☐ about the history and tradition of ethnography

☐ how ethnography applies to research in health care

☐ what are focused ethnography, institutional ethnography and ethno-nursing

☐ how to design an ethnographic study

KEY TERMS

Culture

Emic

Ethnography

Etic

Key informant

Observation

Participant observation

Photovoice

Postmodern ethnography

Thick description

INTRODUCTION

Ethnography is a research method that focuses on the scientific study of the lived culture of groups of people. The word is derived from two Greek words: εθνος (*ethnos*), meaning nation or people, and Γραφειν (*graphein*), meaning to write. It was first coined in 1834, and the method enjoyed considerable popularity and growth during the 19th century as a tool of colonial expansion through the auspices of the Royal Anthropological Society in Great Britain and the Smithsonian Institute in America (see Ellen 1984 for a brief survey of the very early history of the method). Although often conceived as a single method—the 'ethnographic method'—with a single object of study—culture—ethnography has historically developed as a suite of techniques of field data collection that include participant observation, key informant interviews, social network analysis (such as genealogical analysis), and social and other mapping. Equally, the focus of ethnographic study has shifted from the totalising gaze of early ethnographers on the culture of native groups in far-flung places. Ethnographers now seek to gain in-depth understanding of people and events within local cultures, whether these are the meaning-making practices of ethnic groups, or those of neighbourhoods, institutions or social groups defined without regard to ethnicity. In recent years, ethnography has begun to focus on the shared meaning-making of groups that transcend local and even geographical boundaries, for example, the ethnography of multiple users in cyberspace. It has become increasingly useful as a tool for developing in-depth understandings of the workings of complex institutions, including those of the health care system (Savage 2000; Coates 2004; Liamputtong 2009).

Ethnography: A research method that focuses on the scientific study of the lived culture of groups of people, used to discover and describe individual social and cultural groups.

A METHOD WITH A LONG PEDIGREE

The notion of culture is central in ethnography and is based on the assumption that any human group that spends time together will develop a culture. Although there are many definitions possible for culture, for the purposes of ethnography we suggest a broad definition, such as that proposed by Spradley and McCurdy (McCurdy et al. 2005, p. 8), who define **culture** as 'the knowledge people use to generate and interpret social behaviour'. In the mid- to late 19th century, early ethnographers such as Sir Edward Tylor, Lewis Henry Morgan and Sir James Frazer worked by analysing the published reports of missionaries, travellers and colonial officials to derive their understandings of these cultures. These researchers were mainly working in the academic tradition of Victorian natural science, and used a comparative method to show how all human societies passed through evolutionary stages. Their studies emphasised the ways in which the customs and beliefs of so-called primitive societies resembled each other, and by tracing a natural evolution to modernity helped to justify colonial interference in these societies. These early ethnographers also began a tradition of exploring health beliefs and practices, particularly through the examination

Culture: The knowledge people use to generate and interpret social behaviour.

of 'magical' and religious beliefs and their relationship to modern science and medicine. At the same time, philosophers working in the French sociological tradition, such as Durkheim, Mauss and Levy-Bruhl, brought considerable scientific rigour to the comparative method and began to write ethnographic work that focused on the unique features of single societies.

In the early 20th century, a new generation of professional anthropologists grew out of the training opportunities afforded by the establishment of schools of anthropology at major universities such as Oxford (1884), Cambridge (1900) and University College London (1908) (Evans-Pritchard 1951). The Cambridge school is credited with some of the earliest ethnographic fieldwork, and advanced the discipline by sending multidisciplinary teams of researchers under the direction of marine biologist A.C. Haddon to remote locations (such as Melanesia and the Torres Strait in 1898) to conduct systematic fieldwork for the first time. At around the same time, Franz Boas began developing and teaching a form of ethnographic field research at Columbia University in the USA from 1899, based on his early experience of geographic studies on Baffin Island in the Arctic. These early university programs trained a generation of professional anthropologists who made significant advances in the development of ethnographic field methods; among them were Bronislaw Malinowski, A.R. Radcliffe-Brown, E.E. Evans-Pritchard, A.L. Kroeber, Edward Sapir, Ruth Benedict and Margaret Mead.

In these earliest renderings, ethnography continued to focus on a range of cultural practices and beliefs, and ethnographers regarded local customs and social issues of small-scale societies as highly important. Malinowski was the first anthropologist to translate an abstract and inclusive concept of culture from a local language into a series of famous studies that coupled intensive field data with conceptual and theoretical insights that are typical of modern ethnography (Hughes 1992; Baillie 1995). Malinowski developed the tradition that ethnography was conducted by living among other cultures for months and even years. He stated that 'the final goal of which the ethnographer should never lose sight…is briefly to grasp the natives' point of view, his relation to life, and to realise his vision of his world' (Malinowski 1922/1961, p. 25). Malinowski's development of the ethnographic method was partly accidental—he became stranded in Melanesia when the First World War broke out and was forced to remain in the field for several years. Because of this forced sojourn, he was able to collect the ethnographic data that formed the backbone of his classic monographs *Argonauts of the Western Pacific* (1922/1961) and *The Sexual Life of Savages in North-Western Melanesia* (1932).

Other anthropologists were working in similar ways at the time. Radcliffe-Brown took the insights of Durkheim's sociological theory and applied them to field data he collected in the Andaman Islands and Central Australia to produce the classic monographs *The Andaman Islanders* (1922/1964) and *Social Organization of Australian Tribes* (1931). Evans-Pritchard, working in the Sudan among the Azande and Nuer tribespeople, combined the methodological insights of Malinowski and the theoretical complexity of Radcliffe-Brown to produce the first anthropological work that concentrated on medical practices and beliefs and is often regarded as the father of medical anthropology. His monograph on Azande religion, *Witchcraft, Oracles and*

Magic Among the Azande (1937), remains an important source of insight for any student applying the ethnographic method to scientific or medical beliefs.

The later work of Margaret Mead opened the door to a new generation of anthropologists who turned the ethnographic gaze back on their own societies. Although Mead began her ethnographic work by examining diverse foreign cultures including those of Samoa (1961), highland New Guinea (1942, 1956, 1968, 1977) and Bali (Bateson & Mead 1942; Mead & Macgregor 1951), theoretical insights from these studies led her to examine similar areas of culture within her own society of the USA (1944). She became interested in education and socialisation (Mead 1951; Mead & Wolfenstein 1955; Mead & American Museum of Natural History 1970), in aspects of race (American Association for the Advancement of Science & Mead 1968; Mead & Baldwin 1971), and in women's place in the family in Western societies (Mead 1949, 1965; Mead & Heyman 1965). Mead's lead in applying ethnographic research methods to contemporary societies and problems was taken up by the sociology department at the University of Chicago—also known as the Chicago or Ecological school—from the 1920s onwards. After the Second World War, the Chicago School began as a series of ethnographic studies known as the Chicago Area Project that contributed significant methodological developments to ethnography via the study of crime and delinquency, particularly through the use of ecological mapping techniques and the use of ecological theory as a frame of reference for their enquiries. Ethnographies such as Suttles' *The Social Order of the Slum* and Hirschi's (1969) *Causes of Delinquency* are examples of Chicago School contemporary ethnographies. In recent years, the tradition of urban ethnography in the classic style continues in the work of researchers like Philippe Bourgois, who has done complex ethnographic research in crack houses in East Harlem and among urban drug users in San Francisco (Bourgois 1995; Bourgois & Schonberg 2009).

The more recent innovations in **postmodern ethnography** continue to focus on conveying the cultural experience of another (Marcus & Fischer 1999; Hammersley & Atkinson 2007). Postmodern ethnography still requires a traditional methodological commitment in realist ethnography to observation and the use of **key informants** as the basis for detailed description and structural analysis of the social world, and the use of cases, particularly conflicts where individual interests seem opposed to social forces, as in the work of Victor Turner (1968). What is also required is an embedded sense of what it is like to live in the social world so described, and here the approaches used most commonly are life history (see e.g. Marjorie Shostak's *Nisa: The Life and Words of a !Kung Woman* [1983] or Vincent Crapanzano's *Tuhami: Portrait of a Moroccan* [1980]), and the life cycle (see e.g. Michelle Rosaldo's *Knowledge and Passion: Ilongot Notion of Self and Social Life* [1980]). Ethnographers use these techniques in combination with each other to provide greater ethnographic richness, as well as to improve the reliability of both data

Postmodern ethnography requires a traditional commitment to observation and the use of key informants as the basis for description and analysis of the social world.

Key informant: An individual who is able to provide in-depth information to an ethnographer, a notion used more often in ethnographic research than other qualitative methods.

and interpretation. For example, the approach of Robert Levy (1988, p. xix) in describing mind and experience in Tahiti involved a period of unstructured household observation and participation in village life, coupled with systematic, relatively formal interviewing of individual informants to establish life-histories. Once his language was adequate to the task and he had achieved a strong degree of acceptance from his informants, he followed up with detailed but unstructured interviews with 20 informants, aimed at eliciting individuals' responses to their life history and to their present life. Bradd Shore (1982, p. xv), working in Samoa to unravel the symbols and meanings that give structure to social relations, based his work on observations over a 7-year period—household surveys, 55 2-hour interviews, a questionnaire delivered to 140 schoolchildren, and analysis of published materials and recordings made of meetings, speeches, songs, plays and other cultural performances. His use of a dramatic incident, a murder, like Geertz's cockfight (1973, pp. 412–53), provided a structure on which to centre his analysis.

ETHNOGRAPHY IN HEALTH SETTINGS

Despite the methodological, theoretical and disciplinary shifts over the past century, ethnography remains embedded in anthropology, and refers to both the processes for accomplishing it—which generally involves conducting fieldwork and always requires the reorganisation and editing of materials for presentation—and the presentation itself, the product of that research, which usually takes its form in prose (Wolcott 1990). Ethnographic approaches have been applied in a range of contemporary settings including hospitals, businesses, schools and communities—regardless of setting, the focus remains on culture. Ethnographic research is as useful to the study of problems defined and dealt with by human groups as it has traditionally been in the study of systems of belief, of religious frameworks or of worldviews. Ethnographic approaches are also useful in the study of the structures that underpin how people organise their accounts of their social world (Wolcott 1990).

Because ethnography is used in a range of settings and disciplines, a range of approaches to ethnography has also developed, including focused ethnography, institutional ethnography and ethno-nursing.

Focused ethnography

Ethnographers do not always have to be holistic, cross-cultural and comparative and do not need to spend extensive periods of time in the field when they wish to explore a problem or are asked a question. The tenets of traditional ethnography do not need to be followed faithfully, especially when researchers are working under the constraints of time and scope (Wolcott 1990).

Focused or 'micro-ethnography' concentrates on a single problem in a particular setting. Rather than attempting to portray an entire cultural system, **focused ethnography** draws on the cultural ethos of a microcosm to study selected aspects of everyday life. It gives emphasis to

> **Focused ethnography** concentrates on a single problem in a particular setting.

particular behaviours in specific settings and allows researchers to work within time and scope limitations by narrowing the focus and providing objectives that are more manageable. Focused ethnography is also known as specific, particularistic, or mini-ethnography (Wolcott 1990; Laine 1997; Morse & Richards 2002).

Traditional and micro-ethnographic approaches can be applied to any social unit or isolated human group that is under enquiry, and is common in nursing (Leininger 1985, 1994; Laine 1997). Ethnographic research in nursing can focus on a hospital, community health centre, nursing home, general practitioner's rooms or a hospital ward, and can assist in helping researchers and practitioners understand 'cultural rules and norms as well as values as they are related to health and illness behaviour' (Morse 1994a, p. 172).

Focused ethnography can be used to explore special topics or shared experiences and is different from traditional ethnography in that the topic is specific and can be identified before the researcher begins the study (Muecke 1994; Morse & Richards 2002). The use of focused ethnography in nursing research and health research is becoming more common. Along with time limitations, limitations in knowledge and experience may preclude the use of a more traditional ethnographic approach. A more focused approach allows the scope of the research to be clarified for the researcher and provides researchers with the ability to enter and experience the richness of the real world of people within a particular setting (Leininger 1985).

Institutional ethnography

Institutional ethnography is a qualitative mode of social enquiry that was developed with the aim of discovering or exposing the chains of coordination and control in a social system or among settings of everyday life (Smith 1987; DeVault & McCoy 2002; Mykhalovskiy & McCoy 2002; Winkelman & Halifax 2007). According to Travers (1996, p. 765), the combination of 'institutional' and 'ethnography' implies the need to move away from the particular to an explanation of the 'intersections of local practices to practices beyond immediate experience'. Although similar to other forms of ethnography, institutional ethnography is not empirically focused on 'experience' or 'culture', but rather on social organisation, and is concerned with exploring and describing social and institutional forces that shape, limit and otherwise organise people's everyday worlds (Mykhalovskiy & McCoy 2002).

Institutional ethnography: Its aim is to discover and expose the chains of coordination and control in a social system or among settings of everyday life.

Institutional ethnography allows the researcher to gain access to the possibility of explaining how institutional processes are embodied in people's everyday experiences (Kirkham 2003). It explores what is happening to people in local settings such as schools or hospitals, but is not limited to the designated organisational spaces. The aim is to explore how and what is happening to people in these settings, and how their experience is coordinated with and organised by organisational activities or work practices (Mykhalovskiy & McCoy 2002). The purpose of institutional ethnography is not to generalise about a group of people but to find and describe the social processes that might have generalising effects (DeVault & McCoy 2002).

Ethno-nursing

Ethnography has been used in a variety of ways to explore nursing and is continually being developed as a method for research (Laugharne 1995). Ethnography has also been used to study groups of students or nurses (MacKenzie 1992; Baillie 1995). For example, MacKenzie's study sought to understand the learning experiences of district nursing students in the community setting and examined their learning using a series of interviews and observations.

Ethno-nursing is defined by Leininger (1979, p. 38) as the 'study and analysis of the local or indigenous people's viewpoints, beliefs and practices about nursing care phenomena and processes of designated cultures'. The use of ethnography as a method for research in nursing allows nursing to be studied within the natural setting and viewed within the context in which it occurs as well as studying areas that have not been previously explored (Baillie 1995). It can be used to document, describe and explain nursing phenomena in relation to care, health, illness prevention and illness or injury recovery using information from nurses, clients and nursing or health institutions (Leininger 1985). It can provide in-depth data and detailed accounts of nursing phenomena or experiences, and it can give a holistic view not otherwise gained through other research methods (Aamodt 1982).

> **Ethno-nursing:** A method where ethnography is used to document and explain nursing phenomena in relation to care, health, illness prevention and so on.

The flexibility of ethnography allows its use in a variety of settings in the nursing discipline, so researchers can explore whole wards or units within the hospital setting. In addition, the use of a combination of data collection methods allows researchers to acquire enough information to present a comprehensive account of the phenomena being studied (Robertson & Boyle 1984; Baillie 1995). The nursing profession needs to develop a meaningful knowledge and theory base in order to allow nursing practice to evolve and the use of ethnography as a research methodology has potential to contribute to this knowledge base (Robertson & Boyle 1984).

DESIGNING AN ETHNOGRAPHIC STUDY

Although the approach of ethnography does not have a primary focus on numeric measurements, it uses both qualitative and quantitative information to search for and find regularities in phenomena. The regularities it searches for are patterns of observed events that can subsequently be analysed in more detail using various tools, including quantitative methods (Hughes 1992). Ethnographic approaches employ various data collection and analysis techniques such as individual and group interviews, key informant and focus group interviews, structured and unstructured observation and unobtrusive methods (including document analysis) (Liamputtong 2009). (See also CHAPTERS 3, 4.)

The standpoint of the researcher in ethnographic studies can be either **etic** (outsider's perspective) or **emic** (insider's perspective).

> **Etic:** An outsider's perspective. In ethnographic studies conducted from the etic perspective, the researcher has no knowledge or experience of the culture they are studying.

> **Emic:** An insider's perspective, that is, conducted in one's own culture, such as an intensive care nurse conducting research within an intensive care ward.

In ethnographic studies conducted from the etic perspective, the researcher has no knowledge or experience in the culture she is studying. Studies conducted from an emic perspective are conducted in one's own culture, such as an intensive care nurse conducting research within an intensive care ward (Byrne 2001). The ethnographer determines the epistemology on which ethnography is based, and this is usually determined by the techniques the researcher uses to acquire knowledge. Knowledge that is acquired through an understanding of meaning of behaviour according to the perceptions and interpretations of those who engage in that behaviour requires a methodology that explains how those engaging in the behaviour construct reality in their own terms (Pelto & Pelto 1978; Schwartz & Jacobs 1979). An etic epistemology assumes that the meaning of behaviour can be best interpreted and explained by the researcher within their own dimensions (Robertson & Boyle 1984; Barratt 1991).

Neither approach should be employed alone, nor does one approach hold a higher or lower scientific status than the other (Robertson & Boyle 1984; de Laine 1997). While the goal of good ethnographic research is to provide an analysis of society from an observer's point of view, human behaviour usually can only be properly understood in context and in the natural setting in which it occurs (Robertson & Boyle 1984; Laine 1997).

DOING RESEARCH

Area of enquiry

In a recent study, Karen Anderson explored the health promotion knowledge and skills taught in a university nursing course and graduate nurses' health promotion practices. Karen writes:

The research was inspired by a need to increase insight into the teaching and practice of health promotion in nursing. Consistent with focused ethnography, my study focused on the subcultural groups of nursing students and graduate nurses and university and health care institutions. It also drew on an aspect of traditional ethnography in that the culture was unfamiliar to me. I was able to use principles of institutional ethnography to explore the designated organisational spaces such as university and hospitals, the social process in these organisations, and how they affect health promotion in nursing.

After conducting a literature review to explore how these areas have been dealt with by previous research, and to refine my research questions and approach, I designed a study in two phases. The first stage looked at how health promotion is taught in an undergraduate nursing degree, and the second focused on how graduate nurses use their health promotion skills in clinical practice.

In the first stage, I collected data through observations of health promotion units in the Bachelor of Nursing degree, document collection and analysis, and interviews with teaching staff and focus group discussion with nursing students. I selected these techniques for the different aspects they would capture of the teaching of health promotion in nursing. To be an unobtrusive observer, I worked on fitting in to my field setting in a number of ways. I made sure my behaviour was appropriate to the personal attitudes, values and beliefs of my informants. It was also about genuinely caring for their experiences, and also using my own personal experiences and history both as a university student and in health promotion to respond to informants. My knowledge of health promotion and experiences as a student assisted in establishing credibility and ensuring that a level of trust and rapport was established. As a researcher, I needed a level of intuitiveness to synthesise the experience of the informants through immediate contact and empathy, and to be receptive to the experiences of those providing the data, to be willing to be taught by the participants and always be open to their feedback. My participants were my co-researchers, so it was vital for there to be a sense of reciprocity. They needed to feel that I was on an equal footing with them and not exerting power over them. Sensitivity was also of importance, and my perceptions and experiences of the field setting needed to be seen, heard and reported accurately. As a participant observer, I was effectively the data collection instrument, so I had to be dynamic rather than static when measuring what was going on around me.

Gaining entry to the field

An important initial step in ethnographic research is gaining entry to the field. This involves more than just getting formal permission to conduct the research. One aspect of gaining entry into the field is identifying gatekeepers, especially within the formal structure of organisations (Hammersley & Atkinson 2007; Liamputtong 2009). Gatekeeping is not a new or unusual phenomenon in health care or health care research. Gatekeepers can allow or deny researchers' access to the setting or to participants, and offer protection to vulnerable people, such as patients, their families, and health care professionals. Gatekeepers can provide protection at an organisational and professional level (Holloway & Wheeler 2002; Lee 2005).

Working with gatekeepers can assist in increasing the trust and rapport with participants. Establishing rapport is an essential part of fieldwork, and develops an affinity between researcher and participants. Such good rapport increases the validity and reliability of the fieldwork, as participants are likely to be more truthful and accurate in their responses (Liamputtong 2007, 2009). Gatekeepers play an important role in initial negotiations to conduct ethnographic research. One of the problems that gatekeepers may pose to research is the need for them to maintain the integrity of the organisation and the picture that the ethnographic researcher might create. As a result, they may block or limit certain paths of enquiry, which could limit the effectiveness of the research, or which may result in the researcher having to choose approaches that are alternatively secretive or deceptive (Hammersley & Atkinson 2007). Such approaches pose ethical difficulties that may discourage the researcher, damage their relationships or reputation, or damage the integrity and reliability of the research. Negotiating the research question and methods so that they satisfy the requirements of the gatekeeper as well as complying with rigorous and ethical research requirements is usually a better tactic (see e.g. Willis & Saunders 2007, p. 102 ff).

Data collection and analysis techniques in ethnography

Regardless of ontological or epistemological framing (see CHAPTER 1), ethnographic research is well served by a range of qualitative techniques for data-collection and analysis, and particularly where researchers are interested in exploring multiple realities and experiences in the terms of those who are living them (Coates 2004; Creswell 2007; Liamputtong 2009). These techniques include observation techniques such as participant and simple observation, a range of interview techniques such as key-informant, life history and diary-interview techniques, focus and other group interview techniques, and case studies. In recent years, ethnographic techniques have also encompassed a range of visual, mapping and sorting techniques. See CHAPTERS 3, 4, 5, 8, 10.

DOING RESEARCH

In the first stage of my research, I made initial contact with the Head of School, Nursing and Midwifery, and the Bachelor of Nursing Course Co-coordinator to identify the relevant nursing units to observe and to identify the unit convenors. I talked to the convenor in order to gain approval to conduct observations in both of the identified units and to approach the other member of the teaching staff. I asked teaching staff in each unit to inform the students of the purpose of the research and observations and to gain their assent to observations being carried out in their presence before the start of observations. I looked for students' verbal assent in the units being observed, as opposed to their informed consent. Participant verbal assent in observational studies where activities or events are being observed and recorded and not participant data is a common and accepted practice.

Initial observations were carried out in each of the units when I first entered the field. Exploratory observations allowed me to observe and capture the big picture of the people and the events in the field. Further observations and a structured audit tool were used to narrow the focus of enquiry to the health promotion topics that were taught in each of the health promotion units. The audit tool was used to explore the health promotion theories and concepts that were taught as well as health promotion skills, student assessments and the links between the units and nursing competencies. Unobtrusive observations were carried out in each of the units. The nature of the lecture environments and class sizes meant that I was able to sit among other students and observe the teaching of health promotion in nursing unobtrusively. All observations in both lectures and tutorials were audio-recorded to increase the rigour of data collected and to aid in analysis.

DATA COLLECTION METHODS

Observation has long been a technical mainstay of ethnographic data collection. Ethnographic fieldwork is typically framed around participant observation, in which 'the ethnographer enters the everyday world of the other in order to grasp socially constructed meaning' (Laine 1997, p. 147). **Participant observation** requires that the researcher both participate and observe, and the focus of this technique may include individual actions and interaction, social relationships and group life, as well as the motives that underlie action and the accommodation of action to the requirements of the social group. Simple observation may be structured or unstructured, and focuses on the external signs of social life in the physical world, the locations and times in which action takes place, and the way that motives and beliefs are expressed through expressive movement and language. See also CHAPTER 10.

> **Observation:** The process of collecting data by looking rather than listening.

> **Participant observation:** A data collection method used in ethnography and behavioural studies. The researcher is more or less embedded with the group being studied so as to observe activities first hand.

Interview techniques range from structured, where questions follow a survey format and leave little room for individual variation, to completely unstructured, where the logic of the interview and the knowledge it generates derive from the social interaction between researcher and participant (see CHAPTER 3). Key informant interviews have a long history of use in ethnographic research and require a research participant to take on the role of skilled and knowledgeable assistant to the researcher by explaining important aspects of what is observed or otherwise learnt from other participants. Life history interviews demand that participants structure their experience according to a chronological narrative logic by relating the history of their involvement in a social group (see CHAPTER 5). A related technique is the diary-interview, where informants are asked to keep a diary of their activities for a limited period such as a week, and are then interviewed about the activities they record in their diaries (see Liamputtong 2007).

Focus and other group interview techniques are typically used to simulate a naturalistic setting for collecting information from a homogeneous group of participants. In focus groups, the group interview concentrates on specific questions, and the researcher provokes a discussion about a matter of interest in order to record how members of the community or organisation typically think about the matter. In focus group techniques, points of agreement and disagreement are of equal interest, and the researcher needs to be mindful of both what is said and what is left unsaid. Group interviews can also be framed around collecting specific information without the requirement for a focused discussion—for example, a group may be asked to brainstorm an issue, or describe or map a typical aspect of their community or organisation. See CHAPTER 4.

Visual techniques, including photo-elicitation techniques like **photovoice**, are increasingly used to elicit contextual information about

> **Photovoice:** By using photography to record the concerns of their community, people who rarely have contact with those who make decisions over their lives can make their voices heard.

Jon Willis and Karen Anderson

health beliefs and practices (Keller et al. 2008; Liamputtong 2010). Typically, participants are asked to photograph important things in their lives, and then explain their choices. Similarly, other creative techniques including poetry, song-writing or autobiography, and the production of visual art works have been used by researchers to explore the unspoken content of cultural beliefs or practices (see Liamputtong 2007). Visual techniques of ethnographic data collection also encompass asking participants individually or in groups to produce maps or diagrams of their communities and its resources. Such techniques have been used to explore, for example, caring relationships within communities, as well as concrete aspects of physical locations, for example the location of local plants or animals (see Sillitoe et al. 2005 for an extensive discussion of these alternative data collection methods).

Case studies in qualitative research are a typical way of recording and presenting ethnographic information. In this technique, in-depth information about a case of interest is collected using a range of techniques, and then woven together to form an in-depth, contextualised and detailed whole. The case of interest may be a person or community, an agency, an organisation or one of their programs, or a particular event, period or incident. The data about the case may include interview data, observational data, documentary data, or impressions and statements made about the case (Liamputtong 2009).

Case study in qualitative research: The study of a particular issue which is examined through one or more cases within a 'bounded system' (such as a setting *or* context).

DATA ANALYSIS IN ETHNOGRAPHY

Data collected through ethnography is analysed similarly to other qualitative approaches (see CHAPTERS 5, 7, 22). Three main approaches are typically used. In the first approach, the ethnographer presents data in the form of a dialogue with key theoretical points that are raised in a literature review, and so is able to confirm, contradict or extend the theoretical insights gained from the literature. The second approach uses categories and themes derived from the field data themselves as a framework for the analysis and presentation of the data, in a manner similar to that described in detail in grounded theory analysis. The third common approach treads a middle ground between these two, and is usually presented in the form of a critical incident from the field data which is then unpacked according to themes and categories derived from the literature review and from a thematic analysis of the field data, including the conditions under which the field data was produced. This third approach is often referred to as cultural analysis or '**thick description**' in deference to Clifford Geertz who originated the approach. His article 'Deep Play: Notes on the Balinese Cockfight' exemplifies this approach (Geertz 1973, pp. 412–53). Since both thematic and grounded theory analysis are covered in detail in CHAPTERS 7, 22, 23, we will only provide a reflective account of an example of the second approach here, in this case from Karen's research.

Thick description: Descriptions that give ample detail and background information so that people's actions can be understood in the context of the experiences and patterns of meaning that influence them.

DOING RESEARCH

Qualitative data analysis involves searching the data for themes that emerge and then become categories for further analysis (see CHAPTER 22). Ethnographic approaches involving descriptive or interpretive research involve formally identifying themes as suggested by the data and demonstrating support for those themes. Thematic analysis techniques are similar to those of grounded theory, but do not include theoretical sampling. The process of thematic analysis involves coding, sorting and organising the data in themes that have not been decided before coding the data. Central to the data analysis process is coding, the process of identifying themes or concepts in the data in an attempt to build a systematic account of what has been observed and/or recorded.

My early analysis of the data involved 'open coding', which meant searching for similarities and differences and making comparisons between events, actions and interactions and labelling these in categories. Open coding at this stage assisted in identifying some of the main themes in the data. *In vivo* codes, which are directly taken from the data using lay terminology, were also coded during this stage of identifying and coding the data. I carried out open coding on interview and focus group transcripts and documents including field notes, unit outlines and classroom handouts, with the assistance of a software program (NVivo) designed for qualitative data analysis (see also CHAPTER 23). I moved between open coding of individual lines and sentences of text with the interview and focus group texts and paragraphs of text with document analysis.

Open coding of the text gave way to 'axial coding', which involved putting the data back together in new ways and making connections between categories. Axial coding involved exploring the codes and examining the relationships between these codes and developing categories and their subcategories. I then reviewed the data, which included revisiting the transcripts of interviews, the focus group and documents including audit notes and unit outlines and listening to audiotapes of interviews and classroom observations in order to verify the links between the codes and to search for any new codes. Finally, I began writing my account.

Qualitative data analysis: Data analysis in qualitative research is an ongoing, cyclical process that occurs from the very beginning of the research itself.

SUMMARY

Ethnography focuses on the description of practices and beliefs of groups of people, understood within the contexts of the shared cultures that they use to structure and derive meaning from their actions and interactions. Understood in this way, it provides unique insights into the ways

Jon Willis and Karen Anderson

that patients understand illness and the struggle for health, the ways that health practitioners organise and justify their actions, and the way societies privilege particular versions of health and illness, while dismissing others. In this chapter, we have explored the origins of ethnography in early 20th-century anthropological practice, and charted its development since then as a methodological tool used in a range of social and health science disciplines. In particular, we looked at the specific uses of ethnography in the area of health through an examination of focused ethnography, institutional ethnography and ethno-nursing. Finally, we examined a range of data collection and presentation techniques including observation, individual and group interviewing, visual techniques and the use of the case study.

TUTORIAL EXERCISES

1   Watch the teen movie *Mean Girls* (Waters 2004), which depicts the culture of American high school social cliques. Imagine that you are new girl and ethnographer Cady Heron and your task is to describe the operation and culture of the clique known as the Plastics.

   (a) Critique the pitfalls of participant observation for the fictional Cady, depicted by Lindsay Lohan in the film. What strategies could you use to avoid these pitfalls?

   (b) You decide to use key informants to help you understand the social processes of the Plastics. What kind of differences in your understanding would you get if you chose the following as your informants: Janis Ian and Damien; Regina George; Gretchen Weiners and Karen Smith; Miss Norbury and Mr Duvall; Regina's mother?

   (c) One of the major documents produced by the Plastics is the Burn Book. How would you analyse the Burn Book to illuminate processes of meaning construction at North Shore High School?

   (d) The revelation of the Burn Book to the student body, Cady's party, the Mathletes' participation in the State competition, and the Spring Fling emerge as critical incidents in Cady's period of fieldwork. Choose one of these incidents and analyse the cultural meanings of the incident.

2   Identify an ethnographic study from the health literature and use it to answer the following questions:

   (a) What is the field site that the author has chosen for the study? How has this choice been justified?

   (b) What techniques does the author use to collect data? How are different perspectives accommodated by each method?

   (c) How does the author describe the process used to analyse the field data collected in the study? How are these data presented?

   (d) How has the author dealt with conflicting or contradictory data in the study?

3   Think about a ethnographic study of your own:

(a)   Describe your field site for this study. Whose culture(s) is/are represented in this field?

(b)   What techniques would you choose to collect data for your study?

(c)   Write a memo describing your study idea and data collection strategy.

FURTHER READING

Atkinson, P., Coffey, A., Delamont, S., Lofland, J. & Lofland, L. (eds) (2001). *Handbook of ethnography*. London: Sage Publications.

Bernard, H. (2006). *Research methods in anthropology: Qualitative and quantitative approaches*. Lanham, MD: AltaMira Press.

De Laine, M. (1997). *Ethnography: Theory and applications in health research*. Sydney: McLennan & Petty.

Gobo, G. (2008). *Doing ethnography*. Los Angeles: Sage Publications.

Jorgenson, D. (1989). *Participant observation: A methodology for human studies*. Newbury Park, CA: Sage Publications.

Liamputtong, P. (2009). *Qualitative research methods*, 3rd edn. Melbourne: Oxford University Press.

Marcus, G. (1998). *Ethnography through thick and thin*. Princeton, NJ: Princeton University Press.

Spradley, J. & McCurdy, D. (1972). *The cultural experience: Ethnography in complex society*. Chicago: Science Research Associates Inc.

WEBSITES

http://eth.sagepub.com

Sage website of journals in ethnography.

http://jce.sagepub.com

Journal of Contemporary Ethnography *website.*

www-rcf.usc.edu/~genzuk/Ethnographic_Research.html>

Genzuk, A Synthesis of Ethnographic Research.

www.aiga.org/resources/content/3/7/4/5/documents/ethnography_primer.pdf

An Ethnography Primer.

www.lboro.ac.uk/departments/ss/visualising_ethnography

Visualising ethnography.

Jon Willis and Karen Anderson

7

Using Grounded Theory in Health Research

Jemma Skeat

CHAPTER OBJECTIVES

In this chapter you will learn:

- [ ] about the aims of grounded theory
- [ ] about the history and modes of grounded theory
- [ ] what steps are taken in a grounded theory study
- [ ] how to do data analysis
- [ ] how grounded theory has been used in speech pathology

KEY TERMS

Coding

Constant comparison

Data saturation

Grounded theory

Memos in grounded theory

Symbolic interactionism

Theoretical sampling

Theory in grounded theory

INTRODUCTION

Grounded theory is a research method that was developed to allow researchers to build theory 'from the ground up'. It stemmed from the research of two sociologists, Barney Glaser and Anselm Strauss, who believed that theories about social processes and actions should be generated systematically through research, and 'discovered' *from* data, rather than hypothesised and tested *against* data (Liamputtong 2009). Glaser and Holton (2004) suggest that in the grounded theory approach 'the mandate is to remain open to what is actually happening and not to start filtering data through pre-conceived hypotheses and biases[,] to listen and observe and thereby *discover* the main concern of the participants in the field and how they resolve this concern' (online document, section 3.2, emphasis theirs). A grounded theory study aims to develop a theoretical model that is well integrated and explains what is happening in the area of interest in a way that is meaningful to the people concerned. This 'grounded' theory can be used as a basis for prediction, explanation, and further research (Glaser 1978).

> **Grounded theory:** A qualitative research approach in which theories are grounded in the empirical data and built up inductively through a process of careful analysis and comparison.

Grounded theory differs from traditional models of positivist research where hypotheses are proposed and then tested (see 'Hypothesis-driven versus grounded theory research' below). The researcher instead attempts to understand and explain things 'from the ground up'; that is, using the data itself. A grounded theory study does not start with hypotheses about causes or outcomes, and instead focuses on explaining and understanding social processes.

Hypothesis-driven versus grounded theory research

Traditional hypothesis-driven approach

A researcher hypothesises that language development in young children is linked to parent interaction styles, with some styles facilitating language better than others. The research study involves training parents to use certain interaction styles and then measuring children's language outcomes.

Grounded theory approach

The researcher starts with no preconceived hypothesis about parent–child interaction styles, but views the action and interaction between parents and children as a social process that is of interest. The researcher decides to observe parent–child interaction, and uses this data to build a theory that explains how this interaction functions, and why and how it is important.

Grounded theory research also differs from some other qualitative approaches because its focus is on discovering *concepts* that explain social processes, actions and interactions, rather than on a full *description* of what is happening. The idea is to understand what is happening at a deeper level than the surface observations or explanations that people provide. The theory that

Jemma Skeat

is developed through the research process shows the concepts that are important within the research area, and the links between these (Annells 1997b; Glaser 1998; Liamputtong 2009).

HISTORY AND 'MODES' OF GROUNDED THEORY

Grounded theory was developed jointly by Glaser and Strauss (1967); it was a method that they 'discovered' while undertaking research into dying. Following their initial joint book describing grounded theory, the original authors went on to detail the method in subsequent publications, but separately. Glaser published many books and journal articles discussing grounded theory and its application, emphasising the differences between grounded theory and other approaches to qualitative research (Glaser 1978, 1992, 1996, 1998, 2001, 2002a, 2002b, 2004; Glaser & Holton 2004). Strauss, writing with a colleague, wrote a textbook aimed at students that described how to undertake a grounded theory study (Strauss & Corbin 1990, 1998; Corbin & Strauss 2008). Glaser and Strauss differ in their approaches to grounded theory in these later texts, both in the practical description of the method and the theoretical foundations.

Some researchers consider the methods of Glaser and Strauss to represent two different 'modes' of grounded theory (Annells 1996, 1997a,b; McCann & Clark 2003b), which Stern (1994) called 'Glaserian' and 'Straussian'. In one of his books, Glaser (1992, p. 2) argued strongly that Strauss and Corbin's work represented 'a whole different method', and not grounded theory at all. Other researchers, however, suggest that Strauss and Corbin's work is an ongoing development of the original idea, rather than a departure (Charmaz 2000, 2006). A more recent development in grounded theory is the work of Charmaz (2006), who developed a 'constructivist' grounded theory approach. This approach emphasises the role of the researcher, suggesting that the researcher 'constructs' the grounded theory through their interaction with participants, rather than 'discovering' grounded theory through data. Liamputtong (2009) suggests that Charmaz's work presents a new angle to grounded theory research; thus three major modes of grounded theory exist, and despite years of critique and debate in the literature, many grounded theorists believe that there is no single 'right' way of undertaking grounded theory. In fact, many authors have commented on the immense flexibility of this method (Annells 1997b; Strauss & Corbin 1998; Charmaz 2000, 2006; Corbin & Strauss 2008; Liamputtong 2009).

Given that there are differences in the specific techniques and approaches taken in Glaserian versus Straussian research, researchers starting a grounded theory project need to consider the 'mode' of grounded theory that they will adopt. Annells (1997b) listed five broad options to consider:

☐ a Glaserian approach (following Glaser's work)
☐ a Straussian approach (following the work of Strauss and Corbin)
☐ using Glaserian or Straussian grounded theory but with a different research paradigm or philosophical approach to the original (see Annells 1997a for a discussion of research paradigms in grounded theory)

☐   using both modes combined together, within a chosen framework

☐   use of own procedures, within the grounded theory framework.

Goulding (2002, p. 48) suggested that grounded theory modes should be chosen on the basis of 'the researcher's personality and preferred modes of working'. For example, those who like being guided by detailed specifics might prefer a 'Straussian' mode, as Strauss and Corbin provide essentially a step-by-step guide to working with grounded theory. But some researchers have noted that this approach may be overly mechanical and structured (Cutcliffe 2000; Hall & Callery 2001; Dixon-Woods et al. 2004). In contrast, Glaser's work emphasises flexibility and letting the theory 'emerge' from the data. However, there is no equivalent 'how-to' textbook for the Glaserian mode, and researchers need to amalgamate the information provided across his many books and texts in order to use this mode. Charmaz (2006) introduces the constructivist approach to grounded theory in a textbook that includes practical examples for new researchers.

Reading through some of the main grounded theory texts, such as Glaser (1978), Strauss and Corbin (1990, 1998), Corbin and Strauss (2008) and Charmaz (2006), may help to identify if one or other approach is a better fit for you. In this chapter, the focus is on exploring some of the common elements and components of a grounded theory study, though some of the differences in the major modes, particularly Glaserian and Straussian, are highlighted, which may help you when considering your choice of modes.

GROUNDED THEORY: PERSPECTIVES AND QUESTIONS

Glaser and Strauss (1967) initially considered grounded theory as appropriate only for sociologists, to be used to explain the processes that occur in social interaction. Since then, the method has been used extensively in many health and non-health fields (e.g. nursing, occupational therapy, speech pathology, education and business management). Despite this broader application, Glaser (1978) and other authors (e.g. Annells 1997b) have argued that the sociological focus of grounded theory is still important: a theory developed using the grounded theory approach focuses on social processes (human actions and interactions), and this focus needs to be maintained regardless of the discipline of the researcher.

As health professionals, social processes of action and interaction define much of what we do, particularly in diagnosis and therapy. Therefore grounded theory has the potential to help us understand the actions and interactions that take place in the clinical setting. Additionally, processes of professional practice, such as understanding how people develop themselves as an 'expert' in their professional role, could also be explored using grounded theory. There are also important questions for us to understand around the social processes that affect clients, for example how families communicate and interact when a child is sick or disabled, or how clients negotiate their way through the health care system.

Jemma Skeat

As an example of the diverse use of grounded theory in health research, some examples of topics that have been explored using this method in speech pathology are shown in Table 7.1. Some of these published studies will be used as examples throughout this chapter to illustrate how various aspects of a grounded theory study are undertaken.

Table 7.1: Published studies using grounded theory in speech pathology

Authors	Focus/topic
Skeat & Perry (2008)	Implementation and use of outcome measures by speech pathologists
Graves (2007)	Factors that influence indirect speech pathology interventions with adults with learning disabilities
Kummerer, Lopez-Reyna & Hughes (2007)	Mexican immigrant mothers' perceptions of children's speech and language difficulties and therapy
Bruce, Parker & Renfrew (2006)	Barriers and facilitators to accessing education for students with aphasia
Markham & Dean (2006)	Parent and carer perspectives on quality of life of children with speech and language difficulties
Slingsby (2006)	How medical and allied health professionals approach care for stroke patients in Japan
Pilling & Slattery (2004)	Development of speech pathologists as managers
Hersh (2003)	Strategies used by speech pathologists for discharging patients with aphasia
Trulsson & Klingberg (2003)	Living with a child with an orofacial handicap
Ukrainetz & Frequez (2003)	Speech pathologists' role in school settings
David and Whitehouse (1998)	Processes underlying a speech pathology service, including assessment and consultation
Nettleton & Reilly (1998)	Learning of speech pathology students while on clinical placements

Symbolic interactionism:
An American tradition that uses qualitative research methods to study the way people make sense of their experiences through common symbols and symbolic processes.

One of the reasons for the emphasis on social processes and action/interaction in grounded theory is that grounded theory was originally shaped by **symbolic interactionism**, a major sociological theory that provides a framework for understanding the nature of action and interaction in the human world. Blumer (1969/1986) describes three components that are central to the symbolic interactionism perspective:

☐ that humans act towards things around them on the basis of the meaning that those things have for them

☐ that this meaning is derived from social interaction; that is, we create our own meanings for things around us through our interactions with other people

☐ that meaning is developed and modified by our own interpretations, and that our actions are influenced by these interpretations.

Research using a symbolic interactionist perspective seeks to understand the actions and interactions that shape our subjective interpretations of meaning, and how these interpretations influence behaviour (Blumer 1969/1986). This is the basis for the original grounded theory method, and still influences how the method is applied today. (Further discussion about symbolic interactionism and grounded theory can be found in Charmaz 2000, 2006; Cutcliffe 2000; Hall & Callery 2001; Stanley & Cheek 2003).

DOING RESEARCH

I chose a grounded theory study for my PhD. The background to this choice was my involvement in research developing and trialling outcome measures by speech pathologists, occupational therapists and physiotherapists (Perry et al. 2004). Outcome measures are generally tools for quantitatively measuring the effectiveness of therapy (e.g. whether a patient has made progress in therapy from the first to the last session). I observed that clinicians sometimes had difficulty with, and sometimes did not like using, outcome measures in clinical settings. I decided that I would try and understand how speech pathologists start using outcome measures as part of their routine practice. My interest was in how change takes place in clinical practice, and how professionals incorporate new elements into existing clinical practice routines. The use of outcome measures was an example of this.

Grounded theory mode

Given the flexibility of grounded theory, the choice of which 'mode' (or combination) of grounded theory to use came down to a personal decision. I was drawn to Strauss and Corbin's work initially because it is written for new researchers and provides a step-by-step approach to undertaking a grounded theory study from start to finish. But I also found that I was overwhelmed by the steps that were needed, and the structured process that was described in this text. A colleague offered me the opportunity to explore Glaserian grounded theory in more detail by lending me a set of Glaser's books. These books are published by a small company and are not widely available, although they can be ordered through online sites such as Amazon.com. Glaser also has several papers published that further describe his approach to grounded theory. I found that there was a simplicity to the way that Glaser describes coding and analysis in his books and papers, which was a huge contrast to the structured approach of Strauss and Corbin. In the end, I chose to use the Glaserian approach in my study. However, this did not stop me from looking to Strauss (1987) and Strauss and Corbin (1998) to understand further some of the steps of grounded theory research.

Jemma Skeat

THE STEPS TAKEN IN A GROUNDED THEORY STUDY

As noted above, there are aspects to grounded theory that make it different from many other types of research. First, it is inductive; the researcher is seeking to 'discover' a theory from data, rather than to test a theory against data. Second, the coding process aims to define underlying *concepts* and links between these concepts, rather than aiming to fully *describe* something. This section will attempt to highlight the techniques that are central to the grounded theory method and that differentiate it from other research methods. Where possible, the way these steps have been applied in various speech pathology studies will be discussed as examples.

Identifying a focus and reviewing the literature

Remember that the aim of the original grounded theory modes (Glaserian and Straussian) is to *discover a theory from data*. This means that the theory will *emerge* from within the data, and will not be hypothesised prior to the research on the basis of the researcher's knowledge, experience or previous research.

Given this key principle of emergence (which Glaser arguably emphasises more than Strauss), it is not surprising that researchers are asked to start grounded theory with only a general topic area in mind, and particularly to keep away from incorporating pre-existing theoretical or conceptual ideas (Glaser & Holton 2004). If research questions are defined, they need to be open to modification throughout the research process, allowing emergent understandings to be incorporated; further, they cannot be driven by theoretical or conceptual hypotheses that would violate the principle of emergence (Strauss & Corbin 1998; Corbin & Strauss 2008).

A literature review is a natural first step for those embarking on research, but in grounded theory this is an area of potential confusion. Strauss and Corbin (1998) suggest that grounded theorists use a literature review as a source for research problems and to aid the 'theoretical sensitivity' of the researcher (see also Corbin & Strauss 2008). That is, the literature is seen as a way of sensitising researchers to concepts that might be of interest to their theory. On the other hand, Glaser (1998) strongly urges researchers to review the literature only once the core category has emerged (i.e. during the final phases of data analysis), and, if possible, not before. Glaser is concerned that if researchers review the literature before the study, they may place too much emphasis on concepts that are found in the literature but that may turn out to be of little importance to the grounded, discovered concerns of the participants in question (Glaser 1978, 1998). Coming from a constructivist perspective, Charmaz (2006) argues that researchers begin a grounded theory study with theoretical knowledge in their area of interest, and that this presents a starting place for their understanding of the area they wish to study. Liamputtong (2009) argues that this starting place, even if guided by theory, is not the same place that a theory ends up in a grounded theory study, as theory is constructed through the research process.

The instructions of Glaser, and to a lesser degree Strauss, can present a concern for those approaching a grounded theory study for a research degree. Many faculties will expect a literature review to be completed before confirming a PhD candidate, for example. But if we take a Glaserian approach, the literature should not be touched until the end of data collection and analysis. Very few published reports of grounded theory studies focus on this early phase of the research process, making it difficult to understand how researchers have dealt with this mandate to leave the literature alone. In 'Doing research' below, there is an account of how I undertook this process in my PhD, which illustrates one approach to meeting the traditional need for an early literature review while attempting to keep to a Glaserian approach. Accessing Masters or PhD theses that use a grounded theory approach from a university library may provide you with other examples.

DOING RESEARCH

Area of enquiry

I considered grounded theory to be an appropriate choice for research because my chosen topic area—the use of outcome measures as a new element in speech pathologists' practice—potentially involved a number of social structures (e.g. professionalism), social processes (e.g. the routines of clinical care), and interactions (e.g. between managers and clinicians).

Using a Glaserian approach, I developed a general area of focus for my research: *the use of outcome measures by speech pathologists in Australian health care settings.* This general area did not include preconceived conceptual or theoretical constructs gathered from the literature; for example, I was not interested only in 'organisational factors' or 'personality factors' that impacted on the use of outcome measures, nor did I assume that concepts like these were important. I developed a very general research question that was used to guide the research but maintained the neutrality and focus on emergence that Glaser always emphasises: *what is the main concern of speech pathologists when considering, or when using, outcome measures in health care settings, and how is this concern addressed?*

Literature review

Taking a Glaserian approach to grounded theory meant that I needed to steer clear of preconceived ideas in the literature. On the other hand, as a PhD student I needed to present a literature review within an internal forum for postgraduate researchers, and to use the literature to justify my research aims and questions. The order of chapters in my thesis was another concern, as most theses begin with a literature review, leading to the aims and methodology. My attempt to meet both of these needs meant two quite separate literature reviews, both of which were presented in my thesis. The first review was undertaken at the beginning of the research process, and focuses on outcome measurement, which includes definitions, history and application to speech pathology. This literature was placed in the traditional section of my thesis, at the beginning, and provided a context for the study. It was the basis for my presentation in the internal forum. At this stage I deliberately avoided literature around the implementation or use of outcome measurement, or clinicians' views about outcome measurement, in any discipline. In this way, I avoided pre-empting my research by reviewing and synthesising literature that addressed the concepts that I would be attempting to discover. A second review that took place later looked at these concepts in detail, and I wove this literature into the description of the theory in my thesis. For example, when describing a concept that was discovered in my theory, I discussed how this concept had been addressed in other literature, examining the use of outcome measures.

Theoretical sampling and data collection

Theoretical sampling:
A technique in grounded theory whereby sampling is guided by the developing theory and not based on statistical or other predetermined grounds.

Grounded theory uses a sampling technique specific to it called **theoretical sampling** (McCann & Clark 2003a; Liamputtong 2009) to identify both *who* and *what* data collection should focus on. Specifically, theoretical sampling is used to identify:

☐ participants—which people to interview or observe
☐ questions or situations—what data to collect from participants.

Theoretical sampling is based on the principle of emergence, which was noted above. Rather than speculating or hypothesising about people, situations or questions that will be the most useful, grounded theory researchers use the developing theory to guide their decisions about sampling (Liamputtong 2009). As the researcher analyses data, questions and hypotheses about the data begin to emerge. Glaser (1998) calls these 'grounded deductions' (i.e. deductions made on the basis of data), which are used to feed back into the data collection process. In this way 'the growing theory leads the researcher on' (Glaser 1998, p. 157). For example, when considering the role of speech and language therapists in schools (e.g. Ukrainetz & Frequez 2003), an emergent category of 'expertise' might lead the researcher to hypothesise that the way clinicians view their own expertise is important, and thus they may seek therapists with different views of their own expertise, or deliberately include questioning about this in subsequent interviews, in order to understand this category further. The research process in grounded theory is therefore cyclical, using an iterative process of data collection, analysis and theory-building (McCann & Clark 2003b). Strauss (1987, p. 21) pointed out that theoretical sampling is 'sampling of incidents, events, activities, populations'. Thus theoretical sampling takes place both in choosing participants (or situations) of interest to the developing theory, and within the data collection itself, for example in the questions that are asked in the interviews. See also CHAPTER 1.

Although it is common to use interviews or observations for a grounded theory study, in reality the options for data collection are much broader, and researchers can use multiple types of data in the one study, as long as the data are sought using the principles of theoretical sampling above (see CHAPTERS 3, 4, 5, 8, 9, 10). An example of this is provided by David and Whitehouse (1998), who explored the consultation process for a speech pathology service by analysing written clinical reports from within the unit, as well as interviews with clinical staff. Glaser (1998, p. 8) suggests: 'The briefest of comment to the lengthiest interview, written words in magazines, books and newspapers, documents, observations, biases of self and others, spurious variables, or whatever else may come the researcher's way in his substantive area of research is data for grounded theory.' Regardless of type, data are incorporated into the emerging theory by constant comparison with other data (described further below). Using diverse data to develop grounded theory allows the researcher to take a broader perspective of the categories and their properties, and makes the theory more broadly applicable (Glaser & Strauss 1967).

Of course, a starting place is needed for data collection. Glaser (1978) speaks of beginning the study by directing sampling towards 'knowledgeable people' in order to find out about the areas of relevance in the substantive area, which Coyne (1997, p. 625) characterises as 'the purposeful selection of a sample in the initial stages' (see CHAPTERS 1, 2, 5, 8). Strauss and Corbin (1998) suggest that researchers may need to begin with a list of questions or concepts to ask participants about. But these should not be rigidly used, and should be developed as the data from previous interviews are analysed, in order to guide the researcher towards asking theoretically grounded questions. Similarly, while one could approach written documents with a set of questions in mind, the researcher needs to remain open to finding new ideas and using these data-driven concepts to guide further sampling.

Sample size and saturation

Sampling in grounded theory continues until a point is reached where no new ideas are coming out of the data to explain the concepts or categories of interest. At this stage, the data are considered to be 'saturated' (see CHAPTER 1). **Data saturation** becomes evident from the fact that data incidents reveal no new concepts, properties or relationships in relation to the main categories of interest, even when sampling is of participants with diverse characteristics and in diverse situations. Charmaz (2000, 2006) points out that the aim of theoretical sampling is about the refinement of ideas and saturation of concepts, rather than necessarily increasing the size of the sample. In fact, the sample size for a grounded theory study is difficult to judge ahead of time, and varies widely across different studies; for example, the number of participants in the speech pathology grounded theory literature ranges from six to 30.

> **Data saturation** occurs when little or no new data is being generated and new data fits into the categories already developed.

DOING RESEARCH

Getting the right sample

I began sampling with the knowledge that my group of interest were speech pathologists who had experience with, or were considering using, outcome measures. As a starting place, I purposely selected two clinicians who I knew had actually trialled the use of an outcome measure in practice. The data from these interviews guided the next steps in sampling by suggesting certain categories that I needed to pursue, such as levels of clinical experience, roles (e.g. managerial versus clinical), settings or clinical contexts, and experience or exposure to outcome measures. As data analysis continued, further concepts emerged to guide data collection choices. I held second and even third interviews with some participants a few months later to explore how the implementation of outcome measures changed over time, which had emerged as important in early interviews. Data analysis also drove the direction of the questions I used in interviews, so that I was able to explore concepts in more depth. In total, the study included nine speech pathology clinicians and seven managers, and used data from 22 interviews. I also went looking for other types of data when needed to develop my emerging theory further. For example, government and professional documents were particularly important for understanding the concept that outcome measurement was 'needed' in some settings in order to meet outside demands.

Data analysis

It should be obvious from the above that data collection and data analysis are iterative; that is, the researcher collects data, analyses and begins to build their theory, and then pursues more data in order to understand more about the theory, analyses these data, and so on. The cyclical process continues until, as described above, the categories are saturated.

Both Glaserian and Straussian approaches have well-described data analysis techniques, but with some differences to their approaches. The major differences are in the phases of coding—Glaser's 'open', 'selective' and 'theoretical' versus Strauss's 'open', 'axial' and 'selective'—and in the way that the final theory is integrated through coding. There is not room here to elaborate on the specifics of both approaches, but this section will describe some of the common general principles of data analysis in a grounded theory study, particularly the coding types and the emphasis on constant comparison, and will provide some examples of coding and conceptual development. See CHAPTERS 22, 23.

Constant comparison and coding types

Grounded theorists aim to understand the concepts that underlie the patterns in the raw data, ordering these into categories and properties, and link these theoretically by describing how concepts and properties relate to one another, and especially to a 'core' category (Glaser 1978, 1998). To do this, they use a strategy known as 'constant comparison' in order to group data bits together, and to understand how these groups work and link together.

Constant comparison is a fairly simple concept. Take some raw data and consider some of the 'bits' or incidents in the data. The quotations below are from participants in a grounded theory study examining patient discharge strategies used by speech pathologists (Hersh 2003, p. 1014):

> You can say reassuring things like 'You can manage all this, this and this, and look how much improvement you've made'. I think that's an important thing.

> You'd say, 'Look, this is the deal. This is where you were and this is what you have achieved. We really haven't changed communication behaviours over the last month, two months…'

> Oh, they often say 'But we usually get together every week'. And I say, 'Yeah, but you're so much better now…'

Constant comparison allows researchers to see patterns in the data. By comparing each incident within a category to one another, the properties of that category begin to emerge.

Now compare them: what is similar, and what is different? In each, the speech pathologist is talking about something they do with clients to suggest that they have made improvement. In the first incident, the clinician suggests to the client that they have made huge improvements and can now achieve a lot more than they could formerly. In the second incident, the clinician shows the improvement to the client, but also suggests that there has been a plateau in the improvement over time. In the third incident, the clinician justifies fewer or more spaced out sessions by telling a client how much better they are. Constant comparison of incidents allows the researcher to see patterns in the data, and in the initial stages of analysis the researcher simply groups like 'incidents' together and gives a name to the group (Glaser 2002a), and this group is called a category. By comparing each incident within that category with one another, the properties of that category begin to emerge. Initial categories may be simply descriptive in nature; for example, the researcher might decide that all three of the above incidents could be grouped together as examples of 'showing the client their progress'. By looking at the differences, different properties of this category might be proposed, such as that 'showing progress' can be about encouraging clients about their achievement or suggesting that they have reached a stage where no more progress is being made.

In the initial phases of grounded theory analysis, **coding** is 'open'. Glaserian, Straussian and Charmaz's modes all use this stage of coding, in which the researcher is simply coding the data into as many categories as possible to see what the data hold (Glaser 1978). The process involves seeing patterns in the data by comparing incidents, and simply naming these patterns (Glaser 2002a). Corbin and Strauss (2008, p. 102) describe this as

Coding: Part of the data analysis process where codes are applied to chunks of data. Coding allows researchers to move beyond tangible data to make analytic interpretations.

Jemma Skeat

a process of 'breaking open' the data: 'to uncover, name, and develop concepts, we must open up the texts and expose the thoughts, ideas and meanings contained therein'. Liamputtong (2009) suggests that open coding is a 'first run' at data analysis, allowing the researcher to make a start in examining what is happening in the data. Charmaz (2006, p. 48) points out that the researcher should himself take an open stance to the data at this point, by being 'open to seeing what you can learn by coding, and where it can take you'.

As the research progresses and more data are added, constant comparison supports the researcher to look deeper into the categories and incidents, and to consider the concepts that underpin these descriptions. Subcategories develop, and the names of categories show a more conceptual understanding of what is happening in the data and what each set of incidents is really about. Using the examples above, Hersh (2003, p. 1014) described the first and third incident above as examples of 'Encouragement talk'. This category is defined by strategies that aim to boost client confidence 'in order to pave the way towards discharge'. In comparison, the second incident was categorised as an example of 'Presenting evidence', a strategy where clinicians use information or data to justify their position in discharging the patient by 'proving' to the client that their progress has reached a certain point. Higher-level concepts might emerge that define several categories and group these together. For example, Hersh found that both 'Encouragement talk' and 'Presenting evidence' were both examples of a more general concept called 'Preparation strategies', that is, strategies used by clinicians to 'smooth the way' for discharge in a relatively covert way. The process of comparing incidents and grouping them together in grounded theory analysis continues, with further data theoretically sampled in order to extend the researcher's understanding of the developing categories and their properties.

Straussian grounded theory takes a specific approach to this deeper phase of coding by suggesting that researchers 'reassemble' the data that has been opened up during open coding (Strauss & Corbin 1998). An **axial coding** phase is suggested, whereby researchers systematically relate categories to subcategories using properties and dimensions. This allows each category to be fully explored and defined. It is perhaps this difference that Glaser (1992, p. 5) most strongly disagreed with about the Straussian approach, suggesting that the use of axial coding as described leads to 'forced, full conceptual description', and not grounded theory.

Axial coding: A phase of the Straussian mode of grounded theory in which categories and subcategories are systematically related to one another.

Coding now moves towards a more 'selective' phase. Categories become more integrated and the properties better defined. The focus for coding begins to narrow down to fewer categories—the ones that seem to be of real importance to the developing theory.

Ultimately, the researcher might discover a 'core category', something that is a recurring 'theme' within the data, which Glaser (2001, p. 199) defines as 'a latent structural pattern... related to most variation in the data of the substantive area, and therefore organises and explains most of the variation in how the main concern is continually resolved'. At this phase of coding, the researcher looks to understand more about the core category and the key categories around it. Not all new data have to be included in the coding from this point, unless they add new information about the categories of interest (Glaser & Strauss 1967).

In Glaserian grounded theory, there is a final 'theoretical' coding phase. At this phase, new data are not being added to the study, as the researcher is just trying to relate the core category and those around it using a theoretical coding family (Glaser & Holton 2004). Theoretical coding families are discussed further below, but basically they provide a framework for the theory, suggesting what the theory is about—for example whether it is a theory of 'processes' or 'types' or 'strategies'. See also CHAPTERS 22, 23 for more information about coding and data analysis in qualitative research.

Use of memos during data analysis

Memos are an important part of the coding process in grounded theory. They are 'notes to self' that the researchers write as they analyse the data and continue data collection, and they help the researchers to look more deeply into the developing categories and properties, and to come up with 'grounded' hypotheses (based on the data) about what is going on. Strauss and Corbin (1990, 1998) and Corbin and Strauss (2008) propose that three different types of memos may be useful: code notes (ideas about categories and properties), theoretical notes (more detailed memos about each category to try and understand how it works and what its properties are), and operational notes (memos about the research process, including where to sample next).

> **Memos in grounded theory:** A note to self that researchers write as they analyse the data and continue data collection. An important part of the coding process in grounded theory.

Glaser simply (1978) suggests that researchers use 'coding memos'—notes about the categories, properties and relationships that the researcher notes as they are analysing the data. They might include suggestions for further data collection or links between categories that the researcher has noticed. They are used to support the researcher to develop their understanding of the concepts within the data. Towards the end of the research process, sorting through memos supports the researcher to integrate the concepts into a theory.

Coding ultimately heads towards developing a theory. So it is worth finishing this chapter by considering what is meant by a 'theory' in grounded theory.

A 'GROUNDED THEORY' (WHAT IS IT?)

Strauss and Corbin (1998, p. 22) define a **theory in grounded theory** as 'a set of well developed categories (e.g. themes, concepts) that are systematically interrelated through statements of relationship'. A grounded theory is a set of categories that are related to one another to form a framework that explains the *main concern* of the participants in relation to the research area, and shows how this concern is resolved or managed (Glaser 1978, 1998, 2002b; Glaser & Holton 2004).

> **Theory in grounded theory:** A set of categories, related to one another to form a framework that explains the main concern of the participants and shows how this concern is resolved or managed.

Jemma Skeat

Theories can assemble concepts together in different ways. Some show these relationships in terms of 'causes' and 'consequences'. A Straussian approach supports this type of theory, as throughout the analysis process the researcher is directed to look at categories and properties to identify conditions, actions/interactions and consequences. Thus when it comes time for the theory to be integrated, the model is usually one that relates the theory in terms of these relationships. But this is just one way that a theory can link concepts together. Hersh's theory of discharge by speech pathologists integrates many *strategies* that clinicians use, all of them having the same goal of 'weaning' clients from therapy. David and Whitehouse (1998) developed a theoretical model of assessment and consultation in their speech pathology service, and their model focuses on the *processes* that take place both before and during clinical contact with clients. As noted above, Glaser (1998) calls these different ways of linking a theory together 'theoretical coding families', and suggests that there could be hundreds of them. A coding family frames the theory; it becomes a theory that hypothesises causes and consequences, or explains interactions, or relates strategies used by participants to manage problems. The right way of linking concepts and properties together to form a theory is driven by the data, and the researcher must look for the one with the best fit.

Not all published studies that use grounded theory techniques present fully developed theoretical models. For example, Kummerer and colleagues (2007) examined Mexican immigrant mothers' perceptions about children's communication disabilities, literacy development and therapy using a grounded theory approach. The results of the study are listed themes that emerged during interviews, but the relationship between these themes is not defined.

The resulting themes of Kummerer's work present some useful insights that can inform clinical practice, but they do not present a theory. The use of grounded theory methods without necessarily aiming for the development of a theory may illustrate the flexibility and usefulness of grounded theory techniques, particularly constant comparison for analysis. But it should be noted that some authors have questioned the accuracy of calling a study 'grounded theory' if a theory is not developed (Becker 1993; Wilson & Hutchinson 1996; Cutcliffe 2000; Liamputtong 2009).

When a grounded theory is developed, it is never a 'final product'; it is dynamic, ongoing, and 'under development' (Glaser & Strauss 1967). Nevertheless, a grounded theory is able to explain and relate concepts that are important and relevant in the area studied. Because the theory defines a set of concepts, and does not just provide a description of 'what happened' in the data, the theory is applicable in different situations. Boychuk-Duchscher and Morgan (2004, p. 606) suggest that, regardless of the approach taken by the researcher (e.g. Glaserian or Straussian), the purpose of a grounded theory study is the same:

> The discovery of enduring theory that is faithful to the reality of the research area; makes sense to the persons studied; fits the template of the social situation, regardless of varying contexts related to the studied phenomenon; adequately provides for relationships amongst concepts; and may be used to guide action.

SUMMARY

Grounded theory is a method that has roots in sociology and symbolic interactionism. While the specifics of grounded theory may be guided by your choice of 'modes', there are common elements that distinguish a grounded theory study from other qualitative or quantitative studies. These include a focus on emergence (rather than predetermined hypotheses), use of theoretical sampling, constant comparison and use of memos during analysis, and development of a theory product.

Grounded theory has been used by health professionals to explore varied topics and areas, from professional issues such as student learning on clinical placements, to client-focused topics such as understanding parent perspectives on living with a child with handicap. It presents a well-described method of developing theory that is relevant to patients, families, and professionals.

TUTORIAL EXERCISES

1   Identify a grounded theory study from the literature and use it to answer the following questions:

   (a) Has the author identified whether they are using a particular 'mode' of grounded theory? If so, which one? If they have not stated that they are using a particular mode, is there anything within the paper that makes you think they are using one mode over another?

   (b) How have the following elements been described in the paper: use of the literature, sampling and saturation, constant comparison, use of memos? Have the authors used all these components in their study? Are there any areas where the author has used different techniques (e.g. a different type of sampling), or where techniques are not described?

   (c) Has the author proposed a theory (i.e. have they related the concepts that were discovered in the data in a way that shows their relationship?) If so, what does the theory propose?

   (d) Visit the website ‹http://gtm.vlsm.org/gnm-gtm2.en.html›, which summarises the theoretical coding families that Glaser (1978, 1998) proposed. Using these examples, can you identify what type of theory is proposed in your paper (e.g. does it explain a process? Is it about types?).

2   Think about a potential grounded theory study of your own:

   (a) What would your area of interest be for this study? How does this area include a focus on social processes (action/interaction)? Who is interacting?

   (b) Where would you direct your initial sampling? How would you identify and contact people for this initial sample?

   (c) Write a memo describing your study idea and initial sampling decisions.

Jemma Skeat

FURTHER READING

Backman, K. & Kyngas, H.A. (1999). Challenges of the grounded theory approach to a novice researcher. *Nursing and Health Sciences*, 1(3), 147–53.

Charmaz, K. (2006). *Constructing grounded theory: A practical guide through qualitative analysis*. London: Sage Publications.

Corbin, J. & Strauss, A. (2008). *Basics of qualitative research: Techniques and procedures for developing grounded theory*, 3rd edn. Thousand Oaks, CA: Sage Publications.

Glaser, B.G. (1998). *Doing grounded theory: Issues and discussions*. Mill Valley, CA: Sociology Press.

Glaser, B.G. & Strauss, A. (1967). *The discovery of grounded theory: Strategies for qualitative research*. New York: Aldine.

Liamputtong, P. (2009). *Qualitative research methods*, 3rd edn. Melbourne: Oxford University Press.

Mellion, L.R. & Tovin, M.M. (2002). Grounded theory: A qualitative research methodology for physical therapy. *Physiotherapy Theory and Practice*, 18, 109–20.

Skeat, J. & Perry, A. (2008). Grounded theory as a method for research in speech and language therapy. *International Journal of Language and Communication Disorders*, 43(2), 95–109.

Stanley, M. & Cheek, J. (2003). Grounded theory: Exploiting the potential for occupational therapy. *British Journal of Occupational Therapy*, 66(4), 143–50.

WEBSITES

http://gtm.vlsm.org/gnm-gtm2.en.html

Theoretical coding families.

www.groundedtheory.com

Barney Glaser's grounded theory institute.

www.groundedtheoryreview.com

Grounded theory journal.

www.qualitative-research.net

Online qualitative research journal that often includes good grounded theory articles.

http://jpmats.com/GT_Axial_Coding.aspx

An overview and illustration of axial coding using the Straussian approach (also see links on the left-hand navigation bar of this page for other stages of coding).

8

Phenomenology and Rehabilitation Research

Christine Carpenter

CHAPTER OBJECTIVES

In this chapter you will learn:

☐ to explore phenomenology as a methodological approach to conducting qualitative research in rehabilitation

☐ to consider the contribution qualitative methodological theory can make to developing a coherent and rigorous study design

☐ to discuss and critique the design and implementation of a phenomenological study

☐ to reflect on the central role of the researcher in phenomenological research

☐ to discuss the contribution of qualitative research to evidence-based practice

KEY TERMS

Bracketing

Descriptive phenomenology

Evidence-based practice in health care

In-depth interviewing

Interpretive or hermeneutic phenomenology

Method

Methodology

Phenomenological reduction

Phenomenology

Purposive sampling

Reflexivity

Semi-structured interview

INTRODUCTION

For the purposes of this chapter, I would like to take the opportunity to revisit and reflect on a phenomenological study I conducted a number of years ago (Carpenter 1994) from the perspective of what I learnt and what I would do differently given the research experience I have since acquired. This study derived directly from my practice as a physical therapist in spinal cord injury rehabilitation. I had been seconded from a physical therapy department to the position of research coordinator for a large study exploring issues of fertility after spinal cord injury. Clients who volunteered to be involved with this study shared with me their experiences of living with spinal cord injury in the community, some for many years post-injury. It was as a result of these privileged conversations that I came to recognise, for the first time in a long career as a physical therapist in rehabilitation, the significant discrepancies between the clients' and rehabilitation therapists' beliefs and understanding of life after spinal cord injury. I realised that, as a physical therapist, I interacted with clients in a relatively limited post-injury time-frame when they were in the process of assimilating the major changes caused to their lives, but that I had little opportunity to understand the impact on their long-term health or quality of life. It was these insights that led me to conduct the study discussed in this chapter.

Perhaps the most essential step in developing a research study is to generate a clear statement of purpose or question that can withstand scrutiny and critique. The decision about which qualitative methodology to choose (if any) reflects the type of question being asked and, in turn, guides and contributes to a coherent and rigorous study design. For example, the purpose of this study was to explore the meaning of the experience of spinal cord injury from the individual's perspective.

Students and practitioners newly engaging in qualitative research are confronted with, as Creswell (1998, p. 4) observes, 'a baffling number' of methodological traditions from which to choose. In addition, the terms **methodology** and **method** are not used consistently across disciplines. In this chapter, I have defined methodology as 'a specific philosophical and ethical approach to developing knowledge; a theory of how research should, or ought, to proceed given the nature of the issue it seeks to address' (Hammell 2006, p. 167). In contrast, method is defined as 'the actual techniques and strategies employed to collect and manipulate data and acquire knowledge' (Hammell & Carpenter 2000, p. 2). In my opinion, 'an informed and explicitly described methodological approach lends coherence and consistency to the research design, and plays an important role in justifying the plan of inquiry' (Carpenter & Suto 2008, p. 46). It guides the research design and the analytic process, and enhances the credibility of the research. Some researchers do not articulate the theoretical approach that guides their study nor do they justify the use of a qualitative approach. A critical appraisal of such studies often reveals a lack of understanding

Methodology: 'A specific philosophical and ethical approach to developing knowledge; a theory of how research should, or ought, to proceed given the nature of the issue it seeks to address.'

Method: The actual strategies and techniques that researchers use to acquire knowledge and collect data.

of the essential epistemological differences between qualitative and quantitative research, misuse of terminology, and a paucity of scientific rigour. Researchers, as Miller and Crabtree (2005, p. 626) assert, have the responsibility of creating 'methodologically convincing stories' by providing a cogent rationale for their research studies. The issue of using methodological theory, however, continues to be vigorously debated by qualitative researchers. There is a concern that expecting researchers, particularly those with less experience, to ground their proposed research in methodological detail is excessive and that instead what is required is that researchers demonstrate a thorough understanding of the essential distinctions between interpretivist (qualitative) and positivist (quantitative) research (Avis 2003; see CHAPTER 1).

PHENOMENOLOGY

Phenomenology is a methodological approach with a strong and dynamic philosophical and epistemological foundation that seeks to understand, describe and interpret human behaviour and the meaning individuals make of their experiences. There are a number of schools of phenomenological thought, the primary ones being descriptive phenomenology and interpretive or hermeneutic phenomenology, which have some commonalities and also distinct features (Dowling 2007). It is worth recognising the distinctions between the two approaches, but a broad concept of phenomenology based on common characteristics is usually applied in health-related studies.

Descriptive phenomenology

Edmond Husserl (1859–1938) regarded human experience as a fundamental source of knowledge and study in its own right (Dowling 2007) and developed phenomenology as an approach to studying 'things as they appear' (Dowling 2007, p. 132) in order to arrive at a rigorous and unbiased understanding of the essential human consciousness and experience. Descriptive phenomenologists such as Giorgi and Giorgi (2003) and Moustakas (1994) have perhaps the closest connections with Husserl's original conception of phenomenology, and focus on creating detailed descriptions of specific experiences of a phenomenon (Carpenter & Suto 2008). Central to **descriptive phenomenology** are the concepts of **phenomenological reduction** (or epoche) and **bracketing**. Phenomenological reduction is the central aim of this type of enquiry—to gain rich or 'thick' information that represents the essential nature of the individuals' experiences and that 'communicates the sense and logic of the phenomenon to others' (Todres, 2005, p. 110) in new

Phenomenology:
A methodological approach that seeks to understand, describe and interpret human behaviour and the meaning individuals make of their experiences.

Descriptive phenomenology:
An approach to studying 'things as they appear' in order to arrive at a rigorous and unbiased understanding of the essential human consciousness and experience.

Phenomenological reduction is the goal of phenomenological enquiry: to search for the multiple meanings attributed to a phenomenon and to provide a comprehensive description of it rather than an explanation.

Bracketing:
The suspension of all judgments and prior ideas 'in order to enter the unique world of the individual whose experience is the focus of the research'.

ways. Bracketing is the process by which the researcher identifies and attempts to hold in abeyance ideas, preconceptions and personal knowledge about the phenomenon of interest in order to authentically listen to and reflect on the lived experiences of participants (Lopez & Willis 2004). The feasibility and relevance of bracketing is the focus of much debate among qualitative researchers. It is important, however, that researchers engaging in phenomenological enquiry have an in-depth understanding of the concept in order to justify its inclusion or not in their study design. Another assumption underlying the descriptive tradition is that there are features of any lived experience that are common to all persons who have had the experience; for example, most people would share commonalties of experience of the concepts of love and grief. The focus or subject of these emotions will differ in many respects but a common *essence*, considered to represent the core nature of the phenomenon, can be discovered. The essence thus refers to the qualities that give an experiential phenomenon, for example spinal cord injury (Carpenter 1994), its distinctiveness and coherence (Todres 2005). Therefore, an attempt is made to refine, as free as possible from cultural context, an understanding of the essential features of a phenomenon (Dowling 2007). In summary, the descriptive phenomenologist develops detailed concrete descriptions of experience.

Interpretive or hermeneutic phenomenology

In contrast, **interpretive or hermeneutic phenomenologists**, for example van Manen (1997), focus on describing the meanings attributed by individuals' 'being in the world and how these meanings influence the choices that they make' (Lopez & Willis 2004, p. 729). Researchers working in this tradition would encourage participants to describe interactions, relations with others, physical experiences and so on in order to place the lived experience in the context of daily life. This might involve an analysis of the historical, social and political forces that shape and organise individuals' experiences. In this tradition, the researcher's presuppositions or knowledge are valuable guides to enquiry, and in fact make the enquiry a meaningful undertaking (Lopez & Willis 2004). The word '**hermeneutics**' 'describes the process of establishing understanding of the text as a whole by constantly interpreting the individual parts in relation to the other parts and each in relation to the whole' (Carpenter & Suto 2008, p. 65) and is a core characteristic of phenomenological data analysis (Rapport 2005).

It is not possible, within the constraints of this chapter, to provide more than this simplified account of these important philosophical traditions. There are, however, a number of additional core concepts and principles characteristic of phenomenological research that differentiate it from other qualitative methodologies, such as grounded theory or ethnography, which readers may wish to explore further.

Interpretive or hermeneutic phenomenology focuses on describing the meanings attributed by individuals' 'being in the world and how these meanings influence the choices that they make'.

Hermeneutics: A theory of the process of interpretation, used in qualitative research to examine the way people develop interpretations of their life in relation to their life experiences.

Life-world: 'The world of experience as it lived', 'our sense of lived life'.

These concepts—the **life-world**, **intentionality** and **multiple realities**—reflect the central interest of phenomenology in the individual experience. The life-world can be described as 'the world of experience as it is lived by individuals' (Finlay 1999, p. 301), or 'our sense of lived life' (Rapport 2005, p. 131). The concept of intentionality reflects the assumption that the life-world 'is not an objective environment or a subjective consciousness or a set of beliefs; rather, [it] is what we perceive and experience it to be' (Finlay 1999, p. 302). The idea of multiple realities is 'that the same objects or situations can mean different things to different people, and that people and the worlds they occupy are inextricably intertwined' (Carpenter & Suto 2008, p. 66).

In summary, the aim of phenomenological research is to reveal the individual's lived meaning of the world; it does not assume understanding, but rather works with developing it, using the terms of meanings constructed by the participant (Carpenter & Suto 2008).

Intentionality: The assumption that the life-world 'is not an objective environment or a subjective consciousness or a set of beliefs; rather, [it] is what we perceive and experience it to be'.

Multiple realities: The same objects or situations can mean different things to different people; people and the worlds they occupy are inextricably intertwined.

DESIGNING AND CONDUCTING PHENOMENOLOGICAL RESEARCH IN REHABILITATION PRACTICE

The aim of my study (Carpenter 1994), as stated earlier, was to explore the experience of spinal cord injury from the individual's perspective. At the time, I identified phenomenology as the appropriate methodological approach but did not attempt to further define the specific phenomenological tradition. In hindsight, I think the study aim is most congruent with descriptive phenomenology. However, the core concepts and principles were appropriately and consistently used to guide the study design and implementation. Ethical approval was obtained from the University Behavioural Sciences Research Ethics Committee.

Participant recruitment

Participants were recruited if they had sustained a traumatic spinal cord injury 2–5 years before the study and defined themselves as 'successfully rehabilitated' or 'back on track'. Initial access to a network of potential participants was gained through the sponsorship offered by a personal acquaintance. He had sustained a spinal cord injury, was educated as a social worker, and was involved in facilitating a peer-support group. His explanation of the study to the group resulted in three people volunteering to be involved. A further seven participants were recruited by a **purposive snowball sampling** technique whereby the first participants interviewed were asked to recommend others who, in their opinion, met the inclusion criteria (see CHAPTERS 1, 5).

Purposive sampling looks for cases that will be able to provide rich or in-depth information about the issue being examined, not a representative sample as in quantitative research.

Snowball sampling: Sampling that relies on existing participants to identify acquaintances who fit the inclusion criteria of a study in order to increase the size of the sample.

Since conducting this study, I have frequently been asked to defend or justify this 'small sample size'. Questions like this reflect the assumptions of representativeness, normal distribution and generalisability that underpin quantitative and survey approaches. Phenomenological research focuses on determining the essence of an experience or phenomenon. This is usually achieved by employing a rigorous purposive sampling strategy and conducting one to three in-depth interviews with a small number of participants. At the time, I justified the sample size of 10 participants by referring to data or theoretical saturation (see CHAPTERS 1, 5, 7). This is a concept originating in grounded theory but which has been more widely adopted by qualitative researchers (Guest et al. 2006; see CHAPTER 7). **Data saturation** is presumed to have occurred 'when all the main variations of the phenomenon have been identified and incorporated into the emerging themes or theory' (Guest et al. 2006, p. 65; Liamputtong 2009; see also CHAPTERS 1, 7). In reality, however, this concept is difficult to nail down, and there is little consensus in the literature. For example, Morse (1994a) recommends that for phenomenological studies, at least six participants are needed, but for Creswell (1998) there should be between five and 25 interviews. In my study, data collection was curtailed more by the practical constraints of conducting research to fulfil the requirements and deadlines of a graduate program, and it is unlikely that true data saturation was achieved. The key question to ask in phenomenological research when making sampling decisions is whether the sample provides access to enough data and with the appropriate focus to enable the research purpose to be thoroughly addressed (Mason 2002). As a result, the initial sample size is an estimate rather than a fixed number. All the participants I interviewed had considerable experience of living with a spinal cord injury, but some were more articulate and had clearly reflected on their experiences. In general, the greater the *quality* of data acquired from each source, the smaller the sample size required (Carpenter & Suto 2008).

> **Data saturation** occurs when little or no new data is being generated and new data fits into the categories already developed.

DATA COLLECTION: CONDUCTING QUALITATIVE INTERVIEWS

Single, fairly lengthy (60–80 minutes) **in-depth interviews** were the chosen approach for my study (see CHAPTER 3). Bearing the aim of the study in mind, I developed a list of possible questions to guide the interview. I began with broad open-ended questions (see Table 8.1) designed to encourage the participants to express their perceptions and understandings in their own words. As the interview progressed, I attempted to ask probing questions and reflect the participants' understanding back to them to ensure a full exploration of the experience. As a result, each interview was unique and did not follow 'a uniform, standardized, replicable process' (Taylor 2005, p. 40). The interviews gave the participants the opportunity to construct or reconstruct

> **In-depth interviewing:** A method of qualitative data collection that does not used fixed questions, but aims to engage the interviewee in conversation to elicit their understandings and interpretations.

their experiences and as such were 'influenced by their ability to articulate, reflect on and recall experiences and the accompanying emotions' (p. 41). The interviews were audiotaped with the permission of each participant and I transcribed these as soon as possible after the interviews. These transcripts formed the main data for this study but were supplemented by 'field notes' and 'analytic memos' (Hammersley & Atkinson 1995). I recorded field notes immediately after each interview and these were included on each transcript. These notes enabled me to capture the meaning and context of the interviews and to reflect on my participation in the interview. Throughout the process of planning the study, interviewing and reading the transcripts and related literature and data analysis, I experienced, in an ongoing fashion, new insights and ideas that I wrote in the form of analytic memos. The compilation of such notes represents the sort of 'internal dialogue' or 'thinking aloud' (Hammersley & Atkinson 1995) that is a core feature of phenomenology.

Sample interview questions

☐ Imagine the years since your injury as a journey. Could you describe what was most significant for you (influenced you the most) during that journey?

☐ Is there a particular feeling you have when you think of the experience of learning to live with a disability?

☐ Have your feelings about the experience of the past few years changed over time?

☐ Has there ever been a time when your way of thinking about the experience of spinal cord injury has seemed different from those around you?

☐ Is there anyone you know who thinks about spinal cord injury and its consequences differently from you (for example other injured persons, health professionals, friends, strangers)?

☐ How do they think about it?

☐ How is that different from the way you think about it?

☐ What would you describe about your experience to someone newly injured or someone who knows nothing about spinal cord injury?

As a physical therapist, I considered myself experienced in conducting clinical interviews or taking histories as part of clinical practice. There is a danger, however, that the substantial differences between clinical and qualitative interviewing may not be recognised (Britten 2000). The aim of clinically oriented interviews is to acquire the information about a specific health problem needed to assess the problem accurately and develop treatment goals with the client. As a result, they are primarily oriented to the health care professional's agenda. In contrast, qualitative interviews are flexible and adaptable and often characterised as a 'purposeful conversation'. My thesis adviser did recognise the danger and insisted that I conduct two pilot interviews before embarking on the main data collection.

Christine Carpenter

The pilot interviews proved invaluable as they gave me the opportunity to assess the effectiveness of the interview questions and my interviewing technique, to manage the details of participant comfort, taping and transcribing, to establish rapport with the participant, and to practise the authentic listening so essential to phenomenological research. The transcripts of these interviews were discussed with my thesis adviser and reviewed by the two participants to refine the interview process further. It became apparent in the pilot interviews that the participants had redefined the direction of the interview, assuming that my primary interest as a physical therapist (which was known by all the participants) was their physical recovery from spinal cord injury in the formal rehabilitation setting. In fact, it was not my intention to explore their experiences in the rehabilitation system but to explore, from an adult learning perspective, individual conceptions of living with a spinal cord injury over time and the meaning these individuals gave to the experience. As a result of insights gained from the pilot interviews, I refocused the questions on the meanings associated with a significant life event and was careful to omit the words 'rehabilitation', 'rehabilitation process', and 'treatment'. I also emphasised my connections, for the purpose of this study, with adult education rather than physical therapy.

THE ROLE OF THE RESEARCHER IN PHENOMENOLOGICAL RESEARCH

The interaction between participant and researcher is a key to the data collection process in phenomenology and is influenced by how the participant perceives the researcher (Carpenter & Suto 2008). In this study, my background in spinal cord rehabilitation meant that I was perceived as an 'expert', or as someone who understood some of the realities of living with a spinal cord injury, or as someone who could be trusted or provide advice. Establishing a genuine rapport in phenomenological interviews is crucial and involves the concept of reciprocity. Reciprocity 'requires, on the part of the researcher, a genuine presence, self-disclosure, respect, and commitment to involving the participants in all phases of the research' (Carpenter & Suto 2008, p. 126; see also Liamputtong 2007).

Positionality

The concept of '**positionality**' is related to the 'position' from which one 'chooses' to speak. The research question or aim is developed from this position and to some extent lends credibility and authority to the study. Addressing my positionality meant giving a full explanation of the experience and knowledge I had accrued, as a physical therapist, about the research topic during a lengthy career in spinal cord injury rehabilitation. I also examined the theoretical lenses, in particular feminism and the client-centred model of practice, that I had developed through clinical practice, professional conferences and an extensive reading of the literature.

Positionality is related to the 'position' from which one 'chooses' to speak. The research aim is developed from this position and lends credibility and authority to the study.

Reflexivity

Reflexivity is an essential strategy that makes explicit the deep-seated views and judgments that affect the research process, including a full assessment of the influence of the researcher's background, assumptions, perceptions, values, beliefs and interests (Carpenter & Suto 2008). To address reflexivity, I systematically and critically reflected on and analysed all the decisions I made during the research process and constructed a reflective account in the form of analytic memos that my thesis adviser regularly discussed with me.

Reflexivity: A strategy that makes explicit the researcher's deep-seated views and judgments that influence and affect the research process.

In reflecting throughout the research process, my own assumptions became explicit: for example, about living with a spinal cord injury, the nature and impact of disability on a person's life, and the role of rehabilitation in assisting a person to get 'back on track' after an injury. I was able to articulate how these had influenced the research design and particularly the data analysis process. I also experienced a major shift in my understanding of the psychosocial and political issues associated with living with disability that has had a long-term effect on my rehabilitation practice and teaching.

The concept of bracketing

The strategies of positionality and reflexivity are common to all qualitative research, whereas the concept of bracketing is characteristic of descriptive phenomenology. In the original study, I did not address the issue of bracketing and I now take the opportunity to revisit this concept in the context of this study. 'Bracketing, as in a mathematical equation, suspends certain components by placing them outside the brackets, which then facilitates a focusing in on the phenomenon within the brackets' (Gearing 2004, p. 1430). Bracketing is not an attempt to be objective but rather to encourage researchers to set aside as much as possible their internal beliefs, experiences, understandings, biases, judgments and assumptions in order that they might authentically listen to the participants' perspectives and describe the essence of the phenomenon being studied.

More recently, I have been involved in 'bracketing interviews'. This is a strategy by which researchers are assisted to explore the impact of their personal and professional experiences during data collection and analysis. I have found it to be particularly useful when engaging in 'sensitive' research where there are concerns about the personal, ethical and professional consequences for the participants, for example in exploring the impact of women's experiences of physical and sexual abuse on their relationships with health care professionals (Schachter et al. 1999).

Using the strategy of bracketing interviews

Bracketing interviews enable the development of a research-focused relationship between the researcher and an experienced 'bracketer' (Rolls & Relf 2006). The bracketer is a person who has an understanding of the advisory nature of the relationship and of the demands of qualitative research. Before conducting bracketing interviews it is important to negotiate the boundaries of the proposed interviews, for example differentiating the purpose of the interviews from other types of support that might be used by the researcher such as mentor or peers, the timing of the meetings, and questions relating to maintaining confidentiality. In my experience, meetings between the researcher and bracketer took place as needed by the researcher and lasted for 45–60 minutes. Each bracketing interview was treated as a form of data collection, with each session being taped and transcribed. In this way, the interviews were 'embedded in the research process' (Rolls & Relf 2006, p. 294). In being involved with bracketing interviews, both as researcher and bracketer, I have been guided by the four-session process described by Rolls and Relf (see 'The sessions of bracketing interviews').

The sessions of bracketing interviews

Session 1: Before data collection phase

The purpose of this session was to establish an agreement about how to proceed and to explore the researcher's 'lack of neutrality' (Ahern 1999, p. 409). The interview focused on accessing and making explicit the researcher's experiences, assumptions and value systems, and the emotions and feelings held about the research topic. The idea is for the researcher to reflect on experiences that might influence her ability to listen authentically to the participants and that might trigger judgmental or emotional responses to what she is hearing.

Session 2: During the research process

This session focused on the experience of being the researcher and the interaction with the participants. Issues explored in this interview related to actual or potential conflicts between the roles of physical therapist or academic and researcher, that is, managing 'boundary crossing' (Rolls & Relf 2006, p. 298). The researcher was encouraged to explore issues of reciprocity; that is, responding appropriately to questions posed by the participants, revealing personal information, and responding professionally and ethically during the study interviews.

Session 3: During the research process

In this session, we explored issues arising from the data analysis process related to representation; that is, accurately portraying the participants' experiences and perceptions (Carpenter & Suto 2008) in the emerging themes and in writing up the research.

Session 4: At the end of the research

Rolls and Relf (2006, p. 301) suggest that this session is useful 'to consider any outstanding issues arising from the research and to review the bracketing process and reflect on its contribution to the study'.

THE DATA ANALYSIS PROCESS

The analytic approach in phenomenology orients the researcher to an 'exhaustive, reflective and detailed analysis of each individual experience' (Carpenter & Suto 2008, p. 128; see also CHAPTERS 5, 6, 7, 22, 23). As Thorne (2000, p. 69) explains:

> Rather than explain the stages and transitions within grieving that are common to people in various circumstances…[phenomenological analysis] might attempt to uncover and describe the essential nature of grieving and represent it in such a manner that a person who had not grieved might begin to appreciate the phenomenon.

My analytic process began as I transcribed the interviews. I was guided by a series of interpretive stages that I have since recognised as having their foundation in the framework developed by the phenomenologist Colaizzi (1978). These stages are described in Table 8.1.

Table 8.1: Application of Colaizzi's phenomenological framework in data analysis

Stages of framework	Analytical process
Stage 1: Acquiring a sense of each transcript	I read each interview transcript several times to get a sense of the data as a whole.
Stage 2: Extracting significant statements	Data chunks or fragments (units of meaning) were highlighted in the transcripts that identified or informed my understanding of each participant's experience of spinal cord injury. I labelled each statement with the participant's pseudonym, page and line number, and then cut them from the transcript copy and assigned them initially to file folders and later on flip chart paper mounted on the walls.
Stage 3: Formulation of meanings	I wrote my interpretation or restatement of the meaning of the significant statements distilled from the transcripts. During this stage I found it essential to consistently reflect on my own assumptions, reactions to the participants' narratives, and the connections I was making with the related literature, and record these insights as analytic memos.
Stage 4: Organising formulated meanings into clusters of themes	Statements and associated formulated meanings that clearly represented a common focus were grouped together as a theme cluster (or what I called a category). This stage of analysis resulted in approximately 16 theme clusters. I presented the analysis at this stage to a colleague, who was knowledgeable in both qualitative research and spinal cord injury, to examine the emerging relationships between categories (a process called peer review) to ensure that the interpretive process was clear and accurately described. The 16 categories were then further consolidated to form 3 main themes—rediscovering self, redefining disability, and establishing a new identity—that were common to all the participants' descriptions of their experience of spinal cord injury.

Table 8.1: (*cont.*)

Stages of framework	Analytical process
Stage 5: Exhaustively describing the investigated phenomenon	The 3 main themes were then described in detail and illustrated by verbatim participant quotes (or data). This initial account was again discussed with my colleague (peer review). Differences in interpretive decisions occurred and these caused me to reflect and re-examine my analytic process.
Stage 6: Describing the fundamental structure of the phenomenon	Colaizzi (1978) advocates that the theme descriptions should be further reduced to a statement of their fundamental or essential structure. It had become apparent to me that the 3 themes were informed by transformative learning theory and I developed an overall explanation of the themes framed by this theory.
Stage 7: Returning to the participants	Colaizzi suggests that the final validation of the data analysis should involve returning to the participants for another interview to ensure that they can recognise their experience in the themes and final statement (a process called member checking). This was not feasible in this study.

STRATEGIES OF RIGOUR

It is generally accepted that without rigour, research, whatever the methodological approach, fails to contribute to the professional knowledge base or to evidence-based practice. A number of strategies have been identified that can be used to enhance the rigour of qualitative studies (see CHAPTER 1). These strategies do not themselves *ensure* the trustworthiness of the research. They need to be selectively employed, adapted and combined to achieve the purposes of specific studies, and their use is justified by linking strategy decisions with the research question, chosen methodology and study design (Carpenter & Suto 2008; Liamputtong 2009). Several strategies of rigour, congruent with the core concepts and principles of phenomenology, were incorporated into the study design (see Table 8.2).

CONTRIBUTION TO EVIDENCE-BASED PRACTICE

Evidence-based practice:
A process that requires the practitioner to find empirical evidence about the effectiveness or efficacy of different treatment options and then determine the relevance of the evidence to a particular client's situation.

Most rehabilitation professionals recognise that the complex issues inherent in rehabilitation practice have not been addressed in the most influential definitions of **evidence-based practice**, such as 'the conscientious, explicit, and judicious use of current best evidence in making decisions about the care of individual patients' (Sackett et al. 1996, p. 30). These definitions are impairment or disease-oriented, focus on a practitioner-centred approach, and promote the idea of a hierarchy of evidence that privileges randomised controlled trials (RCTs) as a sort of 'gold standard'

Table 8.2: Selected strategies of rigour

Stage of research process	Strategy	Justification
Study design	Rationale provided for methodological decision	This contributes to the integrity of research.
Study design	Establishing a detailed audit or decision trail	A detailed account of how the research was conducted; includes tracking the decisions made in recruiting participants, ethical considerations, collecting data and the analytic approach taken in transforming the data to findings.
Data collection	Data saturation	As discussed earlier.
Data analysis process	Member checking	Also called member validation, it 'is a process whereby the researcher seeks clarification and further explanation from the participants…It reflects some core values of phenomenology [and qualitative research in general] related to accurate representation, privileging participants' knowledge and decreasing the power imbalances between researcher and participant' (Carpenter & Suto 2008, p. 153). There is no definitive procedure for member checking and it can occur at virtually any stage of the process.
Data analysis process	Peer review	This person is asked to review the data (transcripts and field notes) or emerging findings at different stages of the analytic process in order to validate or question the analytic linkages being made between the data, categories and emerging themes.
Data analysis process	In-depth rich description	If diligently maintained, field notes and analytic memos (or reflective journal) contribute to the rigorous analysis process.
Presentation of findings	Reflexivity	An essential activity in phenomenology contributing to bracketing.
Presentation of findings	Representation	The researcher has a duty to portray participants' experiences and opinions fully and accurately. Participants should recognise these representations in their own experience.
Presentation of findings	Providing evidence to support interpretations	Participant verbatim quotations are important in revealing how meanings are expressed in the participant's own words rather than the researcher's words, and inform and support the researcher's interpretive decisions.

Christine Carpenter

(Hammell & Carpenter 2004; see CHAPTERS 1, 15, 17, 18). Evidence-based practice can perhaps be better described as an approach to decision-making in which the practitioner uses the best available research evidence, in consultation with the client, to decide which option best suits that client. There is, however, an increasing call in the health care literature to include greater methodological diversity, notably by recognising the importance of the evidence generated by qualitative and mixed methods research (Gibson & Martin 2003; Hammell & Carpenter 2004; Johnson & Waterfield 2004; Grypdonck 2006; Rauscher & Greenfield 2009), developing more effective approaches to establishing the level of qualitative evidence (Kearney 2001; Cesario & Santa-Donato 2002), and synthesising the qualitative evidence that is available (Finfgeld 2003; Walsh & Downe 2005).

In order for qualitative research to make a significant contribution to professional knowledge and evidence-based practice, the findings of rigorously designed studies need to be disseminated by presentation in professional and public forums and publication in peer-reviewed journals (Carpenter & Suto 2008). This contribution can take a number of forms: by providing evidence to support best practice and clinical reasoning, by aiding in program planning or evaluation, and by advancing conceptual development. A number of recent rehabilitation-oriented studies illustrate these forms of contribution to evidence-based practice.

Client-centred practice, defined as a collaborative approach to practice that encourages client autonomy, choice and control and that respects clients' abilities and supports their right to enact choices (Sumsion & Law 2006), is increasingly discussed as an appropriate model for effective rehabilitation practice. But relatively little research has explored the experience and meaning of client-centred practice from the client's perspective. Cott (2007, p. 1411) conducted a qualitative study using focus groups to 'understand the important components of client-centred rehabilitation from the perspective of adult clients with long-term disabilities'. This study was the first in an ongoing program of research conducted in partnership with policy-makers with the purpose of defining and promoting client-centred rehabilitation in Ontario, Canada.

Other studies focus on helping physical therapists understand patient perceptions and beliefs about rehabilitation interventions. Cooper, Smith and Hancock (2009) conducted **semi-structured interviews** with 25 people who had received physiotherapy for chronic low back pain (CLBP). The purpose of their study was to explore the extent to which physiotherapy facilitated patients with CLBP to self-manage following discharge, their perceptions of their need for self-management interventions or support, and their preferences in terms of delivery. Their findings highlighted areas in which effective self-management could be better facilitated. In another study, Cooper, Jackson, Weinman and Horne (2005) recognised that while most patients who have experienced a myocardial infarction (MI) were offered the opportunity to attend a cardiac rehabilitation program, many failed to do so. To address this clinically oriented problem they conducted

Semi-structured interview: An interview where the researchers have prepared some questions beforehand and use them to elicit information, but at the same time allow the participants to elaborate on their responses.

a phenomenological study to elicit patients' beliefs about the role of cardiac rehabilitation following MI. Semi-structured interviews were conducted with 13 patients after discharge from hospital following MI before they were scheduled to attend a cardiac rehabilitation program. The findings showed that patients were uncertain about the relevance and appropriateness of these programs for them, held erroneous beliefs about the purpose and nature of the cardiac rehabilitation program, and lacked accurate knowledge about MI. This type of information helps rehabilitation practitioners to plan and evaluate cardiac rehabilitation programs in collaboration with those patients who would benefit from attending them, and this in turn contributes to the effectiveness of these interventions.

The interdisciplinary team concept is central to the culture and philosophy of rehabilitation (Martone 2001), but research has focused on the roles and potential areas of conflict between team members (e.g. Caplan & Reidy 1996; Dalley & Sim 2001). More recently, qualitative study findings have highlighted the patient role in the rehabilitation team. Suddick and de Souza (2006) undertook an exploratory study to investigate therapists' experiences and perceptions of reasoning behind the team approach in neurological rehabilitation. Five occupational therapists and five physiotherapists from three different teams (community, rehabilitation centre and stroke unit) were interviewed. It became apparent that interdisciplinary teamwork and patient-centred approaches were not consistently adopted and there was no consensus on whether patients were included on the neurological team. Pellatt (2007) conducted semi-structured interviews with five doctors, five physiotherapists, three occupational therapists and 20 patients in a spinal cord injury unit to identify whether there was agreement between health professionals and patients about the role professionals play in rehabilitation. This study is a component of a larger study exploring patient participation in spinal cord injury rehabilitation. This type of information has important implications for rehabilitation practice, particularly given the more client-oriented policies being adopted by governments (see Department of Health 2001, 2005b).

Qualitative research can also contribute to the development of professional theories and conceptual understanding of practice (see CHAPTER 1). From a theoretical standpoint, Romanello and Knight-Abowitz (2000) discussed the integration of an ethics of care approach into physical therapy practice. Proponents of an ethics of care approach to clinical practice focus on the relationships, involving care, responsibility, trust, fidelity and sensitivity, that characterise specific patient situations (Beauchamp & Childress 2001). It is an ethical theory that has primarily been developed in relation to nursing practice. Greenfield (2006) and Greenfield and colleagues (2008) subsequently used a phenomenological approach to explore the meaning of caring in practice from the perspective of experienced and novice physical therapists. The findings of these studies (1) integrate theory with practice; (2) highlight caring as a core professional value that is learnt experientially; and (3) reveal the importance of incorporating effective role-modelling and critical reflection strategies in educational programs. The authors suggest that future studies are needed to explore patients' perceptions of professional caring.

Christine Carpenter

This type of theory-driven research makes an impact on education and practice and is necessary to advance knowledge within the physical therapy profession.

In Sandelowski's (2004, p. 1382) opinion, 'qualitative research is the best thing to be happening to evidence-based practice'. But conducting the research is only the first step. Qualitative researchers must also be accountable for moving research findings into practice and this means translating the knowledge represented by their findings into practice, encouraging understanding and critical appraisal of qualitative research (Letts et al. 2007a,b), and conducting meta-syntheses (the term more commonly used in the qualitative research literature than systematic reviews) of qualitative research.

SUMMARY

In this chapter, I have discussed several issues and these include:

- [ ] the contribution the use of qualitative methodology can make to the study design and to the coherence of the research
- [ ] phenomenology as a methodological approach by briefly reviewing two dominant philosophical traditions—descriptive and interpretive—and the common characteristics of this type of qualitative research
- [ ] an example of a phenomenological study to illustrate how a study can be implemented including participant recruitment, data collection and analysis
- [ ] the concepts of reflexivity and positionality as related to the notion of 'bracketing', which is a feature of the phenomenological approach
- [ ] the contribution qualitative research can make to evidence-based practice using examples related to rehabilitation and physical therapy.

TUTORIAL EXERCISES

1   Think of a situation in your work or student experience that could be explored using a phenomenological research approach and develop a concise statement of purpose for an exploratory study.

2   If you were conducting this study how would you describe your 'position' in the research and how might you, in the role of researcher, influence the data collection and analysis?

3   If you wanted to include 'bracketing interviews' in the design of your study consider who you would ask (and why) and what you would tell them about the role of the 'bracketer'.

4   How would you involve the participants in enhancing the credibility of your study?

FURTHER READING

Arber, A. (2006). Reflexivity: A challenge for the researcher as practitioner? *Journal of Research in Nursing*, 11(2), 147–57.

Braun, V. & Clarke, V. (2006). Using thematic analysis in psychology. *Qualitative Research in Psychology*, 3, 77–101.

Dowling, M. (2007). From Husserl to van Manen: A review of different phenomenological approaches. *International Journal of Nursing Studies*, 44(1), 131–42.

Gibson, B.E. & Martin, D.K. (2003). Qualitative research and evidence-based physiotherapy practice. *Physiotherapy*, 89(6), 350–8.

Lopez, K.A. & Willis, D.G. (2004). Descriptive versus interpretive phenomenology: The contributions to nursing knowledge. *Qualitative Health Research*, 14(5), 726–35.

Moustakas, C. (1994). *Phenomenological research methods*. Thousand Oaks, CA: Sage Publications.

Smith, J.A., Larkin, M. & Flowers, P. (2009). *Interpretative phenomenological analysis: Theory, method and research*. London: Sage Publications.

Todres, l. (2005). Clarifying the life-world: Descriptive phenomenology. In I. Holloway (ed.), *Qualitative research in health care*. Oxford: Blackwell, 104–24.

WEBSITES

No websites have been consulted for this chapter, but the reader might like to look up the sites of the following societies and journals.

http://britishphenomenology.com/default.aspx

This is the home page of the British Society for Phenomenology. The webpage includes the society's meetings, Journal of British Society for Phenomenology, *and links to other sites for phenomenology and continental philosophy.*

www.spep.org/

The Society for Phenomenology and Existential Philosophy is a professional organisation devoted to supporting philosophy inspired by Continental European traditions.

www.csudh.edu/phenom_studies/

The Centre for Philosophy and Phenomenological Studies aims to promote through electronic media philosophical enquiries and exchanges of philosophical findings as well as pedagogical pursuits by interaction with both undergraduate and graduate students in the field of phenomenological research in the widest possible sense.

Christine Carpenter

www.phenomenologycenter.org/

This is the homepage of the Center for Advanced Research in Phenomenology. The website is coordinated by Drs Lester Embree and William F. Dietrich, Department of Philosophy at Florida Atlantic University. This extensive site offers many valuable sources about phenomenological research.

www.srs-mcmaster.ca/Default.aspx?tabid=630

The Occupational Evidence-based Research Group at McMaster University has a number of very useful resources including critical reviews of quantitative and qualitative research articles. Accessed 17 April 2009.

9

Using Clinical Data-mining as Practice-based Evidence

Martin Ryan and David Nilsson

CHAPTER OBJECTIVES

In this chapter you will learn:

☐ how data-mining is used as a research technique

☐ about its advantages and drawbacks in relation to other research methods

☐ how a health-based case study illustrates the application of data-mining

KEY TERMS

Clinical data-mining

Data-mining

Practice-based research

Research-based practice

Secondary data analysis

Unobtrusive method

INTRODUCTION

Academics are always searching for ways to encourage health and welfare practitioners to engage in research in order to research their own practice and ultimately to build practice knowledge and improve practice. Social work is no exception in this regard. Social workers are often immersed in their heavy client workloads and have little time to think about research, let alone carry it out. Therefore any research method that has the advantages of practitioners generating their own research questions for a research project, using already collected data, doing the bulk of the research themselves and also being useful for practice has considerable benefits. The research method that is the subject of this chapter, **clinical data-mining** or CDM, has all of these advantages.

Clinical data-mining provides practice-based evidence that underscores the importance of experiential knowledge in clinical decision-making and its contribution to establishing broad-based best practice models.

DATA-MINING: DEFINITION

Data-mining is the process of extracting and analysing data to uncover hidden patterns and useful information. It is used commonly in retail, marketing and fraud detection. Clinical data-mining has been defined by Epstein and Auslander (2001, p. 1) as the 'location, retrieval, codification, computerisation, analysis and interpretation of available clinical information for studying client characteristics, social work interventions and client outcomes'. As clear and concise as this definition is, it does not mention a key element of CDM, that it is a form of research most often done by practitioners themselves, rather than external researchers. It also mentions possible foci for such research but neglects to note the significant point that for this method practitioners can generate their own research questions or hypotheses that are designed to address practice issues and are aimed at informing their practice and that of other practitioners. So more precisely, a definition of CDM should be the use of available client and agency information in social work to answer research questions about practice, particularly as related to intervention and its outcomes.

Data-mining: The process of extracting and analysing data to uncover hidden patterns and useful information.

Practice-based research is inductive (concepts derived from practice wisdom) and relies on instruments tailored to the needs of social practice.

Data-mining is essentially a form of **practice-based research** using **secondary data analysis** (analysis of data collected for purposes other than for a specific piece of research) (Kellehear 1993; Smith 2008). Within the qualitative approach, data-mining sits neatly within the **unobtrusive methods** (Kellehear 1993; Liamputtong 2009). In contrast to evidence-based practice (see CHAPTERS 16, 17), CDM is striving to provide practice-based evidence, that is, evidence or information derived from practice. Such evidence 'highlights the importance of experiential knowledge in clinical decision-making and its contribution to establishing broad-based best practice models' (Merighi et al. 2005, p. 710).

Secondary data analysis: An analysis of data collected for purposes other than for a specific piece of research.

An **unobtrusive method** does not require direct contact with informants but uses data that has been published or is available in libraries, the press, or other media.

CONTEXT FOR ITS USE

Social workers in all settings inevitably, and often perhaps to their annoyance, collect and record large amounts of information in a range of forms on client characteristics and their presenting and ongoing problems, as well as their own interventions, and the responses and outcomes for clients as a result of these interventions. This data is primarily used for clinical, administrative, supervisory purposes and for accountability to funding bodies. Such information, while often voluminous, is easily accessible and non-intrusive, yet its utility to social work research is often overlooked or even rejected.

It is often rejected for research purposes because using such data would not be seen as 'proper research'. But this information can be used to answer valuable questions for social workers such as: What are the characteristics of the clients we are seeing? What is happening when they are being seen? What are we actually doing for them? What is it that seems to work in producing better outcomes for these clients? What produces more negative outcomes?

There are numerous examples of CDM studies involving a range of areas, for example: termination in an adolescent mental health service (Mirabito 2001); liver transplant mortality (Epstein et al. 1997); characteristics of end-stage renal dialysis patients (Dobrof et al. 2001); assessing a hospital support program for family caregivers (Dobrof et al. 2006); and social work practice with renal dialysis patients (Auslander et al. 2001). More broadly, social work documentation can be a rich source of research material and has been used as a means of research in social work practice in studies such as those by Floersch (2000, 2004) and Cumming and colleagues (2007).

COMPARISON WITH OTHER RESEARCH METHODS

The evidence-based practice (EBP) movement has been a major influence on the conduct of both research and practice in health for the last 20 years (Nathan et al. 1999; Sackett et al. 2000; Nathan & Gorman 2002). Social work has been slower to come on board in adopting EBP (Murphy & McDonald 2004; Ryan & Sheehan in press), often because of a series of legitimate concerns about this approach to research (Gibbs & Gambrill 2002; Plath 2006). EBP emphasises the importance of practice being based on, and supported by, sound empirical research, with the preferred 'gold standard' to such research being the conduct of randomised controlled trials (RCTs) (see CHAPTERS 1, 15, 16, 17).

Epstein (2001, p. 17) characterises **research-based practice** (RBP), like EBP, as having the following emphases:

☐ It is deductive (derived from theory).
☐ It seeks causal knowledge, therefore it gives priority to experimental, randomised control group designs.

> **Research-based practice** is deductive (concepts derived from theory), and relies on standardised, quantitative research instruments.

☐ It is prospective.

☐ It relies on standardised, quantitative research instruments.

☐ While it is collaborative, research requirements tend in the main to outweigh practice considerations.

On the other hand, practice-based research (PBR), which includes clinical data-mining, according to Epstein (2001, p. 18), has the following essential attributes:

☐ It is inductive (concepts derived from practice wisdom).

☐ It makes use of non-experimental or quasi-experimental designs.

☐ It seeks descriptive or correlational knowledge.

☐ It may be either retrospective or prospective.

☐ It may be quantitative or qualitative, but tends to rely on instruments tailored to the needs of social practice rather than external standardised research instruments.

☐ It is collaborative in nature and practice requirements tend to outweigh research considerations.

Epstein (2001, p. 18) goes on to emphasise that the fundamental distinction is between 'research *on* practice (RBP)' and, for PBR, 'research *in* practice'. For the former, the starting point is 'the research canon', and for PBR it is 'practice wisdom', that is, what practitioners know based on reflection on their experience of practice.

The crucial distinction is not between RBP being quantitative and PBR being qualitative. While RBP, which includes CDM, privileges a quantitative approach, CDM has a preference for seeking quantitative data, but is amenable to the combination of quantitative and qualitative data, and also to qualitative data on its own (see CHAPTER 1). CDM incorporates the ideas of Argyris and Schon (1974) on the reflective practitioner (see also Schon 1983), and their ideas are not incompatible with those of some of their successors (see Fook 1996; Fook & Gardner 2007) on reflective research and critical reflection.

CLINICAL DATA-MINING: ITS ADVANTAGES AND DRAWBACKS

Clinical data-mining has a number of key advantages for social work practitioners wanting to research their own clinical practice. As Epstein and associates (1997, p. 225) point out:

> In comparison with studies based on original data generation, available information studies are likely to raise fewer ethical problems, are faster and less costly to complete, are less disruptive to existing staff and patient care routines, and make use of compliance on outcome indicators that are likely to be more agency and practice relevant.

To this list could be added the advantage that the analysis of available information is non-intrusive, which is ensured as long as the identity and identifying information of the client is carefully protected. This means that no ethical problems are presented and the research can be considered to be non-reactive (Kellehear 1993; Liamputtong 2009; see also CHAPTER 2).

On the other hand, CDM does have its problems. Finding information that will actually answer your research questions may be the first hurdle that will need to be overcome. Even if the information is there, it may not provide information on your chosen key variables because data on them simply has not been collected, which may well serve to highlight problems and issues with an agency's current collection of information. At the least, CDM can serve to highlight such omissions.

Of even more concern from a research purist's perspective is the reliability and validity of available information (see CHAPTER 1). Numerous questions can be raised about the data in relation to these two matters: Is what is written here actually what practitioners have done? Have things been done that have not been recorded? Do practitioners consistently do things or assess things in the same way? If more than one practitioner has entered data, have their assessment and recording practices been consistent? These are obviously legitimate concerns that need to be at least acknowledged as limitations in reporting the results of research using CDM.

Other drawbacks are that CDM can be labour-intensive and dirty (quite literally, as David Nilsson will inform you later in this chapter). Locating old client information, retrieving it and then going through it carefully seeking your particular foci of interest can take many hours of painstaking and laborious work. The work involved may mean that strategic decisions have to be taken in relation to sampling, that is, which pieces offer the most complete and relevant source of data.

Despite the drawbacks, we believe that CDM is a legitimate way of conducting research that is relevant and useful to social workers. As Epstein (2001, p. 23) writes, 'problems of data quality…can be dealt with like any other applied research problem, i.e. with strategic compromise'.

CLINICAL DATA-MINING: THE PROCESS

The following steps are involved in the process of actually carrying out CDM (based on Epstein 2001, p. 28):

1 Locate a research site to inspect and take small samples of all available information sources to ascertain what kinds of actual information are generally available to you.

2 Assess the degree of accessibility, credibility, connectivity and (if handwritten) the actual legibility of this available information.

3 Determine the unit of analysis you are going to examine, the time-frame, and the likely staging of this information-gathering.

4 Carry out a literature review to help conceptualise appropriate research questions and/or hypotheses, as well as identify concepts, theories/models and methods of data analysis in the current literature.

Martin Ryan and David Nilsson

5 'Conduct a detailed inventory of potential variables, distinguishing between predictors (e.g. demographics, health and psychosocial risk factors, resiliency factors), intervening variables (e.g. medical and psychosocial interventions) and dependent variables (e.g. mortality, morbidity, quality of life, client/patient satisfaction, etc.).'

6 Develop initial data extraction forms with a listing of all possible variables and categories in them.

7 Conduct studies of samples of key variables to ascertain their validity, reliability, accuracy and completeness until satisfactory levels are reached or some variables are excluded.

8 Construct finalised forms for data retrieval and then extract the data from the records.

9 Create your own database (whether written or computerised, e.g. on Excel spreadsheet or SPSS [Statistical Package for the Social Sciences] data file) and enter the data. Run frequencies on variables to ascertain which are suitable for the descriptive, bivariate or multivariate analysis (see Chapter 24).

10 Conceptualise, plan and conduct further studies based on the available data.

In relation to this research process, Epstein (2001, p. 29) identifies six important methodological lessons he has learnt in doing his CDM work:

1 Have workers who are most familiar with the information/cases carry out data extraction in order to maximise validity and reliability.

2 Check for an agreement on key variables through multiple data sources (triangulation).

3 Identify strength, resilience and recovery factors as well as deficits and risk factors within the available information.

4 Describe in detail what is involved in the 'black box' of social work intervention.

5 Choose realistic intervention outcomes for your data.

6 Involve social workers at each stage and task (excepting tedious drudge work like data entry) of the CDM research process. This enhances involvement and utilisation of collected information and findings and their later application.

CLINICAL DATA-MINING: A CASE STUDY

This case study is based on a small piece of research that was undertaken at the Royal Children's Hospital in Melbourne within the Diabetes Unit where the second author, David, previously worked as a social worker. The social work service to this unit focused mainly on two key areas: (1) assisting newly diagnosed children and their families with adjusting to this significant event, and (2) assisting children and their families who were experiencing difficulties since diagnosis (either at the outpatient clinics or through an unplanned readmission to hospital).

The Diabetes Unit included a strong multidisciplinary focus with twice-weekly psychosocial ward rounds, one of which focused on children in the adolescent ward. One morning as we were waiting to commence the adolescent ward meeting the medical consultant let out a loud sigh upon reviewing the inpatient list. He had recognised the names of two teenagers whom he noted seemed to keep coming back with disconcerting regularity despite the best efforts of medical staff and the diabetes clinical educator. We had dubbed such patients as 'frequent fliers'.

The consultant began musing about whether there was something we were missing in relation to these clients. He noted that there were a number of other adolescents like these ones who seemed to be 'frequent fliers'. Was there some social or psychological aspect that was driving the frequent readmissions? He then turned and asked David: 'As a social worker what do you think? Is there something else we should be doing?' David had to confess that he really was not sure, but maybe he could look into it and get back to him. And so began an exploratory research process.

The first step David took was to review the medical records of the two teenagers on the ward. In doing so, however, he realised that he was unsure what he was looking for. He decided that it might be better to look at the published literature to get some clues. In undertaking a literature review David was surprised at how little literature there seemed to be on this area, especially in regard to the local Australian context. The international literature did, however, identify a range of factors that possibly contribute to poor diabetes control that can be broadly divided into individual factors and family-related factors. Family-related factors included non-traditional family structures, family cohesion, family stress, family conflict (including teen–parent disputes and sibling rivalry), family resources, parenting skills, and parental self-esteem. Individual (intra-psychic) factors that were identified as possible contributors included learning difficulties, psychiatric status, personality characteristics, body image, health locus of control, knowledge of juvenile diabetes, coping styles, stress, and the effects of recent personal life events.

The literature identified a condition termed 'brittle diabetes' (Tattersall 1985), which referred to patients with extremely unstable diabetes control that can lead to longer-term medical complications and that encompasses about 1 per cent of juvenile cases (Moran et al. 1991). While many studies were aimed at understanding the relationship between psychosocial factors and diabetes control, the true nature of these relationships remained unclear. A number of studies also identified potential relationships between intra-psychic and social and/or environmental factors and diabetes control (see Simonds 1977; Kovacs et al. 1985).

In order to answer the medical consultant's broad question, David needed to come up with a plan to systematically review the available evidence at the hospital—a research project was conceived. The research questions emerged directly from the medical consultant's enquiry. Who are these 'frequent fliers' and how many of them are there in the clinic population? Do they have psychosocial factors in common that may affect their diabetes management and if so what are they? Could we provide some useful psychosocial interventions to overcome these factors and could we use these factors to screen for earlier identification of potential problems and provide preventive interventions?

While a number of possible factors had been identified through the literature review process, David also wondered if there might be factors unique to this hospital clinic or to

Australian children with diabetes. He felt it was important to be open to other possibilities so decided to incorporate a grounded theory approach in which the researcher uses inductive rather than deductive reasoning (Strauss & Corbin 1998; see also CHAPTER 7). David aimed to be open to new and unique possibilities by attempting to approach the data without any preconceived ideas. This was quite difficult after having already consulted the available literature.

In thinking about how he might answer the research questions, David had to consider how he would gather relevant data. Existing hospital records provided an obvious source of readily available data. These included the patients' medical records, social work files, and the case records from a separate in-house mental health service. Clinical data-mining offered a logical way of exploring existing information without having to undertake time-consuming and intrusive interviewing or surveying. This was also a good fit with the exploratory intention of the research. It seemed important to identify more clearly which particular factors might be impacting on this group of patients so that future research could more appropriately focus on the most pertinent issues.

The next step was to identify how many and which patients were experiencing multiple readmissions to hospital. Fortunately, hospitals have excellent recording systems and David requested a report from the Hospital Records Department on average readmission rates for the diabetes clinic over the preceding 3-year period. He discovered that the average readmission rate was 0.85 (i.e. less than one readmission per patient over the 3 years). In order to select an appropriate sample, he needed to identify a cut-off point that represented an unusually high number of readmissions. After consulting with other diabetes team members, he and the team decided that four or more readmissions within the 3-year period would represent a substantially higher than expected readmission rate (i.e. on average more than 1 per year per patient).

A review of the diabetes clinic database using this criterion revealed that out of the almost 750 diabetes clinic patients, only 18 (2.4%) had four or more hospital readmissions over this period. These 18 patients represented 8.7 per cent of the total number of patients requiring a readmission, but the total combined number of bed-days (610) used by these patients represented a disproportionate 21 per cent of total bed-days for all readmitted diabetes patients.

Reviewing the demographics of this small group of patients revealed that all but one was a teenager. Ages at the time of data collection ranged from 10 years 8 months to 19 years 8 months. There were 16 females (66.6%) and six males (33.3%). The females were on average older (median age 18 years 9 months) than males (median age 13 years 10 months).

With the sample group identified, the next step was to review all available related hospital documents. The medical records were stored in the basement of the hospital and over a couple of weeks David reviewed files each evening. This was a slow and methodical process as many of these patients had extensive medical records comprising several volumes. Each section was read to see what psychosocial issues or themes might be present that could impact on the patient's condition.

At this time, David developed a mysterious rash on his forearms which he was certain must be some exotic infection, but a doctor quickly identified this as being bites from paper mites in the dusty old files. It turns out that data-mining can actually be dirty work that uncovers a range of unexpected findings. The file reviews revealed that psychosocial difficulties were indeed prevalent within the sample and 17 patients (94.4%) were previously known to the hospital mental health program and 16 (88.8%) had social work files.

When reading the files, David took notes of all the psychosocial issues identified and then constructed a list of issues in common. Where issues were similar they were collapsed into themes. This thematic analysis (see CHAPTER 22) resulted in 13 key themes being identified for this group of patients:

1   Patient identified as having learning difficulties

2   Patient identified as having a psychiatric condition

3   Patient identified as having body image issues

4   Non-traditional family structure (e.g. single parent and/or divorce/blended family)

5   Marital conflict

6   Parental psychological problems (e.g. anxiety and/or depression)

7   Financial difficulties

8   Family communication difficulties

9   Parent–child relationship problems of overinvolvement (e.g. enmeshment, overindulgent, or overcontrolling practices)

10 Parent–child relationship problems of underinvolvement (e.g. lack of interest, neglect, rejection)

11 Sibling relationship difficulties

12 Multiple other losses experienced by patient

13 General family stress reported.

With the key psychosocial factors identified, David then created a matrix table to map the relative frequency of each factor against the sample of 18 patients. Analysis of these results revealed a range of interesting findings and confirmed the 'practice wisdom' that these cases involving multiple readmissions were indeed complex and multi-factorial in nature.

These patients had on average 5.2 different identifiable psychosocial factors associated with their readmissions. Some noticeable differences emerged when the results for females were analysed separately from those of males. Issues of greater relative prevalence for females included parent–child relationships of overinvolvement, general family stress, parental psychological problems, and sibling relationship difficulties. For males, these were identified: parent–child relationships of underinvolvement, learning difficulties, marital conflict, psychiatric disorder, non-traditional family structure, family financial difficulties, and family communication difficulties.

While these results were not statistically significant because of the small sample size and it was not possible to infer causality within the data, they did provide some valuable insights into this client group and identify some useful factors for targeted social work intervention and further investigation.

One such factor is that of learning disorders. While the number of patients with identified learning disorders (n = 7) did not reach statistical significance, the proportion in this sample (38.8%) appears greater that that expected in the general population and was indeed actually higher than results found in another more general psychological study (Northam et al. 1995) on the same clinic population. This would seem to suggest that patients with learning difficulties may have an increased risk of developing diabetes control problems, leading to more frequent readmissions to hospital. Schade and colleagues (1985) have noted that learning deficits and communication disorders are difficult to detect and therefore may go undiagnosed for long periods. It is possible that undetected, these deficits may compound the effects of other psychosocial factors and negatively impact on diabetes control. Targeted screening for learning difficulties of patients who have more than one unexpected readmission to hospital may allow early remedial interventions.

Another psychosocial factor that could warrant closer evaluation is that of parental psycho-logical problems, which were identified in 61.1 per cent of the sample. Again, this was substan-tially higher than that found in Northam and colleagues' (1996) study in which parental mental health problems ranged only between 22 and 24 per cent. As this was the second most frequently occurring factor, it might be useful to undertake remedial interventions or provide appropriate referrals in relation to parental mental health issues. Support programs and/or education sessions might appropriately address issues such as managing feelings of anxiety and depression.

Other frequently occurring factors also appeared to relate to family functioning. These were non-traditional family structure, general family stress, marital conflict, and parenting problems of overinvolvement. Parent-focused interventions might again provide an important avenue for addressing the underlying problems associated with frequent patient readmission for poor diabetes control. Given also the large proportion of families with a non-traditional family structure, it might be appropriate to establish specialist mutual support groups focusing on the particular challenges for sole parents and parents of blended families.

The findings of this study also suggested that educational initiatives for parents may need to focus on gender differences: girls in the study appeared to be more sensitive to general family stress and sibling relationship difficulties, whereas boys appeared to be more sensitive to marital conflict, financial difficulties, non-traditional family structure, family communication problems, learning difficulties and psychiatric disorders. The other key gender difference was that girls were relatively more affected by parenting issues of overinvolvement and boys by parenting issues of underinvolvement.

This information indeed provided a very useful focus for discussions in subsequent parent education groups. The social worker was able to facilitate discussion about some parents' expectations for boys to manage all by themselves and for girls to be looked after and fussed over more.

The psychosocial factors that were identified in this study could be conceptually categorised with three different intervention foci: patient-focused, family relationships-focused, and parent-focused. There are a range of alternative therapeutic possibilities including individual therapy or casework with patients or parents, group work with adolescents or parents, and family-centred therapy. Since the majority of patients had multiple factors that spanned more than one category, it would seem unlikely that any singular intervention approach would 'solve' these problems and these patients would more likely benefit from a multimodal approach to address these complex interrelated issues.

The findings of this study provided at least a partial answer to the questions of the medical consultant (who was actually a little surprised at how comprehensive the investigation had been after his off-hand enquiry). The diabetes team discussed these findings and how we might incorporate them into our practice. One of the changes that the team made was to revise their adolescent group education program in light of some of the issues identified so that they better addressed family-related issues as well as individual ones. The team also incorporated a new parents group that was run in tandem with the adolescent group.

This relatively simple data-mining exercise provided valuable new insights into a difficult client group, not only for David as a social worker, but also for his multidisciplinary colleagues. He subsequently went on to publish this as an article in the journal *Social Work in Health Care* (Nilsson 2001).

The example of David's study clearly suggests that data-mining provides a logical, practical, inexpensive and non-intrusive method of investigating a difficult practice issue and offers new and useful information to improve professional practice.

SUMMARY

In this chapter, we have outlined the nature and process of clinical data-mining for social work practitioners, as well as providing a case study of its use. Clinical data-mining has considerable potential for generating practice research based on currently available clinical information that has relevance and direct utility to social workers. With increasing computerisation of records in health and human service agencies, large and small, there will be greater opportunity for social workers to mine these rich sources in order to generate practice knowledge able to assist in producing better client outcomes.

TUTORIAL EXERCISES

You are a social worker who works as a case manager in a mental health service. You have noticed among your caseload that some clients do considerably better than others. You are keen to learn about what factors predict positive outcomes for clients across the agency, including your own. Your agency collects basic demographic information and records case notes on all clients.

1   How might you go about exploring this information through data-mining to discover why some clients do better than others?

2   What are some of the possible ways of de-identifying identifiable client information in the use of clinical data-mining?

3   How could information from social work case records be triangulated when doing clinical data-mining research?

FURTHER READING

Epstein, I. (2001). Using available clinical information in practice-based research: Mining for silver while dreaming of gold. *Social Work in Health Care*, 33(3/4), 15–32.

Epstein, I. & Blumenfield, S. (eds) (2001). *Clinical data-mining in practice-based research: Social work in hospital settings.* Haworth Social Work Press, an imprint of Haworth Press Inc.

Fook, J. (ed.) (1996). *The reflective researcher: Social workers' experiences with practice research.* Sydney: Allen & Unwin.

Kellehear, A. (1993). *The unobtrusive researcher: A guide to methods.* Sydney: Allen & Unwin.

Nilsson, D. (2001). Psycho-social problems faced by 'frequent flyers' in a paediatric diabetes unit. *Social Work in Health Care*, 33(3/4), 53–69.

Smith, E. (2008). *Using secondary data in educational and social research.* Maidenhead, UK: McGraw-Hill Open University Press.

WEBSITES

No websites specifically related to clinical data-mining for social workers could be located, but the websites below provide information on data-mining more generally, which may be useful for readers.

http://en.wikipedia.org/wiki/Data-mining

Data Mining (Wikipedia).

www.anderson.ucla.edu/faculty/jason.frand/teacher/technologies/palace/datamining.htm

Data Mining: What is Data Mining.

www.maths.anu.edu.au/~johnm/dm/dmpaper.html

Data Mining from a statistical perspective.

http://hi.uwaterloo.ca/hitalko/Futures-2005/Dreyer2.pdf

Clinical Data Mining Challenges.

10

'Clear at a Distance, Jumbled up Close': Observation, Immersion and Reflection in the Process that is Creative Research

Mark Furlong

CHAPTER OBJECTIVES

In this chapter you will learn:

☐ what is the place of observation in health and human service research

☐ about commonalities and differences in the terms 'observation', 'clinical observation' and 'participant observation'

☐ how to give an outline of the key decision points in establishing an observational protocol

☐ what is involved in undertaking immersive observational work

☐ how to build in transparency

KEY TERMS

Clinical observation

Constructivism

Fieldwork

Observation

Observationally based research

Participant observation

Positivism

Practice-based research

Thick description

INTRODUCTION

Over several decades, Sigmund Freud published a series of case studies—Dora, Little Hans, and Anna O (among others). These accounts were drawn from his personal therapeutic practice and remain remarkable in several ways. For example, these reports are a model of dispassionate, yet intuitively deep, observation (Freud 1974). What is also noteworthy is that these accounts have a rank that has consolidated even as the technology now available to researchers in the therapeutic domain is vastly more sophisticated. Despite the advantages this new methodology brings, what Freud was able to construct from his private practice in a one-on-one consulting room has never been disproved.

In a different field, Erving Goffman studied social phenomena as varied as urban subcultures and in-patient psychiatric units. Based on one of his field engagements in *Where the Action Is* (1969), Goffman reported on inner-city 'con-men' and detailed how these men earned a dangerous living exploiting others—the 'suckers' who were the targets of their game. Not only was Goffman able to capture the liveliness of this subculture, but he explicitly identified a set of quasi-secret practices for a general audience. For instance, he clearly described how these con-men employed a well-practised technique—'cooling the mark'—that minimised their exposure to the risk of violence from those they had cheated (Goffman 1969).

There is perhaps no better example of influential, **observationally based research** than the work of Jean Piaget. From his observations of his young children within the family home, Piaget envisaged his theory that the infant's cognitive development proceeded by way of

Observationally based research is exemplified by the work of Jean Piaget, who from observation of his own children developed the theory that the infant's cognitive development proceeded by particular stages.

particular stages. And, lest it appear that this class of contribution is now exhausted, there continue to be examples of projects based on clinical and/or direct observation that press for recognition. Among others, Suzy Orbach (1984, 2009) contributed to, perhaps has even significantly reshaped, a field of enquiry and understanding.

Without recourse to high-profile research grants, and arising from a vigorous dialogue between her clinical observations as a practising psychotherapist and a critical engagement with feminist and sociological scholarship, Orbach has produced a body of important and influential work. Her research first came to public prominence with *Fat is a Feminist Issue* (1984), and more recently (2009) she has published a critically acclaimed update of her earlier work, albeit one that has yet to be tested in the court of longer-term opinion. Arlie Hochschild (1990, 2003) offers another example that I will return to shortly.

These examples are not intended to promote grandiosity in emerging researchers. Rather, the intention is to emphasise the possibility that individuals, or small groups of individuals, can make useful contributions even if one is not a high-profile researcher in a grandly funded research institute (mindful that this is more possible in some fields than others). It is important to be clear: modestly scaled qualitative projects continue to be able to capture macro-, as well as microscopic, detail and can have an impact in many ways.

'OBSERVATION', 'CLINICAL OBSERVATION' AND 'PARTICIPANT OBSERVATION'

In order to offer material with the widest possible relevance, in what follows the general term 'observation' has been preferred to its cousins 'clinical observation' and 'participant observation'. Before addressing the technical aspects of this term, the relationship between these three related terms will be clarified.

'Observation' is a word with a particular history and a set of (more or less) active uses. Some of these uses remain reminders of older, more formal language practices ('Do you observe the rites of Lent?'). Another example, one that is common but somewhat contradictory, is 'I'm not making a judgment; I'm only offering an observation'. These more esoteric uses to one side, the word 'observation' generally denotes the act of watching, an act that is distinct from doing, interfering or ignoring.

Against this background, the word is generally encountered in health and human service practice in this way: doctors and nurses professionally observe the patient's vital signs—blood pressure, heart rate and so forth. Professional and lay persons alike, we are all acculturated to expect that **clinical observation** is a fundamental dimension in the delivery of proper health care practice. Alongside this dominant use, there are two other relatively common uses of the word that should be noted: many disciplines have students undertake an 'observational placement'; also, trainees in some specialities may experience an 'infant observation' (or the like).

Yet there is another class of observation that might also be included: what of home visits, outreach work, community development, indeed the full spectrum of professional actions that take place beyond the consulting room and the laboratory? There is much data that can be identified by, for example, youth workers and nurses in their everyday ward duties. Using a convention familiar to sociologists and anthropologists, researchers in these settings are said to be engaged in **fieldwork**. If the interest is in research, a bridge between these different practice locations is to introduce the idea that these actors are undertaking a particular kind of **participant observation** within their specific fieldwork settings (see also CHAPTER 6). This term is associated with a mode of data-gathering, one that is probably most identified with the research process rather than with professional practice.

In one sense *clinical observation* belongs to the broader field of practice. Yet the term 'practice' is itself ambiguous as even the most expert and esteemed professors and consultants never proceed beyond practice—even the experts never proceed from practice to perfection. Pre-dating the

---

Observation: The process of collecting data by looking rather than listening.

Clinical observation: Data that the professional has identified from direct observation of empirical aspects of the practice field, either from their immediate perceptions or by means of instrumentation.

Fieldwork: A period of data collection commonly employed in the ethnographic method. Fieldwork may take a year or longer. The researcher usually stays in the community being studied throughout the period.

Participant observation: A data collection method used in ethnography and behavioural studies. The researcher is more or less embedded with the group being studied so as to observe activities first hand.

Mark Furlong

notion of the 'scientist-practitioner' (Long & Hollin 1997; Shapiro 2002), this convention persists and witnesses the belief that professional practice is always a form of research.

TRY IT YOURSELF

1   What is your reaction when you read the statement 'clinical experience suggests there are several different categories of families that do not respond to treatment' (Jones 1987, p. 410)?

2   Do you accept this statement because it has been published in a peer-reviewed journal and/or because it sounds scientific, or would you be sceptical because of the rhetorical nature of the statement?

3   What is the effect of describing something as 'clinical'? Does this form of words tend to equate what is the product of the laboratory with what happens in the (mixed-up) world of practice?

Participant observation began as a particular research method but it has qualitatively evolved to such an extent that it is now difficult to define. Rogers and Bouey (2005, p. 232) suggest that it is now best characterised as a 'mindset' or an 'orientation'. Schematically, it is possible to distinguish three styles of participant observation:

☐   the person who has no role other than to observe
☐   the person who is already known by those to be observed
☐   the active participant who has at least one role in addition to that of observer.

It is with respect to this last style that practice research can be located. In one sense, all practice research is a form of participant observation; and in another sense, it is dissimilar. If the dissimilarity is considered first, the fact that the presence of the observer has an effect on what is observed—what is termed 'reactivity'—has traditionally been regarded as an effect that should be minimised. This is obviously quite different from the practice purpose that the practitioner-scientist has: one seeks to be effective in bringing about a change.

So is it possible to locate practice research in such a way as to have reactivity seen as a positive aspect of, rather than as an interference to, the research aspect of the practitioner-scientist mission?

> Participant observation research uses reactivity as a tool in the research process. How those who are being observed react to the researcher and/or to the observer form part of what is learned about them, their social system, and their view of the world… The personal reactions of the researchers to those they observe are also data that inform them about people and situations they study. (Anastas 2005, p. 228)

In this sense, with all the advantages and disciplines that this use of multiple observational streams involves, practice research can be regarded as a legitimate heir to the legacies of both professional practice and scholarly research. For the very reason that the work professionals do is called 'practice', it follows that **practice-based research** has an important place in building knowledge (Reid 1994; Shaw & Gould 2001; Anastas 2005; see also CHAPTER 9). Further, Dattilio (2006, p. 208) argues that case-based material has an important place in the process of educating practitioners and, if the enquiry is well designed, case-based studies can produce findings that 'can serve as the basis for drawing causal inferences in clinical cases'. See Chapter 9 for more detail of this method and example.

> **Practice-based research** is inductive (concepts derived from practice wisdom) and relies on instruments tailored to the needs of social practice rather than external standardised research instruments.

THE TWO FACES OF OBSERVATION: DO YOU 'TAKE' OR 'MAKE' OBSERVATIONS?

Broadly, the use of observation in research has two faces. The first, concerns **positivism** where observation is used as a method of data collection: vital signs are individually recorded, specified behaviours are carefully noted, intervals between instances calculated, and so forth (see CHAPTER 1). In this use, observations tend to be 'taken' within structured research settings—as occurs in regular primary health practice and behaviourally based psychological practice. In this use, the researcher's attention is required to be convergent (rather than divergent and associative) as the task is to reliably *measure* data (see CHAPTER 11).

> **Positivism:** An approach to research that believes social science research methods should be scientific in the same way as the physical sciences.

The second use of observation, and the use that will be emphasised in this chapter, aligns with practices in social science enquiry where the aim is to understand—to derive meaning—rather than to strictly measure. This position is referred to as **constructivism** or *interpretivism* (see CHAPTER 1). This use is identified with anthropology and sociology, and also with practice-based research (like Orbach's and Freud's), where observations are 'made', rather than 'taken'. That is, researchers operating in less controlled environments, often naturalistic field settings, seek a more or less immersive engagement with the data—a dynamic encounter that seeks to be inductive and open-ended rather than convergent in its focus. The aim of the enquiry is to understand: What are the implicit norms and rules that are in play in this classroom? What schemas for decision-making seem to be guiding the participants in this gang? What sense can be made of this particular gesture in this performance?

> **Constructivism:** An epistemology that says that 'reality' is socially constructed. Constructivist researchers believe that there are multiple truths, individually constructed, and that reality is a product of our own making.

Once immersed, as Goytisolo (cited in Bauman 2005, p. 1091) notes, 'intimacy and distance create a privileged position [where] both are necessary'. This uncomfortable position is the condition that offers the possibility of constructing a new, or at least revised, sense of meaning. This reading is not taken, or found. Rather, it is constructed—perhaps, dimly sensed, then more clearly put together before being provisionally held, and then interrogated. This is not to say that the researcher is operating *de novo*: as was the case with Freud or Goffman, the researcher's attention has been primed by their tacit and/or formal hypotheses, their training and professional experience, their acculturation into particular patterns of gendered thought, and so forth. This set is what is used to make sense of their data, a sense that favours particular forms, structures and patterns of connection.

Thick description:
Descriptions that give ample detail and background information so that people's actions can be understood in the context of the experiences and patterns of meaning that influence them.

In the task of making and interpreting observations, one's attention is not only directed to what is 'out there' because it is also important to monitor one's inner experience: What am I being invited to think? How am I feeling—am I confused, angry, bonded or distanced from the other? This ethos aligns with Geertz's idea of **'thick description'** (1973) where the project is not 'an experimental science in search of law but an interpretative one in search of meaning' (cited in Rapport & Overing 2000, p. 351). In this spirit, as Anastas (2005, p. 229) notes:

> Recording the subjective reactions of the observer brings them into awareness and makes them a part of the data to be used in understanding the events studied. Thus, the observer and the observed not only interact with each other; they are both 'inside the frame' of the research study itself.

As well as honouring the inner experience of the researcher, the effort must be made to de-centre one's received ideas, one's cultural training and, in one particular sense, one's very observations themselves (White 2001). Towards this end, reflective observations offer a particular, though not exclusive, line of data—a second level of reflections on what is initially observed. Other streams of data can include the whole mixed-model repertoire: interviews with participants, written archives, photographs—there is frequently an enormous array of inputs available—among which 'observations' constitute only one source (see CHAPTERS 6, 20, 21).

These two observational faces look in two quite different directions. This difference in orientation literally creates distinct, even antagonistic standpoints (Hartsock 1987). For example, behaviourally focused observational approaches require that the design standardise operational definitions for the variable that is to be monitored and carefully control the period of observation and, if at all possible, the observational context itself. In contrast, more exploratory, open-ended projects tend to gather observations over far longer periods in a manner that is more immersive; *in situ*, and when writing one's field notes, it is important to be 'opportunistic' (Jorgensen 1989), to be open to the possibility of the unexpected. This divergence reflects the different purposes of these two approaches to observation. It follows that what is strength for one is a drawback to the other:

> The more focused an observational system is, the less possible it is to notice phenomena that were 'unexpected'...[because having] specific notions of what will form the variable of interest would likely preclude the observer's being sensitive to the unexpected. (Anastas 2005, p. 218)

This second face of observation aligns with 'the distinct turn of the social sciences towards more interpretive, postmodern and criticalist [*sic*] practices and theorizing' (Guba & Lincoln 2005, p. 191). This turn, it should be noted, presents a distinctly different trajectory from the path taken with observations that follow the behavioural tradition.

Without excluding the behavioural, what this chapter emphasises is the use of observation in the former sense; that is, the observational techniques used engage with social meanings. This emphasis is useful if the interest is in phenomena that are difficult to measure—such as subjective states (psycho-social adjustment; caregiver burden), or interactions between people (patterns of sociality; therapeutic engagement)—where there is limited scope for standardised observational recording. Where it is complex, even ambiguous, it is always possible to 'pick the low lying fruit', that is, to record what is easy to see and define, but this leaves the realm of meaning unexplored. Such meanings may relate to data that is derived from, and that pertains to, both clinical settings and naturalistic environments. Using self and other observations can therefore be a useful component in projects that seek to link 'narrative, generalization and case-based research…where we encounter real people and through them, social dilemmas and realities [in order to] construct typical stories' (McDonald 1999, p. 10).

FIVE EXAMPLES OF OBSERVATION

Observations offer certain advantages. For example, it is possible to gain more from observation than could be gleaned from a survey (see CHAPTER 13) or an interview (see CHAPTER 3) because people providing self reports, however genuinely undertaken, are sometimes blind to what can be observed but not noticed by participants. In 'Doing research' below, a number of examples are presented where observation has been an important aspect of a design.

DOING RESEARCH

Example 1: Building case studies

As well as their use in educating professionals, well-chosen case-based material can have the effect of humanising 'cases and clinicians' (Furlong 1998). For example, in her research on clients with complex needs, Jan Keene (2001) used a single case study chosen from a large sample as a powerful exemplar of the findings her study highlighted. This case study described a man who was experiencing homelessness, mental health issues, multiple substance abuse problems, including heroin addiction, and who was subject to a probation order. This man saw workers in homelessness, mental health and community support agencies as well as a general practitioner, police and a probation officer. In this case study, Keene noted this man's frustration and humiliation at having to give an account of his situation to so many different professionals. Taken within the context of the overall study, the use of this case study focused the findings of her report from the abstract into the particular. Second, the case study had a powerful rhetorical effect as it personalised the issues so as to elicit the empathy of the reader. Keene's research has had a far-reaching impact and has been cited as having had a strong effect on policy.

Example 2: Behavioural observation

Against the background of deinstitutionalisation for people with intellectual disabilities, Jim Mansell and Julie Beadle-Brown (Mansell & Beadle-Brown 2004; Beadle-Brown et al. 2007) have used complex behaviourally based observational studies to investigate, among a larger range of questions, how decisions are made in residential care, how staff respond to challenging behaviours and, at a higher order of complexity, how models of collaborative care can be refined and validated. As with all behaviourally based observational studies, a focused effort is made to standardise the observational regime, a requirement that includes the intensive training of observers themselves. The work of Mansell and Beadle-Brown has been influential in conceptualising, developing and reviewing person-centred planning in learning disability services in the UK and beyond.

Example 3: Field observation

Kevin McDonald (1999) set out to examine the experience of unemployed young persons living in an outer-urban environment with low socio-economic status. This enquiry was guided by an explicit ideological–conceptual stance, a stance that made it appropriate to use a mixed-mode design: in-depth interviewing complemented an extended period of observational data-gathering. Case studies were then used in the final report in order to present powerful exemplars from this project to a research (or policy, or general) audience. This case study material documented, personalised and also dramatised the study's findings, and the report of the project, *Struggles for Subjectivity*, derived much of its power from what the researchers had directly observed and reported. Like Goffman's work (1969), these case studies crystallised a defining interplay, a key moment in the dialogue, between the intent of the study and the teeming rough and tumble of a dense data mass. See also CHAPTER 6.

Example 4: Observing the domestic

Over more than 25 years, Arlie Hochschild (1990, 2003) has been investigating the domestic and intimate dimensions of modern life. In these investigations, a key focus has been the changes that are occurring to households with the rise in the out-of-home employment of women. Using direct observations over an extended period, together with interviewing and other data-gathering tactics, Hochschild not only developed a 'first-hand' knowledge of what the participants said of their situations, but was also able to observe closely what went on.

From these investigations, Hochschild has concluded that women are carrying a kind of 'dual labor'—in both the general economy and within the household. Complementing the impact her conclusions had academically, she has had a broader impact, for example she developed the now popular notion of 'emotional labor'. In her work, she has persistently used observational methods to develop complex and critical knowledge of central social questions, particularly how gender roles remain iniquitous. In terms of engaged, empirical social research, Hochshild's work offers a fine model.

Example 5: Open-ended observation in long-term family work

Moving from a sociological to a more narrowly clinical milieu, Amaryll Perlesz, Dianna McLachlan and the current author (see Perlesz et al. 1992; this research persisted after the current author left the team, e.g. Perlesz et al. 2000; Butera-Prinzi & Perlesz 2004) conducted an extended research program guided by two complementary purposes: (1) to investigate the effectiveness of a therapeutic service offered by a multidisciplinary team to persons who had suffered a head injury, and conjointly to these persons' families; and (2) to refine a model of practice that might better guide the therapeutic practice that was being offered, that is, to further develop theories for practice. At particular points within this program, behavioural observations were made: ratings were scored on specific, standardised scales for pre- and post-treatment scales. In addition, several further levels of observational targets were privileged. These included paying attention to what is often referred to as 'family structure'—the alignments, coalitions and shut-outs that are present between family members: what were initially present, if these changed, and so forth.

With the aim of developing theories for practice even further, an unconventional body of data was also accessed: members of the therapeutic team were also encouraged to track their own inner experience. At least in part guided by a postmodern understanding of counter-transference (Smith et al. 1994), rather than try to diminish, ignore or deny our 'irrational responses', team members gave their feelings, thoughts and reactions an honoured and deliberately central place. This observational material was openly discussed and recorded. Moreover, animated by a collaborative practice and research ethic, an attempt was made to develop an account of practice and family adaptation that was inclusive of family members (see Perlesz, Furlong & the 'D' Family 1996).

When we felt overwhelmed, we did not take this as a signal that we were unprofessional or permanently enmeshed. Rather, staying closely attuned to the details that self-observation revealed, we saw that our reactions offered access to a particular, albeit oblique, kind of knowledge. Observing this subjective realm threw a reflective light upon the relationship between personal experiences—the private troubles that overtake family members and clinicians alike—and the research themes that were identified (and later theorised). These themes, to misappropriate C. Wright Mills's (1967) famous phrase, can be rendered as the public issues, the parallelisms, that were present.

Mark Furlong

In summary, given a purposive intellectual context, particular classes of observations will tend to occur. The task is then to identify and document these (irrespective of whether they seem to make sense or not). When identified, these 'data pictures' can be externalised, which gives them a clarity and a status that enables them to be rendered as items that can then be interrogated. Whether they have been sparked in a conventional clinical context, or have been generated within a naturalistic field, observations occur with respect to an 'object'—a specified item or criterion, a category of item or criterion, a class of categories or, perhaps most productively, with respect to a relationship between categories. This relationship may be an expected one—it may tend to reinforce what is already thought—yet it may also concern what is an unexpected variable, category or relationship.

KEY DECISION POINTS IN THE USE OF OBSERVATION

Formally, the process is to ensure that a three-step sequence is taken: first, there is the observational subprocess itself; then a recording of the relevant phenomena takes place; and then this data is coded. Each of these steps has its discipline (and its uncertainties). The rules that guide this process have been generally stated (even as these rules can only be implemented subject to the specific requirements of the particular project in question). Summarising from Jorgensen (1989), Anastas (2005), Grinnel and Unrau (2005) and Rogers and Bouey (2005), it is necessary to carefully consider the following dimensions.

The observational context and its relationships

Mindful that practical issues are likely to compromise the research ideal, decisions must be made about:

- the period of observation (is it continuous?; by interval? and so on)
- the nature of the setting (controlled? contrived? naturalistic?)
- the relationship between the researcher and those observed (is it 'obtrusive' or 'unobtrusive' data collection?; what of issues of ethics and consent?).

Broadly, behaviourally focused research will insist on a strict policing of the observational period(s) and of the setting, whereas projects that are field based will tend to be more open-ended and opportunistic with respect to setting.

It could also be said that projects that align with the latter orientation will struggle more ambiguously with the conventions of informed consent. That is, it is important to pay sensitive attention to being ethical and respectful and to address the issue of reactivity—how the research/researcher impacts on the field that is being observed.

Decisions need to be made as to whether reactivity—the pattern of reciprocal influence that takes place between the research and 'subject' participants—will be minimised, noted and/ or deliberately used as a data source. A consideration of the division of labour that will best suit the purposes, resources and design of the project is also necessary: Will the person who is the observer-recorder be different from the person of the researcher? If it is practice research, how will the roles of the professional and researcher be balanced? How will the recipient of the service know what role 'their' practitioner is taking and how will this uncertainty affect the (multiple) interactions that take place?

The object(s) of observation and their recording

Deciding on the *who*, the *what* and the *how* of the observational process requires a subprocess in itself. For example, will it be possible to record, using audio/video means, the raw observations? Moreover, depending on the nature of the data that is sought, it may or may not be possible (or even desirable) to count instances of a particular variable because counting requires operationally well-defined criteria (mindful that such criteria definitively shape what is then allowed to be recorded). If it is a separate person who is to do the observing and the recording, how will this person be trained? How will the tendency towards 'calibration drift' (Anastas 2005, p. 219) be countered?

More generally, should the design have a positive regard for flexibility, for noting the outlier and the unexpected in the recording process, or would this compromise the standardised observational discipline that is required? Mechanical recording devices are likely to be methodologically reliable—yet what is able to be rigorously measured is not necessarily the data that is of most value. For example, interpersonal variables may only be apparent to human observers. Similarly, subjectively experienced variables can probably only be identified from self reports.

These two general concerns will now be examined with respect to behavioural observation, and then a field-based, more open-ended program.

Behavioural observation

Observations will seem random, even disordered, if there is no specific field of attention to orient and organise. What is required is a stable figure and ground configuration within which a certain class of perception can occur. It is this stability of reference that contextualises an observation and endows the proposition with a quality of sense (or the opposite). In this style of observation, there are boundaries that define relevance, even accuracy. Sometimes referred to as *structured observation*, what is at issue is that there has to be a target, or targets, of observation which have to be clearly located within a nominated field of reference. This field has temporal, spatial and conceptual characteristics—the gestalt of which can be said to be the 'ground' in relation to which the object, or objects, of observation are placed. The object, or objects, is then isolated to become the focus to which the observer's attention is directed.

Mark Furlong

For example, if the intention is to study communication, specifically if the operational question is concerned with accurately counting the number of each kind of communication expressed by a subject (who in this case is a counsellor), a stable set of categories are required to be fixed, for example 'guiding statements', 'minimal encouragers', 'self-disclosing statements' (see 'Try it yourself' below). And, consistent with the need to ensure reliability (see CHAPTER 1), observers can be trained to be able to consistently identify, and then record, each of these items. In this process, the act of making, and then recording, observations is never spontaneous: it is an action that is highly conditional because it must conform to a stable protocol.

TRY IT YOURSELF

The key task for observational research is to be able to observe-record-code: to know what you are looking for, to be in a position to observe this variable and then to document it when or if it occurs. For example, if you were a researcher who wanted to examine what tutors or seminar leaders said in their sessions, you would need a list of categories that is sufficiently inclusive, and yet where each is well defined. The following list of eight types of speech have been used for this task: information statements; questions (open/closed); minimal encouragers; paraphrasing; guiding statements; self-disclosing statements; interpretations; challenges.

- ☐ Spend sufficient time to make sure that these categories are understood.
- ☐ Allocate two observers to use these categories.
- ☐ Have these observers (unobtrusively) record this data.
- ☐ After 10 minutes, each observer will present their 'findings'.
- ☐ As a large-group discussion, consider the issue of 'inter-rater reliability' (consistency of findings between two observers) (see CHAPTER 11).

Open-ended and immersive observation

There is another class of enquiry, indeed a dimension to most enquiries, that demands a quality that is different from the routine exercise. Mindful that a genuine 'ah-ha' experience, the 'eureka moment', is as rare as the four-leaf clover, observers involved in open-ended and more immersive projects must be on alert for the unexpected—for the outliers, contradictions and other observations that contest assumed notions and accepted coding patterns. In brief, there is often value in feeling disoriented and confused and a benefit in phenomena seeming to be 'out of sorts'. For example, some statements a counsellor may be observed to make could have an impact that lies between, perhaps even inverts, the simplicity that each statement is an example of 'guiding statement', an 'interpretation, and so on (see 'Try it yourself' above). For example, what is said in the form of a question can have the force of an instruction, or an injunction.

It is in this interrogation of standard procedures and received understandings that, as Bateson (1973) notes, the disciplines of rigour and imagination wrestle. In this contest, observations that seem striking, perceptive or intuitive are put into play. Rather than seeing such ideas as inspired, these 'new' ideas are, in one sense, not remarkable at all. They merely represent the introduction into a routinised dialogue between foreground and background of a relevant level of context. Such an introduction denaturalises the conventional configuration. In so far as the research is inductive, this class of 'readings' is desired as it can be beneficial to disturb the taken-for-granted configurations of figure and ground. There is an implicit politics in the question of focus: the field of attention can be altered by modifying the depth of field, or by altering the lens from a convergent focus to one that has a wider angle of view—but such a change involves making pragmatic, as well as ideological, decisions.

TRY IT YOURSELF

Using the same basic information as you used in the exercise above, discuss the ambiguity of verbal communication. For example, aren't some questions really statements if the tone of voice is considered? What of the authority position of the speaker: how does this shape how questions are interpreted?

This discussion introduces the question of validity with respect to a 'simple' observational domain.

Now, in small groups (no more than four students) construct at least three categories of (1) verbal communication, and (2) non-verbal communication where each has an operational definition. Spend at least 10 minutes doing this.

What you 'construct', or 'find', in this exercise are categories of communication of a different order from the eight verbal categories listed above. This kind of inductive enquiry is analogous to an observational process that is open to 'unexpected', rather than predefined, categories of data. That is, depending on the purpose for the study, it is not always clear, or desirable, to know in advance what the categories of observation should be.

THE PROCESS OF OBSERVATIONALLY BASED RESEARCH

The work of Freud, Goffman, Piaget and Orbach was mentioned in the introduction to this chapter. All these researchers have made a large impact, and all used a 'low-tech' approach. What is also shared is that these success stories did not achieve their (now) accepted findings without a powerful experience of struggle—a period of difficulty, confusion and self-doubt. Following the discussion of the experience of immersive observation mentioned above, the experience of confusion that often is part of the research exercise itself is now considered.

The title of this chapter: 'Clear at a distance, jumbled up close' is taken from the autobiography of the renowned anthropologist Clifford Geertz (1995, p. 78). Geertz used this visual metaphor to characterise a repeated experience, one he believed was characteristic of the anthropological project itself: in prospect, what one is about to study is seen in clear relief.

Mark Furlong

The 'out there' seems explicit, knowable, even patterned. Yet as one approaches, then becomes close to and, finally, finds oneself deeply engaged with what was previously 'out there', one finds that this sense of perspective has been disrupted.

This loss of perspective can feel quite shocking. At times this disruption can result in a sense of dislocation that is thoroughgoing. One remembers that the experience had been of seeing clearly, yet this memory prompts a wincing realisation: what one had taken to be an accurate perception—of overview, of knowing, even of sharp insight—has been overthrown. Rather than persist, these preconceptions disintegrate, resolving into the awareness that what was (seemingly) really out there was in fact more a product of one's hubris than of reality.

This descent into uncertainty may be, for Geertz, unsettling, but he would have it no other way. For Geertz, this contradiction enlivens the anthropological research project. Unless one comes to feel out of one's depth, not knowing, perhaps even overthrown in the exchange between 'where you are coming from' and 'what it is you are participating in', there can be no possibility of developing a new synthesis as an observer. We are pattern-makers, so we should take note of the initial picture that we construct, mindful that this is a 'hypothesis' that must be vigorously contested in any thoroughgoing episode of research practice.

For the purpose of the current contribution, what Geertz contends is essential to the anthropological project is similar to the dynamic that can be identified in all immersive observationally based practice research. Am I of this, above this, outside of this, inside this, lost in this?—these experiences are the moments of force that drive the process that makes personally engaged observational enquiry a fertile practice. However structured, or however intuitive, are your observations these experiences cannot be readily transposed into a new code, even a preliminary hypothesis, unless they are perturbed and allowed to jostle.

A sense of confusion can be said to be a necessary condition for production of new knowledge, yet it is not a sufficient condition. This latter condition involves the application of a discipline and a rigour in the service of generating new knowing or, more accurately, more possibilities in knowing. This may sound odd, even pretentious, but observationally based enquiry involves both serious art and intense intellectual play.

Observation has an honourable history

Isaac Newton watched an apple fall from a tree—and then used this observation in formulating the law of gravity. This story reminds us that observation has long played an important role in empirical research. This role continues in health and human service practice as the instruction to each professional to be a practitioner–scientist gains greater prominence. What this chapter has suggested is that each professional is a particular kind of practitioner–scientist: we are all *participant-observers* who act far more at the 'action' end of the continuum than the 'pure observer' end.

As first created in the 19th century, *participant observation* was a research method used by dispassionate outsiders, typically white males, to study exotic native societies naturalistically.

These scientists 'went native' in far-off settings over prolonged periods in order to understand exotic groups objectively, as well as from the natives' perspective. According to Tedlock (2005, p. 467), these ethnographers 'demonstrated their observational skills in scholarly monographs and their social participation in personal memoirs', a convention that posited a division between objective ethnographic data (observations) and subjective autobiographical data (the memoirs).

Such a division makes little sense today. As Denzin and Lincoln (2005, p. 641) declare:

> Nothing stands outside of representation. Research [necessarily] involves a complex politics of representation [where the] socially situated researcher creates, through interaction and material practices, those realities and representations that are the subject matter of inquiry.

The problem of representation is, at least in part, brought into focus in an iconic image of the anthropologist Bronislaw Malinowski (see the third website at the end of this chapter). In this image Malinowski is pictured typing diligently inside his tent, while the natives, whose lives he is so famously in the process of documenting, stare in at him. Some time ago, during the golden age of naive modernism, the image of the isolated anthropologist embedded in dark jungles seemed admirable, even heroic; now, it appears contradictory, ironic or even bizarre. However well intended this great man was, there is less objectivity present in his project to represent the other as exotic than there is colonial conceit.

Of course, the matter of observation always engages with the problem of representation. Whether observation is described austerely as *clinical*, or is presented as *naturalistic* in character, what is placed in view is inevitably ambiguous. This is the case whether the object of observation is minutely targeted and is said to be capable of being reliably measured, as is found in the examples of acute behavioural observation proposed by Mansell and Beadle-Brown (2004), as it is with observational data taken naturalistically from supposedly unobtrusive methods. At both ends of the observational spectrum, questions of meaning cannot be avoided. If it is the apparently objective observational research that is examined, tightly defined categories of attention have been stipulated and data is gathered with respect to the number of members of each behavioural grouping, each of which is counted within a nominated period of structured observation. In this situation, decisions have already been made, about what is pattern and cluster, signal and noise. Classification has taken place before observation. Or this active process takes place later, and/ or in a continuing process. Yet as with observations taken on the basis of a priori decisions, those classifications that are constructed because they come to be experienced as meaningful, or even transformative, only attain this privileged status on the basis that certain criteria have been met.

What is required in such cases is that this criterion—the basis for the classification—is transparently set forth. All too often, in qualitative enquiries the researcher's enthusiasm, and/ or absence of patience or skill in deconstructing their sense-making leaves the reader sceptical that the dots have been joined arbitrarily. It is a rigorous, laborious and often boring task to clearly externalise the decision-making processes upon which an analysis depends.

Mark Furlong

Whether their object is the minute gesture or the larger social gestalt, observations can be used to illustrate, even document, a point, but they can never be said to speak for themselves. A picture is said to convey a thousand words yet these words come from many mouths and never form a coherent, consensual story over time and culture: think of the Mona Lisa, perhaps the world's best known image, which has been interpreted in many different ways across its 500-year history—as unremarkable, chubby-cheeked working woman; as mysterious temptress; as ironically subverted icon.

Summary

It is now the conventional view that war correspondents can never be truly neutral. Rather, the credibility of a report is conditional on the reporter deciphering, and then reporting, the kind of embeddedness that locates their point of view to the reader. Similarly, observations in the health and human service sector can aspire to a condition of importance in so far as their 'back story' is made convincingly. In both contexts, a clear case has to be made that the observer has rigorously disinterred their agenda, biases and criteria for decision-making. Single practitioners, even institutional groups of practitioners, are never in charge of the larger process that judges one research finding 'evidence' and another 'opinion' (Phillips 1973). This being clear, each practitioner-scientist can demonstrate a quality of transparency—which is the quality that most allows scrutiny and therefore the possibility of trust. This is what science is about: the discipline of organised scepticism.

Tutorial exercises

Geertz's notion of 'thick description' was taken from the English philosopher Gilbert Ryle, who examined how even simple behaviours, such as winking, can be ambiguous to interpret (Rapport & Overing 2000, p. 349). In order to deepen your appreciation of this point, and to practise a simulated observational exercise, the following exercise can be attempted (30–45 minutes).

☐ Nominate two people in your tutorial to take part in a simple role-play.
☐ These two people should then leave the main group and secretly plan how they wish to behave when they return to the main group. They could plan to be a 'couple who are flirting', 'two old friends', 'a mother and her teenage daughter', and so forth.
☐ While the two role-play persons are out of the room preparing, the remaining group members should divide into groups of three or four and choose a focus for their particular observations, e.g. instances of eye contact; hand gestures; the raising and lowering of volume and pitch. You should plan to carefully record these observations.
☐ After returning to the main group, the two role-players should interact for, say, 3–5 minutes without introducing their scenario (preferably while being videoed).

☐ Each of the observing teams should record what they see in as much behavioural detail as possible.

☐ After taking time at the end of the role-play for each team to review what they had observed, each team will present their findings in two stages: first, to present the behavioural data they observed, and second, to interpret what they thought the nature of the relationship was between the role-play pair—and to say why they had reached this conclusion.

☐ After each of the teams have reported back, the role-play pair should clarify to the group what scenario they had enacted and then comment on the meanings that the observing teams had put forward.

☐ If the role-play interaction was video-recorded, replay the tape, stopping and starting in order to review and clarify the observations that had been reported.

FURTHER READING

Anastas, J. (2005). Observation. In R. Grinnell & Y. Unrau (eds), *Social work research and evaluation: Quantitative and qualitative approaches*. New York: Oxford University Press, 213–30.

Rapport, N. & Overing, J. (2000). *Social and cultural anthropology: The key concepts*. Routledge: London.

Tedlock, B. (2005). The observation of participation and the emergence of public ethnography. In N.K. Denzin & Y.S. Lincoln (eds), *The Sage handbook of qualitative research*. Thousand Oaks: Sage Publications, 467–78.

Websites

uk.geocities.com/balihar_sanghera/qrmparticipantobservation.html

This website offers an account of the history of, and some useful hints on using, participant observation. This material is written in an informal and accessible way and is recommended if you wish to deepen your understanding.

www.qualitative-research.net/index.php/fqs/article/view/466

This website has a link to a dense, yet a most rewarding, article on participant observation. This contribution not only presents clear background material concerning observation, but it also offers a number of 'how to' pointers and several valuable exercises.

http://classes.yale.edu/02-03/anth500a/projects/project_sites/99_Song/default.htm

This website has the picture of Bronislaw Malinowski referred in the chapter.

Mark Furlong

Part III

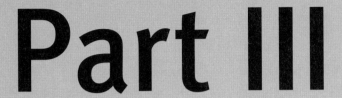

Quantitative Approaches and Practices

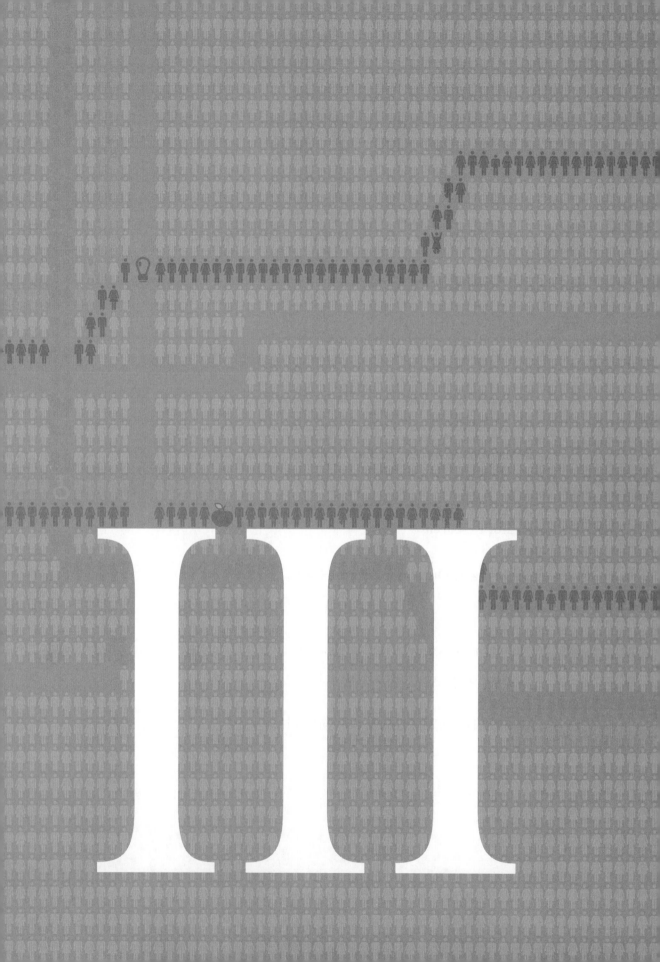

11

Measure Twice, Cut Once: Understanding the Reliability and Validity of the Clinical Measurement Tools Used in Health Research

Christine Imms and Susan Greaves

CHAPTER OBJECTIVES

In this chapter you will learn:

☐ about two different methods of test development: Classical Test Theory and Item Response Theory

☐ what research studies are required to develop a valid and reliable measure

☐ how to apply criteria to evaluate methods used to validate an outcome measure or assessment tool

☐ how to critically appraise the methods used to establish reliability of a measure

☐ how to interpret reliability statistics

☐ how to identify the key criteria for selecting an assessment for use in clinical practice or research

KEY TERMS

Assessment

Interval data

Measurement

Nominal data

Ordinal data

Ratio data

Reliability

Theoretical assumption

Validity

INTRODUCTION

This chapter aims to provide readers with a basis for choosing and appropriately using measurement tools for either research or clinical practice. This knowledge will support the clinician's own practice and assist in interpreting the quality of research they read from the perspective of measurement selection.

Accurate, reliable and meaningful measurement is essential for providing an authoritative basis to explain and support research and to offer recommendations (American Educational Research Association 1999). The choice and use of appropriate measurement tools should be fundamental to logical, empirically based research in health (Bond & Fox 2007). As clinical practice is an iterative process of assessing the need for intervention, applying an intervention, evaluating its effect and adjusting, continuing or ceasing the intervention, accurate assessment and measurement are equally important in the clinical context. Valid and reliable measurement is one of the foundational requirements of evidence-based practice (see also CHAPTERS 1, 15, 16, 17).

Assessment: Also referred to as an evaluation, which is used to describe the process of gathering quantitative data in general.

Measurement may be used to describe the use of an instrument that is capable of measuring the magnitude of the attribute under evaluation using a calibrated scale.

Throughout the literature, varying terms are used to describe the process of gathering data, such as evaluation, assessment and measurement, and the instruments used to gather data such as assessment, outcome measure and measurement tool. In this chapter, we will use **assessment** or evaluation to describe the process of gathering data in general. **Measurement** will be used when the instrument or tool meets the requirements for being a measure; that is, it is capable of measuring the magnitude of the attribute under evaluation using a calibrated scale.

DOING RESEARCH

The *Melbourne Assessment of Unilateral Upper Limb Function* (The Melbourne Assessment, Randall et al. 1999) and the updated *Revised Melbourne Assessment* (Randall 2009) are used throughout the chapter as the primary examples demonstrating specific aspects of measurement theory and test development research. The Melbourne Assessment was developed out of a clinical and research need to quantitatively measure quality of movement of the upper extremity of children with cerebral palsy and other neurological impairments (Johnson et al. 1994). The tool was developed in the late 1980s when there were no valid, reliable measures of the construct *quality of upper limb function*, although there was a need to measure the construct before and after intervention that aimed to change upper limb movement (Johnson et al. 1994).

How do we measure?

Measurement involves the process of description and quantification. It involves recording physical or behavioural characteristics by assigning a value to aspects such as the quality, quantity, frequency or degree of these attributes. Some attributes, such as joint range, can be measured directly. But many characteristics, such as quality of movement, are not directly observable; they are more abstract. Abstract characteristics are evaluated by conceptualising a relationship between the original characteristic and a construct that is assumed to represent it. Thus we measure the 'effect' of that characteristic (Portney & Watkins 2000). For example, range of movement around one joint is directly observable and can be measured, though not with perfect precision, using a goniometer. As quality of movement is not directly measurable, it was conceptualised within the Melbourne Assessment as comprising range of movement around multiple joints, fluency or smoothness of movement, accuracy of movement, and dexterity of grasp and release (Randall et al. 1999). So these attributes were observed and scored during the assessment on the assumption that quality of movement affects them.

Numerical values are typically used to describe the frequency or degree of the attributes assessed. These numbers help us score the level of the performance succinctly. However, not all numbers that are assigned during an assessment have mathematical properties. Specific criteria, called levels of measurement, have been defined to differentiate between types of numbers (Stevens 1946, as cited in Bond & Fox 2007).

Nominal data occur where objects or people are assigned to named categories according to some criterion, for example male/female, and these categories may be given arbitrary numerical values. For example boys = 1, girls = 2. In terms of the definition of measurement given above, these data are observations, not measurements.

> **Nominal data** occur where objects or people are assigned to named categories according to some criterion, for example male/female.

Ordinal data also occur where objects or people are assigned to categories, but in this case the categories can be rank-ordered on the basis of predetermined level. Common examples are the Likert satisfaction scales ranging from very dissatisfied = 1, dissatisfied = 2, neutral = 3, satisfied = 4 and very satisfied = 5. While the rank order describes an increasing amount of the attribute (in this case satisfaction), the intervals between ranks may not be consistent or even known. Ordinal data also have limited statistical flexibility; the data remain as observations, not measurements as per the definition above, because we are unable to determine the magnitude of the difference between values. The scale is not calibrated (Bond & Fox 2007).

> **Ordinal data** result when observations are rank-ordered and values are assigned sequentially to reflect the logical ordering of categories, e.g. Likert scales, which rank responses from low to high.

Christine Imms and Susan Greaves

Interval data also have the property of a rank order and in addition, distances or intervals between the units of measurement are equal. For example, the thermometer measures temperature in equal interval units called degrees. A difference of 1°C is exactly the same at any point on the scale. This scale, however, does not have a true zero. 0° does not mean an absence of temperature; rather, it is the point at which water freezes—the zero is criterion-referenced. Interval-level data meet the criteria for measurement because it is possible to define the distance between values and therefore identify how much one individual or group differs from another.

> **Interval data** have the property of a rank order, and in addition, distances or intervals between the units of measurement are equal.

Ratio data have the same properties as interval-level data, and in addition, have an empirical (absolute) rather than an arbitrary zero. For example, range of movement as measured by a goniometer has equal intervals between units of measurement (in degrees) and an absolute zero: 0° flexion means there is no flexion around that joint and 20° is half the range of 40°. This is the highest level of measurement, and data from ratio scales have the greatest statistical utility because of their mathematical properties.

> **Ratio data** have the same properties as interval-level data, and in addition, have an empirical rather than an arbitrary zero.

There are many examples of tools using ordinal-level data where equal distances or intervals are assumed. For example, the original Melbourne Assessment comprises 37 items on which performance is rated using ordinal scales (Randall et al. 1999). These ordinal data are then summed and converted to a percentage score as if they were interval data. Interval-level data are the minimum requirement for many statistical analyses, and Bond and Fox (2007) assert that it is not appropriate to pretend that ordinal data are the same as interval-level data. See also CHAPTERS 13, 24, 25.

HOW ARE ASSESSMENT TOOLS DEVELOPED?

Developing valid and reliable tools demands considerable time, effort and fiscal resources. Many aspects of this complex process will become apparent through this chapter. We will begin by describing some of the basic concepts within two models of test development, classical test theory (CTT) and item response theory (IRT). Both models initially involve processes designed to select items that measure a construct of interest. This will be described later in the chapter.

Classical Test Theory has for many years underpinned the way that measurement instruments have been developed. The foundation of this theory rests on the premise that the total test score, or raw score (X), is made up of a true component (T) and a random error component (E), so that $X = T + E$. There are three assumptions within this theory: (1) true scores and error scores are uncorrelated (not related to each other); (2) because random errors are normally distributed, the expected mean value of the error is zero; and (3) random error scores are uncorrelated. Generally speaking, the aim of CTT is to understand and improve the reliability of an assessment tool (Kline 2005).

Item Response Theory, also referred to as Latent Trait Theory, is model-based measurement. This means that the test that is being developed must fit the mathematical model to be valid. In IRT, the amount of an underlying ability or 'trait' is dependent on both the person's responses to test items and the level of difficulty of the administered items (Embretson & Hershberger 1999). IRT is based on two 'hard' assumptions. First, the scale is unidimensional; that is, all the items in a test evaluate one single latent trait or ability. Second, the probability of success of people with the same amount of the trait on any one item is independent of their probability of success on any other item. This is called local independence.

One IRT model used frequently in the rehabilitation sciences is the Rasch measurement model (e.g. Fisher & Fisher 1993; Krumlinde-Sundholm & Eliasson 2003). The Rasch model conceptualises a measurement scale like a ruler. On the right-hand side, items are ranked along the measurement scale according to their difficulty. Less difficult items are located at the bottom of the scale; the most difficult items are at the top. People (on the left-hand side) are located on the same measurement scale according to their ability or their level of the trait of interest. People with a low ability are located at the bottom of the scale, and those with higher ability are located at the top. The Rasch model then has two additional assumptions:

- All people are more likely to achieve easier items than more difficult ones.
- All items are more likely to be achieved by people with high ability or more of the trait than by those of low ability or less of the trait.

The location or position of items and subjects along the measurement scale is estimated by the model from the proportion of responses of each person to each item. The Rasch model uses a logarithmic transformation of the raw scores into log-odds information units called logits. The scale resulting from the analysis has the properties of an interval scale with known and equal distances between the units, and is therefore a measure.

The Rasch measurement model was used to revise the scale attributes of the original Melbourne Assessment in the mid 2000s. The result of this revision is a valid interval-level measure comprising four subscales. Figure 11.1 shows the person-item map from the range of movement scale of the Revised Melbourne Assessment 2009 (Randall 2009).

The premises underlying CTT and IRT are different and therefore the processes used to validate tools also differ. A summary of the advantages and disadvantages of each method is presented in Table 11.1.

Christine Imms and Susan Greaves

Figure 11.1: Person-item map from the range of movement subscale of the Revised Melbourne Assessment (unpublished data, personal communication M. Randall 27 March 2009). Location = logit scores for the subscale; ° represents one person; Items indicated by test item on score sheet; Item 11 (reach to brush from forehead to back of neck) is the most difficult item; item 1.1 (reach forward) is the easiest item.

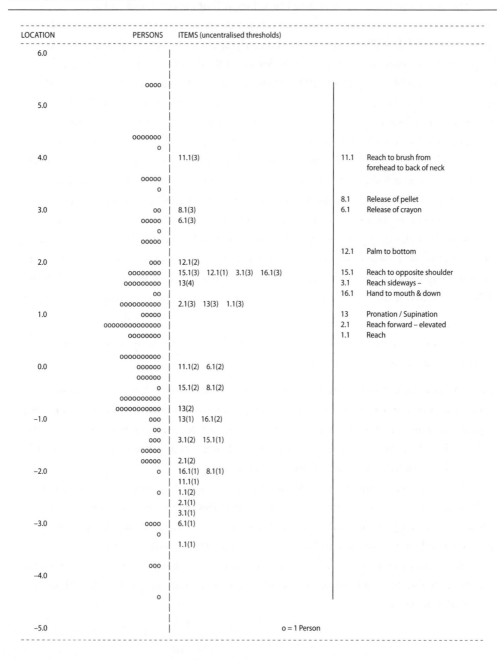

Table 11.1: A comparison of advantages and disadvantages of two methods for developing scales

Theory	Advantages	Disadvantages
Classical Test theory (CTT)	Procedures are based on a number of 'weak' assumptions (e.g. that random errors around a true score are normally distributed) that allow for easier analysis and interpretation. Relatively easy to interpret. Analyses can be performed with smaller representative samples of individuals. In analyses undertaken with very large samples, violating assumptions around the use of ordinal-level data is reported to have a minimal effect on the results.	Item and scale statistics are both sample-dependent, and should only be interpreted for that sample. It is difficult to separate the properties of the test from the attributes of the individuals taking it. That is, it is not possible to separate the ability of the person from the difficulty of the items. It is often assumed that scores from scales can be treated as interval data. However, items are commonly ordinal and the distance between response options may not be equal. Interpreting changes in scores using ordinal data is difficult, other than identifying the direction of change. Inferential analyses using ordinal data should be undertaken using non-parametric statistics. Different forms of a test are considered parallel only after considerable effort to demonstrate their equality.
Item Response Theory (IRT)	The scale derived from IRT analyses is an interval-level measurement, and parametric statistics can be used legitimately. It allows for test-free and sample-free measurement. That is, individuals can be compared even if they take different items from a test, and the scale can produce stable item estimates regardless of the sample of people used to calibrate the items. The hierarchical structure developed during Rasch analysis provides a clinically useful 'item map' by ranking items from difficult to easy. This can be used to monitor progress and develop programs that target clinically relevant areas of difficulty.	The 'hard' assumption of unidimensionality of the scale items may be difficult to achieve. Complex constructs such as quality of life or those affected by a number of potentially unrelated facets cannot be combined into an overall score. While the scale can be initially developed using relatively modest sample sizes, validation of the measure often requires large samples (e.g. 400–500 people) to provide a stable measure.

Christine Imms and Susan Greaves

RELIABILITY

Reliability refers to the extent to which a measurement instrument is dependable, stable and consistent when repeated under identical conditions (McDowell & Newell 1996).

Reliability: The extent to which a measurement instrument is dependable, stable and consistent when repeated under identical conditions.

Establishing the reliability of an assessment tool is an essential component of determining the instrument's adequacy (Streiner & Norman 2003; see also CHAPTER 1).

The need to evaluate reliability is based on the premise that measurement instruments possess some *measurement error*, and that humans are fallible when measuring and can produce inconsistent responses. This discrepancy is described within CTT as the observed score comprising a true score and an error component. As it is not possible to know the true score, the true reliability of a test cannot be known. Rather, we estimate reliability based on the statistical concept of variance; that is, a measure of the variability among scores within a sample. Reliability is expressed as a ratio of the true score variance to the total score variance:

$$R = \frac{\text{True Score Variance}}{\text{True score variance} + \text{Error variance}} = \frac{T}{T+E}$$

Variability (error) in measurement can come from many sources (Streiner & Norman 2003). The most likely sources are variation in performance of the individual, which might be related to mood or concentration, or simply because individuals are not machines and do not act in precisely the same manner on all occasions. Variability can also be related to the rater, for example inconsistent application of scoring criteria or minor variations in administration of test items. Variation for some attributes can also be related to factors such as time of day, stress or prior activity. Generalisability studies allow researchers to examine the effect of multiple sources of error concurrently (Streiner & Norman 2003). It is more typical, however, to find research about single sources of error such as intra-rater, inter-rater and test-retest studies.

☐ *Test-retest* reliability describes the extent to which a stable evaluation of the attribute or behaviour can be obtained on two different occasions when no change is expected.

☐ *Intra-rater reliability* describes the extent to which the same person can rate the same performance consistently.

☐ *Inter-rater reliability* is the extent to which different people rate the same performance consistently.

Intra-rater reliability is higher than inter-rater reliability. And for this reason, repeated measures in research and in clinical practice should be undertaken by the same rater whenever possible. In self-rated measures, intra- and inter-rater reliability estimates are not relevant, and in these circumstances, test-retest reliability is estimated.

Reliability estimates can be understood in terms of consistency and agreement. In general, a high level of consistency is required for instruments that are used to discriminate between individuals, and a high level of agreement is required for measures that aim to evaluate change.

☐ *Consistency:* Many reliability coefficients are based on correlation. Correlation reflects the degree of association between two sets of scores, or the consistency of position within the two distributions. The statistic is called a correlation coefficient.

☐ *Agreement:* While correlation tells us about the *relationship* between two sets of scores, it does not tell us whether the actual values obtained by the two measurements are the same. To do this, we need to consider the agreement between scores (Terwee et al. 2007).

Intraclass Correlation Coefficients (ICCs) provide an estimate of reliability using indices of both consistency and agreement, thus taking into account the magnitude of the difference between scores as well as the relationship (Streiner & Norman 2003). ICCs are the appropriate statistic when calculating reliability for continuous data. They range in value from 0.0 to 1.0, with higher values associated with higher reliability. When data are nominal (simple agreement or disagreement between scores) the Kappa coefficient is appropriate. When data are ordinal, weighted Kappa is the appropriate coefficient.

Measures of agreement such as Bland and Altman's limit of agreement (LOA) plots (Bland & Altman 1986) and standard error of measurement (SEM) are expressed on the actual scale of measurement, which can aid clinical interpretation. An example using the LOA method is shown in Figure 11.2.

Figure 11.2: Bland and Altman plot of intra-rater reliability data from the original Melbourne Assessment showing difference between occasions on the Y axis and the mean of the difference on the X axis. Although a slight bias towards higher scores on the second occasion is evident, clinically, the mean difference between occasions of –1.41 points in a scale of 100 points appeared negligible.

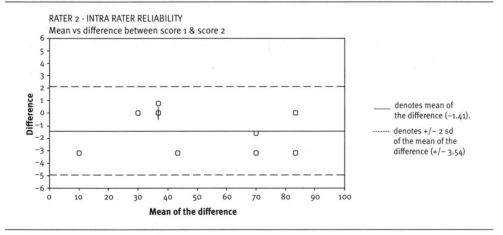

The standard error of measurement (SEM) can be calculated using the standard deviation (σ) and the reliability coefficient (R) as follows: SEM $= \sigma \sqrt{1-R}$. The SEM can be used to draw a confidence interval around an individual's observed score (Xo). This would be shown as $Xo \pm Z$ (SEM) where Z is the value from the normal curve associated with the desired confidence interval (e.g. 1.96 for 95% confidence interval) (Streiner & Norman 2003). Using the Melbourne Assessment as an example, an SEM of 2.56 points for total raw scores of trained raters (Cusick et al. 2005) means that an individual's observed raw score has a 95 per cent confidence interval of $\pm$ 5.02 raw score points. This gives an indication of how much error we might expect within the scoring of the individual's performance on the Melbourne Assessment on that occasion.

Internal Consistency is a measure of the extent to which individual items in a scale are correlated with each other and the total scale score (Streiner & Norman 2003). Thus it provides evidence of homogeneity or unidimensionality of the scale. This is an important property of tools that aim to measure hidden constructs. In the Rasch measurement model, this is a required property of the tool. In CTT, some tools aim to measure constructs that are *caused* by a range of unrelated attributes (e.g. quality of life measures) and these tools are not required to have high internal consistency (Streiner & Norman 2003).

VALIDITY

Establishing the **validity** of an instrument, or the extent to which an instrument measures what it is intended to measure, is vital (Streiner & Norman 2003; see CHAPTER 1). Evaluating the validity of a tool is especially important when we are measuring constructs that are not directly observable, as is often the case in allied health.

Validity: The degree to which a scale measures what it is intended to measure.

Population: In statistical research, the group, or cases, from which the sample in a research project is selected.

Validity is not inherent to an instrument, but rather evaluated within the context of the test's intended use and specific **population** (Streiner & Norman 2003). Validity is not an all-or-none concept; evidence that supports an instrument's validity is gathered over time. Methods used to evaluate various forms of validity are summarised in Table 11.2. Types of validity that are evaluated generally form under the following categories:

- *Content validity* refers to the extent to which an instrument covers all the important aspects or domains of interest that it intends to measure, and does not include items that are irrelevant to what is being measured. For example, the procedures used to develop the original Melbourne Assessment enhanced the content validity of the tool. The authors reviewed the literature on upper limb function, as well as clinical assessments of related upper limb constructs, and held workshops with expert clinicians. Item generation and selection were based on clearly defined criteria relating to the construct and the intended population (Randall et al. 1999).
- *Face validity* indicates that an instrument *appears* to evaluate what it is supposed to and seems plausible to the users of the tool (assessors and respondents). This judgment is made

after the assessment tool has been constructed. It should not be considered sufficient evidence of a test's validity and is not always required, for example in instruments that are designed to obtain information about socially undesirable behaviours (Portney & Watkins 2000; Streiner & Norman 2003).

☐ *Construct validity* reflects the ability of an instrument to measure an abstract concept. Establishing construct validity involves three steps: (1) explicitly describing the theoretical concepts and how they relate to each other; (2) developing an assessment tool that can measure the theoretical construct; and (3) testing the relationship between the constructs and the observed behaviours that represent it (Streiner & Norman 2003). In IRT, the third step is evaluated by how well the data gathered using the tool fit the measurement model and thus provide evidence that performances reflect a single underlying construct (Bond & Fox 2007).

☐ *Criterion validity* concerns the correlation of one tool with another, ideally a 'gold standard' that has been widely used and accepted in the field of interest. One difficulty with this form of validity is the availability of tools that truly are gold standards.

☐ *Concurrent validity* is evaluated by administering both the test of interest and the gold standard at the same time, with an expectation that scores are highly related. Although no gold standard is available, concurrent validity of the Melbourne Assessment with the Quality of Upper Extremity Skills Test, which theoretically evaluates a similar construct, showed high positive correlations between scores (Pearsons $r > 0.8$), providing evidence that both tools evaluate similar constructs (Klingels et al. 2008). When tests are diagnostic, that is, designed to determine if a condition is present or not, then a specific type of criterion validity study is conducted to test the accuracy of the test in comparison with a gold standard. Data from these studies are not simply correlation statistics, but also describe the sensitivity, specificity, positive and negative predictive values and likelihood ratios. Greenhalgh (2001) gives a good overview of these studies and the data generated.

☐ *Predictive validity* is established by evaluating performance using the instrument at a specified time-point (e.g. baseline, diagnosis, discharge) and following the target group over time until the outcome to be predicted occurs. These studies determine the accuracy of the measurement tool to predict future outcomes (De Bie 2001).

Responsiveness concerns the ability of an instrument to measure change following an intervention or over time (Streiner & Norman 2003; Terwee et al. 2007). Methods for evaluating responsiveness as well as the terminology reported in the literature are quite varied and include terms such as 'minimal clinically important change' and 'smallest detectable difference' (Beckerman et al. 2001; Hajiro & Nishimura 2002; Terwee et al. 2007). Within some of the definitions of these terms is an evaluation of how much change is required to be classified as 'important,' and correspondingly, who should be the judge of the importance, the clinician or the client and under what circumstances (Hajiro & Nishimura 2002).

The underlying test property that contributes to the ability of a tool to be responsive is reliability (Beckerman et al. 2001; Streiner & Norman 2003). Tools with high reliability, thus low measurement error, are likely to be more responsive (Streiner & Norman 2003). One method of evaluating the ability of a tool to detect change is the estimate of the smallest detectable difference (SDD). The SDD is equivalent to calculating a confidence interval around the standard error measurement that takes into account both measurement occasions (SDD = SEM×1.96×√2) (Beckerman et al. 2001; Klingels et al. 2008). Tools with high levels of reliability, however, will not necessarily be responsive; the ability of a tool to detect change must also be evaluated within research. Typically, this involves using the tool, along with other instruments known to be responsive, within a clinical trial in which change in the attribute is expected.

Table 11.2: Examples of validation processes used in CTT and IRT

Form of validity	Classical Test Theory	Rasch measurement model
Content validity	Involves a range of methods for generating and selecting items for a scale. For example, a panel of experts may generate and view the items and decide if they satisfy the content domain. This often requires several revisions of the test following pilot testing with a specific sample. Qualitative studies may be used to generate items from key informants, or content analyses undertaken of observations of performance.	Similar to CTT
Criterion validity (concurrent and predictive validity)	Correlation between the target test and a criterion test either conducted at the same time or at a future point in time. For diagnostic tests, accuracy, sensitivity and specificity are evaluated in comparison to a gold standard.	Differential Item Functioning (DIF) analysis: this determines whether items in the scale function the same way regardless of the characteristics of the person taking the test. Test Linking: a process of determining whether two tests, or alternative forms of the same test, measure the same construct.
Construct validity	Factor analysis: an analytical method aimed at reducing the number of categories of measurement, e.g. combines multiple items into groups of factors that measure common variables. Known Groups Method: a method of determining whether a test can discriminate between a group known to have a disorder and a group that does not, or between groups with known levels of the attribute. Hypothesis-testing	Internal scale validity assesses how well the items in the scale fit the Rasch model (fit statistics). Principal components analysis: another term for one form of factor analysis. Rating scale structure: a method of determining the order of score thresholds for each item.
Internal consistency	Cronbach's Alpha: an estimate of the correlation between items within the scale.	Person separation index: an estimate of reliability examining how well persons can be differentiated on the scale.

Note: Sources of information include Portney & Watkins 2000; Streiner & Norman 2003; Bond & Fox 2007; Fawcett 2007; Holmefur 2009.

CRITERIA FOR SELECTING TESTS AND MEASURES IN RESEARCH AND PRACTICE

Theoretical assumptions underlying choice of tests and measures

Determining what is to be measured should be guided by the **theoretical assumptions** that underpin the research or practice appropriate to each health discipline. The International Classification of Functioning, Disability and Health is a universal model that describes the relationships between a health condition, body structures and function, activity performance, participation, environmental and personal factors (WHO 2001). If the intention is to improve participation, then participation must be carefully defined and measured. If the intention is to investigate relationships between constructs within the model, for example the relationship between impairments of body function and participation, then both elements must be evaluated. Careful consideration of the theoretical assumptions under investigation (in practice and research) is an essential component of all test selection.

> **Theoretical assumptions** are hypothetical statements that explain, or are used to predict, certain phenomena. Theoretical models are diagrammatic explanations of hypothetical relationships.

The reason for measuring (or purpose of research or assessment)

Criteria to consider when selecting the measure or test to be used in research or clinical practice are related to the aim, the construct or attribute to be measured, and the population in whom it is to be measured. The tests listed below describe the different purposes for which assessments and outcome measures can be validated (Hanna et al. 2005). For each of these purposes, the level of measurement required for valid interpretation might differ. Tools may be validated for more than one purpose.

☐ **Descriptive tests** describe the difference between individuals within a group. An example of a descriptive measure is the Gross Motor Functional Classification System (Palisano et al. 2008), which classifies the gross motor function of children and youth with cerebral palsy into five different levels of ability based on their self-initiated movement.

> **Descriptive tests** describe the difference between individuals within a group.

☐ **Discriminative tests** distinguish between individuals with and without a characteristic or trait. For example, the Alberta Infant Motor Scale (Piper & Darrah 1994) discriminates between infants with normal or atypical motor development.

> **Discriminative tests** distinguish between individuals with and without a characteristic or trait.

☐ **Predictive tests** aim to assess individuals in terms of their likely future outcomes. For example, hospital admission scores on the Functional Independence Measure were used to predict length of stay and discharge scores (Heinemann et al. 1994).

> **Predictive tests** aim to assess individuals in terms of their likely future outcomes.

Christine Imms and Susan Greaves

Evaluative tests are
designed to measure change
over time and are often
called outcome measures.

☐ **Evaluative tests** are designed to measure change over time and are often called outcome measures. To accurately measure the amount of change, evaluative tools need to collect data at interval or ratio levels, for example the Assisting Hand Assessment (Krumlinde-Sundholm & Eliasson 2003).

The construct or attribute of interest

Carefully defining the construct of interest assists with determining how complex it is and whether a single item or measure can adequately capture the phenomenon or whether multiple behaviours must be measured. Complex constructs may need to be measured by more than one tool. However, it is important to have strong reasons for the inclusion of each measure, to not select too many measures, thus avoiding redundancy of measurement and burden for the client or research participants. It is at this point that a systematic and comprehensive search for existing measures should be undertaken.

Required properties of the tool

VALIDITY FOR PURPOSE

A tool is valid for your purposes when (1) it measures the attribute or construct of interest appropriately, that is, there is evidence of the tool's content, criterion or construct validity; (2) it meets the measurement property requirements for your research or practice needs, that is, it is descriptive, evaluative, discriminative or predictive as needed; (3) it was developed for, or subsequently validated for, the population of people for whom you wish to use it. For example, the original Melbourne Assessment is not valid for children under 5 years of age; the Revised Melbourne Assessment, which was developed in response to a growing research need for a measure that spanned a wider age range, is valid for children as young as (but not younger than) 2.5 years (Randall et al. 2008); (4) the tool is used as it was designed to be used, that is, the tool is administered and scored as instructed. This means that items cannot be extracted and used in isolation, or in combination with items from another tool, without further research into whether valid inferences can be made from the results.

RELIABILITY

If possible, researchers and clinicians should select tools with evidence of reliability in their population of interest because reliability estimates vary depending on the population in whom they are determined (Streiner & Norman 2003). Although a tool may have demonstrated reliability, there is no guarantee that the same degree of reliability will be achieved in every situation. Researchers often perform pilot studies to establish the reliability of a measurement tool before the commencement of data collection. Additionally, the actual reliability is only as good as the person administering and scoring the test. To be reliable, the user must undertake appropriate training and administer and score the test or measure as prescribed.

CLINICAL UTILITY

There are a number of characteristics that influence the clinical utility of a tool (Law 2004; Fawcett 2007), each of which need to be considered when selecting tests and measures. Criteria to consider include:

- ☐ clarity of instructions for administering the assessment, which also affects validity and reliability of administration of the tool
- ☐ format in terms of whether the tool is a self-report survey, interview, observation of performance or administered test; some formats are more invasive than others and require higher levels of active participation from the individual and special equipment, all of which must be considered
- ☐ time to complete, including both administration and scoring
- ☐ examiner training and/or qualifications required to administer or interpret results and cost in time and money
- ☐ cost of the tool including any equipment or software, score sheets and other expendable items
- ☐ amount of effort required by both the clinician and the client or research participant
- ☐ acceptability of the test to the clinician and the client or research participant.

CRITERIA FOR EVALUATING STUDIES THAT EXAMINE THE MEASUREMENT PROPERTIES OF A TOOL

Like any other type of research, the utility and believability of the results of measurement studies depend on the methods used to obtain them. Thus the discerning reader will make a judgment about the internal validity of the study before examining the actual data reporting on the results. (Reminder: internal validity of a study is the extent to which bias is reduced by the design and methods used within the study.) Table 11.3 gives a series of questions that can guide the reader in their consideration of validity studies. This table provides some commonly agreed criteria, where they exist, against which to examine the results. The questions in this table and the one following have been developed using criteria reported in the literature, but the lists are not validated measures of the internal validity of measurement studies and the questions should only be used to guide the reader's thinking.

Christine Imms and Susan Greaves

Table 11.3: Criteria for evaluating studies that examine the validity of measurement tools

Criteria	Yes / No / NA / NR	Describe and evaluate quality
Content validity studies: Examine the extent to which the concepts of interest are comprehensively represented by the items in the outcome measure or assessment tool		
Design Did the study ask a clearly focused question about the content validity of the tool?		
Were the study hypotheses clearly stated?		
Was the measurement theory clearly stated?		
Was the measurement aim of the tool clear?		
Were the concepts to be measured clearly identified and defined?		
Method Was the target population clearly defined?		
Was there evidence that the participants represented the target population?		
Were item selection processes described and adequate in relation to relevance and comprehensiveness?		
Results Did the resulting scale appear to meet the measurement aims?		
If face-validity was desirable, was it present?		
Were floor and ceiling effects avoided? (i.e. <15% of respondents achieved highest or lowest scores [a])		
Construct validity: The ability of an instrument to measure an abstract construct		
Design Were the constructs of interest to be measured clearly identified and defined?		
Was an appropriate theory used to explain the construct of interest?		
Were specific hypotheses about expected relationships generated and the design of the study appropriate to these hypotheses?		
Was the measurement theory clearly stated?		
Construct validity—Classical Test Theory		
Method Was the target population clearly defined?		
Was there evidence that the participants represented the target population?		

Criteria	Yes / No / NA / NR	Describe and evaluate quality
Were specific hypotheses about expected relationships between test scores and scores on related instruments generated a priori (before the study)?		
Was the tool administered as intended?		
Were raters blind to the hypotheses of interest?		
Were comparison measures administered independently—i.e. raters were blind to results of other assessments?		
Were comparison measures valid, reliable and appropriate for the hypotheses within this study?		
Analyses		
Were factor analysis (exploratory or confirmatory) and/or internal consistency evaluated?		
Were expected correlations between measurement tools stated prior to analyses?		
Results What were the results?		
Were at least 75% of hypotheses supported?[a]		
Were Cronbach's alpha scores between .70 and .95?[a]		
Were derived factors supported by confirmatory factor analyses?		
Construct validity: Rasch measurement model		
Method Was the sample generally appropriate?		
Was the sample size adequate for the purpose of the study? (For studies regarding content validity, 10 subjects for each point on the rating scale. For definitive item calibrations, 400–500 subjects are required)[b]		
Was the tool administered as intended?		
Was the Rasch measurement model used to establish construct validity by establishing that data (person and item responses) fit the model?		
Results Was it possible to order items from easiest to hardest and persons from least to greatest ability?		
Were fit statistics (infit and outfit) provided and did items and persons meet criteria for particular model and software used?		

Christine Imms and Susan Greaves

Table 11.3: (cont.)

Criteria	Yes / No / NA / NR	Describe and evaluate quality
Were person and item reliability indices provided and were they high, indicating sufficient items to estimate person ability and sufficient persons to estimate item difficulty with precision?		
Were item difficulty and person ability estimates provided in logits with error estimates in a figure (item-person map) +/- tables?		
Was item difficulty relatively stable when applied to different groups? (item invariance)		
Was person ability relatively stable when measured using a subset of items? (person invariance)		
Was potential differential item functioning investigated to determine whether item difficulty estimates differed for subgroups of persons (e.g. boys/girls, different age groups)?		
Criterion validity: The extent to which an assessment tool produces results relative to other measures		
Design Did the study ask a clearly focused question about the criterion-related validity of the tool?		
Were the study hypotheses clearly stated?		
Was the design of the study appropriate to the purpose of the study? For example predictive validity with long-term follow-up, diagnostic validity using prospective evaluation against a gold standard, concurrent validity against a relevant gold standard.		
Were the concepts to be measured clearly identified, defined and measured appropriately?		
Method Does the tool have an acceptable level of reliability to justify this evaluation?		
Was an appropriate spectrum of participants included in the study?		
Were raters blind to key clinical characteristics of the participants?		
Was the tool administered as intended?		
Was the gold standard actually a gold standard?		
Was every participant administered both the comparison measure and the gold standard?		

Criteria	Yes / No / NA / NR	Describe and evaluate quality
Was the evaluation using the comparison tool independent to evaluation on the gold standard?		
In diagnostic studies were sensitivity, specificity, likelihood ratios and predictive values evaluated?		
Results Were the study hypotheses supported?		
What were the overall accuracy, sensitivity, specificity and predictive values for the tool?		
Did the authors provide confidence intervals to assist in interpreting the precision of their estimates?		
Does the tool have acceptable characteristics for its purpose?		
Longitudinal validity: Responsiveness—the ability of the assessment tool to detect change		
Method Does the tool have an acceptable level of reliability?		
Was the method for evaluating responsiveness clearly described and justified?		
Results Smallest detectable change (related to reliability) was less than minimally important change (judgment) Or, Minimally important change was outside the limit of agreement [a] And/Or Was there a strong positive relationship between change scores on the tool and those evaluated on an external measure?		

NA = Not applicable; NR = Nor reported; Criteria from [a] Terwee et al. 2007, [b] Bond & Fox 2007; Sources include Fritz & Wainner 2001; Greenhalgh 2001; Streiner & Norman 2003; Bond & Fox 2007; Terwee et al. 2007.

Table 11.4 gives a series of questions about the internal validity of reliability studies, and where they are available, provides some commonly agreed criteria against which to examine the results. Like all statistics, reliability coefficients are estimates and confidence intervals should be reported. In addition, like any other estimate, the precision (width of the confidence interval) is strongly influenced by the size of the sample from which it is calculated; that is, the number of observations per subject. While there are reported guidelines for acceptable levels of reliability (for example, Terwee and colleagues [2007] recommend ≥ 0.7), it is important to remember that different degrees of reliability may be required in different circumstances and varying degrees of reliability may be possible across different populations.

Christine Imms and Susan Greaves

Table 11.4: Criteria for evaluating studies that examine the reliability of measurement tools

Criteria	Yes / No NA / NR	Describe and evaluate quality
Design		
Did the study ask a clearly focused question about the reliability of the tool?		
Was the measurement aim of the tool clear?		
Method		
Was the target population clearly defined?		
Was there evidence that the participants represented the target population?		
Was the population of raters clearly defined?		
Was there evidence that the raters represented the target population of raters?		
Was there an appropriate number of raters for the purpose of the study?		
Was the tool administered as intended?		
Were the raters blind to the key clinical characteristics of the participants?		
Did raters complete the evaluations independently?		
For test-retest reliability, was the time before readministration appropriate? Consider potential learning effect, rater memory and/or likelihood of change to influence scores?		
Were analyses of consistency and agreement both undertaken? Was an ICC calculated for consistency (reliability) of scales with interval or ratio data? Was the Kappa coefficient provided for nominal data, or weighted Kappa for ordinal measures?		
Did analyses of agreement include estimates of the SEM or Bland and Altman's limits of agreement?		
Was person separation reliability provided for measurement analysed using the Rasch measurement model?		
Results		
Consistency; ICC's or weighted Kappa's ≥ 0.7[a].		
Agreement: The smallest detectable change (which is calculated as equal to $1.96 \times \sqrt{2} \times$ SEM) is smaller than the minimal important change or minimal important change is outside limits of agreement[a]		

NR = not reported; NA = not applicable; [a] = Criteria from Terwee et al. 2007. Sources include Streiner & Norman 2003; Terwee et al. 2007.

SUMMARY

Health professionals use tests and measures frequently in practice. We use the data obtained to support practice, to understand the condition of the client, to determine intervention choices and to measure change. We must know how, and for what purpose, a test or measure was developed so we can choose the right measure for our intended use. Understanding the psychometric properties of the tool is crucial to knowing how much trust we can place in the findings. Reading validity and reliability research critically will enable you to determine the relative validity and reliability of a tool. Conducting rigorous research when investigating the psychometric properties of a tool is an important contribution to the knowledge base of health professionals. Selecting (or developing) psychometrically sound measures when conducting other forms of research is essential to our ability to develop knowledge in the field.

TUTORIAL EXERCISES

1. UNDERSTANDING VALIDITY

Locate three assessments that are relevant to your profession or field of study. Decide:

☐ The primary or main purpose of the assessment tool. This may be defined in the manual or in papers describing the assessment tool.

☐ Is there a secondary purpose for which the assessment tool has been validated and/or used?

☐ What measurement properties are necessary to make this a good assessment tool for its intended purpose? To what extent does this tool have these measurement properties?

2. HOW RELIABLE ARE YOU?

This is a short exercise in evaluating intra-rater and/or inter-rater reliability.

☐ Using a goniometer, measure the range of elbow flexion and hip extension in at least 10 individuals on two occasions.

☐ Record your measurements but do not look at them again.

☐ At least 30 minutes later, measure both joints again.

☐ Using the limits of agreement method, plot the level of agreement between occasions of scoring for both joints. Use a hand-held or computer-based calculator for calculating means and standard deviations. Draw a plot similar to that shown in Figure 11.2 by hand.

Christine Imms and Susan Greaves

☐ What do the results tell you about your reliability?

☐ Can you identify sources of error? Could you have performed the measurement differently to reduce your error?

3. EVALUATING MEASUREMENT PROPERTIES

Select a test or measure used within your field of practice. Locate the primary publication(s) describing the tool (maybe the test manual).

☐ Using Table 11.3 and/or 11.4 to guide you, evaluate the quality of the research undertaken to develop the tool.

☐ What forms of validity were studied and how? What types of reliability were tested and how? Can you trust the findings?

☐ What were the results of the validity and reliability studies? How do these results influence the confidence with which you would use the tool?

FURTHER READING

Bond, T.G. & Fox, C. (2007). *Applying the Rasch model: Fundamental measurement in the human sciences*, 2nd edn. New Jersey: Lawrence Erlbaum Associates, Inc.

De Bie, R. (2001). Critical appraisal of prognostic studies: An introduction. *Physiotherapy Theory & Practice*, 17, 161–71.

Fawcett, A.J.L. (2007). *Principles of assessment and outcome measurement for occupational therapists and physiotherapists: Theory, skills and application*. <http://library.latrobe.edu.au/record=b2264691~S5>, accessed February 2009.

Greenhalgh, T. (2001). *How to read a paper: The basics of evidence based medicine*. London: BMJ Books.

Streiner, D.L. & Norman, G.R. (2003). *Health measurement scales: A practical guide to their development and use*, 3rd edn. Oxford: Oxford University Press.

Terwee, C.B., Bot, A.D.M., de Boer, M.R., van der Windt, D.A.W.M., Knol, D.L., Dekker, J., et al. (2007). Quality criteria were proposed for measurement properties of health status questionnaires. *Journal of Clinical Epidemiology*, 60, 34–42.

WEBSITES

www.canchild.ca/Default.aspx?tabid=192

> *This provides a set of guidelines and a structured rating form (Law 2004) that assists clinicians when considering the properties of assessment tools. These guidelines and a downloadable form are available on the CanCHILD website (Centre for Childhood Disability Research).*

www.phru.nhs.uk/Pages/PHD/resources.htm

> *For those who wish to critique research that investigates the accuracy of an assessment tool, the Critical Appraisal Skills Program (CASP) of the UK NHS Public Health resources unit >) has a downloadable Diagnostic studies appraisal guide, available at:*

www.phru.nhs.uk/Doc_Links/Diagnostic%20Tests%2012%20Questions.pdf

www.rasch.org

> *This is a very good web-based resource for understanding the Rasch measurement model. The reader is first guided to the Definitions of measurement section and research papers that are available on the site.*

www.socialresearchmethods.net/kb/index.php

> *For further reading available online, this web-text provides definitions and examples of a number of research methods. W.M.K. Trochim (2006)* Research methods knowledge base. *The Measurement section of the text provides additional detail about validity, reliability, scaling and measurement issues. This section of the book is located at:*

www.socialresearchmethods.net/kb/measure.php

Christine Imms and Susan Greaves

12

Single-subject Experimental Designs in Health Research

Miranda Rose

CHAPTER OBJECTIVES

In this chapter you will learn:

☐ how to define single-subject experimental designs (SSEDs), describe their basic components, and outline their origins

☐ how to describe SSEDs within the context of other research designs used to investigate treatment efficacy

☐ how to highlight the phase and stage of research and the type of research questions SSEDs are best suited to

☐ how to summarise basic statistical and visual analysis techniques commonly employed in SSEDs

KEY TERMS

Alternating treatment design

Meta-analysis

Multiple baseline design

Multiple probe design

Randomised controlled trial

Single-subject experimental design

INTRODUCTION

Every day, health and welfare practitioners make therapy and management strategy recommendations to their clients, patients and colleagues in health care and welfare teams. Increasingly, with the advances of evidence-based practice, practitioners want to base their recommendations on high-quality research evidence rather than rely solely on their own clinical experience or advice from more experienced colleagues (Reilly 2004). When contemporary health science students are asked to think about the type of research evidence on which practitioners base their treatment recommendations, students will often mention the so-called 'gold standard' of scientific treatment evidence, the **randomised control trial** (RCT) (see CHAPTERS 1, 8, 15, 16, 17).

> **Randomised controlled trial:** A clinical trial where participants are randomly assigned to groups in order to receive different interventions. This randomisation removes many of the effects that may bias the true result.

Many health and welfare students have had formal education and incidental community exposure to the concepts and methods involved in RCTs. For example, students usually know about the classic drug trial RCTs where participants are either treated with the drug under investigation (e.g. a blood pressure medication) or given a control placebo drug. Differences in the group (treated versus placebo) results (usually the group average score/ mean) are analysed for their statistical significance (in terms of how likely any differences in group results were obtained by chance) and recommendations are made about the effectiveness of the drug under investigation. See CHAPTER 15 to learn more about RCTs.

Some of the important issues about RCTs are now listed:

☐ Researcher bias and contamination are minimised through the random allocation of experimental participants to either treatment or no-treatment groups and the researchers are blinded as to which participants are receiving the experimental or the control treatments.

☐ Large samples of participants are recruited so that the sample might more likely be a true representation of the overall population of interest rather than a special, unrepresentative subgroup, and therefore the results of the study are generalisable to similar groups of people beyond those investigated in the study.

☐ The behaviours or physical measures (e.g. blood pressure, grip strength) being studied are carefully defined and the measurement devices used to take the pre- and post-treatment measures are valid and reliable.

☐ Other factors/variables that might influence how participants respond to treatment are carefully defined and controlled (e.g. other medications, diet, exercise, age, gender).

☐ Replication of the trial is possible because the study protocols are so well defined and clearly described.

Miranda Rose

DOING RESEARCH

Chris

Chris, a physiotherapist working in a rehabilitation centre, has been using two types of treatment for strengthening hand grip in patients with hemiparesis following stroke. A search of the scientific treatment literature fails to show any strong evidence for either of these treatments. Chris knows that many of her physiotherapy colleagues use the two techniques and report good results. She has also seen positive results in patients with both of the techniques. However, she is concerned about having a stronger evidence base to support the use of the techniques in her clinical practice. She would also like to know if one of the techniques is more effective than the other. How could she get the evidence she needs?

David

David is an occupational therapist and academic staff member undertaking research at a university. David wants to investigate the efficacy of sensori-motor integration treatment for pre-school children with general developmental delay. One option is for David to design a large-group comparison study where participants are randomly allocated to either a treatment or a control group. However, David knows that it is very difficult to recruit large numbers of children with developmental delay, so he thinks a group comparison study will be very difficult to mount. What other research design options does David have?

ARE RCTS AND GROUP DESIGNS ALWAYS THE DESIGNS OF CHOICE?

While the above characteristics of RCTs are usually true, I argue that there are some serious limitations in using RCTs for investigating the effectiveness of many physical and behavioural treatments that might be recommended by health and welfare practitioners (e.g. relaxation therapy for stress disorder; massage for chronic knee pain; word meaning therapy for aphasic word retrieval errors; diary use for memory loss after head injury). An RCT is generally not a suitable research design when:

☐ the conditions we are treating are complex and multifaceted and the client/patient group has a high degree of variability. For example, people with aphasia (a language and communication disorder following brain damage) present in extremely variable ways with a huge range of severity and type of symptoms. Therefore treatments for aphasia need to take account of the large range and type of aphasic symptoms: one size (therapy) does not fit all! Such high variability in the client group creates two major problems in employing an RCT to investigate treatment effectiveness:

    ☐ RCTs generally require large numbers of participants in order to be effective. When client/patient conditions are complex and multifaceted and there are many variables that require control, it is even more important to have a large number of participants so that the power of the study is high. Unfortunately, when investigating complex conditions, it is very difficult to recruit a large group of participants with the same type of impairment.

☐ In RCTs, the difference between the response of the experimental and control groups to the treatment is examined with a powerful parametric statistical test (such as Student's t-tests or an analysis of variance) (see CHAPTER 24). These statistical tests have a set of requirements (assumptions) about the nature of the data. One assumption is that the amount of variability in the groups being compared is similar (this is called the assumption of homogeneity of variance or equality of variance; you can look this up in any textbook on parametric statistics, for example Portney and Watkins [2009], or on websites devoted to explaining statistics in plain language such as <http://davidmlane.com/hyperstat/A45619.html>). When the samples being studied have unequal amounts of variability we violate one of the assumptions of using the parametric statistical test. There are some mathematical ways to attempt to overcome this problem. However, when we start to compare the mean differences of two groups with very different amounts of variability, the overall results become difficult to interpret and apply to the 'average' client we might be seeing in the clinic or workplace (see also CHAPTERS 24, 25).

☐ We are trying to carry out research in the clinical/working environment versus experimental environment and we do not have the funding for a large-scale clinical trial or group study of treatments for complex conditions that require hundreds or even thousands of participants. In the clinical setting, we may also not have the flexibility to adapt our treatment protocols beyond the current accepted regimens.

☐ There are simply too few individuals with a particular rare condition that can be recruited for a group study.

☐ The nature of the study is too onerous to expect large numbers of individuals to want to participate.

☐ The therapeutic procedures are too expensive to run across large numbers of participants.

☐ The investigation of a treatment is in the early phases of development. In the early stages of research (called Phase One research) into a particular treatment, we are often unsure about how potent the new treatment will be and what sort of treatment effects we will obtain. This lack of knowledge makes it very difficult to make a sensible calculation about the number of participants that need to be recruited in order to make the study powerful and meaningful. There is a danger of designing the study on too large a scale and spending unnecessary money and resources on it, or equally making the study too small and finding that the results are not meaningful. In Phase One research, we are often unaware of what variables require control and what factors determine candidacy for treatment. Therefore in

Miranda Rose

the early stages pilot-level research work is undertaken to answer some of these questions. Sometimes small-group comparison studies (rather than large RCTs) are carried out.

☐ It is important to observe how participants respond to treatments across time (e.g. how quickly or slowly they respond, how variable the response is across time, that is, the nature of their learning/change). In RCTs, measures of participants are typically taken once before the treatment and a second time when the treatment finishes. This enables a simple 2-snapshot window into the response to treatment. With the large numbers of participants required for RCTs, taking multiple measures of each participant across time becomes impossible or unrealistically expensive to mount (see CHAPTER 15).

Fortunately, there are alternatives to RCT and large-group experimental designs for investigating the effectiveness of various treatments. One powerful alternative is the single-subject experimental design (SSEDs). SSEDs are being increasingly reported in the health science experimental literature so it is important for students to gain an understanding of their strengths and limitations. Further, many clinicians who undertake research in the clinic or workplace use SSEDs so routinely that students will be exposed to them during their clinical practice experiences.

WHAT ARE SINGLE-SUBJECT EXPERIMENTAL DESIGNS?

A **single-subject experimental design** (SSED) is an experimental research method that focuses on a single individual and their response to treatment(s) across time. SSEDs always have at least a baseline phase (usually denoted as the A phase) where measurements of the behaviour (or system) to be treated (the dependent variable) are taken on several occasions during a no-treatment phase. This tells us what the participants' abilities are like before treatment commences and if there is any variability in the pre-treatment ability across time. SSEDs always have a treatment phase (usually denoted as the B phase) where measurements

---

Single-subject experimental design: An experimental research method that focuses on a single individual and their response to treatment(s) across time.

Meta-analysis: A statistical technique that combines the results of similar studies into a single result that provides an estimate of the overall effect.

---

continue to be taken while the behaviour is treated (see the first two panels in Figure 12.1 for an example using mock data). There are an enormous range of SSED designs beyond this basic and quite weak A-B design, some of which are quite sophisticated and will be explained in the next section. In many studies, the researchers carry out a series of SSEDs so they can replicate the findings from a single SSED (it worked for this person; does it work for a second, third etc.?) and create better evidence for generalising the findings beyond a particular individual. In studies where several SSEDs are reported, the data is first analysed individually. Sometimes the strength of the treatment effect demonstrated in each individual study is combined in a **meta-analysis** to create an overall effect size for the particular series of SSEDs.

Figure 12.1: Example of A-B-A-B withdrawal design

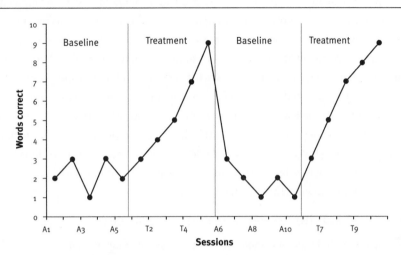

Terms used for SSEDs

Several terms have been used interchangeably for SSEDs. These include:

☐ single-case designs or single-case experimental designs
☐ single-subject designs
☐ interrupted time series designs
☐ N of 1
☐ small N designs.

SSEDs versus case studies: they are not the same!

There is an important distinction to make between two terms (and two types of research) that students and practitioners often use interchangeably but which in fact produce very different levels of research quality. These terms are *SSEDs* and *case studies*. In well-designed SSEDs, there is careful and rigorous control of the behaviour or attribute that is being treated (the dependent variable) (e.g. muscle strength, finger dexterity, picture-naming skills) and of the actual treatment being investigated (the independent variable) (e.g. strength training, dexterity training, word retrieval training). There is also a significant attempt to minimise the influence of any other variables that might influence the outcomes in treatment, such as improvements resulting from clients who simply get better over time, differences in skills between the treating therapists, and the varying motivation of the participants at different stages of the experiment. This careful control of experimental and extraneous variables means that the word 'experimental', in the term *single-subject experimental design*, is warranted. In other words, the investigator starts with a testable hypothesis, operationally defines the dependent and independent variables, carefully measures them, and attempts to minimise bias in the study.

In case studies, however, clinicians report detailed observations and measurements from a particular patient/client/case usually in natural situations without directly manipulating or controlling variables. Therefore SSEDs are true empirical research designs because when carried out well, we can be reasonably certain that any treatment effects demonstrated are a direct result of the treatment and not a result of some confounding variable. In case studies, on the other hand, it is very difficult to know what caused any observed and documented changes in behaviour. Case studies are useful in highlighting the clinical and research field possible therapeutic effects that require more rigorous investigation. Unfortunately, many people use the terms 'case study' and 'single-case design' or 'single-subject experimental design' interchangeably. It is important to consider whether a study you are reading is actually a case study or a true single-subject experimental design because the strength, utility and generalisability of the evidence they produce are very different.

When is an SSED the research design of choice?

SSEDs are the research design of choice when any of the following are true:

- ☐ The investigation of the effectiveness of a treatment is in the early stages (Phase 1 studies).
- ☐ The nature of the condition or the treatment is complex and the participants that can be recruited to research investigations are highly variable.
- ☐ The treatment is being investigated in the context of a rare condition.
- ☐ We want to understand the nature of the participant's response to the treatment (how fast, how variable) across time, not just at two discrete points (before and after treatment). In other words, we are very interested in the process of change across time, its patterns and variability, not just that change does or does not happen.
- ☐ The research is occurring in real-life clinical or community settings (Morgan & Morgan 2009; Portney & Watkins 2009).

DOING RESEARCH

Chris

Chris wants to determine if one of the treatments she is using is better than another for the post-stroke patients she treats in the rehabilitation centre. When she did a literature search of the scientific treatment literature she couldn't find evidence about either of the treatments. Chris is working in a clinical environment without access to large-scale research grant funds or research staff. Is a SSED appropriate to help her investigate her clinical question?

David

David wants to investigate the efficacy of a treatment for general developmental delay in pre-school children. The children with developmental delay present with delays of various types and severity, and as a group are quite heterogeneous. As there is such a large degree of variability in the children, David knows he would need to design a group study with a very large N (number of participants) in order to take care of the number of variables he would need to control for in the study. David knows it is very difficult to recruit such large numbers of children with developmental delay and also that he can't easily recruit large numbers of very similar participants. Would a series of SSEDs be an appropriate research design option for David?

WHEN DID SSEDS DEVELOP? ARE THEY A POPULAR DESIGN?

Many students and practitioners have commented to me that SSEDs are a 'new' or extremely 'novel' research design. In fact, today's range of SSEDs originated in the early experimental work carried out by the famous behavioural scientist B.F. Skinner in the 1940s. Skinner and his colleagues were interested in the ways in which animals learnt over time and therefore the researchers needed an observational and investigative strategy that would allow multiple samples of behaviour to be analysed (Ittenbach & Lawhead 1996). Skinner was frustrated at the popular methods of the era, which involved group analysis of behavioural data. Skinner felt the group aggregating of the data created smooth learning curves that actually obscured the complexity and individual variability associated with true learning. At the time, there was a strong movement in the field of psychology towards group analysis techniques and parametric statistics (such as t-tests, and ANOVAs; see CHAPTER 24), and the individual analysis methods of the behaviour analysts were seen by some as less powerful and inferior. This meant that often the research work of the behaviour analysts was not accepted for publication in the major psychology journals of the time, leading Skinner to start the now prestigious *Journal of the Experimental Analysis of Behaviour* (*JEAB*) in 1958. *JEAB* continues to publish work where the data are analysed individually rather than aggregated (Morgan & Morgan 2009). The power struggle between researchers using large-group studies with parametric statistics and small observational studies with no or non-parametric statistics continues to this day.

Between 1939 and 1963, Dukes (as cited in Ittenbach & Lawhead 1996) reported that 246 single-subject research papers were published, paving the way for the fields of education and psychology to emphasise the SSED in present-day treatment/intervention research. More recently, the disciplines within allied health and nursing have taken to SSEDs enthusiastically. For example, over the past decade in the subdiscipline of aphasia treatment research in speech pathology, SSEDs have become the dominant research design. While in many evidence hierarchies SSEDs are ranked at level 3 or 4 of a 4-tier system (e.g. the NHMRC evidence hierarchy), Guyatt et al. (2000), writing in the *Journal of the American Medical Association*, rank an RCT using SSEDs at the top of their evidence hierarchy. Clearly, there are differences of

Miranda Rose

opinion in scientific circles concerning the strength of evidence obtained from well-conducted SSEDs and series of SSEDs, some of which still reflect the power struggles within scientific circles dating from Skinner's time.

TYPES OF SSEDS

As I have mentioned earlier, there are a variety of SSEDs structured to meet the particular type of the research question, the nature of the treatment type(s) and the participant characteristics being investigated. I have suggested earlier that the basic A-B design is descriptive rather than a truly experimental design (McReynolds & Kearns 1984). The A-B is a weak design because it is difficult to be sure that any change in behaviour noted in the B phase actually relates to the treatment and not to some other confounding variable such as general stimulation or natural recovery. A stronger, more commonly employed SSED is the A-B-A or A-B-A-B or withdrawal/ reversal design. The logic of the A-B-A-B design is that after treatment stops the behaviour under observation (e.g. number of angry outbursts in the classroom) will return to baseline or near baseline levels. Once treatment commences again in the second B phase, changes in the behaviour will occur that replicate those seen in the first B phase, thus supporting the view that it was the treatment that resulted in the behaviour change. Figure 12.1 shows an example of an A-B-A-B design. The participant's response to baseline, treatment, and withdrawal phases is shown by graphing the dependent variable (in this example, the number of words spoken correctly) along the y-axis and time (in this case the treatment session) on the x-axis.

As I have suggested earlier, however, in the social and health sciences it is rare for treatments to result in transient change. As many of our treatments result in more permanent or longer-lasting change, the A-B-A-B design is inappropriate as it is unlikely that the behaviours measured will in fact return to baseline levels after the treatment stops. Further, it is often unethical to withdraw treatments. Fortunately, there are several more sophisticated SSEDs to choose from that take account of the more permanent changes in behaviour and states that are frequently achieved in our treatments. The next section describes two of the more commonly employed SSEDs: multiple baseline experimental designs and alternating treatment designs.

Multiple baseline experimental designs

When it is unlikely that treated behaviours will return to baseline levels after withdrawal of the treatment, multiple baseline designs are frequently the design of choice. In **multiple baseline designs**, the effects of treatment are replicated across several participants or across different target behaviours. The design also allows for replication across different treatment conditions within a single participant so that the relative effectiveness of one treatment over another can be investigated. In multiple baseline designs, baseline data is first collected and graphed across each condition (see Figure 12.2 for an example). Treatment is then applied to one condition while the other conditions are kept untreated.

Multiple baseline design: In this design, the effects of treatment are replicated across several participants or across different target behaviours, and participants act as their own controls.

Figure 12.2: Example of a multiple baseline design (dotted lines in panel 1 = celeration lines)

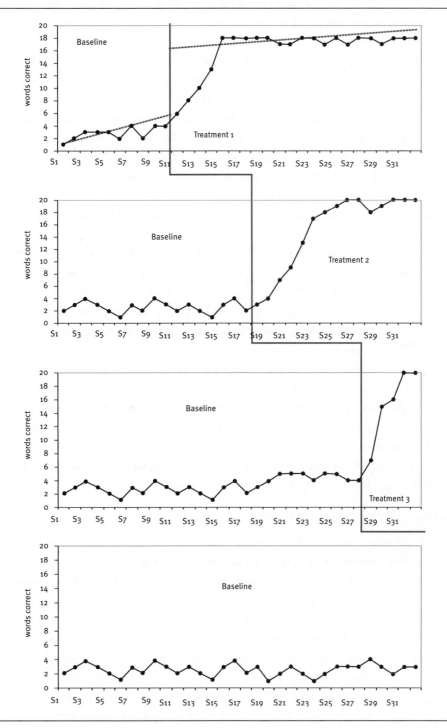

Once a set criterion is reached or a set number of treatments have occurred, treatment is applied to the second condition while the third (and perhaps fourth) is kept in baseline. Again, treatment continues until a set criterion is reached or a set number of treatments have been given. Finally, treatment is applied to the third condition. In this way, we can see the effects of the three treatment types in a stepwise manner while the other behaviours are kept in untreated baseline states. The multiple baseline design allows the researcher to see change in a treated behaviour while there is no or limited change in another related behaviour, making it more certain that any change seen in the first condition is a result of the treatment rather than an extraneous variable. In this way, participants act as their own controls. Further, because measurements are taken and graphed across time the researcher gains a clear view of the nature of any learning taking place in one condition as compared to another, allowing for assessments of the efficiency of the treatments and stability of any treatment effects.

A variation of the multiple baseline design is the **multiple probe design** (Horner & Baer 1978). Sometimes it is clear that a component of behaviour of interest (e.g. finger grip strength of a patient with right hemiparesis following stroke) is a vital component of a larger behaviour (such as holding and writing with a pen). When this is the case, it seems rather pointless to repeatedly measure the participant's capacity to write a sentence if they are yet unable to grip a pen. Similarly, sometimes it seems pointless continuing to repeatedly measure a behaviour that is proving to remain incredibly stable during a study. The researcher has to weigh up the risks of taking unnecessary measures of behaviour and therefore adding an unnecessary burden to the participant, plus added costs associated with extra analysis and reliability measures, versus losing experimental control if an inadequate number of baseline measures are taken. The multiple probe design offers a cost-effective alternative to the multiple baseline design in these situations. Not all probes are taken in every session but rather some are taken at a predetermined and less frequent schedule or once a requisite skill is obtained.

Multiple probe design: A cost-effective alternative to the multiple baseline design. Some probes are taken at a predetermined and less frequent schedule or once a requisite skill is obtained.

Alternating treatment designs

Another useful design when wanting to compare multiple treatments or placebo treatments is the **alternating treatment design**. Here, two or three treatments of interest are provided in rapid succession and in an alternating format, within a session, in a session-by-session format or in a day-by-day format. The results are graphed together to show clearly the difference in rate and stability of learning in each treatment condition (see Figure 12.3 for an example). Strictly speaking, in alternating treatment designs there is no need for the baseline phase. But by including a baseline phase, interpretation of the results is easier because we can clearly see any treatment effects (in comparison to pre-treatment results), and this is particularly so if the effects of the treatments being compared are similar.

Alternating treatment design: Two or three treatments are provided in rapid succession and in an alternating format. The results are graphed together to show the difference in rate and stability of learning.

Figure 12.3: Example of an alternating treatment design (adapted from Rose & Douglas 2006)

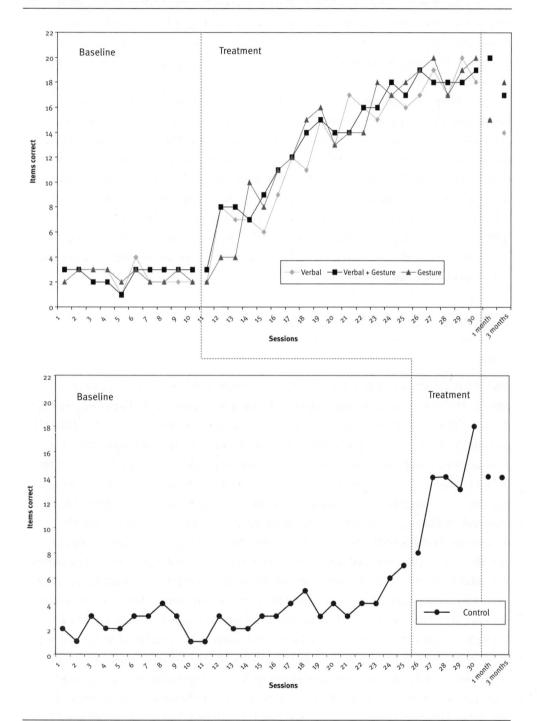

One advantage of the alternating treatment design is that comparative results can be obtained more quickly than in multiple baseline or sequential designs (such as A-B-C-D-A designs). However, in order to take account of any potential order effects (where the order of the treatments is important), systematic counterbalancing or randomisation of treatment sequence is required. The design is not suitable when we are expecting generalisation (or leakage) from one treatment to another.

An example of an alternating treatment design is provided here from a study we did investigating the comparative effects of three types of treatments for a word production impairment (in this case an acquired apraxia of speech) in a man following a left hemisphere stroke. The treatments were a verbal (talking only) treatment, a gesture (hand movements only) treatment and a combined verbal + gesture treatment. Figure 12.3 shows the participant's response to the three treatments and a comparison to the baseline phases and an untreated control group. Each of the three treatments was given in every treatment session, each treatment to one of three carefully matched sets of 20 words. A fourth set of words was never treated and formed the control set. The order of the three treatments was rotated each session to control for any possible order effects.

DOING RESEARCH

Chris

An A-B-C-A design, where B is the first treatment phase and C is the second treatment phase, would be an appropriate design for Chris to investigate the relative effectiveness of the two different exercise treatments (treatment M and P) for hand grip strength. Following an initial stable baseline period where measures of hand grip (e.g. maximum squeeze pressure on pressure meter; maximum time for holding a 1 kg weight) are taken on three of four occasions, hand grip treatment M is implemented for, say, 10 sessions. The hand grip strength measures are continuously probed throughout the design and graphically displayed. Following 10 sessions of treatment M, 10 sessions of treatment P would commence. Then the final A phase occurs, where the hand grip measures are taken to demonstrate whether improvements in the grip strength are maintained or decline during the withdrawal phase. Comparisons are then made of the progress achieved during each of the treatment phases. The design could be strengthened by including a second probe measure of an impaired skill/behaviour not expected to be directly affected by the grip strength training but possibly affected by general therapeutic stimulation or spontaneous recovery of the nervous system after stroke, such as sitting balance. If positive changes are demonstrated in grip strength probes during the therapy but not the sitting balance probes, it is clearer that the specific treatment caused the changes in grip strength rather than other extraneous variables such as general stimulation. The design would need to be replicated across several participants, alternating the order of the treatments M and P to take account of any possible order effects.

David

David could definitely use a series of SSEDs to investigate the effectiveness of the treatment for general developmental delay. Depending on how potent he thought the treatment was and assuming there would be some return to pretreatment behaviours during a withdrawal phase following a short burst of treatment, he could use an A-B-A-B design. In the first burst of treatment some improvement in target behaviours may be obtained, but insufficient to reach desired criteria. Then, with a second burst of treatment where target levels of behaviour might be reached, he could demonstrate the effect of treatment over and above the baseline and withdrawal levels. However, if the treatment was potent and it was not expected that behaviours would return to baseline levels during withdrawal of treatment, a multiple baseline across behaviours design would be suitable. After a baseline phase measuring ball-catching skills, pencil grip and focused attention span during a storybook reading task, treatment would focus on, say, ball-catching skills first, while pencil grip and focused attention in a storybook task were kept in baseline. Then treatment would move to one of the remaining behaviours while the other two remained in baseline, and so on. The order of the treatments (for pencil grip, ball-catching, storybook attention) would need to be randomised across the series of participants to minimise potential order effects.

ANALYSIS OF SSED DATA

Visual analysis methods

The participant response to treatment (and during baseline and no treatment phases) is usually graphed on a standard case chart (e.g. Figures 12.1, 12.2, 12.3). The dependent variable (behaviour or physical attribute being measured) is graphed on the y-axis and the time-frame of the treatment (sessions, number or days, weeks etc.) is graphed on the x-axis. Visual inspection of the graphed results is by far the most popular analysis method (Portney & Watkins 2009). A visual analysis is made of the changes in the performance curves from baseline to intervention phases and between intervention phases. Three important aspects to review in the visual analysis are:

- the level of the graphed data (e.g. low, middle, high)
- the slope (or trend) of the graphed data (e.g. rising/accelerating; falling/decelerating; flat) and thus the rate of change
- the stability of the graphed data (degree of variability and pattern in the data).

These three aspects are reviewed within and across each phase of the study (e.g. baseline, treatment, withdrawal, maintenance and so on).

When relying on visual analysis techniques, it is important during the initial baseline phase that the participant response is either stable or moving in the opposite direction to what is expected during the treatment phases. For example, if we expect an increase in scores during treatment, then it is preferable to have a flat or falling baseline. Then during the treatment phase if the scores rise, it is clear that the positive changes occurring during the treatment phases are not simply extensions of what was beginning to occur during the baseline. For example, when a slowly rising (accelerating) baseline meets a slowly accelerating treatment phase the researcher is left wondering if the trend established in baseline (accelerating) is simply continuing during treatment, and therefore that the treatment is not having a significant effect. Often researchers decide on achieving a pre-set criterion of baseline stability (e.g. no more then 5% variability) before commencing a treatment phase. If the stability criterion is not met, a different behaviour (dependent variable) may need to be observed, measured and recorded or else the study results will be difficult to interpret.

Fortunately, visual analysis can be improved by several design features and graphing techniques:

- ☐ Baseline and treatment phase lengths should be roughly equivalent.
- ☐ Measures of the behaviour being studied (dependent variable) such as counts, percentages, times correct are plotted on the y-axis while the time measures such as day, week, month are plotted on the x-axis.
- ☐ Celeration lines can be drawn for each phase. The celeration lines estimate the slope of each data phase and provide a visual aid to compare the slopes across the phases (Portney & Watkins 2009). These lines are drawn by calculating the median scores in each half of each phase, drawing a horizontal line through the median scores in each half phase, drawing a vertical line through the middle score of each half phase, and then connecting the two points of intersection between the horizontal and the vertical lines (see example in the first panel of Figure 12.2).

Statistical analysis methods

It is important to realise that visual analysis has its critics. Threats to the reliability of visual inspection have been clearly documented (Matyas & Greenwood 1990). When there is high variability in the data or there are accelerating baselines, statistical methods are likely to be more reliable than visual inspection methods. A full description of possible statistical analyses is beyond the scope of this chapter, but Portney and Watkins (2009) provide a clear basic summary, Franklin and colleagues (1996) provide a more extensive discussion, and Howard and associates (submitted) have summarised the major issues and made useful suggestions about statistical analysis of SSEDs. See also CHAPTER 24. One thing to remember is that a combination of visual and basic statistical analyses may be powerful. For example, when visual inspection leaves some uncertainty, we can supplement the visual analysis with simple non-parametric tests. In a study we carried out to investigate the effectiveness of three treatments for aphasic verb retrieval impairments, we compared the last baseline score and last treatment score in each condition with the non-parametric McNemar's test (Rose & Sussmilch 2008). In a more elaborate statistical analysis of the response to treatments for noun retrieval impairment, we used curve-fitting techniques (Rose et al. 2002).

Some authors have attempted to integrate the results from several different SSED studies, all investigating treatment for a particular condition (e.g. aphasic word retrieval difficulty). Meta-analysis of single-subject experimental data is possible, particularly when using the overall effect sizes of interventions from each study. However, there is considerable controversy about how to validly calculate effect sizes from SSED data. Innovative methods are emerging and these offer hope for greater strength of evidence from series of SSEDs in the very near future (see Beretvas & Chung 2008 and Portney & Watkins 2009 for more details).

Reliability of the data

As SSEDs are true experimental designs, researchers must meet data reliability and validity standards expected in empirical research (see also CHAPTERS 1, 11, 13). The reliability of the data is checked by having a second rater re-rate the behaviours measured in the dependent variable (e.g. number of positive statements per 20-minute conversation) as well as the fidelity of any treatment provided. In treatment fidelity checks, a second rater views videotape of the treatment sessions or live treatment sessions, and analyses how accurately the researcher employed the treatment protocol as specified in the study.

SUMMARY

Single-subject experimental designs are a type of experimental research design well suited to and commonly employed for the investigation of treatment efficacy. This is particularly so for the investigation of complex multi-step treatments or for populations with a low overall incidence or high complexity and variability. SSEDs are very well suited to clinic-based research. A well-designed SSED with replication across participants or within one participant across behaviours or conditions provides evidence with strong internal validity. A series of well-designed SSEDs investigating a particular treatment for a particular condition, and then subjected to a meta-analysis, provides very strong evidence. There are a variety of SSEDs to suit a range of treatment efficacy questions including alternating treatment designs, multiple baseline designs and multiple probe designs. While visual analysis of the graphic display of participant response to treatments is common, the use of statistical analysis techniques is becoming more widespread. Further, statisticians are currently developing valid ways to carry out meta-analyses of series of SSEDs, which will assist in providing highly powerful treatment research evidence in the very near future.

Miranda Rose

TUTORIAL EXERCISES

1   You are a health practitioner who recently attended a seminar where a new treatment for memory loss following acquired brain injury was presented. The treatment was derived from sound theoretical principles but has no current scientific evidence supporting it. The treatment involves learning and implementing several different strategies. It is suggested that clients require at least 10 hours of treatment before they begin to acquire any of the strategies taught. Every year, you and your colleagues treat several clients with acquired brain injuries who have memory loss. The clients are diverse in their presentation and in other post-brain injury physical and cognitive difficulties. You want to know if the new memory treatment is any more effective than another treatment that has been used in the clinic for some years, similarly with little published research evidence. Discuss ways in which you could go about designing a research study to answer your question concerning comparative treatment efficacy.

2   Discuss the strengths and weaknesses of using a randomised control trial versus a series of single-subject experimental designs to investigate the effectiveness of a behavioural treatment to improve eye contact during adult–child interactions for pre-school children with autism. You might want to split the tutorial group into two teams: one team prepares the arguments for using an RCT while the other team prepares the arguments for using SSEDs. You could then hold a formal debate (three students elected per team) to compare and contrast the arguments.

FURTHER READING

Portney, L. & Watkins, M. (2009). *Foundations of clinical research: Applications to practice*, 3rd edn. New Jersey: Prentice Hall Health.

Morgan, D. & Morgan, R. (2009). *Single-case research methods for the behavioural and health sciences*. Los Angeles: Sage Publications.

WEBSITES

davidmlane.com/hyperstat/A45619.html

   A website providing interactive tutorials on basic statistics by Associate Professor Lane, Psychology, Statistics and Management at Rice University in the USA.

13

Surveys and Questionnaires in Health Research

Margot Schofield and Christine Knauss

CHAPTER OBJECTIVES

In this chapter you will learn:

- ☐ why we use surveys and questionnaires
- ☐ what are the main survey designs
- ☐ how measurement theory is applied to survey research
- ☐ how surveys are designed
- ☐ how survey questions are constructed
- ☐ what are the main methods for administering surveys

KEY TERMS

Cross-sectional survey

Interval data

Likert scale

Longitudinal cohort survey

Measurement errors

Nominal data

Ordinal data

Questionnaire

Ratio data

Reliability

Standardised scale

Survey

Surveys to test intervention effects

Validity

Verbal rating scale

Visual analogue scale

INTRODUCTION

Surveys are a common descriptive research method in the health and social sciences (Sarantakos 2005; Neuman 2006; de Vaus 2007). Survey respondents are asked a series of questions in a standard manner so that responses can be easily quantified and analysed statistically. This enables the researcher to describe the characteristics of the sample being studied and to make generalisations to the larger population of interest. Surveys are particularly useful for collecting information about research phenomena that are not directly observable or measurable (Bowling 2002). They are also useful for collecting data from people who are widely distributed geographically, since direct contact between researcher and research participant is not necessary (Sarantakos 2005). Survey responses are derived primarily from self-completed surveys or through interview.

A **questionnaire** is a specific type of written survey made up of a structured series of questions. Questionnaires usually have highly standardised response options so that data can be easily analysed and compared across individuals or groups (Bowling 2002). Surveys and questionnaires can also include more open-ended questions that invite respondents to write their own free responses to the questions. Many surveys include a mix of both open and closed response options (de Vaus 2007).

The accuracy of information obtained through survey methods depends on many factors such as the way the sample is selected and recruited, and how the questions are designed, asked and recorded. The validity of the data obtained also depends on the sensitivity of the questions asked, the motivation of the respondents to answer truthfully, and their ability to answer the questions accurately. Surveys can be a very efficient method of obtaining information about individuals but, like all research methods, have a number of limitations that researchers should attempt to minimise.

> **Survey:** A descriptive research method where respondents are asked a series of questions in a standard manner so that responses can be easily quantified and analysed statistically.

> **Questionnaire:** A specific type of written survey made up of a structured series of questions. Questionnaires usually have highly standardised response options so that data can be easily analysed and compared.

WHY DO WE USE SURVEYS AND QUESTIONNAIRES?

Surveys are a popular research method because they tend to be the most economical and efficient way of collecting data about a range of personal characteristics, health symptoms, history and behaviours. Large amounts of data can be collected in a fairly short time and responses can be recorded in ways that are easily entered into data files for analysis. The capacity to ask many questions around a particular research topic also allows for more sophisticated research questions to be asked and multivariate analysis to be undertaken on the data.

One important assumption underlying the use of survey research methods is that the survey respondents themselves are the best source of accurate information about these questions. This method is thus particularly useful for collecting information about social and psychological concepts such as beliefs, attitudes, opinions, expectations, knowledge, and satisfaction with health care (Bowling 2002). For such research questions, the individual is usually the best source of such conceptual information.

In determining whether a survey is the best method of collecting information about a particular research question, the researcher must decide whether a subjective response will yield more accurate information than a more objective form of measurement. For instance, if you want to determine the extent of high blood pressure in a sample, you are likely to get a more accurate response by objectively measuring the blood pressure with a validated blood pressure monitor than by simply asking the sample (see CHAPTER 11). Similarly, for some problems, accuracy of response may depend on who is asked. For instance, asking a young child about the severity of their behaviour problems may not be the most accurate method. It may be better to ask teachers and/or parents to rate the child's behaviour over time.

There are, however, a range of practical and methodological reasons why a survey may be the method of choice, even for research topics where more objective methods are likely to yield more accurate data. For instance, if we take the blood pressure example, the choice of method depends on what we actually want to know about the blood pressure. If the question is, 'What is the incidence of high blood pressure in a particular sample?', then an objective measure will be the best method, since there are likely to be many people with high blood pressure who are unaware of this until tested, and the research question calls for a precise estimate of the incidence (see 'Doing research' below).

If the question seeks to understand the knowledge, attitudes or behaviour of people who have previously been diagnosed by their doctor with high blood pressure, then a survey may well be the method of choice. In making this decision, we would need to assume that people will know that they have been diagnosed with high blood pressure. There will be some error attributable to this assumption. However, this error will be outweighed by the benefits of economically identifying those who have been diagnosed with the condition, and then administering a range of self-report measures. This is because the research question seeks to understand self-reported information associated with those who know they have high blood pressure.

DOING RESEARCH

Survey design is linked to research question

Example: Research on high blood pressure

The decision to choose a survey design depends on the aim of the study. Some examples are shown below.

Study Question: What is the incidence of high blood pressure in a population?

Study design: The best method of answering this question is not through a self-complete survey, rather by taking objective measures of blood pressure from a random sample of the population. This is because many people may have high blood pressure but might

Margot Schofield and Christine Knauss

be unaware of it. Therefore the most accurate method to answer the research question is to measure actual blood pressure using the most reliable measuring instrument for this purpose. If a survey was undertaken, it is likely that the incidence of high blood pressure would be seriously underestimated.

Study Question: Among people diagnosed with high blood pressure, what are their attitudes towards medication?

Study design: A self-complete survey would be an appropriate method to answer this research question, since the sampling frame is limited to those who know they have high blood pressure, and the main information sought, attitudes towards medication, requires a self-report response.

WHAT ARE THE MAIN SURVEY DESIGNS?

There are three main study designs in which surveys and questionnaires are used. The first is in *cross-sectional research* where the primary purpose is descriptive. The second is in longitudinal cohort research, in which the primary purpose is to track changes over time. The third study design is *experimental or intervention research* in which the primary question is whether a particular intervention or experiment produces change in outcomes. Each of these is described in more detail and the role of surveys explained.

Cross-sectional surveys

A **cross-sectional survey** gives a profile of the sample at one point in time. It cannot make inferences about past or future and relies largely on descriptive and correlational analyses (see also CHAPTER 14). An example of such a survey is the National Health Survey undertaken by the Australian Bureau of Statistics (ABS), shown in 'Doing research' below (ABS 2006a). On a smaller scale, typical cross-sectional surveys commonly employed in health services include surveys of variables such as symptoms, pain, patient satisfaction and patient quality of life. In the broader community, surveys of health risk behaviours, health screening behaviours and use of health services or medications are common.

A **cross-sectional survey** gives a profile of the sample at one point in time. It yields a profile of the sample at that time and allows associations between variables to be explored.

DOING RESEARCH

Example of cross-sectional survey

National Health survey 2004–05

The Australian Bureau of Statistics has conducted cross-sectional National Health Surveys every few years to track the state of health of the nation and trends in health service use. The 2004–05 survey results were published in 2006 (ABS 2006a).

The survey was designed to obtain national benchmarks on a wide range of health issues and to enable changes in health to be monitored over time. These National Health Surveys are cross-sectional surveys in that a new sample is selected for each administration. A comparison of trends can be made across time however, because large representative samples are chosen on each occasion.

Research topics

The National Health Survey collected information about:

☐   the health status of the population
☐   health-related aspects of lifestyle and other health risk factors
☐   the use of health services and other actions people had recently taken for their health.

Examples of particular health issues included:

☐   long-term illnesses experienced
☐   mental well-being
☐   injuries
☐   consultations with doctors and other health professionals
☐   health risk factors such as alcohol consumption, smoking, exercise, body mass and dietary practices.

Sample

Approximately 25 900 people from all States and Territories and across all age groups were included. The strategy included interviewing one adult (aged 18 years or more) and one child (where applicable) from each sampled dwelling.

Source: ABS 2006a

A cross-sectional survey can tell us what proportion of a sample or population reports certain symptoms, diseases, or characteristics, and whether these are more prevalent among certain sections of the population. For instance, the ABS survey found that 62 per cent of males and 45 per cent of females were classified as overweight or obese based on their Body Mass Index (BMI, a measure of relative weight based on height and weight ratio).

Longitudinal surveys

Longitudinal cohort surveys administer the same set of questions to individuals on repeated occasions and seek to understand how individuals or groups change over time. They could be undertaken simply to monitor changes in health or some other variable over time, or to measure outcomes of certain interventions or treatments. A study demonstrating the first purpose, to monitor change over time, is the Australian Longitudinal Study on Women's Health. This large-scale prospective

Longitudinal cohort surveys administer the same set of questions to individuals on repeated occasions and seek to understand how individuals or groups change over time, allowing the researcher to predict outcomes.

study has surveyed the same three cohorts of women (young, mid-aged, and older women) every 3 years since 1996 and monitored changes in health status and health care use over time (see <www.alswh.org.au>). See also CHAPTER 14.

Figure 13.1: Example of Longitudinal Postal Survey: Australian Longitudinal Study on Women's Health

Cohort	Year of Surveys				
	1996 98, 98, 00,	01, 02, 03,	04, 05, 06,	07, 08, 09	...... 2015+
Younger	⊠ ⊠	⊠	⊠	⊠	
Mid-aged	⊠ ⊠	⊠	⊠	⊠	
Older	⊠ ⊠	⊠	⊠	⊠	
	S1 S2	S3	S4	S5	

One advantage of longitudinal survey studies is that a greater range of research questions can be asked, predictive questions can be tested and more complex statistical analyses can be undertaken. Researchers can ask, for instance, about which factors at an earlier point in time can predict certain health outcomes at a later point. Such studies are able to shed light on both protective factors and risk factors for later illness or death. For instance, cohort-based studies have shown that certain diets are associated with development of cancer later in life (Bingham et al. 2003), and that smoking is linked to lung cancer (Doll et al. 2005).

Surveys to test intervention effects

Surveys to test intervention effects are administered before and after an intervention to test for changes in self-reported outcomes such as symptoms, subjective well-being, knowledge and attitudes, or health behaviours. This is similar to the previous longitudinal survey category in that measures are administered on repeated occasions with the intention of analysing scores for difference over time. However, in intervention studies, the measures are aligned to the purpose of the intervention or treatment and are designed specifically to test whether the intervention has produced hypothesised changes. For instance, if a particular treatment aims to improve certain symptoms, then a survey can be used to test whether these self-reported symptoms decrease in the projected time-frame after treatment. Surveys can be used alone or in conjunction with other diagnostic or objective measures.

Surveys to test intervention effects take measures before and after a treatment or intervention to determine whether the intervention produces change in outcomes.

HOW IS MEASUREMENT THEORY APPLIED TO SURVEY RESEARCH?

Before describing the process of constructing survey questions, it is important to have some understanding of measurement theory, that is, the set of rules that govern the way questions are constructed and responses recorded. See also CHAPTER 11.

Measurement can be defined as the process of assigning a number or symbol to an attribute or variable according to a rule. It is a central aspect of research since it enables us to obtain data. Common measurement methods used for the collection of data are surveys, direct observation or interviews. Before we are able to measure a variable or construct, we have to operationalise it. In the process of operationalisation, the researcher must define how the variable or theoretical construct will be measured.

The researcher must also distinguish between different types of measures or data collection techniques. We can use measures that produce quantitative or qualitative data. Quantitative data are numerical values and qualitative data are pictures or words. The choice of your measure depends on the research question and topic (see also CHAPTER 1). Since this chapter focuses on quantitative measurement as applied to survey research, we first describe the difference between discrete and continuous measures and then the four levels of measurement.

Discrete and continuous measurement

Variables can be differentiated as discrete or continuous. A discrete variable uses only whole numbers or units. Number of children is an example of a discrete variable. Height, weight and age are examples of continuous variables because there are values between units. Somebody can be 17.4 years old or 1.63 m tall, but a family cannot have 1.4 children. There are variables with two values such as gender (female and male) or variables with multiple values such as age or marital status. Age is a continuous measure, whereas marital status is a discrete measure—there is a fixed number of categories and one cannot gain a score between those categories.

In terms of the broadest definition of measurement, there are four different levels of measurement or four different types of measurement scales—nominal, ordinal, interval and ratio (see also CHAPTERS 11, 24). Each of these is described in the following section.

Nominal data/categorical measurement

For **nominal data** or categorical measurement, we have different categories and allocate a value to each category representing a variable. Examples of nominal measuring are the allocation of a value to gender categories, country of birth, first language or religion (see Table 13.1). If the variable is gender, you could allocate the value 1 to female and 2 to male. The categories that individuals are allocated to are distinct and not continuous. It would not make sense to have the value 1.4 in relation to the variable gender.

Nominal data occur where objects or people are assigned to named categories according to some criterion, for example male/female.

Margot Schofield and Christine Knauss

A further characteristic of nominal/categorical measurement is that the category values are not in a particular order. Therefore we can freely decide if we allocate the value '1' or the value '2' to female. The value simply describes the category and the difference of the variable but does not stand for a specific quantity. The numbers have no quantitative meaning. The fact that a nominal/categorical scale cannot be ordered and has no quantitative meaning has consequences for the analysis. It would not make sense to calculate an average. For nominal/categorical data, we can report frequencies or percentages of individuals. For our example with gender this would mean that we might report that the sample consisted of 10 females and 10 males or of 50 per cent women and 50 per cent men.

Ordinal measurement

Ordinal data result when observations are rank-ordered and values are assigned sequentially to reflect the logical ordering of categories. For variables like satisfaction with a treatment or degree of racism, the different attributes represent relatively more or less of the variable. We could assign a value to an individual that would stand for their degree of satisfaction with a certain treatment. The more satisfied the person is with the treatment, the higher the value. According to the values, the individual could be rank-ordered. We would know that some individuals reported more satisfaction with treatment than others. The categories of the variable can be clearly ordered but are also distinct and not continuous. Therefore it does not make sense to calculate a mean score for ordinal measures because the differences between the scores on the scale do not have meaning. If the value '1' stands for *satisfied with the treatment* and the value '2' for *very satisfied with the treatment*, we would not be able to interpret the difference between the two values in terms of people who answered with '1' being two times more satisfied than people who answered with '2'. The differences between the values are meaningless. The value just describes the rank order for ordinal measurement and therefore the value '2' stands for a higher rating than '1'.

> **Ordinal data** result when observations are rank-ordered and values are assigned sequentially to reflect the logical ordering of categories, e.g. Likert scales, which rank responses from low to high.

Interval/ratio level measurement

The **interval/ratio** scale is used in measuring variables for which the interval between the values on the scale has meaning. The distance between the attributes expresses meaningful standard intervals. Familiar variables for interval/ratio measurement are height or temperature. The distance between 10 and 15 cm is the same as between 15 and 20 cm.

Ratio scales have the same characteristics as interval scales, but they have a true zero point representing the absence of the variable measured. For example, for the variable height, zero stands for the absence of height. A further example of a ratio measurement is IQ. The differences between the values have meaning. Therefore the difference between an IQ of 90 and 100 would be the same as that between 100 and 110 as there is a true

> **Interval data** have the property of a rank order, and in addition, distances or intervals between the units of measurement are equal.

> **Ratio data** have the same properties as interval data, and in addition, have an empirical rather than an arbitrary zero.

zero point. In the measurement of temperature, however, zero does not stand for the absence of temperature and it is therefore an interval measurement, not a ratio one.

The choice of an appropriate method of data analysis depends on the level of measurement. If you are planning to calculate a mean, an interval or ratio measurement level is required (see Chapter 24). It is important to keep in mind that the necessary level of measurement for your research question needs to be chosen before you start your research because it is not possible to convert a lower-level measurement to a higher-level measurement. If you have decided to choose an ordinal measure it will not be possible to convert it to an interval measure.

Table 13.1: Levels of measurement

Level of measurement	Example	Possible Values
Nominal/categorical	Gender	1 = Female 2 = Male
Ordinal	Satisfaction with treatment	1 = not at all satisfied 2 = slightly satisfied 3 = moderately satisfied 4 = very satisfied
Interval	Body temperature	36.9 degrees 37.3 degrees
Ratio	Weight	60.5 kg 75.7 kg 85.3 kg

HOW ARE SURVEYS DESIGNED?

Surveys are usually designed with three components: a cover (invitation) letter, some instructions on how the survey should be completed, and the set of questions to be answered.

Participant Information Letter

The Participant Information Letter aims to inform the respondent about the purpose of the survey and about the researchers conducting the study, as well as to engage their interest and motivate them to respond. Ethical guidelines governing institutional research specify a number of aspects that must be covered in an Information Letter to ensure informed consent (see CHAPTER 2). Typical content of a participant Information Letter includes:

☐ a clear statement of the aims and significance of the research
☐ the names and contact details of the research team
☐ the funding source of the research
☐ reasons why respondents should complete the survey
☐ what is involved in completing the survey, such as maximum time
☐ assurances of anonymity and confidentiality

☐   statement that participation is voluntary and participants can withdraw after agreeing
to participate

☐   information about how the survey results will be used

☐   information about how to gain further information or make a complaint.

Instructions

The instructions are important to ensure that participants know what they need to do and that
the survey is completed correctly. It is usual to encourage participants to attempt to answer
all questions. If the survey is largely about attitudes, the instructions might emphasise that
there are no right or wrong answers and their opinion is what is required. Participants can
be informed about how to answer particular types of questions, and examples of correct and
incorrect responses may be given. The instructions section should indicate how respondents
should return the completed survey, for example 'Please return the completed questionnaire
to the Researcher in the enclosed reply-paid envelope within two weeks'. Each question should
also have instructions to clarify the type of response option: for example *Tick one box only*, or
Tick all that apply, or *Select the response that most closely reflects your views*.

What steps are involved in constructing the survey?

Constructing a survey involves much more than designing individual questions. It involves
consideration of the overall structure, flow and coherence of the survey, and testing out the
adequacy of the developed questions. Typical steps, modified from Sarantakos (2005), include:

1. PREPARATION

The researcher defines the survey objectives and key constructs to be measured, searches for
relevant measures and assesses their reliability and validity, and whether they meet the needs
of the study. If an appropriate measure is found, the researcher decides whether it requires
adaptation. Note that if questions are adapted, this may diminish validity or reliability.

2. CONSTRUCTING AND CRITIQUING THE FIRST DRAFT

The researcher selects the available measures and/or constructs questions to address the key
variables to be measured. It is usual to include a number of questions that describe the socio-
demographic characteristics of your sample. The researcher then reviews the draft questions to
determine whether they adequately capture the constructs, and whether they meet the general
rules for questionnaire construction such as being relevant, unambiguous, and in plain language,
and whether they are logically ordered.

3. EXTERNAL REVIEW AND REVISION

After revision, the draft survey is then reviewed by other experts in survey construction or the
research topic, and feedback obtained. On the basis of feedback received, the researcher revises
the questions and perhaps reorders items. If substantial changes are required, it should go back
to external review before moving on to the next step.

4. Pre-test or pilot test of the revised survey

Once a satisfactory revised draft is available, the researcher should pilot-test the whole instrument with a small sample similar to the intended study sample. Respondents may be asked to provide feedback specifically on how they experienced the survey and whether they thought any questions were ambiguous or difficult to answer.

5. Further revision based on pre-test

Pre-tests or pilot studies will usually lead to further revision of the survey. If a major revision is required, further external review and pilot-testing of the revised version may be required.

6. Second pre-test or pilot test

The revised survey instrument will then undergo further pilot-testing of the survey or pre-testing of the revised component to determine if any further revisions are required before the final draft of the survey.

7. Formulation of the final draft

At this point the researcher stands back and considers the feedback from the various sources outlined above, together with a review of the overall study objectives and methodology, and makes the final changes. Often at this stage, issues of survey length, flow, coherence, structural components, layout and presentation will be reviewed. Any acknowledgments and instructions must be incorporated. A final proofread is required before finalising for printing.

Survey format

Researchers must decide how to present and order the questions within the questionnaire in a way that will enhance its acceptability and ease of completion. Questions should be presented in a logical order with a sense of a smooth transition from one section to the next. The overall design and logic of the survey is related to the likelihood of achieving a higher response rate. Furthermore, the order and logic will affect the meaning given to certain questions.

There are various approaches to the ordering of items within a survey. One common approach is the **Funnel format**. Other formats include the **Inverted Funnel format** and **Mixed format**.

Funnel format

In this model, the questions move from a broad focus to more specific content, from non-sensitive questions to more sensitive questions, and from more impersonal to more personal. The rationale of this is that it is best to warm respondents up with general non-threatening questions first, and as they become more engaged with the survey they will be more inclined to answer more personal questions. This also allows people time to reflect on topics at the more general level and then at a more personal level and suits respondents who are likely to think at a more abstract level.

> **Funnel format survey:** Where the questions move from a broad focus to more specific content, from non-sensitive questions to more sensitive questions, and from more impersonal to more personal.

Inverted funnel format survey: Where the questions move from more specific to more general, from more sensitive to less sensitive, and from personal to impersonal.

Inverted funnel format

In this format, questions move from more specific to more general, from more sensitive to less sensitive, and from personal to impersonal. This format may be useful for respondents who are primed to answer personal questions and where limited time demands that the more specific questions need to be focused on first.

Mixed format survey: Where the questions are organised in sections or domains and particular formats are applied within domains.

Mixed format

This is particularly relevant for longer surveys covering a number of domains. Here the questions are organised in sections or domains and particular formats are applied within domains. For instance, a funnel format may be used within each section, so that overall the survey moves from general to specific, and this pattern is repeated through various sections of the survey.

Structured and semi-structured formats

A structured format means that there is a set ordering of questions for respondents to work their way through. Every respondent is thus responding to the same set of questions in the same order and usually with set response options. This helps to avoid differences in responses that may be due to ordering effects. Semi-structured questionnaires are usually used in interview format and allow for a more flexible ordering of items and often involve more open-ended response formats.

TRY IT YOURSELF

Survey topic in area of interest

Think of a research question or topic in your area of interest that would be suitable to study using a survey format. Define the research question.

_____

_____

Structured questions

How would you phrase the main questions for a structured questionnaire and what response options would you provide?

_____

_____

_____

_____

Semi-structured questions

How would you phrase the questions in a semi-structured, more open-ended way?

_____

_____

_____

_____

Length of the survey

The length of the survey is an important consideration, and response rate is likely to decline with increasing length. It is therefore important to be disciplined in determining how essential each question is for the study. One strategy is to rate all the proposed questions as essential, desirable or optional, and then decide how many questions or what the maximum period is for completion of the questionnaire. If items must be removed, the rating system will suggest which ones to remove. If items are removed, the overall flow and transition must be reconsidered. In general, 15–20 minutes is considered the maximum length for general surveys unless participants are likely to be highly motivated.

Strategies for helping respondents navigate the survey

For longer surveys, strategies to enhance respondents' navigation through the survey include putting clear and engaging headings at the start of each section so that there is an overall sense of structure to the survey.

It can also help to provide feedback at certain points, which tells respondents how far they are through the survey. For instance, in a long survey, respondents might be told when they reach the halfway point and might be encouraged to have a break or a cup of tea before going on to the next section. Some researchers may also include a tea bag! Small gestures acknowledging the burden on respondents can increase completions and goodwill.

Internet-based surveys will usually include a little graph on each page showing the percentage of the survey completed. This provides more regular reinforcement, goodwill, and encouragement to respondents.

HOW ARE SURVEY QUESTIONS CONSTRUCTED?

Types of question content

Questions can be classified in a number of ways depending on the type of content and the type of response options. Dillman and colleagues (2008) suggest that there are five main types of question content: behaviour, beliefs, attitudes, knowledge and attributes.

Margot Schofield and Christine Knauss

Behaviour questions ask about what people do, for example, 'Do you currently smoke cigarettes?'

Belief questions ask about what people believe to be true or false about topics. An example would be to ask them whether they think smoking is harmful to health, or whether they think peer pressure or parental example is more influential in determining smoking uptake among adolescents.

Attitude questions seek to establish what respondents think is desirable. An example would be to ask respondents whether they agree with a statement such as 'Airports should provide a smoking room for smoking travellers', or 'Hospitals should refuse to perform cardiac surgery on smoking patients'.

Knowledge questions seek to determine what people know about particular topics. In relation to assessing knowledge about smoking, we could ask what they know about the harmful health effects of smoking on women, or the effects on unborn babies of mothers' smoking during pregnancy.

Attribute questions seek information about more objective characteristics of respondents such as their age, gender, occupation and place of residence. Many of these attribute questions can be sourced from major published surveys such as those run by the ABS in Australia.

The types of question that ask about more subjective information such as beliefs, attitudes, values, perceived quality of life, pose particular design challenges. Because these questions are less objective, researchers often use a standardised scale since these have been shown to increase reliability and validity (McDowell 2006), and there may be some normative data that you can compare with the results you obtain. Standardised scales are discussed in more detail in the next section.

Standardised scales

A **standardised scale** provides a scientific form of health assessment that is useful for measuring subjective constructs such as pain, mood and level of symptoms.

Reliability: The extent to which a measurement instrument is dependable, stable and consistent when repeated under identical conditions.

Validity: The extent to which the scale measures what it is supposed to measure (content and construct validity).

Standardised scales provide a scientific form of health assessment that is particularly useful for measuring subjective constructs such as pain, mood and level of symptoms. Standardised scales are made up of a series of self-report questions, ratings or items that measure a specific concept, and where the response categories are in the same format and can be summed or aggregated in some weighted form. The scale can then produce a number on a standard interval or ratio scale such as 0 to 100, to reflect a level of functioning, symptoms, pain, affect or beliefs. The process of standardisation means that the number assigned can be compared statistically either within or across individuals or groups. They can be used to test for change over time, for instance as a result of treatment, or to look for differences between groups.

The concepts of **reliability** and **validity** are important for standardised scales (see also CHAPTERS 1, 11, 12). Reliability refers to the ability of the scale to provide consistent stable information across time and across respondents. For instance, if someone completes the scale today and again in two days' time, do you get essentially the same responses? Validity refers to the degree to which the scale measures what it is supposed to measure (content and construct validity). For instance, does it have a good correlation with another 'gold standard' measure?

Standardised rating scales cover a wide range of purposes. Some of the commonly used ones are diagnostic scales, symptom-based scales, quality of life scales, functional level scales, and client satisfaction scales. There are also a wide range of scales that assess psychosocial factors such as attitudes and beliefs, social support, optimism or loneliness. Many scales have a number of subscales as well as an overall scale score. An example is the widely used Quality of Life scale, the Medical Outcomes Study Health Survey Short-Form 36 items (SF-36). This is a well-validated scale comprising eight subscales as shown in Table 13.2.

Table 13.2: Standardised scale. Medical Outcomes Study Health Survey Short Form (SF-36)

8 subscales	2 component scores
Physical functioning	
Role physical functioning	
Bodily pain	Physical component summary
General health	
Vitality	Mental component summary
Social functioning	
Role social	
Mental health	

Source: Ware, Kosinski & Keller 1994

There are good sources available that provide an overview of established scales for health research (Sajatovic & Ramirez 2003; Bowling 2002; McDowell 2006). These can help researchers to select appropriate measures for different studies since they include information on the content, scoring, validity and reliability of many different health measures. A thorough overview of constructing standardised scales can be found in Osterlind (2006).

Constructing your own survey questions

If you decide that there are no established questions for your purpose, you will need to construct your own questions. This is a complex task (de Vaus 2007) but can be guided by a number of important principles as outlined in 'Doing research' below.

DOING RESEARCH

Principles for constructing survey questions

- ☐ Use simple, everyday language typical of the respondent group
- ☐ Avoid jargon, technical terms and abstract concepts
- ☐ Avoid ambiguity and double-barrelled questions
- ☐ Avoid double negatives
- ☐ Avoid making suggestive statements or assumptions about respondents
- ☐ Provide sufficient instructions and probes
- ☐ Pre-coded questions should offer sufficient response categories
- ☐ When asking people to record past events, provide a temporal frame, e.g. 'Over the last four weeks', 'In the past year'.

Response formats

Questions can be classified as open or closed questions depending on how respondents are asked to respond. Open questions simply ask the question and invite respondents to provide an answer in whatever way seems most appropriate to them. This can yield rich data that may be missed if only closed response options are provided, but responses need to be coded before analysis can be undertaken, a time-consuming process. Closed questions provide a set of predetermined response options and respondents choose which option applies to them, an economical method.

Some of the main types of response formats are summarised in 'Doing research' below. At the simplest level, there are *Yes/No* or *Yes/No/Don't know* response formats. These are closed questions and provide little room for participants to give finely discriminated responses. They are particularly suitable for questions where there is a relatively straightforward factual response such as 'Have you smoked in the last week?'

Verbal rating scale:
Used where a question is asked and a range of verbal response categories are provided for the participant to circle the one that most closely represents their view.

Verbal rating scales are commonly used where a question is asked and a range of verbal response categories are provided for the participant to circle the response that most closely represents their view. This is an example of categorical or ordinal data. To make such responses suitable for statistical analysis, the verbal categories are assigned to numbers that can be entered into data files—as shown in the Verbal + Numeric Rating Scale in 'Doing research' below. Note that these numbers represent a rank-ordered scale, not an interval scale.

Likert scale: used to measure subjective variables such as attitudes. The researcher generates a number of statements and wishes to measure the extent to which participants agree or disagree.

Likert scales are used to measure subjective variables such as attitudes. The researcher generates a number of statements (e.g. attitudes) and wishes to measure the extent to which participants agree or disagree with the statements. The scales typically ask each respondent to rate each item on a response scale that has discrete options such as a 1-to-5 (or 1-to-7) response scale. A typical Likert scale is a 5-point scale. This can be unidirectional or have positive and negative (opposing) directions.

Visual analogue scales provide the opportunity for respondents to rate items on a continuous line between two end points. Typically, respondents are asked to mark a position on the line that goes from 0 to 10 or from 0 to 100. This has the advantage of providing an interval measure that can be analysed using a wider range of statistical tests. The continuous nature of this measurement scale differentiates it from discrete scales like the Likert scale, verbal or numerical scales, and may produce a more sensitive and differentiated response under certain circumstances (Grant et al. 1999).

> **Visual analogue scales** provide the opportunity for respondents to rate items on a continuous line between two end points.

DOING RESEARCH

Response formats

Yes / No / Don't know

In general, would you say your health is good?

Yes	No	Don't know

Verbal + Numerical rating scale (*categorical*)

In general, would you say your health is:

Excellent	Very Good	Good	Fair	Poor
1	2	3	4	5

Likert scale (*ordinal*)

In general, would you say your health is good?

Strongly Agree	Agree	Neither Agree nor Disagree	Disagree	Strongly Disagree
1	2	3	4	5

Visual Analogue scale (*interval*)

In general, how would you rate your health?

Mark a position on the line from 0 (very poor) to 100 (extremely good):

0 _____ 100

Open-ended question

In general, how would you rate your health?

_____

_____

_____

Margot Schofield and Christine Knauss

Designing response options to closed questions

While closed questions are helpful in producing numeric data for analysis in the most efficient way, it can be problematic to define what the appropriate response categories are. In designing response categories, it is necessary to ensure that categories are mutually exclusive, and that all or most options are catered for. An example of designing response options for marital status is given in 'Doing research' below.

DOING RESEARCH

Response formats

Suppose you want to know about marital/relationship status. You could look up the ABS question format and find that this is more complex than you first thought.

The ABS distinguishes between 'Registered marital status' and 'Social marital status'. The standard question for **Registered Marital Status** is:

Q. What is your present marital status?

☐ Never married

☐ Widowed

☐ Divorced

☐ Separated but not divorced

☐ Registered married

However, it is clear that this question alone will not tell you anything about the large number of people who live in de facto relationships, nor will it tell you about people who live in same-sex relationships. The ABS has developed a complex series of interview questions to explore the 'Social Marital Status'. To simplify this for a survey, one could add some additional response options to the basic ABS response options.

Question option for 'Social marital status' (modified from ABS format)

Q. What is your present marital status? (*Mark one only*)

☐ Never married

☐ Widowed

☐ Divorced

☐ Separated but not divorced

☐ Married (registered)

☐ De facto relationship (opposite sex)

☐ De facto relationship (same sex)

This example illustrates that even what we might think of as a relatively straight-forward objective piece of information such as marital status can be quite complex to think through and ensure that all possible response options are included. Failure to do this will mean that a proportion of people answering your survey will feel that none of the response options provided apply to them. Furthermore, you will be losing valuable information.

Measurement error

Despite our best efforts to enhance validity and reliability, errors can occur at different stages of the research process and for different levels of measurement. Mistakes can happen, for example by choosing the wrong sample, by having errors in the measurement process or by interpreting the results in an invalid way. **Measurement errors** happen when we do not measure accurately or when we measure a different variable than intended. Measurement errors can be either systematic or random depending on whether or not they have a constant pattern. To minimise or avoid measurement errors it is important to ensure that the measures used have acceptable reliability and validity, which means that they measure accurately and that they assess the variable they intend to assess. See also CHAPTERS 1, 11, 12, 25.

> **Measurement errors** happen when researchers do not measure accurately or when they measure a different variable from the one intended. They can be systematic or random depending on whether or not they have a constant pattern.

Sources of measurement error in surveys

Because survey measures rely on self-report, there are certain types of measurement error that need to be considered. Survey measures may contain errors due to poor memory, failure to understand the question or response options, a desire to give a socially acceptable response, or through having response options that do not match the respondent's response.

Some measurement errors can be identified by including more than one way of measuring variables that are susceptible to error. For instance, self-report measures can be supplemented by having more objective measures and assessing whether there is evidence of systematic error. One example of this is shown in 'Doing research' below, where self-reported weight category is compared with BMI.

DOING RESEARCH

Self-report measurement error

Perceptions of weight

In the 2004–05 National Health Survey, self-reported (subjective) classifications of one's weight as normal, overweight or obese were compared with the more objective weight measure of Body Mass Index (BMI), calculated by a formula based on the ratio of weight to height. It was found that the majority of adults considered themselves to be of acceptable

Margot Schofield and Christine Knauss

weight (63% of males and 59% of females), while 32% of males and 37% of females considered themselves to be overweight. However, these self-report categorisations were significantly below the proportions classified as overweight or obese based on their BMI: 62% of males and 45% of females. Only half of adult males who considered themselves to be of acceptable weight were classified to the normal BMI category, compared with 76% of females. Thus we can conclude that self-reported weight perception has a high degree of error and that females are better than males on the whole at estimating their weight categories.

Source: ABS 2006a

Asking retrospective questions produces another common source of error. People often have difficulty remembering when health events in the past occurred, and memory tends to degrade over time. Measurement error due to memory problems can be improved by including certain prompts to improve memory.

DOING RESEARCH

Strategies to enhance accuracy of survey responses

1. Ask respondent to take accurate measurements

Survey measures of weight: Certain measures are known to be less reliable using self-report. Weight is one of these. For instance, people may not know how much they weigh if they have not weighed themselves recently. Not all scales will produce exact measurement, so even among those who have weighed themselves recently, there will be some variation in accuracy. A further source of measurement error is that respondents may be motivated to provide a biased response. Weight is a construct that has important social meaning, and many people will attempt to minimise their weight, so underreporting of weight may be a problem.

How the question is asked has an important influence on the response obtained. If a self-report method is the only practical option, and the survey is a mail or online survey that people can complete at home, the question could ask them to go and weigh themselves before answering the question.

2. Ask question in various ways

Self-report of alcohol use: Alcohol use is typically underreported in surveys for both social desirability reasons and because of poor memory. Measurement is also problematic because intake is likely to vary substantially over time, and alcohol content varies substantially across different types of drinks. Various methods have been developed to enhance accuracy.

☐ Present diagrams explaining the concept of '*standard drink*', which links standard alcohol content to different glass sizes for different types of drinks.

☐ Ask separate *quantity and frequency* questions.

☐ Ask people to keep a *diary over a 2-week period*. This method helps to even out large variations in use over time. For instance, alcohol use is typically higher on weekends, or linked to certain events such as parties.

☐ Ask separate question about *binge drinking*, e.g. more than five drinks on one occasion.

4. Use scales for subjective constructs

Standardised scales with multiple items can increase accuracy and differentiate concepts for more subjective constructs such as attitudes, mood, stress and quality of life. This is also an example of asking questions in various ways. The more often the person responds to a particular kind of item, the more that construct is likely to apply for them. This works because very small variations in wording can influence how the person responds.

5. Keep the survey as short as possible

Accuracy of responses might also be influenced by the length of the survey. If a survey is too long, participants might lose motivation and give inaccurate answers towards the end of the survey.

HOW ARE SURVEYS ADMINISTERED?

There are several key methods for administering surveys: self-completion questionnaire, group self-completion, mail self-completion, internet-based self-completion, face-to-face interview, telephone interview and internet interview.

☐ *Self-completion questionnaire:* Participants are asked to complete the survey instrument and instructions are provided.

☐ *Group self-completion:* A researcher may administer a survey to a group, such as a class of school students. Participants will each complete their own survey, but the process is facilitated and the researcher is present throughout.

☐ *Mail self-completion:* Surveys are mailed out to participants who are asked to complete the survey and mail back—usually in a reply-paid envelope provided by the researcher.

☐ *Internet-based self-completion:* Participants are invited to complete an internet-base survey and are provided with the web-link for accessing the survey. The steps involved in internet surveys are outlined in 'Doing research' below.

☐ *Face-to-face interview:* The researcher may conduct a face-to-face interview using an interview schedule (list of questions or topics). The responses may be recorded manually or tape-recorded and later coded.

Margot Schofield and Christine Knauss

☐ *Telephone interview:* Telephone interviews are like face-to-face interviews but conducted over the phone. Computer-Assisted Telephone Interviews (CATI) are a popular method whereby the survey is programmed into the computer and an interviewer reads through the questions and types in the respondent's answers. This enters numeric or verbal answers directly into data files.

☐ *Internet interview:* Internet interviews are similar to telephone interviews but conducted using internet-based voice software such as skype, or msn messenger and with the interviewer either typing in responses or voice-recording the interview using the computer software program.

DOING RESEARCH

Internet survey example

1 *Formulate your research question:* For example, 'How is dieting behaviour related to satisfaction with weight and shape in university students?'

2 *Choose a survey-hosting website:* There are many different survey-hosting websites available such as

   ☐ www.advancedsurvey.com/surveys/
   ☐ www.keysurvey.com.au/
   ☐ www.survey-online.com
   ☐ www.surveymonkey.com

   which offer slightly different services and have different prices. Therefore it is important to check which one covers your requirements and offers the necessary features.

3 *Define your sample and clarify how you can recruit participants:* If you want to email the sample a link to the survey, you have to make sure you are allowed to contact the participants by email (e.g. privacy laws). Unless you already have access and permission to use the email addresses, you will need to gain permission from an authorising body. In our case, we would have to seek permission of a particular department or faculty of the university.

4 *Create your survey:* Before you build your survey online, you should decide about your measures.

5 *Build your survey online:* It is usually straightforward to build an online survey and some hosting websites have help programs and helpful tutorials. Furthermore, you can look at example surveys for possible styles, designs and types of questions.

6 *Pilot the online survey:* Feedback from a pilot sample will enable you to revise and improve the online survey.

7 *Send an invitation to participate to your selected participants:* One advantage of an online survey is that you can send your sample an invitation to participate with a direct link to the survey.

8 *Download your data:* Importing the data into a statistics program such as SPSS may be a time-consuming and difficult step. You can download the data as a spreadsheet or as an Excel file. To import into an SPSS file you must write a syntax because all your data will usually be in a text format.

SUMMARY

This chapter has described key issues in the design and conduct of surveys and questionnaires. Besides information about different types of surveys, about the necessary steps when designing a survey, and about standardised scales, practical examples were given to illustrate how and why surveys can be used. The topics covered provide a grounding for new researchers to understand when surveys may be useful and how to go about designing a survey suitable for their research question. A list of additional references and websites is provided to encourage readers to explore this topic further and incorporate surveys into their research.

TUTORIAL EXERCISES

You are asked to evaluate the effectiveness of an intervention that is offered to adults to improve level of experienced stress by practising relaxation techniques. Write your answers for the following questions:

☐ What is your research question?
☐ At what time-points would you ask participants about their level of stress?
☐ What survey administration method would you choose?
☐ What kind of measures would you choose and how would you go about choosing them?
☐ How would you get information about validity and reliability of your chosen measures?
☐ What principles do you need to keep in mind if you decide to write your own questions?
☐ What type of sample would you choose and how would you recruit your participants?

Margot Schofield and Christine Knauss

FURTHER READING

Bowling, A. (2005). *Measuring health: A review of quality of life measurement scales*, 3rd edn. Maidenhead, UK: Open University Press.

de Leeuw, E., Hox, J. & Dillman, D.A. (2008). *International handbook of survey methodology*. New York: Lawrence Erlbaum.

de Vaus, D. (ed.) (2007). *Social surveys 2*, 4 vols. London: Sage

de Vaus, D. (2004). Structured questions and interviews. In V. Minichiello, G. Sullivan, K. Greenwood & R. Axford (eds), *Handbook of research methods for nursing and health science*, 2nd edn. Sydney: Pearson Education Australia, 347–93.

Dillman, D.A., Smyth, J.D. & Christian, L.M. (2008). *Internet, mail, and mixed-mode surveys: The tailored design method*, 3rd edn. Hoboken, NJ: John Wiley.

Fowler, F.J. (2009). *Survey research methods*, 4th edn. Thousand Oaks, CA: Sage.

Lavrakis, P.J. (2008). *Encyclopedia of survey research methods*. Thousand Oaks, CA: Sage.

Sue, V.M. & Ritter, L.A. (2007). *Conducting online surveys*. Thousand Oaks, CA: Sage.

WEBSITES

www.socialresearchmethods.net/kb/survey.php

This site of the Web Center for Social Research Methods provides a comprehensive overview on survey research methods.

writing.colostate.edu/guides/research/survey/pop2f.cfm

This site contains an annotated bibliography of survey research.

www.pollograph.com/kb/docs/designing-a-survey

This site helps you to design an online survey—Pollograph.

www.alswh.org.au

The website of the Australian Longitudinal Study on Women's Health.

www.advancedsurvey.com/surveys

www.keysurvey.com.au

www.survey-online.com

www.surveymonkey.com

These are survey-hosting websites.

14

How Do We Know What We Know?
Epidemiology in Health Research

Melissa Graham

CHAPTER OBJECTIVES

In this chapter you will learn:

☐ how the principle questions in epidemiology can be used to answer population health questions

☐ to distinguish between observational descriptive and analytical epidemiological study designs

☐ how you can use sources of population health data to answer questions about population health

KEY TERMS

Analytical cross-sectional studies

Analytical epidemiological studies

Case-control study

Cohort study

Cross-sectional study

Descriptive epidemiology

Ecological study

Epidemiology

Exposure

Incidence

Longitudinal studies

Measures of association

Morbidity

Mortality

Observational epidemiological studies

Outcome

Population

Population-based health data

Prevalence

Prevalence rate ratio

INTRODUCTION

We often hear health research and statistics quoted in the media. For example: 12 000 Australian women are diagnosed with breast cancer each year; babies die in public hospitals, during labour or shortly after birth, at three times the rate they do in private hospitals; one Australian woman dies every 11 hours from ovarian cancer; and cervical cancer is linked to deprivation. Where do these numbers and statements come from and what do they mean? These numbers are derived from population data that we employ in **epidemiology**. Epidemiological approaches can help us to understand these patterns of health states and make sense out of their meaning.

Epidemiology is concerned with the study of the distribution and determinants of health states in populations.

Population: In epidemiology, 'population' is used to describe all the people who live in a defined area or country.

Population-based health data: 'Ongoing systems that collect and register all cases of a particular disease or class of diseases as they develop in a defined population.'

Epidemiology is concerned with the study of the distribution and determinants of health states in **populations** (Last et al. 1995). Epidemiology can help us to determine the extent of ill health or disease in the community; identify the cause of ill health and the risk factors for disease; understand the natural history and prognosis of ill health; investigate disease outbreaks or epidemics; evaluate existing and new preventive and therapeutic programs and services; and provide the foundation for developing public policy and regulation (Gordis 2009). Essentially, this means that epidemiology can provide the answers to questions asked in the health sector such as: How much disease is there? Who gets it? Where are most people affected? When did they have it? What happens over time? More importantly, it is how we as health professionals apply this to prevent and control health problems. The main aim of this chapter is to introduce you to population data to help us answer the questions of 'who', 'where' and 'when'. Before we examine sources and types of **population-based health data**, let us look at the underpinning principles of observational descriptive and analytical epidemiology and how this data is generated—study designs.

THE WHO, THE WHERE AND THE WHEN

Population health statistics can provide us with useful information. When we hear health statistics or when we think about health and illness within our society, we often ask who are sick, where are they and when were they sick? These questions form the underlying principles of epidemiology and help us to answer many more questions about the population's health and well-being. Returning to our definition of epidemiology, we see that epidemiology is the study of the distribution and determinants of health states or events in specified populations (Last et al. 1995). Health states or events are the diseases or conditions of interest. So in epidemiology, when we investigate the distribution or pattern of a particular health state in a particular population, we are actually trying to answer the questions of 'who', 'where' and 'when'. However, in epidemiology these questions are known as person (who), place (where) and time (when). Let us now consider each of these questions and how they help us to understand the patterns of health within populations.

Person

Let's say that we are interested in how many women have cervical cancer. The first question we ask ourselves in epidemiology is who has the condition or health state of interest; in this case 'who' has cervical cancer? This question can be simply answered by counting the number of persons, in this case women who have cervical cancer. But often a simple count is not enough to answer our question adequately. This is because to say that X number of women have cervical cancer does not really tell us if this is only a small group of women in the population or a very large group of women. In this case, we may need to relate the number of women who have cervical cancer to the size of the population through the calculation of risks or rates (we will revisit and explore risks and rates later). Since populations are not usually a homogeneous group, we may want to express our counts in terms of the characteristics of the population. Commonly used characteristics of the population to describe subgroups include age and sex. In our example, we are only interested in women. In this case, it would also be useful to group our population of women by age—for example, women aged 40 years or more in 5-year age groups (i.e. 40–44, 45–49, 50–54 and so forth). Other characteristics commonly used include socio-economic characteristics such as education, occupation or income; demographic characteristics such as geographic location, marital status, or parity; or characteristics of health-related behaviours such as smoking, alcohol consumption and physical inactivity. Now that we know 'who', let's turn to the next question: 'where'.

Place

Following on from our example above, we may also wish to compare the number of people (women) with the health state (in this case, women who have cervical cancer) by place. By describing the geographic distribution of a health state, we can delineate those who may benefit from health-related interventions and provide information about possible determinants, risk or protective factors. Useful descriptors of place include place of residence, schools and workplaces, or birthplaces. Administrative descriptors of place such as local government area, city, state or country may also be useful. In our example, we may wish to look at the number of women who have cervical cancer in Australia or Victoria.

Time

So far, we have identified that we are interested in how many women aged 40 years or more in Australia or Victoria have cervical cancer. Now, we turn to time—the 'when' question. What time-period are we interested in? Ever? A specific year? Or a time-range such as 2006 to 2007? The time variable can helps us examine trends in health states over time and enable us to identify any changes in the patterns of the health state of interest. For example, has there been an increase or decrease in the health state at different points in time? Time can also help us

Melissa Graham

predict what may occur in the future and provide clues to what is causing a change in the health state's occurrence. Finally, by examining patterns of health states over time we can examine the effectiveness of policies or programs that have been implemented to address the health state.

Now that we have identified the building blocks of epidemiology enquiry, let's look at the types of epidemiological study designs we can use to best answer our person, place and time questions.

OBSERVATIONAL STUDIES: DESCRIPTIVE VERSUS ANALYTICAL EPIDEMIOLOGY

Observational epidemiological studies aim to collect information about people's exposure and health outcomes as these naturally occur within the population.

Unlike experimental epidemiology, **observational epidemiological studies** do not seek to intervene or change people's exposure status. Rather, the aim is to collect information about people's exposure and health outcomes as these naturally occur within the population. Observational studies can be considered as either descriptive or analytical.

Descriptive epidemiology

Descriptive epidemiology describes morbidity and mortality within the population using person, place and time variables.

Descriptive epidemiology focuses on describing health states and events and their distribution. So they describe **morbidity** and **mortality** within the population using person, place and time variables. Descriptive studies do not have an a priori hypothesis that investigators set out to answer; rather they focus on observing and describing what exists in the population. Given this, descriptive studies are helpful in determining the extent of ill health or disease in the community and studying the natural history and prognosis of disease. Descriptive studies are often carried out using pre-existing population health data.

Morbidity: The state of one's health, that is, illness, disability, chronic disease and so forth.

Mortality: Death.

There are two common types of descriptive epidemiological studies: cross-sectional studies and longitudinal studies (see also CHAPTER 13).

A **cross-sectional study** provides a snapshot of the frequency and characteristics of a disease in a population at a particular point in time.

CROSS-SECTIONAL STUDIES

A **cross-sectional study** involves the measurement of exposure and outcome simultaneously within the population of interest. Cross-sectional studies are often described as providing a snapshot of the frequency and characteristics of a disease in a population at a particular point in time. They are also referred to as **prevalence** studies. While cross-sectional studies are particularly useful for describing characteristics of the population, their main limitation is that **exposure** and **outcome** are measured at the same point in time and as such it may not be possible to distinguish whether the exposure preceded or followed the outcome, and thus cause and effect relationships are not certain.

Exposure: A potential risk or protective factor for a health state: an actual exposure (environmental pollution), a behaviour (cigarette smoking) or an individual attribute (age).

Outcome: The health state that is under investigation and of interest.

Prevalence

Prevalence is the frequency of existing cases of a health state in a particular population at a specific point in time or time-period. Prevalence is calculated as:

$$P = \frac{\text{Number of people with the health state at a specified time}}{\text{Number of people in the population at the specified time}} \times 10^n$$

There are two types of prevalence: point prevalence and period prevalence. *Point prevalence* is the frequency of existing cases of a health state in a specific population at a point in time. *Period prevalence is* the frequency of existing cases of a health state in a specific population during a defined time-period (Szklo & Nieto 2007).

A large-scale population-based cross-sectional study (Australian Study of Health and Relationships) conducted in 2000–01 aimed to describe a range of sexual health factors such as contraceptive practices (Smith et al. 2003) along with socio-demographic characteristics. This descriptive cross-sectional study found that 35.4 per cent of women and 44.6 per cent of men always used a condom with casual partners and 30.7 per cent of women and 28.9 per cent of men never did. In relation to heterosexual intercourse, men (90.4%) were significantly more likely than women (84.0%) to report having ever used condoms (de Visser et al. 2003). This study also found that condom use was significantly related to age, with lower use of condoms among older women and more common for women who spoke a language other than English at home (Richters et al. 2003). As you can see, this example describes the distribution of condom use among a defined population at a specific point in time.

As cross-sectional studies are undertaken at a single point in time they do not provide information on time trends. One way of obtaining information that includes the passage of time is the *repeat cross-sectional study*. This is similar to a cross-sectional except instead of taking a single sample from a population at one time-point, a new sample is drawn from the population of interest at each time-point. Unlike longitudinal studies, repeat cross-sectional studies collect data from different individuals at each time-point. The most common form of cross-sectional study is the survey (see CHAPTER 13). For example, the Australian Bureau of Statistics conducts regular repeat cross-sectional population health surveys known as the National Health Survey, which 'collects information about the health status of Australians, their use of health services and facilities, and health-related aspects of their lifestyle' (ABS 2006a, p. 8). The purpose of the survey is to 'obtain national benchmark information on a range of health issues, enable trends in health to be monitored over time, and provide information on health indicators for national health priority areas and for important subgroups of the population' (ABS 2006a, p. 7). Findings from the National Health Survey can be accessed via the ABS website (<www.abs.gov.au>) in report format, aggregated (summary) data, or through the confidentialised unit record file (CURF). Access to CURF data requires approval as it is de-identified individual-level data.

Melissa Graham

LONGITUDINAL STUDIES

Longitudinal studies are similar to repeat cross-sectional studies. But instead of drawing a new sample from the population at each time-point, the same group of people is followed over time. Longitudinal studies are useful to identify new cases (**incidence**) of a health

---

Longitudinal studies follow the same group of people over time. They identify new cases of a health state in a defined population and period.

---

state in a defined population and time-period. For example, an Australian longitudinal study that examined predictors of early motherhood found women who become mothers early tend to live in rural areas, have low levels of education, are married or in a de facto relationship and not in paid employment (Lee & Gramotnev 2006). As you can see from this example, longitudinal studies allow us to follow a defined group of the population (women) over time to see if the socio-demographic characteristics of these women predicted the health state (early motherhood) of interest. As such, we have described the distribution of the health state for women ('who') over 'time' in Australia ('where'). See also CHAPTER 13.

Incidence

Incidence is the number of new cases of a health state in a particular population at a specific point in time. There are two types of incidence: cumulative incidence and incidence rate. *Cumulative incidence* measures the risk of a person developing the health state in a defined time-period. Cumulative incidence can be calculated as:

$$CI = \frac{\text{Number of people with new health events during a specified time period}}{\text{Population at risk}} \times 10^n$$

Incidence rate is a measure of the rate at which new cases of the health state occur in the population during a specified time (Oleckno 2002). Incidence rate can be calculated as:

$$IR = \frac{\text{Number of people with new health events during a specified time period}}{\text{Total person-time at risk}} \times 10^n$$

Analytical epidemiology

Analytical epidemiological studies are designed to test hypotheses about associations between an exposure of interest and a particular health outcome. Thus analytical studies aim to identify or describe cause-and-effect relationships or associations between exposure and

---

Analytical epidemiological studies are designed to test hypotheses about associations between an exposure of interest and a particular health outcome.

---

outcome factors. So in addition to person, place and time variables, analytical studies can help us answer 'why' questions. Analytical studies can help identify if there is an association between two factors (such as cause and effect) and the strength of the association. In order to analyse associations between factors of interest, analytical studies involve planned comparisons between groups and generate **measures of association**.

Measures of association

These determine strengths of associations or relationships between exposures and outcomes. The measure of association used depends on the study design. *Relative risks* are a common measure of association and are primarily used for the analysis of associations in cohorts studies. Relative risk is also known as risk ratio and can be calculated as:

$$RR = \frac{\text{Incidence in the exposed}}{\text{Incidence in the non-exposed}}$$

Another commonly used measure of association is the odds ratio. The odds ratio is mainly used in case-control studies and is the 'odds' of exposure among the cases compared to the 'odds' among the controls and can be calculated as:

$$OR = \frac{\text{Odds of exposure among cases}}{\text{Odds of exposure among controls}}$$

There are four main types of analytical studies: cross-sectional studies, ecological studies, case-control studies and cohort studies. The primary objective of analytical epidemiology is to identify reasons or causes for observed patterns of health states by studying associations between factors (exposures and outcomes) (Szklo & Nieto 2007). This means that to begin with, we must identify the factors of interest in our analytical study: the outcome factor and the factor that may be related to (or be causing) the outcome of interest (exposure). The 'outcome of interest' is also often referred to as the dependent variable. Other authors use the term 'disease'. In epidemiology, however, not all outcomes are diseases and in fact some outcomes may be desirable or favourable health states. As such, it would be unfortunate and inappropriate to label these outcomes as disease. Therefore the terms health state or outcome are used throughout this chapter.

Analytical cross-sectional studies

Previously, I discussed cross-sectional studies as being descriptive, but cross-sectional studies can have analytical purposes as well as, or instead of, descriptive aims. Like descriptive cross-sectional studies, **analytical cross-sectional studies** involve taking a snapshot or cross-section of the population at a particular point in time. However, unlike descriptive cross-sectional studies, which do not involve looking at associations between exposures and outcomes, analytical cross-sectional studies aim to address questions about associations between exposures and outcomes. In analytical cross-sectional studies the exposure and outcome

Analytical cross-sectional studies studies aim to address questions about associations between exposures and outcomes.

Melissa Graham

are both measured at this time-point and as such share the same limitations as descriptive cross-sectional studies. So analytic cross-sectional studies allow us to describe the determinants (the 'why' question) of a health state and measure associations using **prevalence rate ratios**. For example, an analytical cross-sectional study that examined the association between highly active antiretroviral therapy (HAART) and sexual intercourse among HIV-positive women found that recent sexual activity was not associated with HAART use. However, HAART users were more likely (OR = 3.64) to practise protected sex, that is, to use condoms (Kaida et al. 2008).

Prevalence rate ratio (PRR)

The ratio of the prevalence in the exposed to the prevalence in the unexposed. The PRR is calculated as:

$$P = \frac{\text{Prevalence in the exposed}}{\text{Prevalence in the unexposed}}$$

ECOLOGICAL STUDIES

Ecological studies are different from the types of study designs we have looked at so far. In most epidemiological studies, individuals are counted and analysed in terms of their exposure and outcome status. In ecological studies, however, aggregates (groups) of individuals, areas or other larger units are analysed. The use of these aggregate measures means that associations can only be described at an aggregate level. For example, an ecological study has shown that areas of greater deprivation or socio-economic disadvantage have higher incidence rates of very preterm births and that this pattern persists over time (Smith et al. 2007). So while this study suggests that there is an association between deprivation and preterm births at an area level, one cannot conclude that this association exists among individuals. Inferring that group-level associations exist at the individual level is known as the ecological fallacy. Ecological studies commonly use pre-existing population health and other data.

CASE-CONTROL STUDIES

Ecological study: An epidemiological study in which the unit of analysis is groups or aggregates rather than individuals.

Case-control study: A study that compares a group of people who have the outcome factor of interest (cases) with a group of people who do not (controls).

Case-control studies compare a group of people who have the outcome factor of interest (cases) with a group of people who do not (controls). Investigators look back through time to identify exposures in the two groups. The two groups are then compared using measures of association, most commonly the odds ratio. For example, a case-control study compared women's birth weight with recurrent miscarriages. It found that women who experienced recurrent miscarriages had significantly lower birth weights when compared to the controls (women who had not had recurrent miscarriages) (Christiansen et al. 1992). So by comparing a group of people with the outcome of interest with a group of people without the outcome of interest and examining potential prior exposures, we can describe the distribution and determinants of health states. In doing so, we are able to establish cause-and-effect relationships because we know that the outcome followed the exposure. In case-control studies, it is essential that the cases and controls are comparable on all measures with the exception of the outcome.

COHORT STUDIES

Unlike longitudinal studies, where people are not categorised as exposed or not exposed, a **cohort study** follows a group (or cohort) of people over time who have been exposed and a group of people who have not been exposed to a possible risk factor for a health outcome. The incidence of the outcome in the exposed group is then compared to the incidence of the outcome in the group who are not exposed. This enables the relationship between the exposure and the outcome to be assessed. Cohort studies can be either prospective or retrospective.

> A **cohort study** follows a group (or cohort) of people over time who have been exposed to a possible risk factor for a health outcome and another group who have not been exposed.

A *prospective cohort study* commences with a cohort of people who do not have the outcome of interest. Participants are classified as 'exposed' or 'not exposed'. All participants are then followed forward in time until an outcome is established. Then, using the appropriate measure of association, the incidence of the outcome in the exposed group is compared to the incidence in the non-exposed group. For example, a prospective cohort study to examine psychosexual function 5 years after surgical intervention (transcervical endometrial resection/ablation [TCRE] or total hysterectomy) for the treatment of dysfunctional uterine bleeding found that psychosexual problems were higher for women who underwent a hysterectomy than for women who did not undergo hysterectomy (McPherson et al. 2005). As you can see, prospective cohort studies allow us to examine the distribution and determinants of health states over time.

Retrospective cohort studies are conducted in the same way as prospective cohort studies except that they measure exposures from the past and outcomes in the present. Since exposures have occurred in the past, retrospective cohort studies often use sources of data collection such as hospital records. For example, a retrospective cohort study was undertaken to compare the management (exposure) and outcomes of pregnancy in Indigenous and non-Indigenous HIV-positive women in Western Australia in 1991 and 2005. One of the outcomes of interest was HIV status of the babies (Gilles et al. 2007).

We have looked at the types of observational epidemiological study designs that generate health statistics we often see in the media, now let's turn to other sources of health statistics—population health data.

POPULATION HEALTH DATA

There are a number of sources of population health data that are freely available both internationally and nationally. Common sources of such data that are routinely collected include census data and disease registries (such as births, deaths, cancer and infectious diseases).

Melissa Graham

The collection of registry data is a national responsibility and often this data is provided to both the United Nations and the World Health Organization (WHO). Other sources of data include regular surveys such as the National Health Survey and hospital records. There are a number of advantages of using existing population health data. For example, the data has been previously collected and as a result it is inexpensive to access. However, a disadvantage of existing data sources is that often the data may be incomplete or of poor quality. This section will introduce you to a selection of population health data sources and some of their potential uses.

The WHO provides access to a range of interactive databases. For example, we can investigate a range of indicators for reproductive health such as fertility, low birth weight prevalence and maternal mortality within a specific country or across countries using the Reproductive Health Indicators database. This database includes data from WHO, United Nations and World Bank. These agencies compile data provided by each country or develop estimates for a given indicator (WHO 2006). Table 14.1 shows a comparison of selected reproductive health indicators across four countries. As you can see, low birth weight prevalence was lower in both Australia and New Zealand in 2000 when compared to the prevalence in both the UK and the USA in 2002. The maternal mortality ratio (annual number of maternal deaths per 100 000 live births) in Australia (8 per 100 000) is about half that seen in the USA (17 per 100 000) for the same year. Fertility rates across the four countries are similar, with New Zealand and the USA reporting slightly higher fertility rates for the period 2000–05 than Australia and the UK.

Table 14.1: Selected WHO reproductive health indicators

Country	Low birthweight prevalence (%)		Maternal mortality ratio (per 100,000)		Total fertility rate	
	Estimate	Year	Estimate	Year	Estimate	Year
Australia	7	2000	8 (5–10)	2000	1.8	2000–05
New Zealand	6	2000	7 (5–10)	2000	2.0	2000–05
United Kingdom (UK)	8	2002	13 (8–17)	2000	1.7	2000–05
United States of America (USA)	8	2002	17 (11–22)	2000	2.0	2000–05

Source: This table was generated from the WHO Reproductive Health Indicators Database <www.who.int/reproductive-health/global_monitoring/RHRxmls/RHRmainpage.htm>.

Another useful WHO interactive database is the Statistical Information System (WHOSIS). This database draws on core health statistics from the 193 WHO Member States (WHO 2008). It allows us to compare indicators across countries. As you can see in Table 14.2, Australia has the lowest percentage of both mammography (the percentage of women aged 50–69 years who have undergone a breast examination or mammography in the past year or past 3 years) and pap smear (the percentage of women aged 20–69 years who have undergone cervical cancer screening in the past year or past 3 years) screening when compared to New Zealand and the UK.

Table 14.2: Selected WHO core health indicators

Country	Women who have had mammography (%)		Women who have had PAP smear (%)	
Australia	57.0	2002	61.0	2003
New Zealand	63.0	2002	77.0	2002
United Kingdom (UK)	75.0	2003	70.0	2004

Source: This table was generated from the WHO Core Health Indicators Database <www.who.int/whosis/en/index.html>.

As well as the National Health Survey previously discussed, every 5 years the ABS conducts the Australian Census of Population and Housing, which provides a detailed description of the population including age, sex, marital status, education, occupation, living arrangements and other characteristics of the population (ABS 2006b). A range of census data products can be accessed at <www.abs.gov.au/Census>. The ABS allows you to search census data by area, topic or product type. Useful products include the Community Profile, CDATA, SuperTables and MapStats. The ABS also provides births data supplied by individual state and territory Registrars of Births, Deaths and Marriages (ABS 2009). Births data are available via the National Regional Profile data cubes (data cubes are aggregate-level data provided in spreadsheet table format). The ABS also provides customised data tables at a cost to researchers.

The Australian Institute for Health and Welfare (AIHW) provides access to a range of data including alcohol and other drug treatment, cancer, chronic disease indicators, mental health, disability, risk factors and National Hospital Morbidity data (AIHW n.d.). These data are drawn from a variety of sources. For example, the National Hospital Morbidity Database (NHMD) is collated from data supplied by the state and territory health authorities. It is a collection of confidentialised summary records for episodes of care in public and private hospitals in Australia. Procedures and diagnoses are recorded using the International Statistical Classification of Diseases and related Health Problems, Tenth revision, Australian Modification (ICD-10-AM) (AIHW 2009). The NHMD allows you to select a time-period, a health condition based on the ICD-10AM (diagnosis) and a procedure. The box 'Doing research' below gives an example of how you can use the National Hospital Morbidity data to understand patterns of health states.

Mortality data for selected causes by age and sex is also available via the AIHW General Record of Incidence of Mortality (GRIM). GRIM allows you to select cause of death, which can be examined by age, sex, time and so forth (AIHW 2008). As you can see from Figure 14.1, maternal mortality has declined from 30.6 per 100 000 women in 1907 to 0.1 per 100 000 women in 2006.

Melissa Graham

Figure 14.1: Maternal mortality trends, 1907–2006

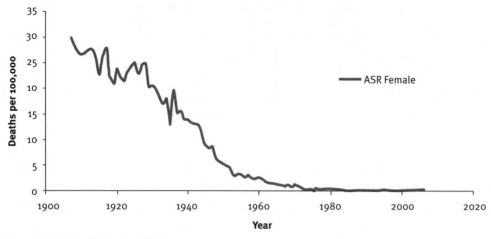

Source: AIHW 2008. GRIM Books. AIHW, Canberra

The Victorian Department of Human Services provides morbidity and mortality data through the Victorian Health Information Surveillance System (VHISS). VHISS is an interactive website that provides access to Burden of Disease data (life expectancy and disability adjusted life years), avoidable mortality and Ambulatory Care Sensitive Conditions (Victorian Department of Human Services 2009). Another source of population health data is the Victorian Population Health Surveys (VPHS). These repeat cross-sectional studies are conducted annually by the Victorian Department of Human Services.

DOING RESEARCH

Hysterectomy in Australia

Let us say we were interested in the incidence of all hysterectomies over time in Australia. Using the National Hospital Morbidity Database, information on all females admitted to hospital for a hysterectomy can be extracted using the *Procedures* data cube. This data cube provides the number of hysterectomies by type of hysterectomy and age from 2000–01 to 2006–07. Each year of data needs to be selected separately. For each year of data we can select the ICD Procedure Chapter in which we are interested—in this case *XIII Gynaecological Procedures* and then *Uterus*. Now we can select the type of hysterectomy in which we are interested—in this case abdominal and vaginal hysterectomy (these need to be selected separately). These interactive data cubes also allow you to export the data into Microsoft Excel. Using ABS population data we are able to find out how many women there were in Australia during the two points in time in which we are interested (2000–01 and 2004–05). We can now use the data from the NHMD (number of people with the health state) and the ABS population data (population at risk) to calculate the incidence of hysterectomy in 2000–01 and 2004–05. The hysterectomy incidence rate was 34.8 per 10 000 females in 2000–01 and to 31.2 per 10 000 in 2004–05. This suggests an overall decrease in hysterectomy of this period. This data also allows us to examine the patterns of hysterectomy over time by age. As you can see in the figure below, women aged 45–54 years had the highest rates of hysterectomy.

Figure 14.2: Incidence rate for all hysterectomy by age over time in Australia

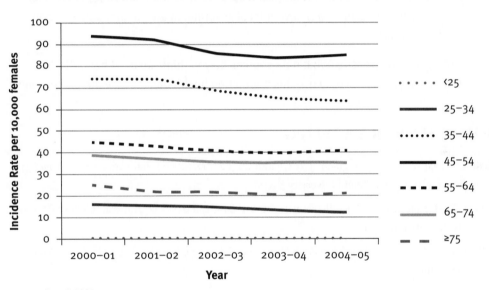

Source: Hill et al. 2007

SUMMARY

In this chapter, I have provided an overview of the underlying principles of observational epidemiology such as person, place and time. Further to this, key measures such as prevalence, incidence and measures of association used in observational epidemiology have been described. I have also outlined and explained the types of study designs used in observational epidemiology, drawing on contemporary examples. Finally, I identified and discussed a variety of sources of population health data that are accessible to health professionals.

Melissa Graham

TUTORIAL EXERCISES

1   A cross-sectional study conducted in 2008 of women aged 30–34 years in Australia found that of the 667 women in the study, 242 did not have any children. Calculate prevalence of childlessness in Australia in 2008.

2   The Births Registry in Victoria, Australia recorded 1652 births to females aged 15–19 years in 2006. The population of females aged 15–19 years for the same year was 169 593. Calculate the incidence of teenage births for females aged 15–19 years in 2006 in Victoria.

3   Explore the Victorian Department of Human Services Health Status of Victorians webpage (<www.health.vic.gov.au/healthstatus/index.htm>). Generate a Burden of Disease Life Expectancy report for your local government area. Now repeat this for Victoria. Is the life expectancy in your local government area higher or lower than that for Victoria?

4   Explore the ABS website. What data sources do you think are most helpful? Why? How do you think you could use this population health data as a health practitioner?

FURTHER READING

Bailey, L., Vardulaki, K., Langham, J. & Chandramohan, D. (2005). *Introduction to epidemiology*. Buckingham, UK: Open University Press.

Bonia, R., Beaglehole, R. & Kjellström, T. (2006). *Basic epidemiology*, 2nd edn. Geneva: World Health Organization.

Oleckno, W.A. (2002). *Essential epidemiology: Principles and applications*. Long Grove, IL: Waveland Press, Inc.

WEBSITES

www.who.int/reproductive-health/global_monitoring/RHRxmls/RHRmainpage.htm

   The WHO Reproductive Health Indicators Database.

www.who.int/whosis/en/index.html

   The WHO Core Health Indicators Database.

www.abs.gov.au

   The Australian Bureau of Statistics.

www.aihw.gov.au

The Australian Institute of Health and Welfare.

www.dhs.vic.gov.au

Victorian Department of Human Services.

www.health.vic.gov.au/healthstatus/index.htm

Victorian Department of Human Services Health Status of Victorians.

Melissa Graham

15

Clinical Trials:
The Good, the Bad and the Ugly

Karl B. Landorf

CHAPTER OBJECTIVES

In this chapter you will learn:

☐ what makes a good trial and what makes a bad trial

☐ the effect of bias in clinical trials

☐ how to minimise bias and other threats to the internal validity of clinical trials

☐ whether the findings of a trial can be generalised to clinical practice

☐ how to report clinical trials

KEY TERMS

Allocation bias

Allocation concealment

Ascertainment bias

Assessment bias

Blinding

Clinical trial

CONSORT Statement

Explanatory trial

Intention-to-treat analysis

Patient-reported outcome

Pragmatic trial

Publication bias

Randomisation

Randomised controlled trial

Selection bias

Stopping rule bias

Types I and II statistical errors

INTRODUCTION

Clinical trials are conducted to determine if an intervention is effective; that is, whether it is beneficial to patients (Peat 2001). Clinical trials can be used to investigate the efficacy of interventions such as a pharmacological or physical treatment (what most health professionals would associate them with), although they are equally appropriate to evaluate other interventions. For example, a clinical trial could be used to evaluate the effectiveness of a behavioural intervention (Carding & Hillman 2001), a health education strategy, or a prevention program (Torgerson & Torgerson 2008). See also CHAPTERS 16, 17.

> **Clinical trial:** A trial conducted to determine if an intervention is beneficial to patients.

Clinical trials can take many forms, from a simple case-series to a more complex, **randomised controlled trial** or RCT. In the pharmaceutical industry, where clinical trials are frequently used, they are often classified into four phases: Phase I Trials—clinical pharmacology and toxicity; Phase II Trials—initial clinical investigation for treatment effect; Phase III Trials—full-scale evaluation of treatment; and Phase IV Trials—post-marketing surveillance (Pocock 1983).

> **Randomised controlled trial:** A clinical trial where participants are randomly assigned to groups in order to receive different interventions. This randomisation removes many of the effects that may bias the true result.

For the novice, it is hard to know which trials to believe and which ones not to believe. Like Clint Eastwood in the classic spaghetti-western film *The Good, the Bad and the Ugly*, consumers of clinical trial research should be able to differentiate 'good' from 'bad', and they should also be able to decide when to dismiss a trial completely because it is truly 'ugly'! Accordingly, students, practitioners and researchers need to arm themselves with relevant knowledge to ensure that they are able to distinguish poor clinical trial research (the bad and the ugly) from high-quality clinical trial research (the good). The aim of this chapter, therefore, is to encourage practitioners to be wise consumers of clinical trials, not necessarily teach you how to conduct clinical trials. To achieve this aim, the following discussion will focus on randomised controlled trial methodology—the best available method to evaluate the effectiveness of an intervention.

Clinical trials can be of high or low quality (even RCTs). Students, practitioners and researchers must be aware of this so they can distinguish the good from the bad. Clinical decisions need to be made using evidence from good-quality trials.

GOOD TRIALS VERSUS BAD TRIALS

So how does a consumer of research determine if a trial is good or bad? Let us return to the example of the simple case series, where a series of participants receive an intervention (treatment) and the effect of that intervention is measured both before and after it is given. While on the surface it appears that this research design makes sense and would be relatively easy to conduct, it unfortunately has many issues that may make the measurement of the effect of the intervention inaccurate. For example, the placebo effect, where a patient responds positively to an inert intervention (i.e. an intervention designed to have no effect) is well known (Torgerson & Torgerson 2008). Many other effects[1] can also cloud the true effectiveness of an intervention; these are likely if the trial is not well planned and controlled.

In contrast, and at the other end of the spectrum, is the randomised controlled trial—where two (or more) groups receive interventions randomly. RCT methodology is currently considered the gold standard[2] for evaluating the efficacy of an intervention because it removes many of the effects that may bias the true result (Straus et al. 2005; Centre for Evidence-Based Medicine 2009). See also CHAPTERS 1, 12, 16, 17. However, even randomised trials, if conducted poorly, can result in inaccurate or biased findings; so thorough planning and execution is essential to ensure valid results.

DOING RESEARCH

An example of clinical trials in health care

Let us consider the results of two clinical trials, both of which I was involved in, that evaluated adhesive tape to reduce pain in the heel of the foot (Landorf et al. 2005; Radford et al. 2006). Taping helps support the foot, which in turn takes force and stress away from the heel. In the first trial, a non-randomised trial (Landorf et al. 2005), a group of 65 participants received foot-taping (i.e. the intervention group) and 40 participants received no taping (i.e. the control group). However, data for the two groups were not collected simultaneously—data for the control group were collected approximately one year after the intervention group data were collected. Consequently, participants did not receive taping randomly and the two groups knew what intervention they received; which means that the intervention group knew they were receiving taping to help their feet, while the control group knew they were not receiving any intervention (i.e. the participants were not 'blinded'). Fortunately, to avoid not treating participants in pain, data were only collected on the control group for approximately two weeks (they then received appropriate advice and free shoe inserts/foot orthoses). In addition to the participants knowing what treatment they were receiving, the investigators knew as well; that is, there was no blinding of assessors in the study.

So what did the results indicate? Well, interestingly, on a 100 mm visual analogue pain scale (a 100 mm line on a piece of paper by which a participant can indicate their pain level, 0 mm = no pain and 100 mm = worst pain imaginable) the intervention group was on average 32 mm better off than the control group at the end of the comparison period. That is, the intervention group's mean pain level was 32 mm lower (i.e. less pain) than the control group's mean pain level. What would the result have been if data were collected on all participants (i.e. both the intervention and control groups) simultaneously and the intervention was truly randomised? In addition, would the result have differed if the participants had been blinded to the intervention in question by adding a placebo or sham treatment? These are important questions because non-randomised and poorly controlled trials tend to overestimate the effect of a treatment (Schulz et al. 1995).

In a follow-up taping study of 92 participants with heel pain (Radford et al. 2006), the investigators incorporated the features mentioned above into a higher quality, and therefore more valid, study. Both the intervention and control groups received sham ultrasound treatment to the painful heel (the ultrasound unit did not actually deliver any ultrasound but appeared to do so). As participants in both groups were unaware that the ultrasound treatment was a sham, even the control group thought that they were allocated real treatment. Importantly, the only difference between the two groups was that the intervention group received taping, while the control group did not. At the completion of the study, the investigators found that the difference in pain on a 100 mm visual analogue pain scale was only about 12 mm, much smaller than the original study that found a 32 mm difference. What could account for this difference and why is it important for the accuracy of clinical trials that evaluate how effective an intervention is? This question leads us to the very essence of why randomised controlled trials are considered the gold standard method for evaluating whether an intervention is truly effective.

RANDOMISED CONTROLLED TRIALS

Randomised controlled trial methodology has been reported in medical science since the 1940s, although its initial use may have occurred 50 years earlier (Doll 1998; Hrobjartsson et al. 1998; D'Arcy Hart 1999). As mentioned earlier, RCT methodology is considered the gold standard when evaluating the efficacy of a treatment (Straus et al. 2005; Centre for Evidence-Based Medicine 2009). There are two key features to an RCT, which in its simplest form includes: (1) there is a comparison of a group receiving an intervention and one that does not; and (2) there is random allocation into those groups (Pocock 1983; Matthews 2006). RCTs where two groups are being compared are sometimes referred to as parallel-group RCTs, as data is collected on both groups at the same time and participants receive only one of two (or more) interventions (Wang & Bakhai 2006). More complex trials can also be performed where multiple interventions are compared (i.e. there are more than two groups).

The main aim of using RCT methodology is to ensure as much as possible that the characteristics of the participants (i.e. the people who receive the interventions) at the beginning of the trial are similar across groups (Friedman et al. 1998). To illustrate why this is important, let us consider an RCT that sets out to evaluate the effectiveness of a dietary supplement on weight loss. It makes sense to ensure that both the intervention and control groups have similar weight at the beginning of the trial. Otherwise, any effect noticed over the course of the trial might be associated with the difference in weight at the beginning, rather than the dietary supplement being tested. If, however, appropriate randomisation and allocation concealment are carried out and the two groups are similar at the beginning of the trial, bias (or systematic unwanted effects) will be minimised (Matthews 2006). Such bias affects the internal validity of a trial, which can make the findings inaccurate. In order to appreciate the power of RCTs, it is important to explore these issues further. Knowledge of such issues provides practitioners with the ability to assess trials for their quality and consequently whether their results are believable.

> **The main aim of using RCT methodology is to ensure as much as possible that the characteristics of the participants (i.e. the people who receive the interventions) at the beginning of the trial are similar across groups.**

Issues that affect the internal validity of a randomised trial

RANDOM ALLOCATION

The key feature of randomised controlled trials is random allocation of participants to groups. This feature, as stated previously, promotes comparability among the study groups (Rosenberger & Lachin 2002), such that known and unknown prognostic variables will be similar (Friedman et al. 1998). Put more simply, **randomisation** is a powerful tool that ensures the study groups are as similar as possible except for the intervention being studied (Matthews 2006). Common methods to achieve randomisation include consulting a random number table (supplied in many statistical textbooks), or more likely nowadays, using a computer program to generate a random number sequence (Jadad 1998). There are different forms of randomisation: simple randomisation, blocked randomisation (where randomisation occurs in equal-sized blocks of participants), stratified randomisation (where randomisation is based on prognostic variables) and adaptive randomisation (where allocation probabilities change as the study progresses) (Friedman et al. 1998). For most studies, simple or blocked randomisation is usually appropriate, but for multi-centre trials randomisation may need to be stratified by centre (Friedman et al. 1998).

Randomisation:
A mechanism where participants are randomly allocated an intervention, e.g. the active test intervention versus a placebo or a sham intervention.

BIAS

In any clinical evaluation, it is essential that the research methodology used ensures that the effect of a treatment is directly attributable to that treatment, and not to extraneous causes (Pocock 1983). For example, one common problem in clinical trials—even controlled trials—is that researchers may unknowingly influence or bias the outcome of a study (Chalmers et al. 1983; Schulz et al. 1995). Such bias can distort the results or conclusions away from the truth, the result being a poor-quality trial that underestimates, or more likely overestimates the benefits of an intervention (Egger et al. 2003). Some of the more common biases that may occur are discussed below.

Selection bias can arise if the investigators systematically manipulate enrolment into the trial (Greenhalgh 2006). For example, selection bias will occur if patients are selected using non-random methods or if they self-select themselves into groups (Peat 2001). This may make the recruits unrepresentative of the population with the condition being studied (i.e. it affects the external validity or generalisability of the trial) (Piantadosi 2005; see also Chapter 11). Selection bias can be minimised by careful sampling procedures and strict adherence to inclusion and exclusion criteria (Peat 2001).

Allocation bias is a type of selection bias. It occurs when the process of allocating participants to groups leads to differences in the baseline characteristics of those groups (Peat 2001). For example, if an investigator recruiting participants thinks a potential recruit may respond poorly to the treatment allocated to them, the investigator may exclude them from the study or postpone their enrolment until they are certain they will receive the intervention they believe to be most beneficial. This may result in differences in the baseline characteristics of participants in the groups to be compared (Chalmers et al. 1983), which is undesirable as the main purpose of randomisation is to ensure as much as possible that the characteristics of the participants at the beginning of the trial are similar across groups (Friedman et al. 1998). Allocation bias can be prevented by appropriate randomisation and concealment of the allocation schedule (*allocation concealment*) from trial staff involved in recruitment and assessment of participants (Schulz & Grimes 2002a). Adequate concealment of the randomised assignment sequence is essential to prevent staff from deciphering the sequence, thus causing bias. Unfortunately, deciphering the randomised allocation sequence is more common than might be expected—staff involved in clinical trials often find it hard to resist 'cracking the code' (Schulz 1995). Trials that have inadequate allocation concealment yield larger estimates of the effectiveness of interventions and are more likely to report significant findings (Schulz et al. 1995; Hewitt et al. 2005). Concealment of a participant's allocation to the intervention or control group can be as simple as it being placed in a sealed opaque envelope that is opened only once the participant is recruited into the trial. A better method is remote allocation where the person recruiting the participant must call a distant and separate randomisation service once the participant is recruited (Torgerson & Roberts 1999). When presenting the findings of a trial, investigators must adequately report how they concealed allocation (Schulz 1996).

Assessment bias may occur if an investigator's assessment of a participant lacks objectivity (Pocock 1983). Subjective outcome measures are prone to exaggerate the effect of the intervention (Wood et al. 2008). For example, if an investigator is aware of the group a participant has been

Selection bias arises if the investigators systematically manipulate enrolment into the trial.

Allocation bias: A type of selection bias that occurs when the process of allocating participants to groups leads to differences in the baseline characteristics of those groups.

Assessment bias occurs if an investigator's assessment of a participant lacks objectivity. Subjective outcome measures are prone to exaggerate the effect of the intervention.

allocated to, they may distort or misclassify the outcome measured (Peat 2001). Bias may also occur from a participant's perspective as well; for example, participants may under- or overreport exposures or not report the outcomes being measured accurately (Peat 2001). Assessments therefore must be accurate and objective, and collected using standardised procedures (Peat 2001). Objectivity is enhanced by blinding assessors and participants if possible (Day & Altman 2000), although this can be difficult with interventions that involve non-pharmacological interventions, such as physical treatments (Boutron et al. 2007).

Ascertainment bias occurs when the results or conclusions of the trial are distorted by the knowledge of which intervention each participant is receiving (Jadad 1998). For example, if the intervention for each participant is known, investigators may alter the types of co-intervention offered to participants or distort the outcomes being measured. Furthermore, if the investigators are unblinded they may alter the way in which they handle a participant who withdraws, drops out or violates the study protocol. For example, the investigator may ignore a participant's breach of protocol or allow participants to withdraw less easily if they know what intervention they have been allocated. Assessment bias, ascertainment bias and inappropriate handling of participants can all be minimised by appropriate blinding (Schulz & Grimes 2002b). Blinding should be reported by investigators, which should include who were blinded (e.g. assessors, caregivers, participants, those involved in data analysis) and how they were blinded, not just the type of blinding (e.g. single-blind, double-blind, and so on) (Schulz & Grimes 2002b; Haahr & Hrobjartsson 2006).

Allocation concealment is different from **blinding**. Allocation concealment refers to the randomised allocation sequence being concealed from those investigators who are involved in recruiting participants, whereas blinding is a technique to prevent assessors, participants or data analysis staff knowing which group the participant is in after they have been allocated.

Stopping rule bias can occur if a trial is stopped inappropriately. For example, it would be inappropriate if investigators are aware of the outcomes of each intervention and continue recruiting only until they obtain a positive (statistically significant) result (see CHAPTERS 24, 25). A pre-specified or a priori sample size (discussed below) should be determined and data collection should generally continue until that target has been reached.

SAMPLE SIZE

Researchers should conduct a prospective sample size calculation to decrease the chance of **Type II statistical errors** (Moher et al. 1994). A Type II error (see CHAPTER 25) occurs when the investigators conclude

Ascertainment bias occurs when the results or conclusions of the trial are distorted by the knowledge of which intervention each participant is receiving.

Allocation concealment refers to the randomised allocation sequence being concealed from investigators who are involved in recruiting participants.

Blinding: A technique used in RCTs to prevent assessors, participants or data analysis staff knowing which group a participant is in after they have been allocated.

Stopping rule bias can occur if a trial is stopped inappropriately.

Type II statistical errors occur when researchers mistakenly conclude that there was no difference, no association and so on when in fact there was.

that there is no significant difference between the groups (i.e. that the intervention being studied is not effective); although there may have been a clinically important effect, the trial did not have a sufficiently large sample size to detect it statistically (Portney & Watkins 2009). Therefore all trials should recruit an appropriate number of patients into the trial to be able to detect clinically important effects (Altman 1980).

Sample size can be estimated using readily available tables (Peat 2001) or calculated using appropriate formulae (Friedman et al. 1998). Appropriate sample size is fundamental to any clinical trial (Cohen 1977). Accordingly, there is an ethical imperative that the investigators conduct an a priori sample size calculation to power the study appropriately from a statistical standpoint (Altman 1980; Moher et al. 1994). Without this, the study might be doomed to failure—that is, it is underpowered—from the start. Researchers should include a paragraph on how the sample size was determined, including accurate reporting of parameters such as the effect size that the study was powered statistically to detect (Charles et al. 2009). See also CHAPTERS 1, 25.

> The **sample size** of an RCT must be determined before the start of the trial, and should be large enough to be able to detect if the intervention being evaluated leads to a clinically worthwhile effect.

OUTCOME MEASURES

Appropriate **outcome measures** should be used to measure the effect of the intervention (Roland & Torgerson 1998). These should include **patient-reported outcomes**, where the patient, rather than the clinician, reports on the impact of a disease or intervention on the status of their health (Willke et al. 2004). Patient-reported health status measurement (or questionnaires), also referred to as health-related quality of life measurement, offers a broader investigation from the patient's perspective of the effect of an intervention, compared to surrogate outcome measures that are usually generated by the clinician (Jenkinson & McGee 1998; Muldoon et al. 1998; Bowling 2005; Landorf & Burns 2009). Clearly, when evaluating the effect of an intervention on a patient, the patient's perspective on whether that intervention is effective or not is most important (see also CHAPTERS 11, 13).

> **Outcome measures** are used to measure the effect of an intervention. They should be both valid and reliable.

> **Patient-reported outcome:** An outcome where the patient, rather than the clinician, reports on the impact of a disease or intervention on the status of their health.

Outcome measures should be both valid and reliable (Portney & Watkins 2008). Researchers should clearly state what outcome measures were used, and give details about the validity and reliability of the measures, particularly if they are not well known (see CHAPTER 11). Primary outcomes should be nominated before the trial begins to avoid selective reporting of outcome measures, which can lead to bias and overestimation of the effectiveness of an intervention (Chan et al. 2004).

The outcomes used in a clinical trial to measure the effect of an intervention need to be appropriate for the condition and participants being studied, and should have proven validity and reliability.

Karl B. Landorf

INTENTION-TO-TREAT ANALYSIS

An **intention-to-treat analysis** should be conducted as the primary analysis. With this type of analysis, outcome measures are obtained regardless of compliance with the trial protocol, and data from all participants are analysed according to allocation, even if the participants had adverse events or unexpected outcomes (Fergusson et al. 2002; Schulz & Grimes 2002c). Intention-to-treat analysis maintains the balance of confounders, which reduces variability between groups (Newell 1992), thus maintaining the comparability of groups originally established by randomisation (Keech et al. 2007). Doing so provides a more pragmatic or real-life estimate of the benefit of a treatment (Hollis & Campbell 1999). Researchers should state in their article whether they have analysed their results using the intention-to-treat principle.

> **Intention-to-treat analysis** is used in RCTs, where outcome measures are obtained regardless of compliance with the trial protocol and data from all participants are analysed according to allocation.

DROPOUT RATE

The dropout rate from a clinical trial must be reported and should be kept to a minimum; trials with substantial loss to follow-up (e.g. greater than 15%) should be viewed with caution (Lang & Secic 1997). Excessive dropout may lead to distortion of results, particularly if more dropouts occur in one group. Accordingly, investigators must ensure that a minimum number of participants drop out of a clinical trial. Researchers must transparently indicate what the dropout rate was in their trial.

Table 15.1: Issues that affect the internal validity of an RCT

Issue	Method to control issue
Groups that differ in their baseline characteristics	Randomisation
Selection bias	Strict adherence to inclusion and exclusion criteria; allocation concealment
Allocation bias	Allocation concealment
Assessment bias	Blinding; objective outcome measures
Ascertainment bias	Blinding
Inappropriate handling of participants not complying	Blinding; intention-to-treat analysis
Stopping rule bias	Blinding; pre-specified sample size calculation
Small sample size	Pre-specified sample size calculation
Inappropriate outcome measures	Use of valid and reliable outcomes that include health status measurements
Non-prespecified data dredging	Trial registration (see below: Reporting RCTs)

Issues that affect the external validity of a randomised trial

Randomised controlled trials can either be explanatory or pragmatic (Schwartz & Lellouch 2009). An **explanatory trial** is one that is highly controlled, thus reducing the number of variables that can affect the final outcome. It therefore has more ability to explain what variable caused the result detected. However, because of the tight controls placed on the trial, the results of an explanatory trial may not necessarily be able to be generalised to everyday practice. In contrast, a **pragmatic trial** is one in which the investigators attempt to mimic common practice, thereby endeavouring as much as possible to make the results generalisable to everyday practice.

> **Explanatory trial:** A trial that is highly controlled and hence reduces the number of variables that can affect the final outcome.

> **Pragmatic trial:** One in which the investigators attempt to mimic common practice, thereby endeavouring as much as possible to make the results generalisable to everyday practice.

Pragmatic trials have become more common over the past decade or so in an effort to make clinical trials more meaningful to clinicians and the public (Zwarenstein & Treweek 2009). If a pragmatic trial is conducted, the participants, interventions, clinicians and study protocols should represent common practice as much as possible to ensure external validity and generalisability (Roland & Torgerson 1998). To assess a trial for external validity, practitioners should ask themselves the following questions: Were the participants in the trial of similar age and sex to those that would normally be treated with the condition in practice (Jüni et al. 2001)? Did they have a comparable severity of disease or number of co-morbidities? Was the intervention equivalent to what would be used in everyday clinical practice? Was the setting alike, that is, was the type of treatment centre or experience of the care providers comparable? Were the type of outcomes used and duration of follow-up similar?

Practitioners using the results of RCTs to inform their clinical decision-making must assess the extent to which each trial can be generalised to their workplace. A demonstrated beneficial effect of an intervention in an RCT in one group of the population (e.g. younger adults) may not exist with another group (e.g. older adults). Therefore a practitioner that predominantly treats older adults may not experience the same beneficial effect of that treatment because the participants from the trial are not comparable with the patients in their workplace. Practitioners need to keep this in mind when reading articles that present the findings of RCTs. They should constantly appraise whether the characteristics of the participants, interventions and settings are similar enough to their situation (Jüni et al. 2001).

To ensure the findings of a clinical trial are generalisable, practitioners need to assess whether the participants, interventions and protocols employed in the trial are similar to their practice.

Karl B. Landorf

Publication bias occurs when a trial is published or not published because of the direction of its findings. Studies that have a positive result are more likely to be published.

Citation bias occurs where articles that have statistically significant findings are cited more often than others.

There is one final matter that practitioners need to be aware of when considering external validity and that is that the RCTs they encounter may be biased from a publication perspective. **Publication bias** occurs when a trial is published or not published because of the direction of its findings (Duley & Farrell 2002). Studies that have a positive result are more likely to be published and trials finding no difference between groups are, on average, less likely, or will take longer to be published (Ioannidis 1998). **Citation bias** also occurs where articles that have statistically significant findings are cited more often than others (Nieminen et al. 2007). Practitioners need to take into account that they may be more likely to come across positive, statistically significant trials and that less positive trials are less likely to be published and cited.

Table 15.2: Components of an RCT that need to be considered by practitioners when assessing how generalisable the findings are to their practice

Component	Issue
Participants	If the patients in a practitioner's workplace have different characteristics to the participants in the trial, they might react differently to the intervention.
Interventions	If the intervention used in a practitioner's workplace is sufficiently different to that evaluated in the trial, the benefits of the intervention may not be the same.
Settings	If the environment and experience of staff in a workplace are different to that of the trial, the benefits of the intervention for patients may not be the same.
Outcomes	If the type and definition of the outcomes used to measure the effect of the intervention in the practitioner's workplace are different to those used in the trial, a different effect of the intervention might be perceived.
Follow-up period	If the standard follow-up period for participants in a practitioner's workplace is inconsistent with that in the trial, the benefits of the intervention may be under- or overestimated.
Publication	Positive, statistically significant trials are more likely to be published and cited, whereas less positive trials are less likely to be published and cited.

Reporting RCTs

The **CONSORT Statement** aims to ensure accurate and complete reporting of the design, conduct, analysis and generalisability of trials, thus ensuring the highest possible standards are met when clinical trials are published.

Bias may also occur during the dissemination process, both on the part of the authors and the readers of articles reporting randomised controlled trials. For example, insufficient information may be supplied in the article for readers to judge whether the study is of adequate quality for the results to be believable. To rectify this, researchers and editors involved in publishing scientific medical research developed the **Consolidated Standards of Reporting Trials (CONSORT) Statement** (Begg et al. 1996).

This statement aims to ensure accurate and complete reporting of the design, conduct, analysis and generalisability of trials, thus ensuring that the highest possible standards are met when clinical trials are published. To facilitate this process, a checklist was also developed with items ranging from the title and abstract, to methodological issues and reporting of results. In addition, a flow diagram was suggested to illustrate the progress of participants through the trial.

The CONSORT statement has since been revised (Altman et al. 2001; Moher et al. 2001a,b) and is widely recognised as the benchmark for appropriately reporting RCTs. It has been endorsed or recommended by many journals including the *New England Journal of Medicine*, *The Lancet* and the *Journal of the American Medical Association* (Laine et al. 2007). Following the CONSORT Guidelines (Moher et al. 2009) will ensure that researchers provide adequate details about a trial, thus providing clinicians and other researchers with sufficient information to judge whether the findings are believable. This is important when making decisions about incorporating findings into clinical practice (Altman 1996). A comprehensive guide to interpreting and reporting RCTs using the CONSORT Guidelines is available (see Keech et al. 2007). See also CHAPTER 26.

A priori nomination of important components of a clinical trial (e.g. inclusion and exclusion criteria, primary and secondary outcomes, data analysis) is now expected. Most health and medical journals now demand clinical trial registration before the trial begins (International Committee of Medical Journal Editors 2009). In addition, the WHO (2009) state that 'the registration of all interventional trials is a scientific, ethical and moral responsibility', and the World Medical Association's revised Declaration of Helsinki (2008, paragraph 19) now states that 'every clinical trial must be registered in a publicly accessible database before recruitment of the first subject'. If not registered, the investigators will have difficulty publishing the results of a trial, particularly in high-impact journals.

Trial registration ensures that investigators commit to certain parameters for the conduct and analysis of their trial. Such scrutiny places tight controls over investigators and minimises the chance that they will cause bias. For example, a prespecified plan for data analysis avoids investigators going on a 'fishing expedition' once the data is collected. Such data-dredging exercises, where the investigators continue to analyse the data until they find significant findings, even from less important secondary outcomes, can lead to bias. Testing multiple non-prespecified hypotheses inflates the **Type I statistical error** rate, resulting in spurious and often implausible findings (Proschan & Waclawiw 2000; Austin et al. 2006) (see CHAPTER 25). Multiple hypothesis tests on subgroups within the participants in a trial can also lead to similar false positive results (Wang et al. 2007). Researchers should state that the trial was registered and include the registration details (i.e. the name or code of the registry and the registration number). To appreciate further the nature of clinical trial registration, the website address of a clinical trial registry is included below under Websites.

Type I statistical errors occur when researchers mistakenly conclude that a finding was statistically significant when it may be a result of chance rather than being a real difference.

Karl B. Landorf

Assessing the quality of clinical trials

With all of the above in mind, the quality of a clinical trial is clearly affected by a number of issues. Good trials are ones where most of these issues have been well thought through and addressed before the trial begins. Importantly, they lack bias and are likely to report a more accurate estimate of the effectiveness of an intervention. In addition, as systematic reviews (see Chapter 18) become more common, thorough quality assessments of the trials included are recommended to minimise bias from poor-quality studies (Egger et al. 2003).

Once a clinical trial is published, though, how does a practitioner determine whether it is good or bad from a quality perspective? Fortunately, methods are available to rate the quality of a clinical trial and there are many quality rating scales already in existence. But even though such scales are often used, there is still some debate about their appropriateness for identifying high- and low-quality trials (Jüni et al. 1999). Two rating scales that are commonly used are the PEDro Scale (PEDro 2009), used for clinical trials involving physical therapies (see also Chapters 17, 18), and the Jadad Scale (Jadad et al. 1996). Both of these scales are more concerned with the internal validity of trials than their external validity or generalisability to clinical practice. Nevertheless, they can be useful in determining the level of believability of the trial from a methodological standpoint.

SUMMARY

In the modern health care environment, practitioners must use the results of clinical trials to guide their practice when they want to know if an intervention is effective. While not always easy to detect on the surface, the quality of a clinical trial can be generally classified as good or bad, and some may even be considered downright ugly! Randomised controlled trials are considered the gold standard to determine the effectiveness of an intervention. However, if an RCT is conducted poorly, it will be prone to bias, which will affect its internal validity. As such, the findings will not be accurate, precise or meaningful.

To avoid such bias, many issues need to be considered when conducting a trial, such as random allocation, allocation concealment, blinding of investigators and participants, use of valid and reliable outcome measures, appropriate handling of participants dropping out of the trial, and appropriate statistical analysis. When using the results of a clinical trial, practitioners must evaluate all of these issues to assess whether a trial is of good quality, and therefore whether its results are believable.

Investigators should report the results of an RCT in line with the recommendations outlined in the CONSORT statement. Doing so makes it easier for practitioners to find key pieces of information easily, so they cannot only determine the effectiveness of the intervention being tested, but also how believable the results are (i.e. is it a high-quality trial?). Finally, practitioners need to assess whether the participants, interventions and protocols employed in a clinical trial are similar enough to their practice (i.e. are the findings generalisable?). By following the guidelines outlined in this chapter, practitioners will be able to avoid incorporating the findings from bad trials into their practice, concentrating instead on findings from good trials.

NOTES

1   Other than the placebo effect, there are many other phenomena that may make the results of a poorly controlled clinical trial inaccurate, such as the Hawthorne effect, regression to the mean, and resentful demoralisation (Torgerson & Torgerson 2008). Such effects need to be controlled for appropriate randomisation, use of placebo/sham interventions, and blinding of investigators and participants.

2   Although RCTs are considered the gold standard for evaluating the effectiveness of interventions, an even better method is the systematic review (Centre for Evidence-Based Medicine 2009; see Chapter 18). A systematic review combines many RCTs that have evaluated an intervention, thereby increasing sample size and improving the precision of the estimate of the effect of the intervention. But to conduct a relevant systematic review one must have RCTs to include in the first place.

TUTORIAL EXERCISES

1   What are the key reasons for conducting a randomised controlled trial?

2   Discuss issues of bias in clinical trials and how they may affect the findings.

3   Discuss the effect a small sample size may have on an RCT.

4   What components of an RCT would you need to consider before generalising the results of the trial to your practice?

5   Evaluate a published RCT to determine if the authors have satisfied the recommendations in the CONSORT Guidelines for reporting RCTs.

6   Assess the quality of a published RCT using the PEDro Scale.

7   Think of an intervention that is used for a common condition you might encounter in practice. Try to design a high-quality RCT that would evaluate the intervention's effectiveness.

Karl B. Landorf

FURTHER READING

Duley, L. & Farrell, B. (2002). *Clinical trials*. London: BMJ Books.

Greenhalgh, T. (2006). *How to read a paper: The basics of evidence based medicine*. Malden, MA: Blackwell Publishing/BMJ Books.

Herbert, R., Jamtvedt, G., Mead, J. & Birger Hagen, K. (2005). *Practical evidence-based physiotherapy*. Edinburgh: Elsevier.

Peat, J.K. (2001). *Health science research: A handbook of quantitative methods*. Sydney: Allen & Unwin.

Torgerson, D.J. & Torgerson, C.J. (2008). *Designing randomised trials in health education and the social sciences: An introduction*. Basingstoke, UK: Palgrave Macmillan.

WEBSITES

www.anzctr.org.au/default.aspx

A website for a clinical trials registry (the Australian and New Zealand Clinical Trials Registry).

www.cebm.net/levels_of_evidence.asp

A website explaining where randomised controlled trials sit in the hierarchy of levels of evidence.

www.consort-statement.org

The website that contains all relevant information about the CONSORT guidelines for reporting randomised trials.

www.pedro.org.au

The website where a copy of the PEDro clinical trial rating scale can be downloaded.

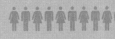

Part IV

Evidence-based Practice and Systematic Review

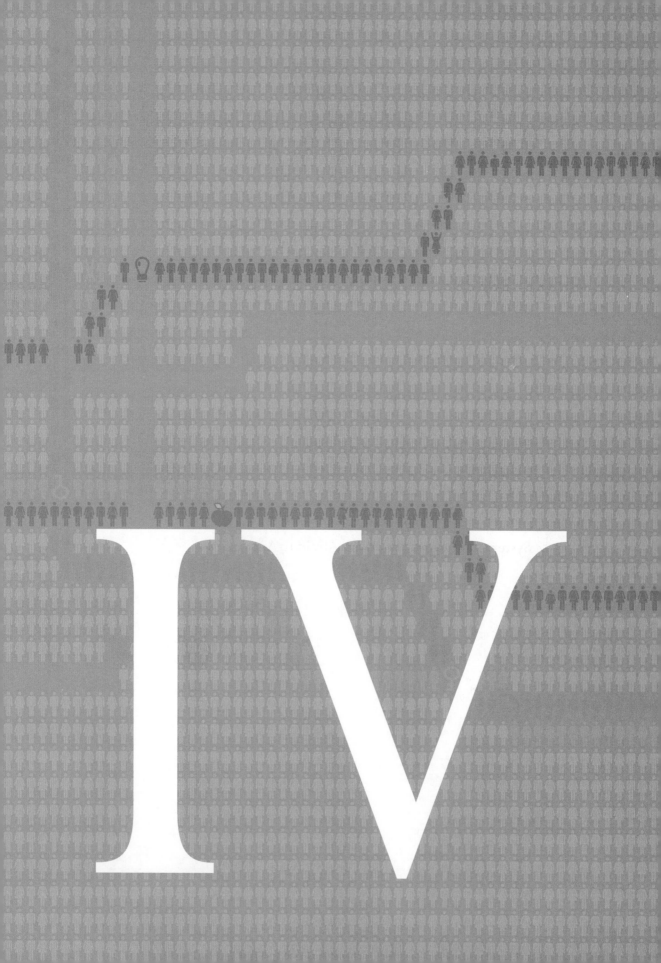

16

Evidence-based Health Care

Deirdre Fetherstonhaugh, Rhonda Nay and Margaret Winbolt

CHAPTER OBJECTIVES

In this chapter you will learn:

- ☐ to appraise clinical guidelines
- ☐ to describe how evidence can be implemented in practice
- ☐ to develop strategies for success
- ☐ how to use audit to implement evidence-based health care

KEY TERMS

Clinical audit

Evidence

Evidence-based practice in health care

Systematic review

INTRODUCTION

'Everyone' is talking the talk of **evidence-based practice in health care**. According to Winbolt and colleagues (2009, p. 442) '[t]he move to evidence-based practice (EBP) has been driven by changing professional, government and consumer expectations as well as a need to

> **Evidence-based practice in health care:** A process that requires the practitioner to find empirical evidence about the effectiveness or efficacy of different treatment options and then determine the relevance of the evidence to a particular client's situation.

justify the care given in terms of effectiveness and cost.' Health services say they 'do' EBP, but do we really know what it is? Are we using the same language and is there a shared understanding of what it means? We would argue for a resounding 'no' to all three questions. In this chapter, we will unpick some of the myths, rhetoric and misunderstandings and try to clear the confusion. Having established what EBP is, we will explore some of the skills you need to determine confidently how good the evidence is and, just as importantly, how to translate it into everyday practice. The importance of leadership at every level will be emphasised.

DEFINING 'EVIDENCE'

When reviewing the literature for this chapter, one thing that became obvious is the confusion over what is meant by evidence-based practice. Indeed, most research papers appeared to confuse 'research-based' practice with EBP (Closs & Lewin 1998; Dysart & Tomlin 2002; Byham-Gray et al. 2005; Ferguson et al. 2008; Scott & McSherry 2008; Rubin & Parrish 2007; see also CHAPTER 9). Reading one, two or a dozen research papers and applying that to practice is *not* EBP. **Evidence** in the definition of EBP has a very specific meaning and is arrived at through a

> **Evidence:** Evidence in the context of EBP is what results from a systematic review and appraisal of all available literature relevant to a carefully designed question and protocol.

very specific and rigorous process. Evidence is what results from a systematic review (see CHAPTER 18) and appraisal of all available literature relevant to a carefully designed question and protocol; it is rated according to a hierarchy that determines 'how good' that evidence is or how confident the reader or practitioner can be in applying it (see also CHAPTERS 1, 15, 17).

Taking this then as the definition of evidence, to what extent do health professionals engage in EBP? It would seem to us that experience, tradition and less frequently research, rather than evidence, informs practice. Surveys often ask questions about the use of research, which is quite different from whether or not practice is evidence-based. Those papers that report health professionals being supportive of EBP often overestimate the extent to which what they do is actually based on the evidence.

TRY IT YOURSELF

Think about your own practice:

☐ What informs your approach?

☐ Do you base your practice on what you learnt at university or on what is tradition in the workplace?

☐ How often do you actually read research papers?

☐ Do you know how to appraise a research paper and determine if it is high-quality research or do you just scan the paper and read the results or the abstract and take them as gospel?

☐ Do you know how to differentiate a systematic review from a literature review?

☐ Could you appraise a systematic review?

EVIDENCE-BASED PRACTICE

There are many definitions of evidence-based practice, but of note is the number that leave out what we see as perhaps most important, and that is *the client*. EBP evolved from evidence-based medicine (EBM) established by Archie Cochrane (1979), after whom the Cochrane Collaboration is named (see CHAPTER 17 for more detail). One of the acknowledged gurus of EBM is Sackett, and if you go back to these authors' definition (1997), which most writers do, you will find they always included clinician expertise and client[1] choice. These aspects of the definition are often ignored, and then EBP is criticised as ignoring clinical expertise and client choice! Sackett and associates (1996, p. 71) define EBM as

> the conscientious, explicit and judicious use of current best evidence in making decisions about the care of individual patients. The practice of evidence-based medicine means integrating *individual clinical expertise* with the best available external evidence from systematic research…and the more thoughtful identification and compassionate use of individual *patients' predicaments, rights and preferences* [emphasis added].

Further to this, Sackett and associates (1997, pp. 2–3) advocate that:

> The practice of EBM is a process of life-long, self-directed learning in which caring for our own patients creates the need for clinically important information about diagnosis, prognosis, therapy and other clinical and health care issues in which we:
>
> ☐ convert these information needs into answerable questions;
>
> ☐ track down, with maximum efficiency, the best evidence with which to answer them;
>
> ☐ critically appraise that evidence for its validity (closeness to truth) and usefulness (clinical applicability);
>
> ☐ apply the results of this appraisal in our clinical practice; and
>
> ☐ evaluate our performance.

EBP reduces inconsistency in practice and increases efficiency and effectiveness, and has thus been accepted by government and funding bodies as essential to better health care (see CHAPTER 17). It is integral to clinical governance, which is now widely accepted as the responsibility of health organisations both nationally and internationally. Many definitions of clinical governance exist, but one that is commonly quoted refers to it as 'the framework

Deirdre Fetherstonhaugh, Rhonda Nay and Margaret Winbolt

through which health organisations are accountable for continuously improving the quality of their services and safeguarding high standards of care by creating an environment in which excellence in clinical care will flourish' (Scally & Donaldson 1998, p. 3). Clinical governance is defined by the Australian Council on Healthcare Standards (2004, p. 4) as 'the system by which the governing body, managers and clinicians share responsibility and are held accountable for patient care, minimising risks to consumers, and for continuously monitoring and improving the quality of clinical care'.

TRY IT YOURSELF

Think about a practice from your workplace:

☐ Why it is practised in that way? If others practise differently in relation to this situation, on what do they base their decisions to practise their way?

☐ If you were required to justify your practice in court tomorrow, what would you use to mount your case?

☐ If your boss asked you to demonstrate that your practice was cost-effective, could you do so?

☐ If your client asked you to indicate other options and provide evidence as to why one option was better than others, how would you go about it?

☐ How do you determine if the practice is 'best practice' and acceptable to your client?

In the unhappy event that you end up in court it would be far more convincing to be able to say: 'I based my decision on the best available international evidence, clinical experience and informed client choice' than 'Well, Your Honour, we have always done it that way and we know what is best for our clients'. You are also more likely to improve your budget situation if you can present reasoned evidence to your boss rather than simply argue from a position of emotion. Your clients have the right to make decisions about their health care and they are usually the best judge of what is best for them in their situation—but they can do this fully informed if you present to them the best available evidence and all options rather than just your opinion.

EBP usually begins with a question or problem from clinical practice. Examples may include:

1   Is this treatment better than usual care?

2   Can this education program improve health outcomes?

3   What are the barriers to reducing falls by 10 per cent?

4   How do older people and their families make decisions regarding end-of-life care?

5   What is the essence of pain?

Each question will be best answered using different research methods. Randomised controlled trials are the ideal way to answer 1 and 2—although ethical considerations may prevent the use of RCTs even for effectiveness questions (see CHAPTERS 2, 15). Grounded theory, ethnography or phenomenology will provide more appropriate answers to questions 3, 4 and 5 (see CHAPTERS 6, 7, 8). Regardless of the question, however, EBP moves from the question to the development of a rigorous protocol that will determine what research will be included in a systematic review.

As you can see from CHAPTER 18, a **systematic review** is a major undertaking of finding all relevant evidence, appraising it and determining what recommendations for practice can be made. From this review it is possible to know what, if any, evidence exists in relation to the question, how credible the evidence is and what recommendations can be made for practice. Good practice guidelines are then based on these recommendations rather than the idiosyncrasies of the organisation or the most powerful ego on the health care team.

Systematic review:
A comprehensive identification and synthesis of the available literature on a specified topic. In a systematic review, literature is treated like data.

Misconceptions of EBP

Some detractors argue that EBP encourages practitioners to follow a kind of recipe book approach. This is clearly not the case. EBP provides the best available research evidence to inform your practice, *but* you must also individualise that evidence using person-centred care and your clinical expertise.

Another common criticism of EBP is that it is restricted to randomised controlled trials and meta-analyses and thus ignores important qualitative research (see CHAPTERS 1, 8). It is the case that EBM privileges RCTs. It is also true that most of the questions medical practitioners ask are about effectiveness of treatments, and these questions are best answered by RCTs (see CHAPTERS 15, 17). However, other health practitioners, such as nurses and allied health professionals, are often interested in questions of meaning and/or how to change practice. The best available evidence must be related to the question asked (see also CHAPTER 1). So, for example, if you want to know how it feels to be told you are being 'placed' in a nursing home, you have a terminal illness, or your baby has died, the best evidence will *not* come from RCTs but from qualitative research (see CHAPTER 1 and chapters in PART II). Arguing against EBP on the basis of how medicine has developed is baseless. The philosophy underpinning EBP cannot be debunked by critiquing how it is operationalised. Rather, non-medical practitioners (and medical practitioners interested in more than effectiveness) need to develop EBP to include the evidence that answers other relevant questions. This is happening. Indeed, the Cochrane Collaboration is also defining evidence more broadly now and exploring ways of evaluating qualitative research.

Further criticisms of EBP have been that clinical expertise and client preference are ignored. This is particularly so when EBP is interpreted and implemented as disease-oriented and the guidelines and clinical recommendations have not been developed to answer the question about the most appropriate treatment or intervention for a particular patient or client at a particular time (Nay & Fetherstonhaugh 2007, p. 458). Evidence about the effectiveness of an intervention, that is, that it 'works' in a controlled population, does not answer the question about applicability or feasibility in a specific client–clinician context.

Deirdre Fetherstonhaugh, Rhonda Nay and Margaret Winbolt

As already noted, EBP does not mean you have reviewed some recent papers from the library and/or a group of experts drew up some guidelines. It also does not mean that you evaluate the care given at your place of work and base your practice on the 'evidence' gathered from that evaluation.

EBP includes client preference and clinician expertise; the best available evidence must relate to the question asked.

DOING RESEARCH

Benevolent oppression

Mrs Angus is living in the community on her own but with some community services. She has mild dementia, arthritis and has had a stroke. She frequently has constipation, for which she has always taken daily laxatives. She has lost 6 kg in the past 3 months. Mrs Angus's daughter Rhonda is concerned that her mother keeps coughing and spluttering and is worried that she will choke and wants the dietician to see her. Rhonda is also concerned about her mother coping at home alone. She cannot look after her mother as she works full time and has young children. Rhonda asks Mrs Angus's GP to organise for her mother to be admitted to a residential aged care facility.

An Aged Care Assessment Service assessment finds Mrs Angus eligible for high care. Despite Mrs Angus's initial refusal to move, Rhonda convinces her mother that she needs 'looking after'. The social worker finds a 'nice place' which is 20 km from where she has always lived, so she has to change her GP. Mrs Angus is admitted to 'care'. The dietician orders vitamised food despite Mrs Angus's insistence that she would rather die than eat 'that mushy junk'. The 'new' GP prescribes the same daily laxatives for her constipation that she has always had and the practitioners give these to her religiously without review or assessment. Mrs Angus dies within a month of admission. Rhonda is distraught with guilt and feels that her mother just 'gave up'. The practitioners try to reassure her that what they all did was best for her mother and at least she died in care and not at home alone.

Benevolent oppression is taking away the rights of the person within a framework of believing it is 'best' for them. In short, it can be seen as 'killing with kindness' (Nay 1993).

This vignette describes a fairly typical situation with which many of you will be familiar. How might EBP have resulted in a better outcome? There is available evidence about the effectiveness of various interventions that could have been implemented to address some of the clinical health issues that Mrs Angus experienced. The implementation of evidence-based practice, however, is not just about instigating interventions because they have been proved effective in controlled populations. Client choice and, where appropriate, the clinician's judgment and expertise[2] are also important components of evidence-based practice. For Mrs Angus, her involvement and preferences would have been crucial factors in the effectiveness of any intervention implemented. Appropriate assessment of swallowing status and the implementation of risk minimisation strategies including modifying the way in which assistance with food was provided, ensuring that Mrs Angus sat upright when eating and drinking and swallowed slowly, may have prevented the automatic vitamising of food that Mrs Angus so opposed (Joanna Briggs Institute 2008).

Constipation is a common and often underrated clinical condition in older people (Department of Veterans' Affairs 2007) which requires assessment, evaluation and reassessment (Registered Nurses Association of Ontario 2005). The aim of any intervention to address constipation should be to restore regular bowel movements, and the choice of interventions should be tailored to the person's needs and situation (Joanna Briggs Institute 2000). Mrs Angus's routine daily laxatives were not effective. Neither the GP, nor the staff administering the laxatives, did an assessment or evaluation that took into account Mrs Angus's individual history and needs, which would have helped to determine an appropriate treatment. While the information provided here is not comprehensive enough to be in any way conclusive, it is likely that Mrs Angus may have been depressed since depression is common in older people (Hay et al. 1998). She was losing her independence and control and others were making decisions for her. The current situation with admission into residential aged care services in Australia requires the Cornell Scale for Depression to be used. It is only a screening tool, but a high score should flag the need for further investigation (Alexopoulos et al. 1988), so that if a diagnosis of depression is made the appropriate evidence-based interventions can be implemented. Mrs Angus may have benefited from such assessment. It is clear that an interdisciplinary approach perhaps involving Mrs Angus, her daughter, the GP, nurses, dietician and physiotherapist would have resulted in a better outcome.

Appraising clinical guidelines

As the example above demonstrates, the application of the best available international evidence, combined with client preferences and choices, can result in better outcomes for clients and their families. The example can also be used to show how good-quality clinical practice guidelines (CPG) developed from systematic reviews of the available evidence can give health professionals access to the evidence in a 'ready to use' format. Essentially, '[c]linical guidelines are systematically developed statements which assist the health professional and the patient to make decisions about what is the appropriate health care in specific circumstances' (Field & Lohr 1990, p. 38). CPGs are beneficial in that they clearly identify what should be happening in a given area of practice, can bridge the gap between research and practice by providing easy access to the evidence, and have the ability to increase consistency of care and health care outcomes. CPGs also have the ability to empower clients as they are readily available and make the evidence understandable to the consumer.

There are, however, some limitations surrounding CPGs. Most of these relate to poor development techniques and flawed or outdated practice recommendations. Factors that may contribute to poor-quality recommendations include a lack of evidence, poor-quality evidence, conflicting evidence, or the evidence not being applicable to the client population for whom the guideline is intended. There are numerous organisations and groups that develop CPGs relating to almost any area of health practice. The use of internet search engines now means that these can be located with ease. But there is little information about the quality of these guidelines or the safety of implementing their recommendations. It is therefore important that health professionals are in a position to assess or appraise the quality of CPGs, and to determine the strength of the recommendations and create confidence in them prior to implementation.

A number of tools have been developed to assist health professionals appraise CPGs, examples of which are the Appraisal of Guidelines Research and Evaluation (AGREE), the National Institute of Clinical Studies (NICS) and the National Institute for Clinical Excellence (NICE).

Regardless of the tool chosen, appraising a clinical practice guideline essentially means identifying whether the key components of a good-quality guideline are present. A good-quality CPG should provide details of:

- the name of the developing organisation
- the names and credentials of the guideline developers
- the development method and any limitations identified by the developers
- the client group or population for whom the guideline has been developed
- the systematic review protocol and search strategy
- funding sources and any potential or actual conflict of interest
- the date it was published
- how the development team plan to review or maintain the currency of the recommendations.

Clinical practice guidelines should also contain clearly worded recommendations for practice, each supported by a discussion of the evidence on which it is based and an indication of the level or grade of the evidence. A brief summary of the recommendations should also be included and many guidelines now contain information written specifically for clients (see Websites below). Taking this further, Vlayen and colleagues (2005) prefer a framework for guideline appraisal that suggests it involves not only ascertaining the presence of the above components, but also establishing the validity, reliability, clinical applicability, clinical flexibility, feasibility and clarity of the guidelines.

This framework can be applied by asking a series of questions of the CPG as shown in Table 16.1.

Table 16.1: Questions to ask of a clinical practice guideline

Development team	Does the CPG: ☐ tell you the name of the organisation that produced the guideline? ☐ tell you who was on the development team? ☐ tell you if consumers were involved in the development? ☐ list who funded the development? ☐ outline any conflicts of interest?	You are looking to establish the credentials of the developing organisation and whether it has the appropriate credentials in guideline development and whether the development team is appropriate to the topic and client population being targeted by the guideline. You are also seeking to ascertain any potential or actual conflicts of interest between the development team, the funding sources and the recommendations.
Clarity	Is the CPG: ☐ clearly worded and user-friendly? Does it: ☐ include a summary of recommendations? ☐ provide information for clients?	The CPG needs to be clearly worded, understandable to the intended audience and user-friendly. CPGs can be lengthy documents and are made clearer if a simple summary of recommendations is included. Information written specifically for clients can promote their understanding of the evidence and can assist decision-making.
Validity	Does the CPG tell you: ☐ how the evidence was collected? ☐ the level of evidence supporting each recommendation? ☐ about the potential risks; costs?	You are asking whether there is sufficient information in the document for you to establish the source/sources of the evidence and exactly how it was collected and appraised, e.g. is the systematic review protocol given? Is the systematic review accessible? You are seeking some indication of any potential risks in implementing the recommendations, either to the client or to your organisation. It is also valuable to know the potential financial costs associated with implementation.
Reliability	Could the CPG development be repeated by someone else?	You are seeking to ascertain if the CPG gives enough detail about the development strategy to enable someone else to repeat it.
Clinical applicability	Does the CPG tell you: ☐ what its purpose and aim is? ☐ the topic it covers? ☐ which client group it refers to? ☐ which professional group it is aimed at? ☐ the ethical considerations?	You need to be sure the CPG is applicable to the client group for whom you wish to implement it. You need to ascertain the exact topic and purpose before considering implementation, e.g. a CPG related to medical management of constipation in children may not be appropriate for nursing management of constipation in an older person living in a residential aged care setting.

Deirdre Fetherstonhaugh, Rhonda Nay and Margaret Winbolt

Table 16.1: *(cont.)*

Clinical flexibility	Does the CPG tell you: ☐ who was included and who was excluded? ☐ does it consider the role of client preferences?	This is linked to clinical applicability in that you can use this information to decide whether a CPG not written specifically for your client group is flexible enough to be adapted for your purposes. It is also important to know whether the guideline development team considered the role of client preference and choice as this will enable you to make decisions about whether the CPG is flexible enough to support these.
Review	Does the CPG provide the issue date and have a plan stating how and when it will be reviewed?	CPGs rely on the latest available evidence and this can become dated very quickly. Outdated recommendations may put both the health professional and the client at risk, so it is important that you know when the CPG was issued. It is recommended CPGs are reviewed and updated if necessary every 3 years (NHMRC 1999).
Feasibility of implementation	Does the CPG give suggested implementation strategies and identify any policy and administration implications?	You are seeking guidance as to any implications that implementation of the recommendations might have on your organisation. You are also seeking the developers' thoughts on how their recommendations might be implemented.
Dissemination strategy	Does the CPG explain how the development team planned to disseminate it?	This provides background information to how the development team intend to promote the CPG.
Evaluation strategy	Does the CPG explain how the development team plans to evaluate it?	This provides information as to how uptake and effectiveness of the recommendations is to be evaluated. It may also assist you in developing an evaluation strategy in your workplace.

TRY IT YOURSELF

Ask the above questions of a clinical policy or guideline from your work area. Would you consider this a good-quality policy or guideline? If not, how could it be improved?

Implementing EBP: issues, strategies and using audit for implementation

Establishing what is evidence-based practice is not the same as implementing it. It is the implementation that creates the challenge for practitioners. In order to implement evidence-based practice, one must first establish what current practice is. This can best be achieved by measuring it against what the evidence advocates should be done according to a meta-analysis or meta-synthesis of the research evidence by undertaking a process called **clinical audit**. Clinical audit is about clinical effectiveness since the evidence against which current practice is measured is what has been established as being effective from the research evidence published in the literature. The ongoing goal of clinical audit is about improving the quality of health care provided.

Clinical audit: A process that provides a systematic framework for establishing care standards based on best evidence. It can identify areas of care that require improvement.

Clinical audit is a process that provides a systematic framework for establishing care standards based on best evidence. It is a practical way to compare day-to-day practice with best evidence care standards and it can identify areas of care that require improvement. Clinical audit can identify the areas of needed practice change in sufficient detail so that it can also be used as an implementation tool for instigating and then evaluating the improvements. Clinical audit can also provide evidence that the care currently being provided is of a quality standard and thereby provides positive feedback, which is just as important as identifying what improvements need to be made. According to Prasad and Reddy (2004, p. 112), clinical audit is 'essential for achieving and maintaining professional credibility, and necessary for defending decisions, policies and action on a scientific rather than an intuitive basis'.

The starting point for clinical audit is evidence-based guidelines from where statements can be converted into audit indicators. An indicator is a broad statement of good practice based on the best available evidence. The next step is to determine what items, namely criteria, are necessary in order to achieve best practice as encapsulated by the indicator. The criteria provide the more detailed and practical information on how to meet the indicator. Criteria refer to the resources (structure) that you need, the actions (process) that must be undertaken, and the results (outcomes) you intend to achieve (Morrell & Harvey 2003, p. 28). Structure criteria are the resources in the system that are necessary for the successful achievement of the indicator. Structure criteria may include a consideration of staffing levels and skill mix; requirements for knowledge and expertise; organisational arrangements and the provision of equipment and physical space; and existing policies, assessment tools, procedures or protocols. Process criteria are the actions and decisions taken by staff in conjunction with those for whom the care is being provided in order to achieve the specified indicator. Process criteria may include assessment, planning, intervening, evaluation and documentation. It is one thing to have policies—process is what you do with them. Outcome criteria are what you expect to achieve by meeting the structure and process criteria. They describe the desired results from the perspective of the recipient of the service or care and they also measure adherence or compliance with evidence-based practice as encapsulated in the indicator derived from the recommendation in the evidence-based guideline. Outcome criteria are typically expressed in terms such as physical or behavioural response to an intervention, reported health status or level of knowledge and satisfaction. All these criteria need to be measurable (Morrell & Harvey 2003).

Deirdre Fetherstonhaugh, Rhonda Nay and Margaret Winbolt

In a guideline about oral and dental hygiene in older people living in residential care facilities, a recommendation statement that advocates an assessment of oral health using the Oral Health Assessment Tool (OHAT) can be converted into an indicator affirming that residents will have their oral health assessed within two days of being admitted to the facility using the OHAT. Table 16.2 sets out the criteria necessary to meet this indicator (Morrell & Harvey 2003).

Table 16.2: Audit indicator

AUDIT INDICATOR		
Residents will have their oral health assessed within 2 days of being admitted to the residential aged care facility using the Oral Health Assessment Tool (OHAT).		
Structure	**Process**	**Outcome**
S1-1 OHAT is available.	P1-1 Registered nurses access assessment tool and undertake assessment.	O1-1 Oral health assessments are undertaken and documented for 100% of residents within 2 days of being admitted to residential care facility.
S2-2 Education program targeted to registered nurses about oral health assessment is available in the residential care facility.	P2-2 Registered nurses are able to attend education sessions.	O2-2 100% of registered nurses working in residential aged care facility have attended education session on oral health assessment.
S3-3 The residential care facility has developed (or has) competencies for registered nurses in oral health assessment.	P3-3 Registered nurses have their competency in undertaking oral health assessments measured.	O3-3 100% of registered nurses working in residential care facility are competent in undertaking oral health assessment.

Each of these structure and process criteria have an associated/defined audit activity such as checking whether the registered nurses have attended the education sessions about oral health assessment. This check is then undertaken and measured against the targeted outcome. For this example, for instance, a check of the number of nurses who had attended the education sessions may reveal that only 80 per cent compliance had been reached. It then needs to be established why the expected outcome as a measure of adherence to the indicator of EBP in this clinical area has not been achieved. Once the reason has been identified, a strategy to rectify this gap can be ascertained and then implemented. For instance, in this example it may be that it is the registered nurses working overnight who have not attended the education because the sessions are only held during the day. Scheduling education at a more appropriate time for night duty staff, training a night staff member to provide the education at night, or organising some 'paid' education time for night staff during the day when they are not working, are all examples of strategies or interventions that could be put into place to improve compliance with the requirements of EBP in this clinical area. A staff member, for example the clinical educator, would be given or take on the responsibility of implementing the strategy within an expected time-frame, then a repeat audit can be undertaken to determine whether improvement in adherence to the required evidence-based indicator has been achieved.

Feedback to all key stakeholders is an essential component of effective clinical auditing. A systematic review on audit and feedback (Jamtvedt et al. 2006, p. 2) concluded that '[t]he relative effectiveness of audit and feedback is likely to be greater when baseline adherence to recommended practice is low and when feedback is delivered more intensively'.

The advantage of using clinical audit as a means of determining adherence to EBP is that it is not just a measure of what is currently happening, but an implementation tool which highlights gaps in enough detail so that strategies for improvement can be identified and then implemented.[3] There is no point offering education if the obstacle to implementation is documentation.

According to Logemann (2004), Byham-Gray et al. (2005), Rubin and Parrish (2007) and Chronister et al. (2008), barriers to EBP being translated into practice typically include:

- [ ] lack of time
- [ ] lack of organisational support
- [ ] resistance to change
- [ ] inability to understand and appraise research
- [ ] lack of access to the internet or inability to navigate it
- [ ] lack of relevant research evidence.

Ideally, addressing these barriers requires an 'all of organisation' approach. If the systems, including documentation, value task completion at the expense of clients and staff, accessing evidence and implementation change will be seen as privileges rather than an expectation of the health care environment. Similarly, when education and research are not built into role expectations, they will be neglected. Most staff still do not have well-developed skills in accessing and appraising evidence—processes and structures that support training, access to the internet and implementation of evidence into practice, at least to the same extent as training in clinical 'problems' and new equipment, will demonstrate to staff that EBP is significant and not just rhetoric.

We found that building research discussions into current practice, rather than making it something separate staff 'go to', can embed it more in everyday practice. For example, case conferences and handover can be simply the handing over of tasks and information *or* they can be an opportunity for discussions about what the best available research evidence offers.

Deirdre Fetherstonhaugh, Rhonda Nay and Margaret Winbolt

Any change will meet with some resistance. But Thompson and Learmonth (2002, pp. 214–15) offer some examples of helpful strategies, and these include:

- identifying all groups involved in, influenced by or able to influence the change
- assessing the characteristics of the proposed change that might influence its acceptance
- assessing readiness and enabling factors for this change
- identifying possible external barriers to this change.

Contemporary leadership is essential. The change literature from diverse fields demonstrates how leadership can 'make or break' an organisation (Covey 2004; Goleman 2006). If change is simply imposed and staff feel devalued, they will resist. Transformational leadership, on the other hand, can excite staff about change and indeed grow leaders at every level. Kitson and colleagues (1998) reported from their research that facilitation is vital, and we would support this contention. Such facilitators are often termed 'local champions' as they keep staff enthused and committed. Some health facilities have formal relationships with universities and this can assist the implementation of EBP, provided clinical staff feel that they have ownership of the process and do not see it as simply the university's project that will stop if the link with the university is broken.

SUMMARY

Evidence-based practice is shown to be much more than just reading the research. As Nay and Fetherstonhaugh (2007, p. 461) suggest, 'EBP involves much more than locating, analy[s]ing, and appraising the best evidence available about the effectiveness of an intervention'. It is argued here that there is a need to increase the extent to which practitioners use EBP rather than experience, tradition or relying on unappraised research papers. Barriers to implementation are common across all health professions and settings. Lack of time is always cited as a major barrier, as is the difficulty practitioners have in appraising research. We acknowledge that practitioners usually do not have time to conduct systematic reviews, develop guidelines and work through all of the steps involved in EBP. But many areas of practice now have guidelines based on the best available evidence and our encouragement would be for practitioners to become expert in finding and appraising these guidelines. The time wasted across the health sector with every organisation, and sometimes every unit within an organisation, developing their own guidelines could be much better spent implementing evidence-based guidelines already in existence. We have provided examples to assist guideline appraisal and offered strategies for implementation. Finally, we argue the significance of transformational leadership to translation of evidence into practice and transforming task and disease-based environments into EBP environments.

TUTORIAL EXERCISES

1 Think about a situation from your experience where some change was proposed. What barriers do you recall to that change? What strategies were used to overcome the barriers? Can you think of others that may have been more successful?

2 Develop a presentation to explain to your colleagues how EBP differs from research-based practice. Convince them as to why EBP is beneficial to an organisation, health professionals and clients.

NOTES

1 Sackett et al. (1997) uses the term 'patient' choice.

2 This can depend on the level of education and expertise.

3 Morrell and Harvey (2003) provide excellent guidance and advice on how to undertake clinical audits.

FURTHER READING

Dawes, M., Davies, P., Gray, A., Mant, J., Seers, K. & Snowball, R. (2005). *Evidence-based practice: A primer for health care professionals*, 2nd edn. London: Elsevier.

DiCenso, A., Guyatt, G. & Ciliska, D. (2005). *Evidence-based nursing: A guide to clinical practice*. St Louis: Elsevier Mosby.

Morrell, C. & Harvey, G. (2003). *The clinical audit handbook*. London: Elsevier Science.

Sackett, D.L., Richardson, W.S., Rosenberg, W. & Haymes, R.B. (1997). *Evidence-based medicine: How to practice and teach EBM*. London: Churchill Livingstone.

Vlayen, J., Aertgeerts, B., Hannes, K., Sermeus, W. & Ramaekers, D. (2005). A systematic review of appraisal tools for clinical practice guidelines: Multiple similarities and one common deficit. *International Journal for Quality in Health Care*, 17(3), 235–42.

WEBSITES

www.latrobe.edu.au/acebac

The Australian Centre for Evidence Based Aged Care (ACEBAC) aims to improve the care of older people by advancing service delivery through research programs that focus on the conduct

Deirdre Fetherstonhaugh, Rhonda Nay and Margaret Winbolt

of systematic reviews; developing and evaluating guidelines for best practice in service delivery and organisation in aged care, based on the systematic review of research findings; conducting international, multi-site programs to implement best practice guidelines; and evaluating the impact of the implementation of best practice guidelines on health and social outcomes in aged care.

www.cochrane.org

The Cochrane Collaboration website provides access to systematic reviews of health care interventions.

www.nice.org.uk

The National Institute for Health and Clinical Excellence in the UK is responsible for providing national guidance on the promotion of good health and the prevention and treatment of ill health in the areas of public health, health technologies and clinical practice.

www.nhmrc.gov.au/guidelines/health_guidelines.htm

This website lists guidelines and provides access to them.

www.joannabriggs.edu.au/about/home.php

The Joanna Briggs website provides access to evidence-based resources for health care professionals in nursing, midwifery, medicine, and allied health.

www.agreecollaboration.org/intr/

This website provides information on the appraisal of guidelines, research and evaluation collaboration.

www.nhmrc.gov.au/nics

The National Institute of Clinical Studies (NICS) works to improve health care by getting the best available evidence from health and medical research into everyday practice. The website provides information on guidelines and gives access to a wide range of resources including reports, newsletters, brochures and websites.

www.york.ac.uk/inst/crd

The Centre for Reviews and Dissemination (CRD) is a department of the University of York and is part of the National Institute for Health Research. CRD undertakes high-quality systematic reviews that evaluate the effects of health and social care interventions and the delivery and organisation of health care.

www.nice.org.uk

The National Institute for Clinical Excellence.

17

Evidence-based Practice in Therapeutic Health Care

Megan Davidson and Ross Iles

CHAPTER OBJECTIVES

In this chapter you will learn:

☐ what evidence-based practice is

☐ about a 5-step approach to evidence-based practice

☐ to discuss evidence hierarchies and evidence quality

☐ to apply the evidence to current practice

☐ to provide a case study for a therapy question

☐ to provide a case study for diagnostic question

KEY TERMS

Clinical practice guidelines

Evidence-based practice

Randomised controlled trial

Systematic review

COCHRANE'S CRITICISM AND SACKETT'S STEPS

Evidence-based practice: The use of best research evidence, along with clinical expertise, available resources and the patient's preferences to determine the optimal management option in a specific situation.

Evidence-based practice is a concept whose modern genesis can be found in the words of Archie Cochrane, a British epidemiologist (1909–88), who said, referring to the profession of medicine, 'It is surely a great criticism of our profession that we have not organised a critical summary, by specialty or sub-specialty, adapted periodically, of all relevant randomized controlled trials' (Cochrane 1979, p. 8). The legacy of Archie Cochrane's criticism is the Cochrane Collaboration, a worldwide multidisciplinary organisation established some years after his death, which is dedicated to doing precisely what he said was needed. The technology of the systematic review (see CHAPTER 18) has transformed health care practice from care based largely on expert opinion and tradition to one in which the question 'what is the evidence?' informs practice decisions. Critical summaries (systematic reviews and clinical practice guidelines) now provide practitioners with readily accessible access to research evidence. The availability of these documents on the web means that patients have almost as much access to the 'critical summaries' as their doctor or therapist.

Although definitions of EBP abound, it is commonly agreed that EBP is the use of best research evidence, along with clinical expertise, available resources and patient's preferences to determine the optimal assessment, treatment or management option in a specific situation (see also CHAPTERS 15, 16).

The underlying assumption of EBP is that if health care is based on evidence about what is most effective, the quality of care will be better than if it is not. Sackett's widely adopted 5-step approach to EBP (Table 17.1) provides a practical framework for teaching and practising EBP (Sackett et al. 2000).

Table 17.1: The five steps of EBP

EBP Step	Knowledge and Skill Required
1. ASK an answerable clinical question.	Recognise a knowledge-gap and formulate a structured question that defines the problem, the intervention and the outcomes of interest.
2. ACQUIRE the best available evidence.	Know evidence sources and types, and search databases.
3. APPRAISE the evidence.	Critically appraise the evidence to determine its validity and clinical importance.
4. APPLY the evidence.	Integrate the evidence with clinical expertise and patient preferences.
5. ASSESS the process.	Reflect on steps 1–4 and identify ways to improve efficiency.

Note: Based on Sackett et al. (2000) and Del Mar et al. (2004)

(Reproduced from Iles & Davidson (2006), Evidence based practice: A survey of physiotherapists' current practice, *Physiotherapy Research International*, with permission from Wiley-Blackwell)

EVIDENCE HIERARCHIES AND EVIDENCE QUALITY

Step 2 of the EBP process is to acquire the available evidence. A brief encounter with an electronic database such as PubMed or even Google Scholar is enough to reveal that there is a mountain of research 'out there'. Without a system to organise the research available, the evidence you need may as well be a needle in a vast electronic haystack. Developing a clearly answerable clinical question (Step 1) to guide your search is the first way to organise your way through the maze of available research papers. However, even the best questions may result in a mountain of evidence. Since time is a barrier to performing EBP for many practitioners (Iles & Davidson 2006), some system is needed to identify which papers should be read, or what evidence is most important or credible.

How much confidence you can have in the results of the research will at least in part depend on the research design. For a question about therapy effectiveness, you are more likely to use a well-designed **randomised controlled trial** (RCT) to inform practice than a single case study, because you can be more confident that the outcomes are actually due to the intervention and can be generalised to patients who are like those included in the study (see CHAPTERS 12, 15). By classifying studies according to the research design, it can be easier to identify evidence that has greater capacity to inform and change practice.

The Centre for Evidence Based Medicine (CEBM) and the National Health and Medical Research Council (NHMRC) provide a hierarchy (levels) of evidence showing the relationship between the research design and the level of confidence that research design conveys (Table 17.2). The higher the level of evidence, the greater the confidence one can have in applying that evidence to clinical practice. Across all research designs, a **systematic review** represents the highest level of evidence and various forms of case study the lowest. Depending on whether the clinical question is about therapy efficacy, diagnostic accuracy or clinical prognosis, the levels in between will look slightly different. Research design alone does not guarantee research quality. **Clinical practice guidelines** generally take into account both the research design and the quality of the research in arriving at a recommendation for clinical practice. Systematic reviews also frequently summarise the strength of evidence based on research design and quality.

An evidence hierarchy allows you to use a 'top-down' approach to the evidence. If you can locate a relevant, well-conducted and reasonably recent systematic review you may not need to search any further. A well-performed systematic review will have gathered, critically appraised and summarised all the relevant research with a minimum of bias, providing the reader with results that can be incorporated into practice with a high level of confidence (see CHAPTER 18).

Randomised controlled trial: A clinical trial where participants are randomly assigned to groups in order to receive different interventions. This randomisation removes many of the effects that may bias the true result.

Systematic review: A comprehensive identification and synthesis of the available literature on a specified topic.

Clinical practice guidelines: 'Systematically developed statements that assist the health professional and the patient to make decisions about what is the appropriate health care in specific circumstances.'

Megan Davidson and Ross Iles

Table 17.2: Hierarchy of evidence

Level of evidence	Research Question		
	Therapy effectiveness	**Diagnostic accuracy**	**Prognosis**
I	Systematic review of Level II studies	Systematic review of Level II studies	Systematic review of Level II studies
II	Randomised controlled trial	Study of sample of consecutive patients; independent, blind comparison with reference standard.	Prospective cohort study
III-1	Pseudo-randomised control trial (allocation not random)	Study of sample of non-consecutive patients; independent, blind comparison with reference standard.	Representative case series; all or none of the people with the risk factor have the outcome of interest.
III-2	Comparative study with concurrent controls (e.g. cohort study; case-control study; interrupted time series)	Study that does not meet Level II or III-1 evidence	Analysis of prognostic factors among participants within a randomised control trial
III-3	Comparative study without concurrent controls (e.g. historical control)	Diagnostic case-control study (includes people with and without the condition)	Retrospective cohort study
IV	Case series (with post-test or pre-post test outcomes)	Diagnostic study with no comparison to a reference standard	Case series or cohort study with persons not at same stage of disease.

Source: Based on Table 1, NHMRC 2008a, p. 6

If no systematic reviews are available on the topic, the next level of evidence should be sought to answer the question. In the case of therapy efficacy, this would be to examine relevant RCTs (see CHAPTER 15). If this level of evidence is not available, the next highest is sought and so on. How much influence the evidence should have when making clinical decisions depends on the level and quality of the evidence. This requires the reader to critically evaluate the evidence (Step 3) to determine its quality and therefore the extent to which it is valid or believable. All evidence should be assessed (i.e. critically appraised) to determine the extent to which the results are free from bias. This can be a time-consuming process, and physiotherapists have identified relatively low confidence in their ability to appraise research (Iles & Davidson 2006). A database such as PEDro (Physiotherapy Evidence Database), where individual studies have been critically evaluated and carry a quality rating, provides physiotherapists who are short of time or expertise with a valuable resource (see also CHAPTERS 15, 18). However, even if the research report has not been pre-appraised, there are a number of tools available that can assist in quality appraisal of research—including the quality scale used by PEDro (see the box 'Quality appraisal tools').

Quality appraisal tools

☐   CEBM has critical appraisal tools for systematic reviews, RCTs and diagnostic studies.

☐   The Critical Appraisal Skills Program (CASP) of the NHS in the United Kingdom provides a number of tools for various study designs.

☐   The PEDro scale.

☐   The University of Glasgow General Practice and Family Care website has a number of quality checklists (see Websites on page 300).

CURRENT PRACTICE

The process of locating, appraising and applying the research evidence is no different between medical practitioners, nurses, dentists, physiotherapists, speech therapists, podiatrists, social workers or any other health professional. But the types of questions that are of primary concern to the different disciplines are diverse, and the body of evidence available to answer questions varies enormously. For the profession of physiotherapy, a relatively large body of relevant research evidence is available and has been collected, appraised and made available as **PEDro**. PEDro contains (at March 2009) 444 clinical practice guidelines, 1967 systematic reviews and 11 752 clinical trials of direct relevance to the discipline of physiotherapy.

> **Physiotherapy Evidence Database (PEDro)** collects, appraises and makes available a relatively large body of physiotherapy research evidence.

Most health practitioners are now trained in the basics of evidence-based practice in their pre-qualification courses. Many therapists who graduated before this was the case have also skilled up during postgraduate studies by taking short courses or by self-directed learning. Despite this, surveys of the attitudes, knowledge and skills of physiotherapists indicate that while attitudes are positive, there is considerable variability in the self-reported knowledge and skills, confidence and competence in evidence-based practice (Jette et al. 2003; Iles & Davidson 2006; Salbach et al. 2007). This pattern of positive attitudes and poor or inconsistent EBP knowledge and skills can also be seen in surveys of other professions from nursing (Pravikoff et al. 2005; Koehn & Lehman 2008) to medical specialists (Poolman et al. 2007; Dahm et al. 2009). Barriers to EBP are typically identified as lack of time, knowledge and skill. Younger, more recently graduated practitioners are often found to have better self-rated knowledge and skills. Physiotherapists and other health professional groups clearly have some distance to go to optimising their practice.

A survey of 124 physiotherapists in Victoria, Australia (Iles & Davidson 2006) found that despite a very positive attitude towards EBP, the five steps of EBP are not frequently practised (i.e. at least monthly). Eighty per cent said they frequently identified a knowledge gap, and

60 per cent said they formulated that gap as an answerable question. Forty-four per cent said they frequently tracked down the relevant evidence to answer the question, but only 10 per cent said they frequently searched the PEDro database, and only 15 per cent the Cochrane library. Although 69 per cent said they read published research reports at least monthly, only 26 per cent critically appraised what they read. Recent graduates rated their EBP skills more highly than more experienced graduates, but did not perform EBP tasks more often. Physiotherapists with higher levels of training rated their EBP skills more highly and were more likely to search databases and to understand a range of EBP terminology than those with lower levels of training. The barriers to EBP were time required to keep up to date, access to easily understandable summaries of evidence, journal access, and lack of personal skills in searching and evaluating research evidence.

A survey by Jette and colleagues (2003) of a sample of 488 physical therapists in the USA also reported positive attitudes to EBP, and better self-evaluated knowledge and confidence among younger/more recently graduated therapists. Salbach and associates (2007) surveyed neurological physical therapists in Ontario, Canada and found that only half the 270 respondents said they had training in searching and appraising research.

THERAPY CASE STUDY

Danny, a physiotherapist who graduated a couple of years ago, is working in the outpatients department at a metropolitan hospital where chronic musculoskeletal conditions are common. He has diagnosed his patient with Achilles tendinopathy and he generally treats this condition with an eccentric exercise program with good outcomes. Danny's patient describes a friend who had the same symptoms and had ultrasound therapy and found the treatment really effective. Danny is not sure how effective ultrasound is in treating Achilles tendinopathy or whether eccentric exercise will give his patient a better outcome.

Recalling his undergraduate training in the 5-step approach to evidence-based practice and using his textbook from the course (Herbert et al. 2005), Danny sets out to determine whether eccentric exercise or ultrasound is the better treatment option for his patient.

Step 1: Ask an answerable question

Danny knows that formulating the question well will help in finding the answer. An answerable question defines the problem or patient group, an intervention and an outcome. Danny decides to use the PICO format (Population, Intervention, Comparison, Outcome) (see CHAPTER 18) to structure his question. Danny writes his question as: 'For people with chronic Achilles tendinopathy is therapeutic ultrasound or eccentric exercise more effective in reducing pain levels?'

Step 2: Acquire the evidence

Danny decides the first place to look is the Cochrane Library as it is a source of high-quality systematic reviews and the most likely place to find level 1 evidence. Searching for 'Achilles tendinopathy' in the title, abstract or keywords (Figure 17.1) yields a relevant Cochrane review,

'Interventions for treating acute and chronic Achilles tendinitis' (McLauchlan & Handoll 2001), but this is focused largely on comparisons of drug therapies. Apart from some benefit from non-steroidal anti-inflammatory drugs (NSAIDs) for acute symptoms, the review concludes there is insufficient evidence to draw conclusions. There were no trials in the review that compared therapeutic ultrasound with eccentric exercise.

Figure 17.1: Cochrane Library search screen

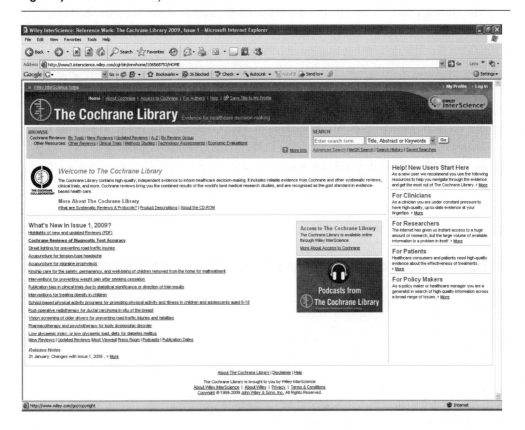

The search of the Cochrane Library also identified three non-Cochrane reviews relevant to eccentric exercise for Achilles tendinopathy (Satyendra & Byl 2006; Kingma et al. 2007; van Usen & Pumberger 2007). The Cochrane Library provides a structured abstract and quality appraisal of non-Cochrane reviews and two of the three reviews have been appraised (Satyendra & Byl 2006; Kingma et al. 2007). This means that Danny probably does not even need to retrieve the published review, but can rely on the information in the Cochrane Library. The Kingma review was considered good quality and therefore its conclusions reliable. The authors concluded that while eccentric exercise for pain in patients with chronic Achilles tendinopathy is 'promising', they could not determine the magnitude of the treatment effects. The mean reduction in pain across all studies for the eccentric training group was 60 per cent (95% CI 29-94) compared to 33 per cent (95% CI: 13-86) in the comparison groups. Danny can see the variation is quite large (the confidence interval is very wide) and that only one of the studies was deemed to be of adequate methodological quality. It does not look as if any of the included studies compared eccentric exercise with ultrasound. Danny decides to look further as there appears to be promising evidence for the effectiveness of eccentric exercise, but it is not clear how effective exercises can be.

The other appraised review (Satyendra & Byl 2006) concluded that eccentric exercises result in statistically significant but modest benefits. Danny notices that the Cochrane Review Database commentary points out some methodological flaws in the review and that the results should be interpreted with caution. Again, it does not appear that any studies comparing eccentric exercise and ultrasound have been included. Danny is happy to find some level 1 evidence providing modest support for his usual treatment approach, but is still not sure how effective eccentric exercise is or whether ultrasound is a viable alternative for his patient.

Danny decides the next step is to turn to PEDro. He knows this is a source of pre-appraised evidence so that will save him some time. He goes to the PEDro website (Figure 17.2) and enters 'eccentric achilles' in the title/abstract search box and selects

Figure 17.2: PEDro search screen

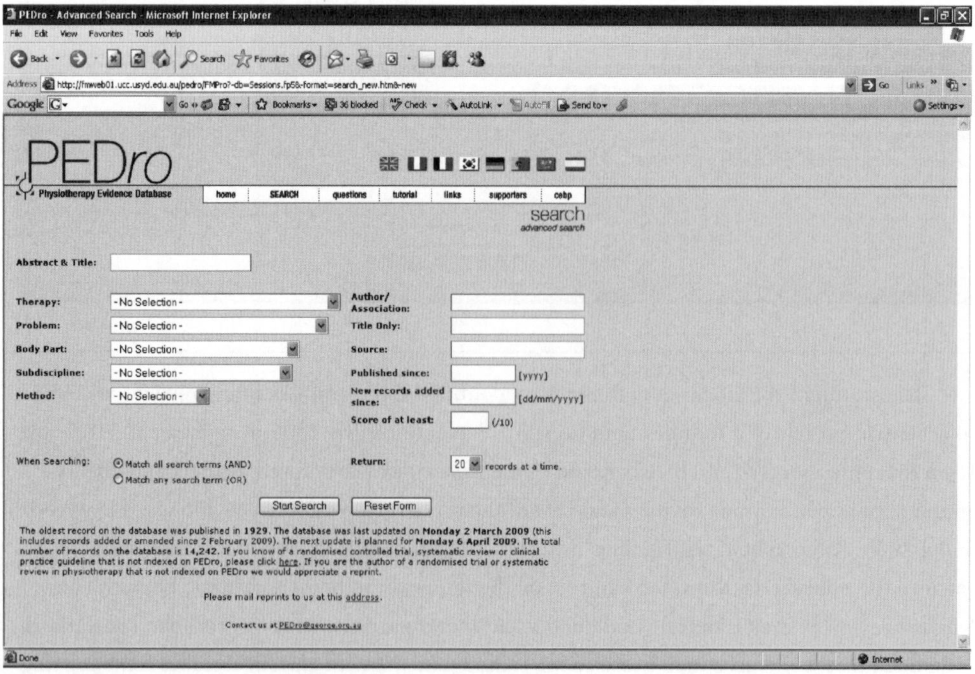

'electrotherapies, heat and cold' from the therapy drop-down menu. Danny is not sure whether achilles tendinopathy would be classified as 'lower leg or knee' or 'foot and ankle' in the body part box so he decides to leave it blank. This search returns 24 records, including five systematic reviews, one of which Danny did not find in his search of the Cochrane database (Woodley et al. 2007). Danny's quick examination of the abstract reveals that this review includes studies of eccentric exercise for Achilles, patellar and lateral elbow tendinopathies with results similar to the other review he had already located. Danny decides not to read further as he really wants to find out about the effectiveness of ultrasound therapy.

One of the clinical trials found—a pilot study comparing eccentric exercise with therapeutic ultrasound for chronic Achilles tendinopathy—appears to be a direct hit (Chester et al. 2008). The abstract is available on PEDro, but Danny wants to examine the full article. He finds the article on the *Manual Therapy* journal website, but finds he needs a subscription for the full article. He therefore decides to use the information found in the PEDro abstract. The PEDro score was 6/10 as the study did not conceal allocation, blind therapists or patients and the analysis was not by intention to treat. Danny is not concerned that therapists or patients were not blinded as this is reasonable given the nature of the interventions. He knows that failing to conceal allocation and perform intention to treat analysis may overestimate the results (Herbert et al. 2005). Regardless, the study found no significant differences between the groups and Danny realises this may be because there were only 16 participants in this pilot study, meaning the trial probably did not have adequate power to detect a difference between the groups, if indeed one existed. Danny notes the statement in the abstract that 'Both interventions proved acceptable to the patients with no adverse effects', and decides there is no evidence directly comparing the two treatments head to head that gives a reason to favour one of the treatments over the other. Danny wonders if there is any other evidence relating to ultrasound treatment for Achilles tendinopathy. He re-searches PEDro by entering 'ultrasound Achilles' in the abstract and title box, but this does not locate any further relevant articles.

Step 3: Appraise the evidence

By targeting pre-appraised sources of evidence, Danny has been able to rely on the appraisal from experts in the area. This has saved him valuable time.

Step 4: Apply the evidence

Level 1 evidence suggested eccentric exercises are an effective treatment, but there was no level 1 evidence for ultrasound as a treatment for Achilles tendinopathy. The only level 2 evidence Danny could find comparing eccentric exercise and therapeutic ultrasound could not determine which was the better treatment. Danny, remembering that an absence of evidence is not evidence of absence (i.e. just because there no evidence to show a treatment is effective it does not mean the treatment is not effective, rather that it is yet to be shown either way), decides to discuss his findings with his patient. Danny tells his patient what he has found. He explains that there is some evidence to support the eccentric exercises as an effective treatment, but almost no research could be found on ultrasound. Danny is enthusiastic about the eccentric exercise program, and the patient agrees to try this approach.

Step 5: Assess the process

Danny reflects on the process and realises that most of the systematic reviews he found in the Cochrane database were listed in the PEDro database. He decides that next time he might begin his search with PEDro.

DIAGNOSIS CASE STUDY

Donna, a physiotherapist who graduated a couple of years ago, is working in a private practice that has a strong relationship with various sports clubs and sees quite a lot of sports-related knee injuries. The practice runs a regular professional development program and as part of this the young physiotherapist has been asked to prepare a session on diagnostic tests for Anterior Cruciate Ligament (ACL) injuries.

Recalling her undergraduate training in the 5-step approach to evidence-based practice and using her textbook from the course (Herbert et al. 2005), Donna sets out to provide the practice with the best evidence available relating to clinical tests for ACL injuries.

Step 1: Ask an answerable question

Like Danny, Donna knows that formulating the question well will help in finding the answer. An answerable question defines the problem or patient group, an intervention and an outcome. In this case, the problem is ACL injury, the intervention is the diagnostic tests, and the outcome is the test accuracy. Donna is familiar with common tests of ACL integrity (Lachman, Anterior Draw, and Pivot Shift tests), but just in case there are other tests that she does not know about, Donna writes her question as: 'What is the diagnostic accuracy of tests for identifying injuries to the Anterior Cruciate Ligament of the knee?'

Step 2: Acquire the evidence

Donna knows that good, recent systematic reviews of original studies are the type of publication at the top of the hierarchy of evidence and will provide the best snapshot of the evidence in the least time. She also knows that an evidence-based clinical practice guideline (CPG) might be worth looking for.

Donna's first thought is to search PEDro, but she is unsure whether this database includes research relating to diagnostic tests. She determines also to search PubMed, which is freely available. Although she knows that she might miss something on the other major databases, such as Embase and Cinahl, her time is limited and she does not have access to these databases.

Donna goes to the PEDro website and types 'diagnosis' into the title/abstract search box, and selects 'lower leg or knee' in the body part box (Figure 17.2). This search returns 35 records, including two CPGs and four systematic reviews. One of the CPGs looks relevant (Arroll et al. 2003) and she notes that its name is 'The diagnosis and management of soft tissue knee injuries: internal derangements'. The link provided does not work, but she notes this is a CPG of the New Zealand Guidelines Group so she locates their website and downloads the guideline, which was published in 2003 and updated in 2007. A quick look confirms that the guideline is evidence-based and endorsed by a number of professional bodies, including the NZ Society of Physiotherapists. The CPG contains a wealth of information and would be a useful resource for the physiotherapists in the practice.

The introduction (p. 17) notes that a 'thorough history and careful clinical examination provide most of the information required to diagnose a soft tissue knee injury'. It also contains the background information relating to screening for red flags—signs and symptoms that indicate a serious condition may be present, such as neurovascular damage, septic arthritis or cancer. The guidelines recommend the use of the Ottawa Knee Rules (OKR) for ruling out a fracture. The practice already routinely screens for fracture using the OKR, and any patient with a positive test result is sent for a plain X-ray.

Accurate diagnosis of the soft tissue injury will allow an appropriate conservative management plan to be devised, or, for conditions not amenable to conservative management, an appropriate referral to be made. Donna notes that the guidelines have recommendations on aspects of the history and which tests are most strongly suggestive of a particular diagnosis. This will be useful information, but Donna would like to have a systematic review with meta-analysis that quantifies test characteristics such as sensitivity and specificity.

Donna next searches PubMed, the freely accessible version of Medline on the web (Figure 17.3). Donna chooses to search using the Clinical Queries approach.

She types 'anterior cruciate ligament' into the Clinical Study Category, selects 'diagnosis' and 'narrow, specific search', which returns 183 total results and seven reviews. Of the reviews, three appear relevant (Jackson et al. 2003; Malanga et al. 2003; Benjaminse et al. 2006). In PubMed, the title of the paper can be clicked on to read an abstract. This allowed Donna to determine quickly which papers were relevant. Opening the abstract also yields a list of 'related articles', and by looking at these Donna found another two relevant articles (Solomon et al. 2001; Scholten et al. 2003). Donna obtains the most recent review first as this should provide the most up-to-date evaluation. She obtains a PDF copy of the article by Benjaminse et al. (2006) from the JOSPT website. The review covers the Lachman, Anterior Drawer and Pivot Shift Tests and includes 28 individual studies. Having obtained the relevant article, Donna knows that she now needs to evaluate the quality of the review before she decides if she can use it with confidence to inform clinical practice.

Figure 17.3: PubMed clinical queries screen

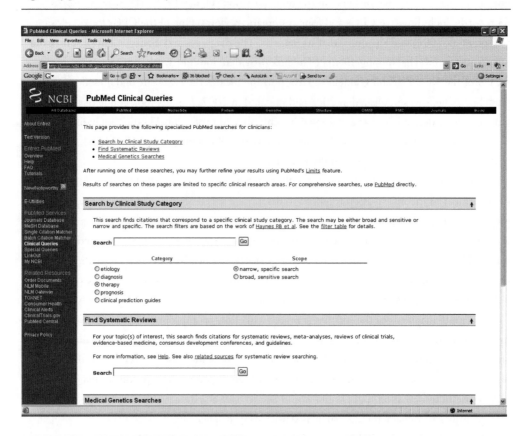

Step 3: Appraise the evidence

In her copy of Herbert et al. (2005, p. 106), Donna sees that she can use the same three questions to appraise a diagnostic test systematic review as for reviews of therapy and prognosis:

1   Was it clear which studies were to be reviewed?
    (a)   Is there a list of inclusion and exclusion criteria that defines the patients or population?

2   Were most relevant studies reviewed?
    (a)   Were key databases searched with sensitive search strategies?
    (b)   Was the search conducted recently?

3   Was the quality of the reviewed studies taken into account?
    (a)   Was there a minimum quality for studies to be included?
    (b)   Was quality evaluated with a scale or checklist and were the quality assessments taken into account in drawing conclusions?

She creates a table (Table 17.3) and reads the paper with a view to finding this information and noting relevant results. Donna concludes that despite the problem of the overall low quality of the reviewed studies, they may still be of some use to inform clinical practice. She knows that biased studies are likely to overestimate estimates of test accuracy. From the paper, Donna extracts only the results relating to performance of the test without anaesthesia, as this is what is relevant to physiotherapy practice. The review presents pooled estimates for the whole group and for acute and chronic subgroups for each of the three ACL tests (Table 17.4). She notes that while the estimates for the whole group are based on more than 1000 for each test, the numbers used to calculate the acute subgroup estimates are quite small, only 27 for specificity of the Pivot Shift, and only 77 for the Anterior Drawer test. This has made the 95 per cent confidence intervals for those estimates quite large.

Table 17.3: Quality appraisal of the Benjaminse review

Was it clear which studies were to be reviewed?	Were most relevant studies reviewed?	Was the quality of the reviewed studies taken into account?
Yes: human; at least 1 test for ACL rupture; arthroscopy, arthrotomy or MRI gold standard; 2 × 2 table could be constructed.	Yes: Medline, Embase and Cinahl to April 2005 plus reference checking and personal contacts.	No. All studies were included. Quality evaluated independently by 2 authors using Cochrane Methods Group approach. Only 3 studies had independent, blind comparison of index and reference tests and only 3 studies avoided workup or verification bias. Pooled sensitivity and specificity was weighted only by sample size.

Table 17.4: Extracted results for whole group and subgroups, without anaesthesia, from Benjaminse review

	Sensitivity	Specificity	LR+	LR-
Whole Group data				
Anterior Drawer	55 (52–58)	92 (90–94)	7.3 (3.5–15.2)	0.5 (0.4–0.6)
Lachman	85 (83–87)	94 (92–95)	10.2 (4.6–22.7)	0.2 (0.1–0.3)
Pivot Shift	24 (21–27)	98 (96–99)	8.5 (4.7–15.5)	0.9 (0.8–1.0)
Acute Subgroup Group data				
Anterior Drawer	49 (43–55)	58 (39–76)	1.4 (0.5–4.4)	0.7 (0.5–1.0)
Lachman	94 (91–96)	97 (93–99)	9.4 (0.4–210)	0.1 (0.0–1.1)
Pivot Shift	32 (25–38)	100 (48–100)	1.3 (0.1–23.7)	1.0 (0.7–1.3)
Chronic Subgroup Group data				
Anterior Drawer	92 (88–95)	91 (87–94)	8.9 (5.3–15.2)	0.1 (0.0–0.5)
Lachman	95 (91–97)	90 (87–94)	7.1 (1.2–40.2)	0.2 (0.1–0.7)
Pivot Shift	40 (29–52)	97 (95–99)	7.7 (1.7–36.4)	0.8 (0.4–1.4)

Step 4: Apply the evidence

Donna notes that the reviewers conclude that the Lachman and Pivot Shift tests are recommended over the Anterior Drawer. The guidelines gave the Lachman test a grade A recommendation (i.e. based on good evidence) that the test is 'reasonably accurate', but recommended that the Pivot Shift test be used only by experienced practitioners because of the complexity of the manoeuvre (grade C recommendation, i.e. based on expert opinion). The guidelines do not recommend the Anterior Drawer, but this is not based on any research evidence.

Donna is therefore confident that the Lachman test is a useful clinical test for acute and chronic ACL tears. It has high sensitivity and specificity and this means that most positive test results will be true positives, and most negative test results true negatives. The Pivot Shift test is very specific in chronic injuries, but the estimate of specificity in acute injuries has a very large confidence band (from 48% to 100%), so she decides this test is most useful as a follow-up test to the Lachman in the assessment of chronic injuries.

Using the guideline, the systematic review, and an article from the *Australian Physiotherapy Journal* (Davidson 2002) on the interpretation of diagnostic tests, Donna draws the following conclusion:

> Where the patient history suggests an ACL injury may have occurred (i.e. sporting injury, audible 'snap' or 'pop', a sense of instability of the knee and swelling following the injury), a positive Lachman test is strongly suggestive of an ACL tear. In chronic injuries, a positive Pivot Shift Test is strongly suggestive of an ACL tear.

Donna suspects that both tests might not be necessary and calculates the pre- and post-test probabilities of an ACL tear. She determines that she would be 50 per cent confident in her diagnosis given a patient history suggestive of an acute ACL injury. She calculates that if the Lachman test was positive, using the positive LR of 9.4 she would then be 90 per cent confident of the diagnosis.[1] If the condition was chronic, a subsequent positive Pivot Shift Test would further increase her confidence to 99 per cent.[2] Donna thinks that in fact the second test is not essential, which will be good news for the practitioners.

Step 5: Assess the process

Donna feels she used her time effectively to answer her research question using high levels of evidence. The next time she has a clinical query regarding diagnostic accuracy she is confident she can efficiently perform the steps required to make the best use of the available evidence.

SUMMARY

By following a stepwise approach to locating, appraising and applying the best research evidence, therapists are likely to arrive at conclusions regarding treatment that ultimately lead to better outcomes for their patients. Evidence-based practice does not aim to base clinical decisions purely on research, but to ensure that the characteristics of the patient and the expertise of the therapist are combined with the most up-to-date and clinically relevant knowledge in order to guide treatment.

While there may be a very large body of research for some questions, several mechanisms exist that can streamline the process. Understanding what type of research design will provide the highest level of evidence can significantly shorten the search for research articles. Knowledge of databases containing pre-appraised literature can mean that therapists need to spend less time determining the quality of the research.

Finally, the best way to make the process more efficient is to practise. The greater confidence in EBP-based skills in recent compared to older physiotherapy graduates (Iles & Davidson 2006) is likely to be not only the result of the teaching of specific skills, but also the opportunity to practise and hone those skills as part of learning. Physiotherapists recognise the importance of evidence-based practice but find the process time-consuming (Jette et al. 2003; Iles & Davidson 2006). If Danny and Donna continue to answer their own clinical questions using the step-wise approach, not only are their patients likely to experience better outcomes, but time will become less of a barrier to practising evidence-based physiotherapy.

TUTORIAL EXERCISES

1   What question regarding the effectiveness of therapy do you want to answer? Write that question in the PICO format:
    P—Population: what group of people are you interested in?
    I—Intervention: what therapy do you want to know about?
    C—Comparison: what do you want to compare the therapy to?
    O—Outcome: what do you expect to be the result of applying the therapy?

2   Using the terms from your research question above, search the Cochrane Library and PEDro for evidence to answer your question.

3   Are there any clinical guidelines that will help answer your question(s)? These can be found in PEDro.

4   Is there any pre-appraised evidence that answers your question(s)? These can be found in PEDro and the Cochrane Library.

NOTES

1   Pre-test probability of 50% converts to pre-test odds of 1 (odds = p/(1-p)), multiplied by the +LR of 9.4 gives a post-test odds of 9.4, which converts to a post-test probability of 90% (p = odds/(1-odds))

2   Pre-test probability of 90% converts to pre-test odds of 9 (odds = .90/(1-.90)), multiplied by
     the +LR of 7.7 gives a post-test odds of 69.3, which converts to a post-test probability of 99%
     (p = 69.3/70.3)

FURTHER READING

Herbert, R., Jamtvedt, G., Mead, J. & Birger Hagen, K. (2005). *Practical evidence-based physiotherapy*. Edinburgh: Elsevier Butterworth Heinemann.

Sackett, D.L., Straus, S.E., Richardson, W.S., Rosenberg, W. & Haynes, R.B. (2000). *Evidence-based medicine. How to practice and teach EBM*. Edinburgh: Churchill Livingstone.

WEBSITES

www.cebm.net/index.aspx?o=1157

The Centre for Evidence Based Medicine.

www.phru.nhs.uk/Pages/PHD/resources.htm

The UK Critical Appraisal Skills Program (CASP).

www.pedro.org.au

The Physiotherapy Evidence Database.

www.pedro.org.au/scale_item.html

The PEDro scale.

www.cochrane.org.au/library

All residents of Australia and New Zealand have access to the Cochrane Library.

www.gla.ac.uk/departments/generalpracticeprimarycare/ebp/checklists/#d.en.19536

The University of Glasgow General Practice and Family Care.

www.ncbi.nlm.nih.gov/entrez/query/static/clinical.shtml

PubMed (Public Medline) Database Clinical Queries.

www.nzgg.org.nz/index.cfm

The New Zealand Guidelines Group.

18

Everything You Wanted to Know about Systematic Reviews but Were Afraid to Ask

Nora Shields

CHAPTER OBJECTIVES

In this chapter you will learn:

☐ what advantages systematic reviews have and their implications for health professionals.

☐ about the constituent parts of a systematic review, including the setting of the research question, search strategies, quality assessment, data extraction and data synthesis.

☐ about practical advice and assistance about how to conduct a systematic review.

☐ what limitations are inherent in systematic reviews and their implications on the conclusions that can be drawn from a review.

KEY TERMS

Narrative review

PICO concept

Quality assessment

Systematic review

INTRODUCTION

A systematic review is a comprehensive identification and synthesis of the available literature on a specified topic (Centre for Reviews and Dissemination 2001). This method can be used to review the literature in any area of health. It is often used to synthesise the results of randomised controlled trials (see CHAPTER 15), but the method can also include research from many types of study designs including diagnostic tests and observational studies (Higgins & Green 2008; see CHAPTERS 11, 12). All systematic reviews adhere to a strict scientific protocol with well-described methods.

A systematic review is a useful process to collate previous literature in an area, either to answer a clinical question or to identify areas for future research. One of the key advantages of systematic reviews is that they can make it easier for researchers and practitioners to cope with the volume of literature available to review, by quickly identifying the relevant information and by excluding literature that is not relevant (Higgins & Green 2008). They are particularly useful for health professionals, as they summarise the key information in an area, allowing clinicians to read one paper that provides data from any number of other papers. High-quality systematic reviews can provide reliable evidence with which to aid clinical decision-making (Cook et al. 1997; see also CHAPTERS 15, 16, 17).

Systematic reviews are different from **narrative reviews** in that they provide an objective or scientific summary of the literature rather than a subjective opinion-based summary (Cook et al. 1997). In a systematic review, literature is treated like data.

Systematic review:
A comprehensive identification and synthesis of the available literature on a specified topic, where literature is treated like data.

A **narrative review** aims to provide 'a critical interpretation of the literature that it covers'. It is now seen as contrasting to, and less focused than, a systematic review.

With narrative reviews there is a risk of 'researcher bias', that is, the author might only review a small amount of the literature or present only one side of the argument because his or her beliefs can influence how he or she appraises the literature. There is also a risk that the breadth and depth of the literature reviewed is reduced or that the reviewer has decided to include some material but not other (Collins & Fauser 2005). This risk of bias is minimised in a systematic review because the methods used are transparent and can be replicated in the same way as an empirical research study. The systematic review process recognises that we are likely to bias the results of a review unless we follow clearly defined rules.

Systematic reviews follow a strict protocol to make sure that as much of the relevant research base as possible has been considered (Moher & Tricco 2008). The review protocol or how you are going to review the literature is decided in advance (a priori). This helps you reduce the biases associated with your selection of the literature you review. The method to be used at each stage of the protocol is defined and reported. The original studies included in a systematic review are appraised and synthesised in a rigorous and valid way and the results are presented in context with other relevant studies.

Systematic reviews can also reveal 'new' evidence, particularly when they include a meta-analysis (see CHAPTER 17). Small studies are often unable to provide a final conclusion on a research question because of a lack of power. However, when a number of these studies are combined (using predetermined set criteria), their results added together can reveal new information. A **meta-analysis** is a statistical technique that combines the results of similar studies into a single result that provides an estimate of the overall effect (Higgins & Green 2008). See also CHAPTER 24 for statistical analysis in quantitative research.

> **Meta-analysis:** A statistical technique that combines the results of similar studies into a single result that provides an estimate of the overall effect.

A STEP-BY-STEP GUIDE TO CONDUCTING A SYSTEMATIC REVIEW

This chapter outlines a six-step approach to conducting a systematic review:

Step 1: Set an answerable question for your review.

Step 2: Decide on a strategy that comprehensively searches for evidence.

Step 3: Define inclusion and exclusion criteria.

Step 4: Assess report quality.

Step 5: Extract standardised data from each report.

Step 6: Summarise or synthesise the findings of your review.

The method for each step of your review process should be determined at the start and is not normally changed once the protocol has been agreed. Any decisions made after this should be fully justified and agreed on by all the reviewers.

Step 1: Set an answerable question for your review

You might assume this is the easiest part of the review process. It is very important to spend some time thinking about the research or clinical question you want to answer in your review, since the question you set will decide how you approach every other step in the process.

A useful process to start you off is to develop a **PICO concept** or logic grid (Moher & Tricco 2008). PICO stands for:

☐ **P**opulation
☐ **I**ntervention or indicator
☐ **C**omparator or control
☐ **O**utcome

> **PICO concept:** **P**opulation, **I**ntervention or indicator, **C**omparator or control, and **O**utcome.

A well-thought-out review question will comprise these four elements.

Your review question should indicate your research population—the relevant participants in the research study—for example adults or children, but it is better to be even more specific, for example adults with multiple sclerosis or children with developmental coordination disorder.

The *intervention or indicator* is likely to be the entity you are most interested in. For example, it might be a treatment technique such as intravenous antibiotics, or a diagnostic test such as amniocentesis, or a construct such as quality of life.

The *comparator or control* is what you are comparing the intervention or indicator with, or what the main alternative is to the indicator or intervention you are proposing. This might be usual care or a placebo in the case of a clinical intervention, or another population, for example comparing children with spina bifida to children with typical development.

The review question also needs to state what *outcome* you are interested in. There might be only one such outcome, for example length of hospital stay, or many outcomes, for example pain and mobility.

In some cases, a fifth component is added to your review questions: *research design*. This element is included if you are limiting the review of the literature to a particular type of study design, such as randomised controlled trials or economic evaluations.

DOING RESEARCH

The following examples are provided to help you set an answerable question for your own systematic review:

Example of a review question about interventions

Are cardiovascular exercise programs beneficial and safe for people with Down syndrome? (Dodd & Shields 2005)

Example of a review question about diagnostic assessment measurements

What is the accuracy of clinical tests to diagnose superior labral anterior and posterior lesions in adults? (Mirkovic et al. 2005)

Example of a review question about incidence or prevalence of a condition

What is the prevalence of and risk factors associated with playing-related musculoskeletal disorders in professional pianists? (Bragge et al. 2006)

Example of a review question about aetiology or risk factors for a condition

Is the self-concept of children with cerebral palsy different from that of children with typical development? (Shields et al. 2006)

Example of a review question about economics

Is the prophylactic circumcision of male newborns economically beneficial to a health care system? (Cadman et al. 1984)

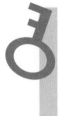

TRY IT YOURSELF

To figure out if your review question is too broad or too narrow, try 'scoping' the electronic databases to get a feel for the extent of the literature in the area. This consists of running some basic searches to get an idea of how much literature might exist; this will help you decide to focus your question if there is a large amount of literature or broaden your question if the literature base is small.

Step 2: Decide on a strategy that comprehensively searches for evidence

The easiest and most common way to find relevant literature for your review is by searching electronic databases (Higgins & Green 2008). This can be supplemented by searching through the key journals relevant to your research question and by using citation tracking of key papers or leading researchers via the Web, through electronic databases, or by contacting the experts in the field. The best search strategies are those that combine these methods to locate literature (Greenhalgh & Peacock 2005; and see CHAPTER 17).

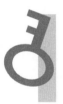

TRY IT YOURSELF

Go and introduce yourself to your local health sciences librarian. Librarians are a terrific resource when trying to locate literature and finding your way around electronic databases and library systems.

WHICH ELECTRONIC DATABASES TO CHOOSE?

There are many electronic databases available for you to search for literature (Greenhalgh 1997). A good place to start is to search either the general medical databases such as PubMed, Embase, Cochrane database or Medline or the general allied health databases such as Cinahl, Amed or Psychinfo.

The next step is to search discipline-specific databases such as PEDro (physiotherapy) (see CHAPTER 17), OT seeker (occupational therapy), ERIC (education) or other speciality databases such as AustSportMed and Sportdiscus, DARE (database of abstracts of reviews of effects), or the Campbell database (education, criminal justice and social welfare).

Finally, you can supplement your electronic searches by:

1   *Manual searching.* Read through the reference lists at the end of the articles you include in your review to help identify any additional references that did not come up in your electronic searches.

2   *Web of Science.* This database is useful for citation tracking backwards and forwards. It provides a list of all references cited by a particular article (this is the same information you get when you search manually), but it also provides a list of articles that have subsequently cited that paper (forward citation tracking).

Nora Shields

3 *Google scholar.* This database performs a function similar to the Web of Science in that you can track articles that have referenced a paper since publication.

4 *Contact key authors in the area.* Contacting the leading researchers in an area can help to validate the articles you have sourced. If there have been any major papers you have missed they will be able to let you know very quickly as they are the people most au fait with that area. They can also tell you about the current research that is being done in the area.

5 *Related articles feature on PubMed.* This can be a useful feature to identify papers that are similar to those you have included in your review.

6 *Manual search of key journals.* Most disciplines will have a key journal(s) associated with that area. Often it is important to hand-search electronic or hard copies of these journals to identify relevant studies in the area, particularly more recent studies that have not yet been indexed on the electronic databases.

7 *Clinical trials registers.* Most journals are moving to the point where they will only publish clinical studies that were pre-registered with a relevant clinical trial register. Examples of clinical trial registers are the Australian New Zealand Clinical Trials Registry and the WHO International Clinical Trials Registry Platform.

TRY IT YOURSELF

Before using an electronic database, make sure you create a personal account for yourself on that database so that you can save and edit your searches.

HOW TO SELECT YOUR KEYWORDS OR SEARCH TERMS

The PICO concept or logic grid used in Step 1 can also be used to help select your key search terms. When choosing your search keywords you need to identify MeSH terms and free text terms. MeSH terms are controlled terms or phrases used to index journal articles and books in the life sciences; they are used to list articles in the respective databases. Free text terms are any additional terms that can be used to describe your key concepts but which are not MeSH terms. It is important to include also your MeSH terms in your free text search as errors are often made when cataloguing the electronic databases.

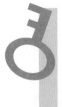

TRY IT YOURSELF

Before running your final searches it is worthwhile checking if the key words you select identify the correct types of literature. If a term returns a large amount of unrelated literature, you might want to reconsider including it as part of your search strategy. Remember that your search terms are like the key to a lock—if you have the wrong key it won't open the lock; if you use the wrong search terms, you won't identify the literature you need.

DOING RESEARCH

Example of a search strategy

You have decided your review question is: What effect does participation in a progressive resistance exercise program compared with usual care have on the body structure and function, activity limitation and participation restriction of people with Down syndrome?

So your PICO concept terms are:

P   people with Down syndrome

I   progressive resistance exercise

C   usual care

O   body structure and function, activity limitation and participation restriction

For each concept you need to write out all other terms and words used for that concept, for example:

P   Down syndrome, Trisomy 21, intellectual disability

I   progressive resistance exercise, strength training, rehabilitation, physical therapy

For each concept you check the corresponding MeSH terms:

P   Down syndrome, mental retardation

I   exercise, physical therapy, rehabilitation

Now you are ready to finalise your concept grid

Table 18.1: An example of a search strategy

	Population		Intervention	
AND ⟶	MeSH	Free text terms	MeSH	Free text terms
OR ↓	Down syndrome	Down syndrome	Exercise	Progressive resistance training
	Mental retardation	Mental retardation	Physical Therapy	Strength training
		Trisomy 21	Rehabilitation	Exercise
		Intellectual Disability		Physical Therapy
				Rehabilitation
				Physical training

Your final search strategy would look like this:

1   exp Down syndrome/ OR exp Mental Retardation/ *(these are MeSH terms)*

2   (Down syndrome OR Mental$ Retard$ OR Intellectual$ Disab$ OR Trisomy 21).ti,ab.
    (these are free text terms)

3 1 OR 2 *(this combines MeSH terms and free text term searches for the same concept)*

4 exp exercise/ OR exp Physical Therapy / OR exp Rehabilitation

5 (exercise$ OR Physical Therapy OR Rehabilitation OR progressive resistance training OR strength training OR physiotherapy OR physical training).ti,ab

6 4 OR 5

7 3 AND 6 *(this combines the two concepts in your PICO system)*

TRY IT YOURSELF

It can be easy to get confused by the 'mechanics of searching' and worrying about whether you need to use the advanced functions the databases offer (like filters or limits). The simplest search strategies are often the best. If you do find you are getting addled by the mechanics of searching, it is best to speak to your librarian. Librarians are the experts in this area and are always happy to help.

TRY IT YOURSELF

Purchase a copy of a bibliographic software program, for example EndNote. It will help you sort through the items identified by searching the electronic databases.

WHAT TO DO WITH YOUR SEARCH YIELDS?

Use a software package such as EndNote to download all unfiltered yields from the databases you have searched. Usually, you can download the search yields directly from the databases. In some instances, you will need to download a filter for that database to your bibliographic management software first; for example, a filter for the PEDro databases is freely available on the PEDro website (see Websites below; see also CHAPTER 17).

It is important to document each stage of the process, so make sure you have noted the number of items identified in each database or search strategy. Remember to keep a copy of the unfiltered final search yield for future reference. When you start to exclude items based on title and abstract, do so using a copy of your unfiltered final search yield.

Continue to document the final strategies employed and note all changes and amendments from the protocol.

Step 3: Define the inclusion and exclusion criteria

HOW TO DECIDE ON YOUR INCLUSION/EXCLUSION CRITERIA

Not every item identified by your search strategy will be relevant to your review question. Therefore you need a way of deciding what is relevant to your review question (inclusion criteria) and what can be left out (exclusion criteria). This step in the process helps you to select the articles that will help you answer your review question (Centre for Reviews and Dissemination 2001).

Your inclusion and exclusion criteria should flow logically from your review question and an easy way to decide on your criteria is to use the PICO concept grid again. Ask yourself:

P   Who should the included studies be about?

I   What intervention(s) should the included studies have investigated?

C   What should the intervention be compared to?

O   What are the outcomes I am interested in?

DOING RESEARCH

Example of inclusion/exclusion criteria

Let us return to our review question, which is: What effect does participation in a progressive resistance exercise program compared with usual care have on the body structure and function, activity limitation and participation restriction of people with Down syndrome?

P   people with Down syndrome
I   a progressive resistance exercise program of six weeks' duration minimum
C   a control or 'usual care' group
O   all outcomes—impairments, functional activities, quality of life, social participation.

So studies will be included in our review if they investigated:

1   people with Down syndrome

2   a strengthening program, which was 6 weeks minimum in duration, compared the intervention with a control group or a 'usual care' group such as usual physiotherapy, participation in their usual physical activity.

Studies will be excluded if:

1   they include people with other forms of intellectual or physical disabilities such as cerebral palsy

2   they involved a single exercise training session

3   full details of the intensity of the exercise program are not included

4   there was no comparison group (so a single group study).

The method by which the inclusion and exclusion criteria are applied is also important. It is always best for at least two assessors to decide independently whether a study meets the inclusion criteria. If they disagree, then they can use a consensus method to make a final

Nora Shields

decision on whether to include a study. This decision is based on a discussion of their reasons for including or excluding a study. Having two reviewers undertake the task helps ensure that studies are not missed by chance. If the consensus method fails to produce a decision then it is possible to ask a third reviewer to adjudicate.

Step 4: Assess the quality of the included studies

WHY COMPLETE QUALITY ASSESSMENT?

Quality assessment is an integral part of the systematic review process (Whiting et al. 2003). As systematic reviews are generally written to assist health care professionals in answering a clinical question, you only want to include the best possible evidence available to help them

Quality assessment: Part of the systematic review process that can guide the interpretation of the review findings and help determine the strength of inferences made from the results.

make their decisions. Therefore an additional inclusion criterion is often included so that only articles that meet a minimum quality threshold are included in the review. The quality assessment process will help you determine whether or not a study meets the set criterion.

The quality assessment process can guide the interpretation of the review findings and help determine the strength of inferences we can make from the results (Crowther & Cook 2007). Considering the quality of the included studies is helpful when interpreting heterogeneous data and helps you decide if the quality of the studies has affected the results. When interpreting the data, we might also place more emphasis on the high-quality studies compared with those of lower quality. In fact, in meta-analysis it is possible through mathematical methods to give proportionally more weight to higher-quality studies (Greenhalgh 1997). Finally, the quality assessment process can help guide future research by determining the limitations of previous research studies and making recommendations for how future studies might eliminate possible sources of bias.

WHAT IS QUALITY ASSESSMENT?

The quality assessment process is used to assess the degree to which each included study has employed measures to minimise bias (Jüni et al. 2001). It is a standardised process, so that we appraise all studies equally. Through quality assessment, we assesses internal validity, or the degree to which the results are likely to approximate the truth and external validity, or the extent to which the effects observed in a study can be applied outside the study.

HOW TO PERFORM THE QUALITY ASSESSMENT?

You start by choosing a quality assessment tool. It is always best to select a quality assessment tool with strong psychometric properties (one that is valid and reliable). Which tool you select depends on the research design of the studies you are assessing. If your inclusion criteria specified a particular study design (for example RCTs), then the quality assessment tool you choose needs to reflect that criterion. There are numerous quality assessments tools for RCTs and observational studies, but not for many other types of studies. See CHAPTERS 11, 15.

Quality assessment is completed at the same time as data extraction (see Step 5) and should be carried out by two reviewers. The reviewers normally assess the included studies independently of each other, to reduce the risk of reviewer bias. They then compare their scores. If disagreements arise, these should also be resolved by consensus (see Step 3). If an agreement cannot be reached, a third reviewer should be called on to adjudicate.

You also need to document the quality assessment process. It is best to use a standard assessment form and remember to keep a record of the process, including, for example, the number of items on which there was initial agreement. This data can be used to calculate a kappa squared statistic, which gives an indication of the level of agreement between the reviewers.

TRY IT YOURSELF

It is always best to choose a validated quality assessment scale if one is available. An example is the PEDro scale for assessing the quality of RCTs.

WHAT TO DO IF THERE IS NO VALIDATED CHECKLIST AVAILABLE?

Selecting a validated quality assessment tool is not always as easy as it seems, particularly if the study designs of your included studies are not RCTs. If there is no standardised quality assessment tool available for you to use, you can either select a quality checklist or you can decide on individual quality components that you feel are important in controlling bias for the particular study designs you are assessing. A quality checklist is a list of quality items suggested by experts in the fields (e.g. see CRD Report No 4, Stage 2 Phase 5).

You can also develop your own quality assessment tool for your review. To do this, you must identify the bias that you wish to assess and then develop an item that assesses only that one source of bias. You also need to define a decision rule for scoring the item. It is acceptable to borrow items from related scales or examine studies where authors have attempted to build an assessment scale. But you should be aware that your new 'tool' will have no validity or reliability unless you specifically undertake some separate research work in this area (see CHAPTER 11).

Step 5: Extract standardised data from each report

Data extraction is the process by which you obtain the information you need to answer your review question from what was reported in the included articles. As with the previous steps, it is important to have a standard process for extracting data and minimising error. This can be done by designing a good data extraction form and by having two reviewers extract the data independently of each other. At a minimum, one reviewer can extract the data if the extraction is then checked by a second reviewer (Higgins & Green 2008).

WHAT SHOULD YOU INCLUDE IN YOUR DATA EXTRACTION FORM?

You need to be careful that your data extraction form is balanced in the amount of data you intend to extract. If you extract too much data, then the process might be wasteful, but include too little detail and you may have to re-extract data later. The key thing to keep in mind is that the information extracted should be related to the research questions posed.

Data extraction forms are often very similar in structure, so if you develop a good data extraction form for one review, you will be able to adapt it for subsequent reviews.

Step 6: Synthesise the findings of your review

HOW TO SYNTHESISE YOUR DATA

Now that you have located all the studies you want to include in your review, and have extracted all the data, how do you go about collating the data and summarising the results? It is probably easiest to start off with a descriptive analysis of your data.

Descriptive analysis is where you provide information about the study characteristics that gives context for the population data and the environment within which the study was conducted. Tables are the easiest way to collate descriptive data and to identify trends in the data. For example, a table can summarise the key elements of the study under the headings sample size, participant details (sex, age, height, weight, employment or schooling characteristics), intervention details (frequency, intensity, duration, equipment used, personnel involved) and outcome measures used. This type of data analysis will help you judge whether the characteristics of the included studies allow for generalisation of the results (see CHAPTERS 24, 25). It will also help to identify restrictions and omissions in the results.

Quantitative data analysis can also be completed by calculating effect sizes and performing a meta-analysis. Before deciding to perform a meta-analysis it is important to determine whether data from the included studies are clinically and statistically homogeneous and whether you have all the data you need. The descriptive data analysis will help you identify clinical homogeneity, and there are statistical methods of identifying statistical homogeneity (see CHAPTER 24). While a meta-analysis may be appropriate in a systematic review, not all good systematic reviews need to contain meta-analyses. If a meta-analysis is appropriate then you need to decide which comparisons should be made and which outcome measures will be used.

Meta-analysis can be a useful tool when there is a large body of smaller studies in an area (Greenhalgh 1997). Combining their data can increase the power of the analysis and therefore improve the precision of estimate of effect. This reduces the uncertainty across several independent studies and can 'reveal' new information. Meta-analysis is based on lots of assumptions, and the variation between studies (clinical heterogeneity) might make the results meaningless. Larger studies can also have a proportionally greater effect depending on the model used to conduct the meta-analysis.

SUMMARY

A systematic review is a comprehensive identification and synthesis of all relevant studies on a review question. It is conducted according to an explicit and reproducible method to minimise the risk of reviewer bias. Systematic reviews help health professionals cope with large volumes of literature by summarising it and providing more reliable evidence that can aid clinical decision-making. They are also used by researchers to identify gaps and strengths of the current literature, assisting research design.

The method of conducting a systematic review should be transparent, easily replicated and scientifically rigorous. The process comprises setting an answerable clinical question, searching for relevant information, deciding which studies should be included and excluded, assessing the quality of the included studies, extracting relevant data and synthesising the findings of the review.

TUTORIAL EXERCISES

What clinical question do you wish to know the answer to? Write it down and develop a protocol for a systematic review that would help you answer that question. Your protocol should include the following:

- ☐ an answerable review question
- ☐ a list of the electronic databases you intend searching, plus the methods you would use to supplement your search strategy
- ☐ a list of your inclusion and exclusion criteria
- ☐ a suitable quality assessment tool
- ☐ a data extraction form for the review
- ☐ a plan for how you intend to synthesise the data.

FURTHER READING

Centre for Reviews and Dissemination (2001). Report No 4: Undertaking systematic reviews of research on effectiveness. University of York. <www.york.ac.uk/inst/crd/index.htm>.

Greenhalgh, T. (1997). How to read a paper: Papers that summarise other papers (systematic reviews and meta-analyses). *British Medical Journal*, 315, 672–5.

Higgins, J.P.T. & Green, S. (2008). Cochrane Handbook for Systematic Reviews of Interventions 5.0.1 [updated September 2008]. <www.cochrane-handbook.org>.

Jüni, P., Altman, D. & Egger, M. (2001). Assessing the quality of controlled clinical trials. *British Medical Journal*, 323, 42–6.

Lau, J., Ioannidis, J. & Schmid, C. (1997). Quantitative Synthesis in Systematic Reviews. *Annals of Internal Medicine*, 127, 820–26.

van Tulder, M., Assendelft, W., Koes, B., Bouter, L. & the Editorial Board of the Cochrane Collaboration Back Review Group (1997). Method guidelines for systematic reviews in the Cochrane Collaboration Back Review Group for Spinal Disorders. *Spine*, 22, 2323–30.

Nora Shields

WEBSITES

www.cochrane.org.au/libraryguide

The website for the Cochrane library.

www.campbellcollaboration.org

The Campbell database.

www.anzctr.org.au

The Australian New Zealand Clinical Trials Registry.

www.who.int/ictrp/en

WHO International Clinical Trials Registry Platform (ICTRP).

www.nlm.nih.gov/mesh

MeSH headings.

www.pedro.fhs.usyd.edu.au/scale_item.html

PEDro scale for assessing the quality of RCTs.

www.cochrane.org.au/libraryguide

The Cochrane library is a collection of databases containing high-quality independent evidence to inform decision-making in health care. This library gives you immediate access to several hundred systematic reviews covering all aspects of health care. It should be your first stop in reviewing the literature to answer a clinical question, as Cochrane reviews represent the highest level of evidence on which to base clinical management decisions.

www.york.ac.uk/inst/crd/index.htm

An excellent resource to help you with writing your systematic review is the Centre for Reviews and Dissemination at the University of York Report No 4: Undertaking systematic reviews of research on effectiveness (2001). A copy of the report is available free at this website.

www.york.ac.uk/inst/crd/pdf/crd4_app3.pdf

This is the Centre for Reviews and Dissemination, University of York website. It gives an example of a data extraction form.

www.consort-statement.org/index.aspx?o=1065

The QUOROM Statement (Moher et al. 1999) was the outcome of a conference convened to address standards for improving the quality of reporting of meta-analyses of RCTs. It is a useful guide when writing a review and can be downloaded from this website.

Part V

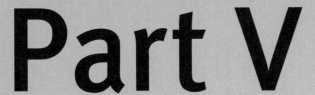

Mixed Methodology and
Collaborative Practices

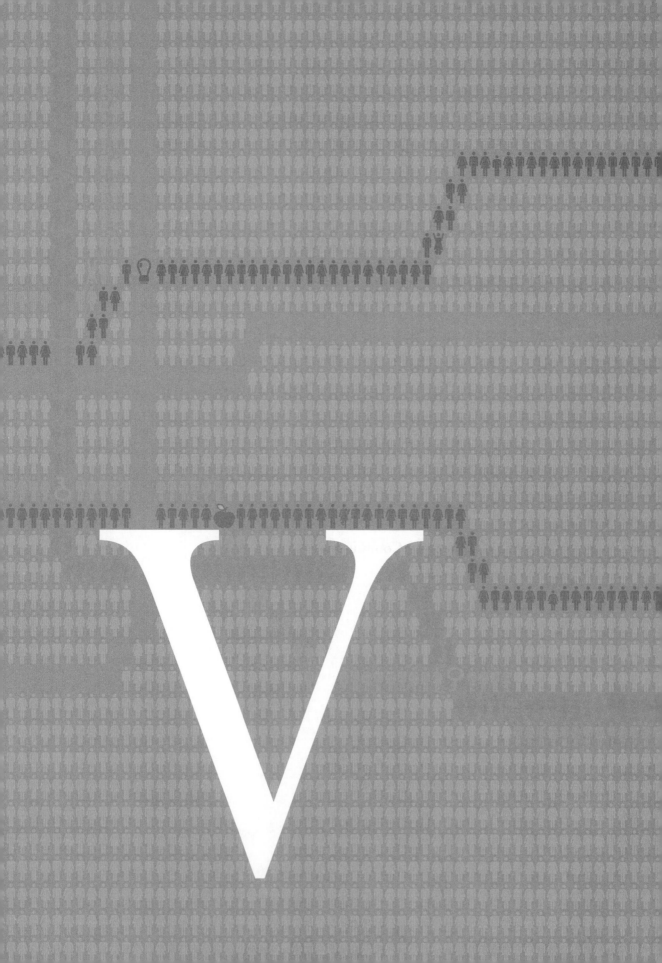

19

Integrated Methods in Health Research

Carol Grbich

CHAPTER OBJECTIVES

In this chapter you will learn:

☐ what are the issues and practicalities regarding the integration or mixing of methods in health research from three perspectives; ontological (theoretical), epistemological (design and data collection)

☐ how to integrate and interpret the results of data analysis

KEY TERMS

Concurrent design

Constructivism

Epistemology

Ontology

Positivism

Pragmatism

Q^2 or Q squared

Sequential design

Triangulation

INTRODUCTION

Within both qualitative styles alone and quantitative styles alone, it is possible to use multiple approaches for data collection, data analysis and data interpretation, but it is the combining of quantitative and qualitative approaches (Q^2 or Q squared) that is of greatest interest currently

Q^2 or Q squared: The combination of quantitative and qualitative approaches in a research study. It is the concept used in mixed methods research design.

(see also CHAPTERS 1, 20). The first question you, as a researcher, need to ask yourself before considering a Q^2 approach is: 'Does my question have both qualitative and quantitative components?' A typical question with a Q^2 possibility might be: 'What is the impact of (x) on the attitudes of (y) towards (z)?' Here it would be useful to get an overall sense of the impact of some change or existing issue on a large group by perhaps using a survey

(see CHAPTER 13) then, in order to find out more detail, adding face-to-face interviews (see CHAPTER 3) or focus groups (see CHAPTER 4) to clarify the in-depth individual views of a smaller sample of this group.

Another indicator that an integrated approach could be useful would be the presence of the potential to measure relationships between variables in addition to gaining the views of a group of people. For example: 'What are the effects of the latest safe sex campaign on the perceptions and behaviours of young males and young females?' Here the question can be broken down into more than one component. For example: 'Are males and females different in terms of behaviours following exposure to a safe sex campaign?', which forms the quantitative component where relationships between variables could be measured; and 'What are the effects of the images and information of the campaign on young males and females in terms of their perceptions regarding safe sex?', which forms the qualitative component to be collected through interviews or focus groups. Implicit in this are also the questions: 'Why are there differences between males and females?' (if these are found) and 'How could a better campaign be constructed?' (if the current one was ineffective).

INTEGRATED APPROACHES

The integration of theoretical ideas, data collection techniques and/or data analytic techniques is generally used to provide answers to more complex questions, to enable the inclusion of a broad overview of larger numbers of people, or to measure relationships between variables in a situation where rich in-depth information is also required.

Other reasons for attempting integration include the bringing together of two or more separate sets of data to illuminate different aspects of a research question, a process called **triangulation**; the clarification of one set of results by or from another; and the extension or

Triangulation: The use of multiple methods, researchers, data sources, or theories in a research project.

development of one set of results into another set.

Integrated approaches offer many advantages to the researcher. For example, you can attempt to answer more complex research questions with greater certainty. You can explore the detail of individual experiences behind the statistics, and conversely statistics can provide an overview and a context for narratives. The approaches help in the development of particular measures or questions. They can track changes over time and allow one data set to feed into the development of another. They can also foster the mix of a range of traditional designs as well as encourage the development of innovative mixes to provide better answers to research questions while enhancing the generalisability of the results.

However, there are also some disadvantages or weaknesses of these approaches. For example, the study will be larger and may take longer or require a larger research team to carry it out effectively. Greater skills are needed to successfully design, undertake, analyse and interpret integrated data sets. One paradigm (see definitions below and CHAPTER 1) may dominate and be treated appropriately, while the other may be glossed over in terms of design, data collection, analysis and interpretation. Last, different weightings of paradigms and techniques need appropriate clarification and justification or the validity of both may be severely compromised (see also CHAPTER 20).

Let me examine in more detail the three major issues of ontology, epistemology and the integration and interpretation of multiple data sets so you can see what is involved.

ONTOLOGICAL INTEGRATION

In research, the word **ontology** refers to the theoretical underpinnings of different paradigms or methodological approaches. Both quantitative and qualitative approaches come from different paradigms—usually defined as agreed upon sets of assumptions or collections of underpinning beliefs about the twin natures of reality and knowledge— and these paradigms guide the research to be undertaken (see CHAPTER 1). The quantitative paradigm (often termed **positivism**) is characterised by a focus on development and implementation of research instruments; 'objective' (distant, non-involved) researchers; deduction (the formation of hypotheses for testing from observable empirical facts); confirmation and explanation of facts as a result of theory and hypothesis-testing; the use of statistical analysis; and an assumption that the results found can be widely generalised and easily replicated. The qualitative paradigm (often termed **constructivism** or *interpretivism*) is characterised by 'subjective' researchers who are the research instruments and whose biases contribute to the construction of perspectives, by induction (creating explanations from diverse observations) or discovery, and by theory or concept development to interpret findings (see also CHAPTER 1).

Those favouring Q^2 approaches have suggested that one way to bypass the complexities of these two differing paradigms and to circumvent the pitfalls inherent in combining the two is to adopt the philosophical position of **pragmatism** (Teddlie & Tashakkori 2003; Johnson & Onwuegbuzie 2006;

Ontology: the study of the nature of being, existence or reality in general.

Positivism: The belief that social science research methods should be scientific in the same way as the physical sciences.

Constructivism: An epistemology that suggests that 'reality' is socially constructed, a product of our own making.

Pragmatism: Reality exists not only as natural and physical realities but also as psychological and social realities, which include subjective experience and thought, language and culture.

Carol Grbich

see also CHAPTER 1). Pragmatism was originally a set of values developed by Charles Pierce, George Herbert Mead, William James and John Dewey in the late 19th and early 20th centuries to enable us to make a connection between the nature of knowledge and the techniques or methods we use to gain knowledge.

Put simply, pragmatism refers to the connection between knowledge and the methods by which this knowledge is gained. In more detail, pragmatism seeks the middle ground in areas that have previously been polarised, as have quantitative and qualitative approaches, particularly in terms of their subjective and objective positions. According to pragmatist positions, knowledge of the world can be obtained by observation, experience and experimentation. In this manner, the focus becomes the research question(s) that requires answers by whatever mix of data collection approaches appear to be most useful. Humans are viewed as interacting with the physical world to create meaning and knowledge, which leads to the development of theories that can be tested on the grounds of how well they can be applied. Each notion or theory or concept can be interpreted in terms of actions and outcomes in the real world and seen as a contribution to a dynamic and changing set of 'truths' or theories. Within the limits of change these results are seen as providing some predictability. Thus the meanings or outcomes of a research study provide a path to be followed in order to produce new explanations or to confirm existing ones. There is an underlying assumption that where problems are uncovered, solutions do exist and can be trialled and evaluated in an ongoing fashion. Morgan (2007) sees the following terminology shift as one way of integrating quantitative and qualitative within a pragmatic paradigm: induction and deduction become 'abduction' (allowing you to move backwards and forwards between induction and deduction, from one set of results to another); subjectivity and objectivity become 'intersubjectivity' (which accepts that there is a real world out there but adds that we all have our individual interpretations of this world); and context and generality become 'transferability' (where you decide how much of your results will be likely to be applicable to another like setting or situation).

EPISTEMOLOGICAL INTEGRATION

Epistemology is related to the methods used to gain knowledge (see CHAPTER 1). Putting together quantitative and qualitative approaches in terms of design is simpler than arguing over the differences in paradigms and relies largely on your creativity. However, there are areas of decision-making you will need to address. The first is your research question(s), which will need to be suitable for integrated approaches. The second is 'which approach is to be the dominant one or are both to be equal?' as this will determine the final weighting of your results and interpretation. The last decision lies with issues of time: should you collect your data sets at the same time (concurrent) or at different times (sequential)?

Epistemology is concerned with the nature of knowledge and how knowledge is obtained.

SAMPLING

The inclusion of both probability and non-probability sampling strategies has opened up options for you as a Q^2 researcher. The usual probability approaches (random, stratified, systematic, cluster and multiple approaches) are joined by the non-probability approaches (maximum variation, homogeneous, typical case, intensity, extreme, snowballing, convenience, opportunistic and multiple approaches) to provide a wide variety of options within the sequential, concurrent and multilevel designs that can be designed from these two options (see also CHAPTER 1). It has been suggested by Collins and associates (2007) that the size of your sample needs to match your method or data collection technique so that your focus groups have between six and 12 participants, your ethnography has a defined culture of whatever number is involved, for example six street youth or 250 people in a tribal group, and your correlational and causal comparative studies have at least 60 (one-tailed hypothesis) to 80+ (two-tailed hypothesis) depending on the desired proportion of the total population available.

DESIGN

There are two major design orientations at your disposal.

Sequential designs

In **sequential design**, one data set follows another and extends or explores the findings from the first set. For example, you could undertake a qualitative study to explore a particular issue or phenomenon and you could create hypotheses from these results that you could test using a survey or experimental design. Alternatively, you could develop a short questionnaire survey to elicit key issues that can then be explored in depth using qualitative approaches of interviewing and observation. Synthesis of the two sets of results is needed to clarify the dual outcomes and to utilise the increased validity these two approaches provide. You can see here that the questions for the second part of the study evolve from the results of the first part (see also CHAPTER 20).

> In **sequential design**, one data set follows another and extends or explores the findings from the first set.

RESEARCH EXAMPLE: SEQUENTIAL DESIGN QUANTITATIVE TO QUALITATIVE

A simple sequential investigation into the role of information in online investment (Williamson 2008) addressed the research question: 'What is the role of information in online investment in Australia?'

The quantitative component involved a broad-based survey overview (predominantly using 6-point rating scales) of the behaviour patterns and habits of 520 investors, accessed through two online companies, the Commonwealth Bank and Sanford Online, who put the survey questionnaire up on their websites. Of the respondents, 200 offered to be interviewed and 29 were chosen to create a geographically representative sample Australia-wide. Interviews were face to face, lasting up to two hours and pursuing in greater depth both the original question areas and the outcomes of the wider survey but compared with their own individual survey profile.

There was considerable value in combining the two methods, especially as both were treated separately and with respect to the differing ontological, epistemological and data-analytic orientations. The equal balance allowed one set of data to feed into another and to complement the original survey finding by providing depth of explanation.

RESEARCH EXAMPLE: SEQUENTIAL DESIGN QUALITATIVE TO QUANTITATIVE TO QUALITATIVE

Baluch and Davies (2008) have used a three-way sequential design: qualitative to quantitative to qualitative in a longitudinal study examining the poverty dynamics and trajectories in rural Bangladesh following the particular government interventions of microfinance in 1994, new agricultural technologies in 1996–97 and the introduction of educational transfers in 2000 and 2003. They used three sequential phases.

Phase 1 involved the collection of qualitative data by 116 focus groups in 11 districts to examine perceptions of change regarding the interventions for 'poor' and 'better off' groups of men and women.

Phase 2 involved a quantitative household survey of 2152 households to compare with an earlier brief survey undertaken by other researchers that had measured the initial impact of the interventions.

Phase 3 involved the collection of 293 qualitative life history interviews in order to understand the processes and institutional contexts that influence livelihood trajectories. The combination of data collection techniques in a sequential manner enabled a better understanding of the changing profiles of risk and opportunities that the poor in Bangladesh face and how these profiles shape the dynamics of poverty much more clearly. The patterns and trends thus exposed have implications for policy.

The combining of the two data sets helped to compensate for the blind spots that often eventuate from a single approach and strengthened the overall research process.

In a **concurrent design** the questions researchers ask would tend to be framed from the start; they could consider using multiple reference points where intact but separate data sets are collected concurrently.

Concurrent/parallel/triangulation designs

In a **concurrent design** your questions would tend to be framed from the start and you could consider using multiple reference points where intact but separate data sets are collected concurrently. For example, you could use dual sites with the same sampling approach but with different designs (one quantitative, one qualitative), then use the synthesised results to build up a complex picture (see also CHAPTER 20). Within the concurrent approach, an internal integration or merging or synergy of data collection approaches occurs. This involves you in processes where aspects of the usually separate techniques intermingle. For example, using both focused (limited response) quantitative and open-ended (qualitative) questions in the same survey allows immediate comparisons and a more holistic view of the questions to be addressed, and also allows you to follow up responses on the spot. Another possibility involves you in asking why your participants have chosen a particular course of action, then counting the responses and presenting these as a percentage of the total, and then establishing variables from this and measuring relationships between these.

DOING RESEARCH

Concurrent design

The Sakai Virtual Research Environment is an open-source virtual collaboration environment initially developed by a consortium of research-intensive universities to encourage collaborative research (Procter et al. 2008). This modular environment (Sakai) can be set up either as a virtual learning or a virtual research environment. Access is controlled and email lists, chat room and 'work sites' are provided. The site collects usage data through log data that provides the user's address and password, their type of Web browser and the page from which they were referred. In addition, the database tables stored inside the virtual research environment provide a record of the 'click stream' showing individual actors chatting, editing pages, viewing documents and so on. In this evaluation quantitative data was collected over time to identify patterns and trends regarding the amount of time spent in a particular arena. To identify differences between individual participants and projects, the 'who', 'what' and 'where' of patterns of use and trends were treated as rudimentary qualitative data to create 'user stories' from within the database of use, and these were expanded to semi-structured interviews both on and off line where participants were asked to comment on and make sense of graphs of their own activity online at the Sakai site.

Using reduced quantitative data as the focus for qualitative enquiry was very illuminating, especially when as part of the evaluation we involved participants in 'sensemaking', that is explaining their own profile data graphs.

Carol Grbich

DOING RESEARCH

Multilevel concurrent design

A triangulation approach can often be seen in multi-site research. In an investigation of strategic scanning in organisations (Audet & d'Amboise 2001), four organisations were selected for cross-case comparison along two polar dimensions: *performance of the firm* and *level of uncertainty in the firm's environment*. Two of the firms selected had high levels of uncertainty—one with a high and the other with a lower performance level, and the remaining two had low levels of uncertainty and either a high or lower performance level. Data comprised semi-structured interviews in all sites with different levels of staff. Interview schedules comprised closed- and open-ended questions relating to the variables that had been identified. Within-case analysis was followed by cross-case analysis of firms with similar performance levels.

The advantage of a detailed research design is that it allows for greater flexibility, but when the diversity of sites is too great the study can head off in unexpected directions that are hard to control in terms of variables.

New and innovative approaches

At present, most data collected is still within the survey/interview/observation/document analysis framework in multiple data sets, with the documents traditionally being written communications or transcriptions, but looking to the field of media images should alert you to what is being attempted in this field. Gamberini and Spagnolli (2003) have brought together both qualitative and quantitative data sets under the heading of an exploration of human–computer interactions, encompassing the digital, physical, real and artificial aspects of this through three triangulated data sets. The first set involves the *split screen technique*, which allows a synchronised visualisation of different environments on the same screen, in this case the real and the virtual environments a participant is involved in on screen. In this way, individual interaction with a computer can be seen on one half of the screen while the other half details the depth view of what is actually happening as the individual interacts with the program. This process can be undertaken by one individual or multiple users by splitting the monitor into further blocks of two screen displays. The second option is the *action indicator augmented display*, which picks up the faster individual interactions with the computer interface, particularly quick hand movements on buttons, which are reflected in arrows at the bottom of the screen. The third is the *pentagram*, which allows transcription of multiple sequences of events in its own timeline. Although these approaches can be used as tools to provide a single conclusion, they can also provide individual or multimedia displays in their own right, allowing the reader to observe all the data collected.

As new and innovative approaches are developed by researchers, it becomes harder to confine these within the boundaries of standard definitions. The example below is one that exhibits both concurrent and sequential approaches in a complex multilevel design.

DOING RESEARCH

Multilevel concurrent and sequential design

A study to investigate domestic violence (Thurston et al. 2008) combined epidemiological, survey and qualitative methods in a longitudinal study in order to evaluate domestic violence interventions in emergency care settings in Canada. The focus was on accessing the factors that influence uptake and maintenance of the intervention at the micro (individual management, staff and patient), meso (organisational and collective) and macro (extra-oganisational) levels.

Data was collected by:

1 observation of the five emergency departments and three urgent care sectors (repeated over several hours) observing environment, employees, patterns and procedures, case meetings and committee meetings

2 105 open-ended interviews with nursing staff and managers in seven hospitals over two phases

3 a review of 5 years of de-identified patient notes

4 a review of relevant media coverage over 6 years

5 a review of site-specific documents, meeting minutes, annual reports etc.

6 a brief questionnaire survey of female residents in shelters for abused women in the city of Calgary

7 10 ethnographic interviews with five different types of health care professionals were conducted to follow up the themes identified in item 2 regarding the nature of their work.

This study has the multiple characteristics of different levels and styles of data collected over time in phases with sequential follow-up.

Further debate is needed on the issue of methodological congruence and method triangulation so that researchers have some guidelines on what will be acceptable as 'sound'.

Carol Grbich

ANALYSIS, DISPLAY, INTERPRETATION AND SYNTHESIS OF RESULTS

Bryman (2007) has identified three major groupings of barriers faced by researchers who have attempted to conduct mixed method research:

- ☐ intrinsic differences between qualitative and quantitative in terms of theory, data sets and the additional time taken to gather these and to merge analyses
- ☐ institutional differences of audience, publication, discipline and funding agencies
- ☐ researcher preference or comfort zone in a particular style.

Of these the merging of analyses in the first point appeared to be the most confronting. So let us see if we can attempt to break down this barrier. The choices in terms of data management are to treat the data sets as separate and to analyse and display them separately. Alternatively, you can analyse them separately but integrate them in terms of display, taking care to weight the display appropriately. The third option is to integrate your data sets in some way so that an amalgam is presented for display.

Separate data sets

The difficulties surrounding presentation of qualitative and quantitative approaches lie in the creation of a very large results section culminating in a final drawing together of the findings in a summary so that the reader can make sense of the diversity presented. An example of this is provided by Duncan and Edwards (1997), who interviewed 95 single or lone mothers in three countries (UK, USA and Sweden) and contextualised these within census data. The results are largely displayed in separate chapters (e.g. a chapter on social negotiation of understandings is followed by one chapter on census data). This approach can leave the reader see-sawing between the different data sets, and making connections between the two data sets may be difficult.

Combined data sets

In contrast to the separation of data sets, it may be preferable to amalgamate the findings in such a way that a neat display of graphical information occurs, followed by a few carefully chosen qualitative quotes that serve to display the homogeneity (or diversity) of the data gathered. The use of matrixes can serve to bring together variables, themes and cases, as can lists, network diagrams and graphical displays. Wacjman and Martin (2002) studied managers in six companies. A questionnaire was completed by a random sample of 470 managers together with interviews with 18–26 managers from each company. The data is presented equally with the quantitative survey results displayed in an extensive single table and the career narratives of 136 managers divided into male and female responses and presented as substantial quotes and commentary. The totality of this approach may well be neater and more powerful in capturing the reader's attention through the different perspectives presented, but it may also result in the complexity of the findings being 'dumbed down' and those findings that are not matched by the other data set somehow dropping off the radar screen.

Integrated data sets

It has been suggested by Dixon-Woods (2005) that several approaches might be appropriate in the transformation and integration of data.

INTEGRATIVE SYNTHESIS

This synthesis is used where the major tool is summarising—collating the key concepts under categories. For example, in a study of doctor–patient interaction the key categories might be doctor–patient interactive style, financial constraints, time constraints and so on. These concepts have already been determined through data analysis and do not need further development at this stage. A theoretical interpretation can then be made to reflect the aggregated emphasis now displayed by the data. Integrative synthesis can be undertaken using a variety of summarising approaches:

- [ ] *content analysis* (a summary of the major content of your data sets by categorising and determining frequency—see CHAPTER 22)
- [ ] *thematic analysis* (summarising your findings via the identification of recurrent themes, although it is useful to know if the generation of these themes have been data- or theory-driven—see CHAPTER 22)
- [ ] *case survey* (summarising the overview of a large number of cases by coding data via a set of closed questions for quantitative analysis—see CHAPTER 13)
- [ ] *qualitative comparative analysis* useful for smaller numbers of cases with Q^2 data (via the construction of a table showing logically possible combinations of pairs of independent and corresponding outcome variables.

These pairs are minimised to the most relevant few. This approach can often be useful in indicating what conditions need to be in place to achieve particular outcomes).

INTERPRETIVE SYNTHESIS

This synthesis is grounded in the data collected and seeks to develop explanatory concepts and theories from data groups that have been analysed but minimally conceptualised. This can be done using:

- [ ] *narrative* form (recounting and describing using data juxtaposition and the creation of interpretive fames—see CHAPTER 5)
- [ ] *grounded theory* (using the constant comparison of data sets and creating grids for cross-case comparisons. Here concepts are clustered into categories and axial coding undertaken for the generation of theoretical explanations—see CHAPTER 7)

☐ *meta-ethnography* involving reciprocal, translational analysis (where metaphors, themes and concepts from each data set are translated into the other sets, contradictions are identified, and lines of argument are developed from the separate data sets)

☐ *meta-study* (carefully critiquing how the theories and methods have impacted on the data collected)

☐ *realist approach* (a theory-directed approach to analysis of all findings from all sources)

☐ *matrix synthesis* (clustering the data into categories and codes in matrices for cross-case comparison).

The processes of integrating data in this way are still subject to the major question: 'Should we attempt to integrate data that has been collected qualitatively or quantitatively within very different paradigms and traditions?' This leads to other questions such as 'Should we even attempt to "quantitise" qualitative data or "qualitise" quantitative data?', and 'Which approach should be treated to these processes first?', 'How should we read the results of integrated studies?', 'Are we reading too much into minimalist quantitative data and losing too much of the rich detail of qualitative data in these processes?' The lack of transparent detail of process and outcome in health research means that we have inadequate information on which to judge these processes.

SUMMARY

The advent of the third paradigm, the Q^2 approach, is an exciting one. The development of pragmatic theory as an underpinning is a sensible move as it opens this new paradigm to considerable flexibility with regard to design and analysis of collected data. The advantages of using an integrated Q^2 approach lie in increasing the numbers of approaches that can be applied to a particular question in the hope that more aspects of the problem can be investigated so that the answer may be more complete. The disadvantages lie in the use of inappropriate questions that may be inadequately operationalised; the use of a range of data collection techniques that may look at such different aspects that comparison becomes impossible; minimal data analysis such that homogeneity of results is achieved but the true complexities are overlooked or smoothed down; and inadequately transparent integration of results so that it is not evident how the different data sets were treated, understood or interpreted.

TUTORIAL EXERCISES

1   Construct a research question that you think will be a suitable candidate for a mixed methods approach and divide it into two questions: one that would enable you to collect qualitative data and one that would enable you to collect quantitative data.

2 Take the following research question and identify which qualitative and quantitative data collection techniques would be most appropriate. Justify your choice. Research question: *Are the current waiting times in the emergency outpatient clinic satisfactory to staff and patients?*

3 You have collected some quantitative data and some qualitative data in an integrated methods study where you have been observing primary health care in action. Your data sets comprise:
— observations of 20 family practices and 1000 patient visits to 40 GPs in a city environment
— medical case notes for each patient
— patient questionnaires after each visit
— billing data for each patient
— a practice environment checklist
— ethnographic field notes.

You then undertake descriptive statistics on the survey and billing data, concentrating on percentages. You also undertake thematic analysis of your interviews and field notes, content analysis of the case notes, and thematic and content analysis of visits and the practice environment. List the ways these various sets of data could be brought together for display and explain which approach you think would be the most effective.

4 The concept of *pragmatism* has been briefly outlined in this chapter. Google 'pragmatism' and see what else the original research theorists who introduced this word have to say about it. How do their views differ from those briefly outlined in this chapter?

FURTHER READING

Brewer, J. & Hunter, A. (2006). *Foundations of multimethod research*. Thousand Oaks, CA: Sage Publications.

Creswell, J. (2003). *Research design: Qualitative, quantitative and mixed method approaches*, 2nd edn. Thousand Oaks, CA: Sage Publications.

Creswell, J., Fetters, M. & Ivankova, N. (2004). Designing a mixed methods study in primary care. *Annals of Family Medicine*, 2, 7–12 . This article evaluates five mixed methods studies in primary care and develops three models for designing such investigations.

Creswell, J. & Plano Clark, V. (2007). *Designing and conducting mixed method research*. Thousand Oaks, CA: Sage Publications.

Dixon-Woods, M. (2005). Synthesising qualitative and quantitative evidence: A review of possible methods. *Journal of Health Service Research and Policy*, 10(1), 45–53.

Kelle, U. (2001). Sociological explanations between micro and macro and the integration of qualitative and quantitative methods *Forum: Qualitative Social Research*, 2(1) February. <www.qualitative-research.net/fqs-texte/1-01/1-01kelle-e.htm>, accessed 1 January 2009. Kelle presents three versions of triangulation design: triangulation as mutual validation, triangulation as the integration of different perspectives on the investigated phenomenon and triangulation in its original trigonometrical meaning.

Teddlie, C. & Tashakkori, A. (eds) (2003b). *Handbook of mixed methods in social and behavioral research*. Thousand Oaks, CA: Sage Publications. This book covers issues and controversies, cultural issues, transformational and emancipatory research, research design, sampling and data collection strategies, analysing, writing and reading and their applications across such disciplines as organisational research, psychological research, the health sciences, sociology and nursing.

WEBSITES

http://mra.e-contentmanagement.com

The website of the International Journal of Multiple Research Approaches.

http://mmr.sagepub.com

The website of the Journal of Mixed Methods Research.

www.eldis.org/static/DOC13680.htm

This makes available Marsland, N., Wilson, I.M., Abeyasekera, S. & Kleih, U. (2000). A Methodological Framework for Combining Quantitative and Qualitative Survey Methods, Statistical Services Centre, University of Reading.

http://66.102.7.104/search?q=cache:Mkq-Qla2cuoJ:www.education.up.ac.za/alarpm/PRP_pdf/Pieterse%26Sonnekus.pdf+pieterse+and+sonnekus&hl=en

This makes available Pieterse, V. & Sonnekus, I. (2003). Rising to the challenges of combining qualitative and quantitative research. Paper presented to Sixth World Congress on Action Learning, Action Research and Process Management (ALARPM) in conjunction with the Tenth Congress on Participatory Action Research, ALARPM, pp. 1–12.

www.npi.ucla.edu/qualquant/?

This is the website of Qualitative Tools for Multimethod Research. It was developed by members of the Division of Social Psychiatry at the University of California's Neuropsychiatric Institute. It includes an introduction which addresses the challenges for those who enter into qualitative enquiry. It also features extensive bibliographies.

20

The Use of Mixed Methods in Health Research

Ann Taket

CHAPTER OBJECTIVES

In this chapter you will learn:

☐ what is meant by 'mixed methods'

☐ about the different types of mixed methods

☐ what uses mixed methods have in health research

☐ about the advantages and disadvantages of mixed methods

☐ what are the challenges in using mixed methods

KEY TERMS

Epistemology

Mixed methods

Ontology

Pragmatism

Triangulation

INTRODUCTION

At the outset, it is important to recognise that there is little consistency in the use of the term '**mixed methods**'; the term can be and has been used in a multiplicity of ways. It is not that some of these uses are 'right' and the others 'wrong', but that there are many different ways in which the term can be productively used when discussing the design or implementation of research. Multiple uses of the term only present a difficulty if we do not scrutinise how each author uses the term (see also CHAPTERS 1, 19).

Mixed methods:
A research design that combines research methods from qualitative and/or quantitative research approaches within a single research study.

The use of mixed methods has proliferated in the past 10–20 years, with a growth in journal articles and books, and now even specific journals devoted to mixed methods research. This chapter considers mixed methods in relation to health research, research carried out with the general purpose of understanding how to promote health more effectively and improve the care and cure of those who are ill. A particular focus for this chapter is research in public health and health promotion.

DIFFERENT TYPES OF MIXED METHOD

The term 'mixed methods' can be understood in a number of different ways. First of all, it can simply refer to a number of different types of methods being used within a single study. Often it is used to refer to mixing qualitative and quantitative methods (see CHAPTERS 1, 19), but it can also refer to mixing different types of qualitative method within a study. Second, it may refer to mixing that occurs at different stages in the research process, for example in data collection, in data analysis or indeed in both these stages. Third, different modes or ways of mixing methods within a single study need to be considered. Sometimes a research study is divided into a number of stages, carried out sequentially, so a qualitative stage may be followed by a quantitative stage or vice versa; for example, a qualitative component such as focus groups may be used to help define and pilot a structured survey schedule. Sometimes the mixing is parallel—a qualitative component in a study runs alongside a quantitative one, without interaction, answering different research questions. Or the mixing may be a 'blend'—two or more interacting strands, answering the same research question(s) (see CHAPTER 19). Below, I elaborate on these with some examples.

The range of situations in which mixed methods can be used is extremely wide. Focusing particularly on health research, Table 20.1 presents some of the most common purposes in which a mixed design may be particularly helpful, and also gives some examples of studies. The list of purposes in this table should be seen as illustrative rather than exhaustive.

Table 20.1: Examples of different purposes for use of mixed methods

Purpose	Explanation	Examples
Understanding health and quality of life	Contrasting findings from qualitative and quantitative approaches can help deepen our understanding of important health outcomes and/or how best to measure or assess them.	Cox 2003 Dunning et al. 2008
Understanding health-related behaviour and its relationships with health and health-related outcomes	Contrasting findings from qualitative and quantitative approaches can help tease out the complex interaction of different factors in accounting for health-related behaviour, and help in exploring the role of factors like appropriateness, accessibility and acceptability.	Sinha et al. 2007 Holroyd et al. 2004 See also case study in this chapter
Designing and developing interventions**	Use of qualitative methods alongside quantitative outcome measures can help to understand how an intervention works, enabling researchers to refine intervention design, often within the early stages of intervention. Formative evaluations often use mixed methods.	Strolla et al. 2006 Westhues et al. 2008 Wilson et al. 2007
Evaluating interventions**	Use of qualitative methods alongside quantitative outcome measures can help to understand which parts of the intervention were important in enabling different outcomes to be achieved, or, alternatively, help to understand failure to achieve outcomes. Use of mixed methods can aid in achieving greater understanding. Process evaluations often use mixed methods.	Moffatt et al. 2006 Beaver & Luker 2005 Beilby et al. 2006
Improving research design	Use of qualitative methods provides a way of improving aspects of a quantitative design. This can apply at different stages, e.g. defining specific hypotheses to test; designing a sampling strategy; designing recruitment strategies; designing survey instruments.	Donovan et al. 2002 Quimby 2006

*** To be understood as encompassing a spectrum from simple interventions right through to complex system-wide interventions*

WHY USE MIXED METHODS?

The simplest, and arguably most important, answer to this question is that use of mixed methods can enable researchers to tackle questions that it would be difficult or even impossible to tackle with a single-method design (see CHAPTER 1). So that, for example, while the randomised controlled trial might be the preferred design for testing hypotheses about the outcomes from particular interventions (see CHAPTER 15), understanding the processes behind those outcomes requires the use of qualitative methods (see chapters in PART II). Yet another example is provided by the value of **triangulation** of different methods of data collection and/or different methods of analysis in teasing out answers to complex questions on health-related behaviours (see CHAPTERS 1, 19). O'Cathain and associates (2007) present an interesting analysis of studies funded by a single commissioner in England between 1994 and 2004. They found that 18 per cent (119 out of 647) of the studies commissioned were mixed methods, and that the main stated reason for using mixed methods research was to answer a wider range of questions than quantitative methods alone would permit.

Triangulation: The use of multiple methods, researchers, data sources, or theories in a research project.

But the necessity of a mixed approach is not the only reason for choosing mixed methods. Another potential reason for their use is promoting choice and empowerment for research participants: offering the choice of how to provide their data (e.g. self-completion schedule versus one-to-one interview versus group interview) can be personally empowering for participants, acting to reinforce their autonomy in choosing how and whether to participate. Providing this kind of choice may assist in reaching different subgroups within the population of interest, thereby enabling research participation, whereas, for example, offering only a self-completion questionnaire at once excludes those with low reading and writing ability.

A CASE STUDY—EXPLORING REASONS WHY WOMEN DO NOT USE BREAST SCREENING

In this section, I consider a single example of a mixed methods study, drawn from recent research. This is a very simple example of a mixed methods study, where data collection and analysis contained both qualitative and quantitative components; it can be regarded as a blended study in the terms discussed above. In this study, the use of mixed methods turned out to be crucial in understanding women's behaviour in using or not using breast screening. Here the focus is on just some of the results of the study, illustrating the usefulness of mixed methods in this case.

Background to the study

The study was commissioned in 2004 by the Department of Public Health in southeast London, UK. This was against a background of concern about low local uptake of breast screening for the target group of women aged 50 to 64. Average uptake was just over 60 per cent for the area as a whole and as low as 54 per cent in some parts; this fell below government targets at the time of a minimum acceptable level of uptake of 70 per cent. The area is characterised by high levels of deprivation, although containing pockets of relative affluence within its urban inner-city setting. It is a culturally and ethnically diverse area: in some parts of the area, half or more of the local population is black or minority ethnic and there are around 130 languages spoken across the area (Barter-Godfrey & Taket 2007).

Study recruitment

A sample of 306 women aged 50–64 were recruited opportunistically from a variety of community sources, including voluntary groups, community sector organisations and faith groups, between July and December 2004. Women were offered the choice of how they would like to give their views: group interview, individual interview (face to face or telephone), or self-completed questionnaire (see CHAPTER 13). The majority (85%) chose to complete the questionnaire themselves and return it by post. Of the 15 per cent who chose to have the questionnaire administered, the majority chose to do this over the telephone; their answers were noted by the researcher taking the call.

Information about the study was presented in English and other relevant languages (Bengali, Arabic, Somali, Turkish, Vietnamese, Albanian, Cantonese, French, Spanish, Portuguese), and questionnaires were produced in English and French (no demand for other languages was expressed). The use of a variety of recruitment mechanisms ensured that the sample contained women from all the major ethnic communities in the area, and diversity in the sample in terms of other socio-demographic characteristics. Women were offered £20 in vouchers for their participation in the study. Ethics clearance for the study was gained from London South Bank University Research Ethics Committee. Participation in the study was entirely voluntary and respondents were assured of confidentiality. No ethical issues arose during the study.

Designing the study

Funds available for the research, as well as the requested timetable for completion, constrained our choice of study design. In particular, this ruled out a totally qualitative design (see chapters in PART II), and also a sequential mixed methods design with a qualitative stage preceding a larger quantitative survey (see CHAPTER 19). The decision was therefore made to use a single schedule, one that was largely structured, for both interviews and self-completion. Themes of interest were initially established by considering the research problem of low uptake of breast screening, using themes already identified in research literature and from an advisory group of relevant professionals. Specific structured questions were selected for each theme, and these are discussed further below.

The schedule explored the health issues that are important for women, their knowledge and beliefs in relation to breast cancer and their use or non-use of breast cancer screening.

Ann Taket

Information about socio-demographic characteristics and aspects of daily life (living situation, work, caring responsibilities) was also collected. Asking about daily life was intended to provide some insight into the daily burden our sample had, in terms of themes of responsibilities and isolation. Most of the questions were structured with a set of responses to choose from, one of which was always 'other', with space to specify further. There were three open questions, placed carefully within the schedule, which provided the main qualitative strand within the study; these are discussed below.

The schedule underwent several stages of piloting before finalisation. Using a small availability sample of women in the right age group, living or working in south London, we tested the acceptability of question topics. Items that were acceptable to the group included asking direct questions about attending and rejecting breast screening. There was a preference for providing alternative answers to choose from rather than being expected to articulate their own reasons for behaviour choice, especially when behaviour did not conform to health promotion messages. Time and resource constraints led us to be highly selective about the questions included in order to keep the instrument to no more than four sides of A4 in its self-completion form. We considered that this restriction in length would also maximise the likelihood of women completing the questionnaire, and improve rates of response. See also CHAPTER 13.

THE QUALITATIVE STRAND

The qualitative strand of the study focused around the comments supplied by respondents against selection of the category 'other' in the closed questions, and answers to three open questions. The first of these was on the first page of the schedule, before any mention of breast cancer or breast cancer screening (these questions appeared on the second page, not visible initially). This first open question asked women 'What are your main health concerns?' Note also that the study was presented under the title 'Women and Health'. This was in order to appeal to the broadest possible section of the target population. We were concerned about the possibility that non-attenders who distance themselves from breast screening and those who do not identify with breast cancer would deselect themselves from the sample if the research was presented as a breast cancer or breast screening study. This was borne out by the lack of reference to breast cancer in the open 'health concerns' section and the small proportion of the sample who held strong beliefs opposing mammography and rejecting breast screening.

The second qualitative section was designed to elicit further information about our respondents' health concerns, this time more indirectly, through two open questions that formed the two closing sections of the schedule. Under the heading of improving local health services we asked: 'What are your suggestions for improving health care service provision, for you and women like you?' Then, finally, under the heading of 'Any other comments', we asked: 'Is there anything else you would like to say about looking after your health or health care provision for women over 50?'

THE QUANTITATIVE STRAND

The quantitative strand of the study focused around the answers to structured questions. These explored a number of different areas. First of these were women's daily life; their health and health-related behaviour; concerns about specific health issues (diabetes, breast cancer, heart disease, osteoporosis), exploring in particular notions of candidacy. 'Candidacy' refers to an individual's personal conception of their being 'a candidate for' developing a particular disease, and explains the causes and prevention of disease in terms of an individual's beliefs about who is affected by it and who is not (Davison et al. 1991, 1992). The second major section related to breast cancer screening, where questions explored past behaviour in some detail (including reasons for attendance and non-attendance), convenience of appointments and finally, future intentions. A third major section explored sources of health advice/information and health service provision, attitudes to looking after their own health, views about health service communications (relevance and clarity), and included asking about attitudes to breast cancer screening in terms of three different dimensions (whether screening was important, reasonable, reassuring).

Analysis and interpretation of data

An SPSS database (version 11) was created for use in analysing the data (see CHAPTER 24). Reponses to the open-ended questions were coded thematically on the basis of the researchers reading through about a third of the sample and noting emerging themes (see CHAPTER 22). Themed responses were included as separate variables in the database with dichotomous coding: theme raised or theme not raised. Some 'flags' were also included in the database, to record issues that were not overtly included in the schedule, such as mental health, literacy and the menopause. The flag system was also used to identify which participants had included narratives supplementary to the direct questions about breast cancer and breast screening, for later use in qualitative analysis.

All the questionnaires and interviews were coded prior to data entry, using the coding schedule. Any items in the dataset that were not obviously allocated to one particular code were discussed between the researchers and coded by consensus about what would best represent the participant's responses. Quantitative data was subject to a range of descriptive and simple inferential statistical analysis and a limited amount of multivariate analysis (see CHAPTER 24). Moving between analysis of qualitative data and quantitative data helped illuminate our understanding of women's behaviours in relation to breast cancer screening.

BREAST CANCER AND BREAST SCREENING—NOT A MAJOR HEALTH CONCERN FOR OUR SAMPLE

One very important finding from the study came in response to our first open question: 'What are your main health concerns?' At this stage, only 4 per cent of our sample mentioned anything that we could link to breast cancer or breast screening as one of their main health concerns. In other words, for our sample, other concerns were more important. This question was deliberately placed before any specific breast screening questions were introduced into the schedule, since we wanted to get some idea of women's specific concerns before introducing the topic of breast cancer or breast screening. Instead, women talked about a chronic medical or physical condition (60% of the sample); an acute medical or physical condition (27%); psychological issues (19%); pain, including pain management (17%); ageing/deterioration (11%); weight loss or maintenance (10%); maintaining good health (9%); menopause (9%); provision of services (6%); concerns not about self (2%). Other issues (not groupable!) were mentioned by 11 per cent of the sample. Twenty-three of our samples (7.5%) did not report any health concerns.

Comments and concerns about breast screening and to a lesser extent breast cancer were made in the undirected open sections at the end of the schedule by 26 per cent of the sample. However, these are mostly comments that supplement the options provided in the screening uptake section of the questionnaire and appear to be prompted by the presence of questions about breast screening, hence the increase from 4 per cent of women raising the issue at the start of the questionnaire and 26 per cent raising the issue at the end. This strongly suggests that breast cancer and breast screening are not high priorities for concern for the women in the sample. Women in our sample did not spend time worrying about breast cancer. They had plenty of other matters of greater concern. We doubt whether we would have identified this without the blended design, where the first open question invited women to speak about whatever were 'their main health concerns' rather than being led by mention of particular topics. As a contrast, an international study (NOP World 2005), carried out at roughly the same time, gives a very different impression. This study, a quantitative one, asked: 'Thinking now about breast cancer, how concerned, if at all, would you say you are about getting it?' In the UK sample, the percentage answering 'very' or 'quite' concerned was 71 per cent for women aged 45–54, and 69 per cent for women aged 55 to 64. This different form of questioning gives quite a different impression of women's concerns; arguably the higher response is led by the question, which invites an expression of concern.

Our finding about the low level of concern with breast cancer at once begins to make the low levels of screening uptake in the population more understandable.

UNDERSTANDING BREAST SCREENING BEHAVIOUR—RATIONAL AND PERSONALLY JUSTIFIABLE

Moving backwards and forwards between the data in the qualitative and quantitative strands of the study enabled us to conclude that the decision to attend or decline screening is rational and personally justifiable, engaging factors linked to emotions and attitude. A few examples are presented here in terms of three patterns of screening behaviour identified in the sample: those who adhere to, reject and are ambivalent towards the screening program.

The adherence group is made up of those who always attend screening, the largest group in our sample, 78 per cent. Our sample was not representative of the population at large in terms of screening behaviour, and this is perhaps not at all surprising; other research in inner cities suggests that literacy, participation and concerns about health are important issues, so people who are non-participative, have difficulties with English language notices or are unconcerned about health issues are less likely to screen (Lai Fong Chiu 2002; Pfeffer 2004) and similarly are less likely to join a health research study such as this. The rejection group is those who have never been to breast screening and have no intention of attending in the future (6%). The third group, which we labelled the 'ambivalent', were those who sometimes attend, sometimes decline (16%). Notice that our study design, achieving a total sample of 306, contained sufficient women in the rejection and ambivalent groups to permit meaningful analysis in those groups. A smaller, purely qualitative study would have been unlikely to achieve this, given that no access to an accurate sampling frame that identified women by their screening behaviour was possible.

Looking into the three groups in turn, first the adherers, some women will always go to screening, they adhere fully to the screening program, and simply receiving the invitation is enough to encourage them to attend:

'I had the appointment so I went. It was just a thing you do like having your eyes tested.'

The second group, the rejecters, simply reject the breast screening program outright; have never been to screening and have no intention of ever going:

'I have never attended screening and would rather not know as nature knows best. In my opinion it is best to leave things alone regardless what the experts say.'

'I do not like the idea of six lots of four x-rays on my breasts by the time I am 65 years old.'

'Breast screening is likely to lead to minor problems being treated with major surgery.'

To a certain extent, some of the issues the women raise can be approached as misconceptions, for example concerns about the radiation, which can be changed through health promotion over time. But for raising uptake at the point of the next invitation, this would be the group least amenable to change.

The third group was those whose behaviour was changeable: sometimes attending, sometimes not. Inconvenience was the most commonly reported reason for not attending an appointment (31% of those who have declined breast screening at least once). Other options, such as 'something came up' (8%), and 'I was unwell that day' (10%) also indicate that the appointment was untimely rather than unwelcome. Inconvenience as a reason to miss breast screening appointments was a prolonged state, rather than a reflection of the specific day or time of day that is offered for the appointment. This can be seen as a reflection of the pressures and demands within the woman's life at the time of the invitation. Less than half of those who missed inconvenient appointments rescheduled them. In the context of other demands competing for the time and resources of these women, perceived inconvenience can de-prioritise attending screening to the point of missing appointments.

Ann Taket

Experiencing or expecting pain is associated with the decision to decline screening and 16 per cent of women who decline screening reported doing so to avoid pain:

'I now do not want to go because the last screening I had was so painful.'

Twenty-one per cent of women who declined screening reported doing so to avoid anxiety:

'I find it quite traumatic going to screening and have to work myself up to it.'

and 14 per cent do so to avoid embarrassment, with 10 per cent feeling uncomfortable getting undressed:

'I feel unable to go as I hate my weight. Silly excuse…but it affects me badly.'

Put this with the role of anticipated regret and worry, and we found that many of the women in our sample are emotionally involved with mammography, and attend screening or avoid it in ways that look after their emotional well-being, aside from their potential physical health.

Positive attitude and perceived personal importance of breast screening were the most important variables in our study. These were the variables that were predictive of consistent attendance compared to inconsistent attendance, *and* consistent declining compared to attendance. At point of invitation, some women are switched off by their own beliefs about screening, whereas others almost automatically attend. For some women, attitude is shaped by previous negative experiences, to the point where they no longer feel that it is reasonable for them to attend. These women may be motivated to return, they have attended before and may be persuaded that the pain or anxiety is worth it, especially to avoid anticipated regret. One implication is that we may need to focus on changing their attitude towards the value of screening. For others, their attitude towards screening is generally positive but is not strong enough to convert it into behaviour, either because there are too many other demands competing for priority or because they never quite get around to it, and so far they have not knowingly suffered for that decision. These women may be persuaded by encouraging them to see attendance as important, given their overall positive attitude.

Thus once we examine the details of women's reasoning around the time they receive the invitation to screening, we find their behaviour perfectly reasonable in response to their particular circumstances at the time. The concept of the decisional balance, an individual's weighing up of the pros and cons of competing behaviour choices, drawn from the transtheoretic model (Velicer et al. 1998), proved useful in understanding women's screening behaviour.

CHALLENGES AND TERRORS OF MIXING METHODS

The case study above illustrates the value of mixed methods within a relatively small and contained study. The qualitative data aided our interpretation of the quantitative findings and vice versa, producing a richer understanding of the complexity of factors underlying low uptake rates for breast screening in the population studied, and providing a number of different insights into the action that could be taken to improve these (see also CHAPTER 1).

In this final section, the challenges of using mixed methods are explored. In some cases the literature presents these issues in such stark and terrifying terms as to imply that they are to be avoided at all costs (together with the use of mixed methods) rather than merely as challenges to be addressed!

The first concern that is sometimes raised is the danger of epistemological confusion. Different methods rest on quite different assumptions about how the world is (**ontology**) and how we can come to gain knowledge of that world (**epistemology**) (see CHAPTERS 1, 19). Some argue that there is a danger in using methods that rely on different epistemologies in a single study. See for example the work of Sale and associates (2002), who would see this as forbidden in certain circumstances. Here a different position is offered, namely that this does not matter, provided that the differences are acknowledged and brought into play when results are discussed and interpretations made. We can label this a position characterised by theoretical pluralism, underpinned by **pragmatism** (in the sense explained so fluently by the American philosopher Richard Rorty; see for example Rorty 1989; see also CHAPTERS 1, 19). Some would argue that this position amounts to wanting to have our cake and eat it too, but on the other hand, is that not a desirable position? The notion that we have to choose a single theoretical position and not deviate from it conveys a kind of rigidity that is no longer expected even within the hard sciences—consider for example the wave/particle duality accepted in terms of theories of light, Heisinberg's uncertainty principle, chaos and complexity theory, to name but a few. For more detailed exposition of this stance see the excellent editorial by Johnson (2008), who labels this a dialectic approach.

Ontology: the study of the nature of being, existence or reality in general.

Epistemology is concerned with the nature of knowledge and how knowledge is obtained.

Pragmatism argues that reality does not exist only as natural and physical realities, but also as psychological and social realities, which include subjective experience and thought, language, and culture.

Mixed methods research is also often regarded as multiplying the work involved, with consequent implications for resources, not only in terms of finance but also in terms of having researchers with the necessary range of skills, particularly since the tendency in the past has been for individuals to focus on either qualitative or quantitative methods in their research careers. Of course, this can be overcome by the use of teams, and so perhaps it is merely that mixed methods research makes studies carried out by a lone researcher rarer (although still does not remove them entirely). Mixed methods research is not necessarily extremely expensive, as the case study above shows. There is, however, a need to consider how a broader range of research methods training could be encouraged for individuals, and this is a matter that is beginning to receive attention.

One final question is whether it is harder to get mixed methods research published. This connects to the related challenge of publishing qualitative research. Journals still tend to specialise in either qualitative or quantitative research. Mixed methods studies, owing to their

Ann Taket

relative rareness, are arguably harder to get through referees, as there may be a shortage of referees with the relevant experience. The growth of specialist journals for mixed methods research, such as the *Journal of Mixed Methods Research* (first published in 2007), and the *International Journal of Multiple Research Approaches* (first published in 2006), provides a partial answer—but does not satisfy those of us who would rather see our research published in health journals to reach our intended audiences. There is also the question of word length. On purely practical grounds, it is far harder to summarise a complex mixed methods design within the same word length that a simpler non-mixed design would take. To satisfy the demands of peer reviewers, the description of method may take so many words as to prohibit the discussion of the results to any great extent!

IN CONCLUSION OR INCONCLUSION?

I make no apology for the pun in the title above. It is difficult to offer hard-and-fast conclusions about the use of mixed methods in health research. There are too many unknowns, which the preceding section has alluded to.

My position is that, increasingly, those of us in the fields of health research, and especially public health and health promotion, will need to become passionate practitioners of mixed methods research in order to answer the complex questions that need to be addressed if we are to successfully design and implement programs to address health inequities in the diverse communities that we serve. However, I see difficulties in always achieving the funding necessary for the extent of such research required. Competitive research funding still disadvantages qualitative and mixed methods designs, perhaps not as much as 20 or even 10 years ago, but still clearly evident. Within universities, where the drivers are for winning the highest category of research funding and publishing in the most highly regarded journals (not usually read by practitioners) this may militate against mixed methods research. On the other hand, I see a positive development in the growth of practitioner-based and community-based research, with the concomitant advantages of ownership and relevance. So perhaps the most fertile base for growth in mixed methods research is within communities of practice.

SUMMARY

The chapter begins by introducing a number of different ways the term 'mixed methods' can be understood. First, it can refer to a number of different types of methods being used within a single study; often it is used to refer to mixing qualitative and quantitative methods. But it can also refer to mixing different types of qualitative method within a study. Second, it may refer to mixing that occurs at different stages in the research process, for example in data collection, in data analysis or indeed in both these stages. Third, we need to consider different modes or ways of mixing methods within a single study: sequential, parallel or blended.

The chapter illustrates the range of situations in which different types of mixed method may be appropriate and discusses their advantages and disadvantages. It considers the different potential reasons for mixing different types of qualitative method. The chapter also discusses some of the issues involved in using mixed methods in health research, illustrated by means of a case study of research carried out by the author. It ends with a discussion of some of the challenges (or fears) expressed about mixed methods.

TUTORIAL EXERCISES

1 Read the following article: Laws, R.A., Kirby, S.E., Davies, G.P.P., Williams, A.M., Jayasinghe, U.W., Amoroso, C.L. & Harris, M.F. (2008). 'Should I and Can I': A Mixed Methods Study of Clinician Beliefs and Attitudes in the Management of Lifestyle Risk Factors in Primary Health Care. *BMC Health Services Research*, 8.
   In your group discuss the following questions:
   — What type(s) of mixed methods are being used?
   — What advantages did the use of mixed methods give?
   — What disadvantages did its use give?

2 Read the following article: Stewart, M., Makwarimba, E., Barnfather, A., Letourneau, N. & Neufeld, A. (2008). Researching Reducing Health Disparities: Mixed methods Approaches. *Social Science & Medicine*, 66(6), 1406–17
   In your group discuss the following questions:
   — What type(s) of mixed methods are being used?
   — What advantages did the use of mixed methods give?
   — What disadvantages did its use give?

3 Compare and contrast the use of mixed methods in the two articles above.

4 You are approached by a community group to help them produce a report about community views on local health services. The community group serves a population diverse in ethnicity, religion, educational achievement and income. Outline how you might use mixed methods to do this, and what the advantages and disadvantages of your proposed design might be.

FURTHER READING

Creswell, J.W. & Plano Clark, V.L. (2006). *Designing and conducting mixed methods research*. Thousand Oaks, CA: Sage Publications.

Greene, J.C. (2007). *Mixed methods in social inquiry*. San Francisco: Jossey-Bass.

Ann Taket

Hall, B. & Howard, K. (2008). A synergistic approach: Conducting mixed methods research with typological and systemic design considerations. *Journal of Mixed Methods Research*, 2(3), 248–69.

Johnson, B. (2008). Editorial: Living with tensions: The dialectic approach. *Journal of Mixed Methods Research* 2(3), 203–07.

Mendlinger, S. & Cwikel, J. (2008). Spiraling between qualitative and quantitative data on women's health behaviors: A double helix model for mixed methods. *Qualitative Health Research* 18(2), 280–93.

Teddlie, C. & Tashakkori, A. (2009). *Foundations of mixed methods research: Integrating quantitative and qualitative approaches in the social and behavioral sciences*. Thousand Oaks, CA: Sage Publications.

WEBSITES

www.fiu.edu/~bridges

    Bridges: Mixed Methods Network for Behavioral, Social, and Health Sciences.

http://mra.e-contentmanagement.com

    International Journal of Multiple Research Approaches.

http://mmr.sagepub.com

    Journal of Mixed Methods Research.

http://qhr.sagepub.com

    Qualitative Health Research.

www.socialresearchmethods.net/tutorial/Sydenstricker/bolsa.html

    Research Design and Mixed Method Approach.

21

Collaborative Participatory Research with Disadvantaged Communities

Priscilla Pyett, Peter Waples-Crowe and Anke van der Sterren

CHAPTER OBJECTIVES

In this chapter you will learn:

- [ ] to understand the key features of collaborative participatory approaches for research with disadvantaged communities

- [ ] when and why to use collaborative and participatory approaches

- [ ] details of the method in practice

- [ ] how to use collaborative participatory research in an Indigenous health context

KEY TERMS

Collaborative participatory research

Community

Indigenous people

Participatory action research

Project agreement or memorandum of understanding

Steering committee or advisory group

PARTICIPATORY APPROACHES TO RESEARCH

In this chapter, we will discuss the use of a collaborative participatory approach for research, particularly with disadvantaged communities. You might have come across terms such as 'collaborative', 'participatory' or 'community-based' research, as well as 'participatory action research' or 'action research'. Each of these approaches promotes the active involvement in research by people who have been conventionally the focus of the research. Such research approaches do not seek to discover widely generalisable findings, but rather to generate understandings specific to particular contexts, and to produce actions and outcomes that are relevant and of benefit to local communities.

The term 'action research' was first coined by Kurt Lewin (1946/1988) in the late 1940s in the USA, and this approach has been widely used in organisational development, workplace relations and education. Participatory research was developed a little later in what were then known as 'Third World' settings by people such as Paulo Freire (1972) in South America. In recent decades, participatory action research and collaborative approaches to research are increasingly used by practitioners in health and welfare, who recognise the importance of consumer or patient involvement in the production of knowledge, for example in developing patient care plans, conducting a community needs analysis or assisting people living with chronic illness (de Koning & Martin 1996; Koch et al. 2002; Stringer & Genat 2004).

Participatory action research: A method where informants become co-researchers and the researcher becomes a participant, using their research expertise to assist the informants in self-research.

Participatory action research (PAR) involves a repetitive cycle of observing, reflecting, planning and acting (see Figure 21.1).

Figure 21.1: The Action Research Cycle

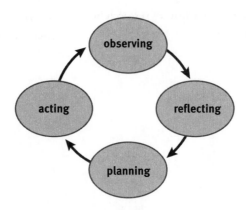

This process is sometimes depicted as a spiral or helix to show that the process occurs repeatedly over time. A PAR project must involve not only research or enquiry and the participation of community members, but also action to improve their situation. Furthermore, the research and action generated from it is ongoing, with continuous evaluation and modification of the action. Many resources are available that describe PAR in greater detail, as well as its application in various contexts (Carr & Kemmis 1986; Hart & Bond 1995; Bray et al. 2000; Stringer & Genat 2004).

DOING RESEARCH

Examples of PAR

Women living with multiple sclerosis (MS) in South Australia:

This project sought to understand the experiences of living with chronic illness. The researcher initially established and participated in a discussion group comprising eight women living with MS and four nursing consultants. This group met for 10 sessions over 6 months. The format of the sessions enabled the sharing of expertise and experiences; in the initial sessions nurses provided information about incontinence, while subsequent sessions opened up opportunities for the women to share their experiences of incontinence or any other matters they wished to raise. Analysis of the themes arising from the group sessions was ongoing, and feedback of each session was given to participants at the beginning of each of the sessions that followed. The women were then involved, both individually and collectively, in developing, planning and implementing actions to address each of the issues raised in the group. Subsequent additional discussion groups were established; and the authors note that the use of a PAR methodology allowed for the development of distinctive group dynamics and outcomes (Koch & Kralik 2001; Koch et al. 2002).

Prevention of schistosomiasis among schoolchildren in Tanzania:

This project sought to investigate sustainable ways to prevent schistosomiasis (a tropical skin disease) by targeting schoolchildren, among whom infection is high. As a result of an initial screening and treatment program, several school and community-based activities were developed. Teachers, children, parents and the broader community became involved in the development and evaluation of health promotion activities. Schoolchildren were trained to conduct household sanitation surveys and were involved in redesigning and readministering modified household surveys. Reflection by participants on the findings of the screenings and household surveys, and evaluations of health promotion activities, led to further activity, including the development of a curriculum for schistosomiasis education in schools (Freudenthal et al. 2006).

Health workers in an urban Aboriginal Medical Service:

Bill Genat and colleagues undertook a participatory action research project with Aboriginal health workers (AHWs) and some non-Indigenous health workers in an urban Aboriginal Medical Service (AMS). At the heart of the research process were two focus groups with these health workers. One group decided they wanted to get better at their work and focus on 'best practice'. They reviewed practices such as home visits, ways to encourage clients to maintain medication schedules and so on. Working collaboratively in the groups, the health workers developed protocols for these practices, implemented the protocols in the field, then reviewed and refined the protocols further in subsequent focus group meetings. The other group decided to focus on increasing the status of AHWs through organisational policy within the AMS. Working collectively, they developed policy recommendations and pursued them with management. The health workers were acknowledged as co-authors of the book that describes this project. These processes constituted the typical action-reflection cycles within an action research project and they were participatory (Genat 2006).

COLLABORATIVE PARTICIPATORY RESEARCH

The practicalities involved in conducting research in most developed countries means that ongoing action and evaluation are rarely incorporated into the research process. The reality is that funding for community-based research projects generally comes from governments or other organisations whose accountability structures result in inflexible timelines. This inflexibility does not allow the luxury of true action research projects where ongoing reflection enables the repetition of the research activity towards a solution.

Collaborative participatory research involves a transfer of knowledge between researchers, community leaders and community members, including knowledge of how to undertake research with community organisations.

We have found that our own research practice can be better described through the use of the term **collaborative participatory research** (CPR), a term that highlights the importance of collaboration and participation. This model recognises that the researcher has certain technical expertise, and that community leaders and community members have knowledge of their community needs and perspectives. Importantly, this approach involves a transfer of knowledge, including knowledge of how to undertake research with community organisations (Nyden & Wiewel 1992). Actions or outcomes that are useful and relevant to the participants, and an ongoing reflection process to continually improve these outcomes, are still desirable but may not be achievable.

Key features of CPR

- ☐ Research is conducted *for* and *with* communities not *on* or *about* communities.
- ☐ Research takes time to build relationships of mutual trust.
- ☐ Researchers are accountable to the community.
- ☐ Benefits of the research are decided by the community.
- ☐ Community members are involved in planning and carrying out the research, in analysing, reporting and acting on the findings.
- ☐ The knowledge and experience of community members are valued.
- ☐ Researchers respect community members' interests, values and perspectives.
- ☐ Research is a two-way partnership of knowledge and skills exchange.
- ☐ Researchers build community capacity by sharing knowledge of how to do research.
- ☐ The research process is empowering.
- ☐ The research is solution-focused.
- ☐ Researchers are committed to social change through practical or policy outcomes.

Twin goals of empowerment and change

Rather than being a method of health and social research, CPR is more an approach to research that has explicit political goals. The first is to empower people through their involvement in the research process and the production of knowledge about their situation and to enable them to identify those aspects of their situation that they would like to see improve. Involvement in the research process may occur at a number of levels: setting the research agenda, guiding and monitoring the research process, or being part of the research team in designing the project, collecting and analysing data, and writing up the findings. In CPR, the location of power in all stages of the research process ideally lies with the research participants. They become agents, stakeholders and co-researchers, and the role of the researcher ranges from director to facilitator or catalyst for action (Stringer 1999; Stringer & Genat 2004). Because of its potential for empowerment and capacity-building, the process of a CPR project is as important as the outcome. Indeed, capacity-building is one of the intended outcomes of CPR.

The second goal of CPR is to carry out research that will bring about changes and improvements in the lives of the participants. As such, it is an approach that seeks to address structural inequality and social injustice. CPR has been used in research with oppressed, marginalised or disadvantaged communities in many contexts, such as people living in poverty in developing countries, refugees, illicit drug users, sex workers and people living with HIV/ AIDS (Warr & Pyett 1999; Maher et al. 2002; Coupland et al. 2004; Liamputtong 2007, 2009, 2010; see also CHAPTER 1). CPR aims to produce tangible outcomes for the communities involved. These may be changes in knowledge, attitudes or behaviour, changes to policy or practice, or improvements to service delivery or in the material circumstances of people's lives.

Priscilla Pyett, Peter Waples-Crowe and Anke van der Sterren

DOING RESEARCH

Examples of CPR in developed and developing countries

In Chicago

A collaborative partnership was established in a disadvantaged area in Chicago between a university-based researcher and a community-based HIV/AIDS organisation. Motivated by social justice and the need for cost efficiency in the delivery of health and social services, the partners shared a commitment to social change. The aim of the collaboration was to influence local policy—to increase understanding of and reduce discrimination against people with or at risk of HIV/AIDS and to increase people's access to a range of local services. The partners established a community-based advisory board, used multiple methods of data collection and provided feedback at a specially convened conference of community leaders. The partners learnt that policy can be informed and influenced by a collaborative and participatory approach to information-gathering and by researchers communicating their findings and practical information to community leaders (Figert & Kuehnert 1992).

In Tanzania

Researchers in Mwanza, Tanzania used CPR to develop appropriate methods, monitoring and feedback processes for conducting a large-scale randomised control clinical trial. They held community workshops with study participants (women working in food and recreational facilities), and managers and project workers in community-based clinics that offered reproductive health services. These workshops enabled the researchers to build a shared understanding with participants of appropriate community structures and approaches for the research trial. They established a Community Advisory Committee based on the guidance given through the workshops. The committee worked closely with the researchers to determine appropriate clinical procedures, mobilisation activities and referral mechanisms for sexually transmitted infection contact tracing and HIV/AIDS-related care. It also served as a mechanism through which the project could be monitored and adverse effects reported and dealt with. CPR also enabled the research team to implement location-specific targeted interventions related to the trial (Vallely et al. 2007; Shagi et al. 2008).

Why use CPR with disadvantaged communities?

With the increasing realisation that health problems are related to social inequalities, health researchers need to engage with disadvantaged and marginalised groups (Liamputtong 2007).

If we are to understand more about the circumstances of people's lives and the pathways to better health and well-being, we need to conduct our research in such a way that it can give people a voice. However, access to marginalised groups is often extremely difficult, particularly when compared to some of the more common subjects of health research, such as the relatively 'captive' populations that can be recruited from schools, hospitals, clinical settings and general households. In addition, the researcher may meet with resistance, since people who are disadvantaged and marginalised often have good reason to mistrust people who represent authority, such as researchers. There is also a high likelihood that the researcher will encounter problems with language, literacy, cultural difference or comprehension (Liamputtong 2009). Finally, relocating members of marginalised communities for follow-up research is also more difficult.

Since the Ottawa Charter (WHO 1986), strategies for health research that emphasise participation have been gaining attention and respectability in both industrialised and less industrialised and resource-poor countries. Such participation, particularly with its combination of insider and outsider knowledge, has the potential to increase the validity, relevance and cost-effectiveness of the research, and to improve longer-term outcomes (de Koning & Martin 1996; Stringer & Genat 2004). The validity and legitimacy of a CPR approach are grounded in the honesty and reflexivity of the research process in declaring agendas, carrying out the research and implementing its goals, and in the honesty, clarity and detailed reporting of the process and context of the research (Hagey 1997; Waterman 1998). CPR is thus becoming increasingly important in the health field (de Koning & Martin 1996; Stringer & Genat 2004; Israel et al. 2005; Minkler & Wallestein 2008).

Ideally, a community group working with a researcher identifies a problem or situation that they want to change, and participates collaboratively in the planning and process of research, the interpretation of results and the development and application of any intervention for change. However, community groups rarely have sufficient resources to carry out research on their own, while budget cutbacks in university, health service and community settings in Australia, as in other industrialised societies, increase the need for more cooperation as a way of using limited resources more effectively. The different perspectives of researchers, health professionals and community representatives on the same health problem or social issue can lead to more productive and rigorous research, more relevant and creative problem-solving, more culturally appropriate interventions and more effective social change.

Collaborative participatory approaches to research are generally used with smaller communities, particular those experiencing disadvantage. '**Community**' can refer to a geographic community or a community of 'interest' or 'identity'. A geographic community might be as large as the population of Australia or as small as a neighbourhood or a suburban street. A community of interest or

Community can refer to a geographic community or a community of 'interest' or 'identity'.

identity may be a group with a shared history or cultural affinity such as age, gender, religion, ethnicity or sexual orientation; or it may be a group that shares an experience of disadvantage such as poverty or homelessness, or a group who are stigmatised by their behaviour, such as sex workers, injecting drug users or people with mental health problems. Any of these communities or population groups may have shared experiences of disadvantage, but we also need to be aware that there may be a diversity of interests, values and aspirations within groups.

People living in geographic communities are relatively easy to locate, access and describe, but groups of people or communities that are linked by shared identity, history or interests are often described as 'hard to reach' for the purposes of research or health promotion. They are also hard to define, or put a boundary around, so it is difficult to draw a representative sample for a research project. Developing collaborative relationships with community representatives of such hard-to-reach populations is crucial to planning research that will include a broader representation of the relevant population (Liamputtong 2007).

Research with marginalised and disadvantaged populations requires a high degree of reflective practice, one that is responsive to the social context of the research (Pyett & VicHealth Koori Health Research and Community Development Unit 2002; Liamputtong 2007). We have to ensure that not only do our actual research processes not cause harm to the groups we are researching, but also that the research is not used to further marginalise these already vulnerable people (Liamputtong 2007; Pyett et al. 2008). CPR involves the community in determining what they see as the benefits from the research.

CPR IN PRACTICE

The key to CPR is the respectful engagement of participating communities throughout all stages of the research process: research design, data collection, data analysis, communication and dissemination, and action and evaluation. Here we discuss how the community can be engaged at each of these stages and some of the issues involved in such engagement.

Research design

A long lead-up time that pays attention to relationship-building and appropriate planning of the research is essential to the success of any CPR project (see 'Doing research' below). The participating community should be involved in developing aims, objectives, appropriate methods for data collection and analysis, and deciding on processes for monitoring the project and for feedback and dissemination of findings. Such participation can be built through appropriate community engagement and consultation, through the development of a memorandum of understanding or project agreement, and through the establishment of an advisory group.

DOING RESEARCH

The importance of a long time-frame

Successful collaborations are often preceded by lengthy periods of consultation and time for the partners to get to know one another. For example, in the Victorian Blood Borne Virus and Injecting Dug Use (BBV/IDU) Training Project box on page 361, the partners knew each other from previous working relationships over several years and this particular project took 12 months' planning and development (Waples-Crowe & Pyett 2005). Similarly, Wand and Eades (2008) report that consultation with health workers began over a year before a student research project in Aboriginal mental health began. Finally, in the human papillomavirus (HPV) project described in the same box (see pages 360–1), one of the key partners had good long-term connections with the local Aboriginal community and an Aboriginal Women's Advisory Committee.

However, you should be aware that some researchers can find it quite challenging to spend the time required to develop relationships, trust and strategies that will facilitate collaboration (see Mayo et al. 2009).

Community engagement and consultation

Ideally, in CPR, the research is community-initiated. But in practice, it is more often the case that a researcher approaches a community with an idea for a research project or the offer of partnering with the community to conduct research that will be of benefit to them. What is most important about the early stages of engaging with a community is that the researcher communicates openly, listens respectfully and responds clearly. The researcher may have previous experience of working with the community or with other community groups, or they may be initiating their first community partnership. It is the researcher's responsibility to be as well informed as is reasonably possible about the community, its organisational structures and relationships, its history and culture, its strength and resilience, as well as its needs and circumstances of disadvantage.

We have written elsewhere about the importance of time in building relationships of mutual trust (Waples-Crowe & Pyett 2005; Pyett et al. 2009). Trust can only develop over a period of time, and this early stage of engagement requires a significant investment of the researcher's time and a demonstration of the researcher's commitment to listen and learn from the community.

Part of the initial engagement will be to establish what level of involvement and responsibility the community wishes to have. We need to be aware that people will have competing time commitments such as paid employment, family responsibilities, child care, household maintenance and educational pursuits, and they may not have the confidence,

Priscilla Pyett, Peter Waples-Crowe and Anke van der Sterren

interest, time or energy for research. Sometimes an underresourced and time-poor community might welcome a researcher who is prepared to do most of the work so long as they are kept fully informed of the process and outcomes of the research. Where possible, however, a greater level of community involvement will enrich the process, increasing the validity and relevance of the findings while also building community capacity.

Initial consultation should include explanations of the need to obtain both funding and ethics approval, and the possibility that these applications may involve long delays or be ultimately unsuccessful. The researcher needs to balance the need for negotiation with communities before applying for funding against the risks of disappointing communities if the funding is not obtained. Since the capacity of communities to participate in research may be limited by lack of skills, resources, time, interest or commitment to the project, we need to build funding and resources into the project to support community participation. These may include skill-building, back-filling organisations for staff involvement in the project, or providing child-minding facilities. Employing community members as part of the research team is a valuable way of facilitating two-way knowledge exchange.

Developing a project agreement

A **project agreement or memorandum of understanding** (MOU) can be drawn up to clarify the roles, responsibilities and expectations of the researcher and the community partners around particular matters such as ownership of data, outcomes, and publications. While MOUs are seldom legally binding, this process is important for the collaborating partners to develop an understanding of each other's values and expectations. The MOU is a useful document to refer to and possibly to amend as the project develops. It is also important to have a process for monitoring and enforcing the principles of the MOU when one of the partners is not adhering to it.

> A **project agreement or MOU** is drawn up to clarify the roles, responsibilities and expectations of the researcher and the community partners around issues such as ownership of data, outcomes and publications.

Researchers can be uncertain where to begin and who to consult (Wand & Eades 2008). As we have argued elsewhere, it is important to identify key stakeholders and consult with them about others who should be included (Pyett et al. 2009). A community organisation may have a clear structure and protocols identifying who should be consulted, such as a director, board of management, executive officers or community liaison personnel. Some communities will not be represented by organisations, but there may be identifiable spokespersons or community elders. Representation is complex and not easily understood by outsiders. As already mentioned, group members are likely to have diverse as well as shared interests and values. This is where relationships are important. Health professionals or welfare workers may be able to identify key community members, but although existing networks can help you get started it is also necessary to consult more broadly. Establishing a steering committee or advisory group can help in identifying who should be consulted and how the community should be represented.

Steering committees or advisory groups

Researchers using CPR often establish a **steering committee or advisory group** to provide advice and guidance on all matters pertaining to the community with whom and for whom they are conducting the research. This is the group to whom researchers or health professionals must refer if they are to identify accurately what the group's needs, interests and priorities are, and the group who must finally judge and decide whether the research has described their situation or met their needs. It should include key stakeholders and experts in particular topics or cultural aspects. These people may be community elders, relevant service providers or health specialists, or people with other relevant technical expertise. Membership may change over the duration of the research as advice may be needed on different aspects of the project. It is a good idea to build in some project funding to reimburse members for their time and travel costs and to provide refreshments during meetings.

> A **steering committee or advisory group** provides advice and guidance on all matters pertaining to the community with whom and for whom the research is being conducted.

Data collection and analysis

We need to be mindful that academic language can be alienating (Pyett et al. 2008, 2009) and we should communicate in ways best suited to the communities we are working with. We find that community groups are more comfortable with more familiar terms such as 'information-gathering' than 'data collection', and 'understanding what we have found out' rather than 'analysis and interpretation'.

While both quantitative and qualitative methods can be used in CPR, quantitative data collection is often more difficult in community-based contexts. Sample sizes are usually small, which means that data analysis may be limited to simple descriptive statistics. Qualitative methods, which rely on face-to-face interaction and that enable more in-depth exploration of issues, are often more appealing and accessible to community groups (see Liamputtong 2007, 2009, 2010; see also CHAPTER 1 and chapters in PART II).

Working with communities to do CPR means that we need to be flexible and open to learning from our community partners. Involving community members in data collection and analysis is not only important for showing respect for their experience and contribution but also because the validity and relevance of the findings will be enhanced by the breadth of their understanding and through the sharing of insider and outsider knowledge (Stringer & Genat 2004; Liamputtong 2009).

Maintaining confidentiality can be problematic when working in small communities. People in the community may recognise research participants or communities mentioned in reports even when names and all obvious identifying characteristics have been removed. It is also often hard to maintain confidentiality *within* the research team when community members are also researchers, and special strategies may need to be developed to protect the confidentiality of participants. For example, standard protocols may need to be adjusted so that names and potentially identifying characteristics are removed from transcripts before other members of the research team have access to the raw data.

DOING RESEARCH

Data analysis

One of us was involved in a project working with members of a consumer advocacy group in which we conducted a number of focus groups with women who had all participated in a similar health screening process. We noticed that in all of the groups, younger women seemed less interested in the discussions than older women. We were not sure if the younger women had fewer concerns about the program or whether the older women were dominating the discussion and inadvertently intimidating the younger ones. So we organised an extra focus group for younger women. In this focus group all the young women had plenty to say, and while their experiences were not dissimilar to the older women, we realised that in the mixed age groups the younger women did not want to be seen to share the attitudes or values of the older women.

Communication and dissemination

In CPR, it is important that the research findings are reported in a way that is appropriate to the community. This may include community reports, community forums, posters, videos, or even more innovative formats such as a dance performance such as we describe in 'Doing research' below (see also Liamputtong 2007, 2009, 2010). It is essential to write clearly, using lay language and avoiding academic jargon or medical terms. Community members and advisory groups should be given plenty of opportunity to read and provide feedback on any publications or other outcomes of the project.

Because we are collaborating with our community participants as co-researchers, we need to include them as co-authors in any publications, even if they do not actually do the writing. Most people in any community other than the academic community do not like writing and are more comfortable with verbal communication. Neither providing access to a community for research purposes nor conducting interviews or administering surveys actually constitute authorship for academic purposes, but in CPR the community members provide far more input. They contribute valuable knowledge about the community, their ideas shape the planning and implementation of the project, their understanding informs the interpretation of data, and in these ways they deserve co-authorship. It is also important to acknowledge the support of community organisations, boards of management and advisory groups as well as funding bodies (see also Pyett et al. 2008).

DOING RESEARCH

Dance as dissemination

One of the most innovative examples of feedback about a research process that we have come across involved a dance performance. Staff of the Aboriginal Community Controlled Health Organisation (ACCHO) and members of the university research team participated in a performance by the local Indigenous men's cultural dance group to illustrate the value of CPR in an applied research setting. The performance was an innovative, culturally appropriate way of disseminating the finding that by working together the ACCHO and the university researchers had improved well-being for community members and contributed to greater harmony within the community. The community set the research agenda and the university researchers facilitated the development of appropriate social health programs and increased the capacity of the community to administer and run these programs. Participants have reported increases in self-esteem, resilience, self-reflection and problem-solving abilities. The programs have expanded from a Men's Group to include a Women's Group, a Youth Group, a diversionary program for court-referred men, and the Indigenous men's dance group, which has performed commercially and aspires to professional status (Mayo et al. 2009).

Action and evaluation

We recognise that it is not always possible to achieve the outcomes recommended through the process of CPR, nor do we always have the time or resources to evaluate outcomes even when they are implemented. Nevertheless, CPR is solution-focused and the goal is to bring about changes for the benefit of the participating communities. Outcomes can be policy-directed or practice-based; they may be health promotion resources, material resources, training and workshops or community forums. The researcher or the community may wish to use the evidence collected for advocacy or service improvement. The process of CPR is an outcome in itself through its potential for community empowerment and providing training for community researchers. There may be unintended consequences from the way the researcher engages with a community. With a CPR approach, it is essential to have some flexibility in order to respond to issues that arise, even though they might be strictly outside the scope of the research.

Actions and outcomes may also be limited by the agenda of the funding body, or by the capacity and resources available within the community to carry out the actions they desire. Alternatively, senior management or Board members may disagree with the recommended actions. A process for managing disagreements should be developed early in the project-planning phase and written into the project agreement or memorandum of understanding.

Priscilla Pyett, Peter Waples-Crowe and Anke van der Sterren

DOING RESEARCH

Limitations imposed by a funding body

Two of us were involved in a project that was funded by a government department and conducted by a community-controlled organisation. Our task was to carry out a research and awareness-raising project around alcohol and pregnancy in an Indigenous community. The community-controlled advisory group recommended setting the research on alcohol within a holistic approach that is compatible with Indigenous views of health and using the findings to develop training for Aboriginal health workers. Representatives of the government department insisted that the funding was allocated specifically for alcohol research and drew our attention to the funding agreement, which required a resource kit to be developed. We were accountable to the Indigenous community but constrained by the funding requirements. Fortunately, we were able to negotiate a compromise where we developed a holistic resource kit and the government department funded a number of regional and metropolitan training sessions that were conducted every time the kit was launched in an Aboriginal organisation.

A COMMUNITY CONTEXT: INDIGENOUS HEALTH RESEARCH IN AUSTRALIA

It is unfortunately well known that in Australia today the greatest inequalities in health and life expectancy are between our Indigenous[1] and non-Indigenous populations. The health status of Aboriginal and Torres Strait Islander people is poorer than the rest of the population in relation to almost every disease or condition for which information is available and across the entire life cycle. According to the latest reports from the Australian Institute of Health and Welfare (AIHW 2008), Indigenous Australians have a life expectancy that is 17 years lower than non-Indigenous Australians (p. 348), they are three times more likely than non-Indigenous Australians to have diabetes (p. 119) and eight times more likely to have end-stage renal disease (p. 139). They are twice as likely to be unemployed (p. 730) and to have completed less than 10 years of schooling (p. 666). Perhaps the most disturbing statistic is that they are 13 times more likely than non-Indigenous Australians to be in prison (p. 884). As the Australian federal government has acknowledged in their 'Close the Gap' policy, there has been little change in any of these statistics in recent decades.

These gross disparities are the consequences of multiple social, economic, political and historical factors that we can only touch on briefly here. As noted by the Council for Aboriginal Reconciliation (1994, p. 19), the 'history of control and exclusion has had a deep and lasting spiritual and psychological impact on Aboriginal and Torres Strait Islander peoples and communities' and this has had 'continuing intergenerational impact'; furthermore, 'Indigenous

Australians continue to be excluded from social and economic opportunities both through individual discrimination and through systematic factors'.

Why CPR is appropriate in this context

A collaborative and participatory approach to research is appropriate to an Indigenous world-view of health and well-being that ties individual health to spiritual and social well-being and to the well-being of their entire community. The National Aboriginal Health Strategy Working Party (1989, p. x) has defined health as 'not just the physical well-being of the individual, but the social, emotional, and cultural well-being of the whole community'. For Aboriginal peoples health is 'not merely a matter of the provision of doctors, hospitals, medicines or the absence of disease and incapacity' but 'a matter of determining all aspects of their life, including control over their physical environment, of dignity, of community self-esteem, and of justice' (p. ix). CPR enables communities to apply these holistic understandings of health, and to promote community well-being by building self-esteem and community capacity in health.

Collaborative approaches that promote active Indigenous participation in research are necessary to further the process of self-determination. **Indigenous people** have a particularly troubled history with researchers, who have often been part of the colonisation, oppression and ongoing surveillance of Indigenous populations in Australia, New Zealand, Canada and North America. Research is still seen as a dirty word in most Aboriginal and Torres Strait Islander communities because it is seen historically as taking knowledge without any benefit to the communities that have been researched (Smith 1999; Humphery 2001; Liamputtong 2010). A great deal of anthropological and other medical and social science research has been undertaken since colonisation, but this has rarely led to any improvement in the lives of Indigenous people, as is reflected in the continuing gap in health outcomes right across Australia. Indigenous people have often been neglected in the research process, treated as subjects rather than active agents (Smith 1999; Humphery 2001; Liamputtong 2010). A recent systematic review of Australian Indigenous child health, development and well-being epidemiological studies conducted in 2006 found that only 28.6 per cent of 217 studies identified reported involvement of Indigenous people in the research process (other than as participants) (Priest et al. 2009). It is this kind of finding that explains why many Aboriginal and Torres Strait Islander communities feel neglected in the research process.

Recognition of the rights of Indigenous peoples to self-determination, together with increasing numbers of Indigenous researchers, have resulted in calls for respectful, reciprocal and equal relationships between researchers and Indigenous communities (National Aboriginal and Torres Strait Islander Health Council 2003; NHMRC 2003). In recent years, many researchers (both Indigenous and non-Indigenous) with the help of Indigenous communities have been trying to address the imbalance from research being 'done to' communities to research been 'done

Indigenous people: The original inhabitants of a country, widely recognised to be disadvantaged across a range of social, political and health indicators.

with' or 'by' communities. For example, the Cooperative Research Centre for Aboriginal Health has developed an Indigenous Research Reform Agenda (see Henry et al. 2002a,b and < www. crcah.org.au/research/approachtoresearch.html>). Publications like the NHMRC's *Values and Ethics: Guidelines for Ethical Conduct in Aboriginal and Torres Strait Islander Health Research* (2003) and *Keeping Research on Track* (2005) provide advice for researchers and Indigenous communities on culturally respectful and ethical research practice. CPR demonstrates several of the core values espoused by these documents: *respect* for the knowledge that community leaders and community members bring to the research partnership; *responsibility* in that researchers are accountable to the communities they research with; *reciprocity* through capacity-building and feedback of research findings to the communities; and relationships of *equality* between the researcher(s) and the communities involved in the research.

Awareness of and respect for cultural issues, cultural diversity and cultural safety are essential to ethical research with Indigenous communities (Ramsden 1990; Coffin et al. 2008). It is the researcher's responsibility to become educated about the history and culture of the local community and to ensure that the research process is culturally secure and adopts appropriate methods (see Liamputtong 2010).

Applying CPR in an Indigenous context

While the broad principles of CPR outlined in the previous sections are equally relevant in the Indigenous health research context, consideration needs to be given to the socio-cultural context, and in particular how the power relations resulting from colonisation influence the way in which relationships are developed and how research is undertaken. For instance, Indigenous cultures are extremely diverse, and have been impacted by colonisation in diverse ways. Colonisation has forced Indigenous people to adapt, and the culture has changed, not disappeared. Some people still live a very traditional life, but many have been dislocated from their traditional homelands and have been influenced by the dominant European culture. Two-thirds of Indigenous Australians live in rural and urban centres, while only 25 per cent live in remote or very remote areas (ABS and AIHW 2008). When approaching an Indigenous community or population group about research, time must be taken to get to know the particular history and culture of the group that researchers will be working with, rather than assuming that all Indigenous communities are the same.

Getting to know the Indigenous community means developing an understanding of which organisations or groups are appropriate to be approached and involved in the research. In Aboriginal health research, this may mean developing relationships with Aboriginal community-controlled health organisations (ACCHOs), or Aboriginal Medical Services, as they are called in some states and territories. Local Aboriginal health organisations are usually members of regional or state-level peak bodies who may also wish to be involved in the research. Aboriginal health organisations are incorporated, community-controlled services committed to a holistic approach to health care, to responding to the needs of the community, and to community participation in decision-making. Aboriginal health workers are integral to service delivery in these organisations, although in many states in Australia they also work in mainstream (i.e. non-Aboriginal) health organisations. Other Aboriginal community-controlled organisations may also be appropriate to be involved in the research, depending on the research topic, for example Aboriginal housing boards, legal services, child care agencies and family violence services. As community-controlled spaces, ACCHOs are central components of self-determination within Aboriginal communities, and as such are logical partners in CPR.

The diversity of Indigenous communities throughout Australia means that it is impossible to provide definitive guidelines for undertaking CPR in these contexts. Instead, we will give two examples that illustrate some of the principles and complexities of CPR in this context, and we draw on one of these projects to offer some practical steps for successful collaboration between mainstream and Indigenous organisations.

DOING RESEARCH

CPR in Indigenous settings

Recruiting Aboriginal women into a study on human papillomavirus (HPV)

Researchers from the Women, Human papillomavirus prevalence, Indigenous, Non-Indigenous, Urban, Rural Study wanted to collect baseline data on 50 Aboriginal women in Dubbo before the introduction of the vaccine for human papillomavirus. Aboriginal women in Australia have lower rates of cervical screening and higher rates of mortality from cervical cancer than non-Aboriginal women. When the standard recruitment process failed, the researchers adopted a CPR approach.

One of the key stakeholders in the research partnership, Family Planning New South Wales (FPNSW), had good long-term connections with the local Aboriginal community and an Aboriginal Women's Advisory Committee. The concept of the research was discussed with the Advisory Committee, who endorsed the project and helped establish a local steering committee. The research team employed an Indigenous health co-ordinator to ensure cultural safety, respect and appropriate research resources for the participants.

But they were still unsuccessful in recruiting women for the study. So the local clinic team, in collaboration with the Aboriginal Health Promotion Officer, developed four key strategies:

1 *Street Walks:* The Aboriginal Health Promotion Officer and a family planning nurse spent time walking the Dubbo main street during business hours, talking to Aboriginal women and distributing flyers about the study and the local FPNSW services.

2 *Attendance at community forums:* The Aboriginal Health Promotion Officer or a clinic nurse attended mothers' groups and playgroups to promote the study and FPNSW services.

3   *Flexible appointments and drop-in clinics:* The FPNSW clinic adopted and advertised additional flexible appointment times and drop-in nurse-run clinic sessions.

4   *Travel and babysitting:* A small reimbursement for out-of-pocket expenses was negotiated for study participants.

With these culturally appropriate, flexible strategies the project team succeeded in recruiting 41 Aboriginal women into the study. Furthermore, increased numbers of Aboriginal women accessed cervical screening in the year following the study (Read & Bateson 2009).

The Victorian Blood Borne Virus and Injecting Drug Use Training Project

The idea for this project was initially the outcome of discussions between workers from one Indigenous and two mainstream organisations who had worked together on a number of projects over several years. The aim of the project was to provide Aboriginal workers throughout Victoria with current information about blood-borne viruses (BBV) and to begin discussion on the emerging issues associated with injecting drug use (IDU) in Aboriginal communities. The training would also aim to break down stigma about IDU and improve the services available to Indigenous users. Funding was provided by the Office of Aboriginal and Torres Strait Islander Health (OATSIH).

A memorandum of understanding was drawn up and signed by senior executives in all three organisations that supported the collaborative arrangements and time necessary for relationship-building and developing mutual understanding. At this stage two further organisations (one mainstream and one Indigenous) were invited to join the project and participate in the planning and delivery of the training.

The five partner organisations attended a 2-day cross-cultural awareness and skill-sharing workshop. This was an important two-way learning experience where the mainstream worker learnt about Indigenous history, values and perspectives and the Indigenous workers learnt how mainstream organisations dealt with the sensitive issues associated with BBV/IDU.

Three training sessions were designed and a resource kit developed. Each of the partners brought unique skills that were recognised and valued by other partners in planning and implementing the program. The training targeted Aboriginal drug and alcohol workers, hospital liaison workers, mental health workers and cultural and spiritual well-being workers. The training was successful in increasing workers' understanding of people with hepatitis C and HIV/AIDS and reducing some of the stigma associated with IDU. The mainstream and Indigenous organisations learnt to respect and trust each other and all were confident of ongoing collaboration (Waples-Crowe & Pyett 2005).

Identifying elements of a successful collaboration

OATSIH became interested in why the BBV/IDU training project succeeded on such a sensitive topic and as a collaboration between three mainstream and two Indigenous organisations, when so many similar partnership projects have failed because relationships have broken down. OATSIH funded a further study to identify the factors that facilitated such a successful collaboration, and two of us were involved in this project (Waples-Crowe & Pyett 2005). We identified 10 steps to guide successful collaboration between mainstream and Indigenous organisations. In disseminating these findings we have sought feedback and have added two further steps that were integral to the BBV/IDU project but that were not identified by the participants themselves.

Steps to guide successful collaboration between mainstream and Indigenous partners

1   The project should be community-initiated.

2   A long time-frame is necessary for developing relationships and planning the project.

3   Mainstream organisations need to take responsibility to get educated about the Indigenous community rather than expecting the Indigenous organisation to explain everything to them.

4   Mainstream organisations need to undertake cultural awareness training for their staff before engaging with Indigenous community organisations.

5   Mainstream and Indigenous partners need to value each other's skills, experience, values and perspectives.

6   Building trust takes time and mainstream organisations need to work within the time-frame of the Indigenous community.

7   It is important to identify all the key partners and formalise partnerships through project agreements or MOUs.

8   Good planning is essential and must involve all partners.

9   The project needs to produce an outcome that is seen as useful to the participants.

10 Supportive work environments are essential and require the support of senior management.

11 Ongoing communication and feedback are important at all times throughout the project.

12 Individuals in both mainstream and community organisations need to show leadership in order to support their co-workers and community members through the collaborative process.

Adapted from Waples-Crowe & Pyett 2005

SUMMARY

The principal benefits of collaborative participatory research are that it is inclusive, and that it builds confidence, capacity and trust. A collaborative participatory approach to research facilitates social change for the benefit of participating communities. It is therefore particularly important that researchers collaborate with marginalised and disadvantaged groups, who have every reason not to trust, who have experienced exploitation and have few opportunities to have their perspective seen or heard. As health researchers, we have a responsibility to give something back to the communities we research. This can be achieved by sharing our findings and validating their experiences, but also, through collaboration, by increasing the skills and the confidence of people with whom we are researching.

In this chapter, we have learnt the importance and value of including disadvantaged communities in the planning, implementation and dissemination of research that affects them. We have seen that CPR is particularly valuable for research with Indigenous communities. We have learnt the importance of time spent in building relationships of mutual trust in order to carry out research that will be relevant and beneficial to the collaborating partners, and we have been introduced to some practical guidelines for undertaking CPR.

TUTORIAL EXERCISES

1   What is the name of the traditional owners of the land you live on? What are some of the Aboriginal and Torres Strait Islander organisations in your local area? They could be in health, housing, social services, child care, land councils, etc. It is important for non-Indigenous people to get some knowledge of the Aboriginal and Torres Strait Islander group you intend to research and this will make approaching community organisations a lot easier.

2   Imagine you are working with Aboriginal and Torres Strait Islander patients/clients and you recognise a health issue or service gap that could be researched. How will you involve Aboriginal and Torres Strait Islander people in planning your project? What organisations would you approach? What steps would you take to discuss how Aboriginal and Torres Strait Islander people want to be involved in the project?

3   Draw up a memorandum of understanding or project agreement. Devise a template for a project agreement or MOU between yourself (or your organisation) and a community group or organisation. What are the important things that would need to be included?

4   Look at the human papillomavirus project described on page 360. Applying the steps outlined in the box, can you identify the CPR strategies that made the project a success? Can you think of anything else the research team could have done to improve their process in a culturally appropriate and ethical manner?

NOTE

1   We use the terms Indigenous, Aboriginal and Torres Strait Islander and Aboriginal interchangeably to refer to all Aboriginal and Torres Strait Islander peoples and communities in Australia. We recognise that communities have different preferences for the way they are named and described but we are unable to refer to individual tribal groups in this chapter.

FURTHER READING

Hart, E. & Bond, M. (1995). *Action research for health and social care: A guide to practice*. Buckingham, UK: Open University Press.

NHMRC (2003). *Values and ethics: Guidelines for ethical conduct in Aboriginal and Torres Strait Islander health research*. Canberra: NHMRC. <www.nhmrc.gov.au/health_ethics/human/conduct/guidelines/_files/e52.pdf>.

NHMRC (2005). *Keeping research on track: A guide for Aboriginal and Torres Strait Islander Peoples about health research ethics*. Canberra: Australian Government Publishing Service. <www.nhmrc.gov.au/PUBLICATIONS/synopses/e65syn.htm>.

Nyden, P. W., Figert, A., Shibley, M. & Burrows, D. (1997). *Building community: Social science in action*. Thousand Oaks, CA: Pine Forge Press.

Smith, L.T. (1999). *Decolonizing methodologies: Research and Indigenous peoples*. Dunedin, NZ: University of Otago Press.

Stringer, E. & Genat, W. (2004). *Action research in health*. New Jersey: Pearson.

WEBSITES

Methodology

www.communitybasedresearch.ca/index.html

A Canadian Centre for Community Based Research is focused on strengthening communities through social research.

www.luc.edu/curl

A website from Loyola University in Chicago that has developed collaborative participatory research relationships with many community organisations.

Indigenous health

www.healthinfonet.ecu.edu.au

The Australian Health Information Network: information on Australian Indigenous people's health, health practice and health policy.

www.crcah.org.au

> *The website for the Cooperative Research Centre for Aboriginal Health.*

www.naccho.org.au

> *The website for the National Aboriginal Community Controlled Health Organisation (NACCHO) and all its state and territory affiliates.*

www.health.gov.au/oatsih

> *The website for the Office of Aboriginal and Torres Strait Islander Health.*

Part VI

Making Sense of Data and Presentation

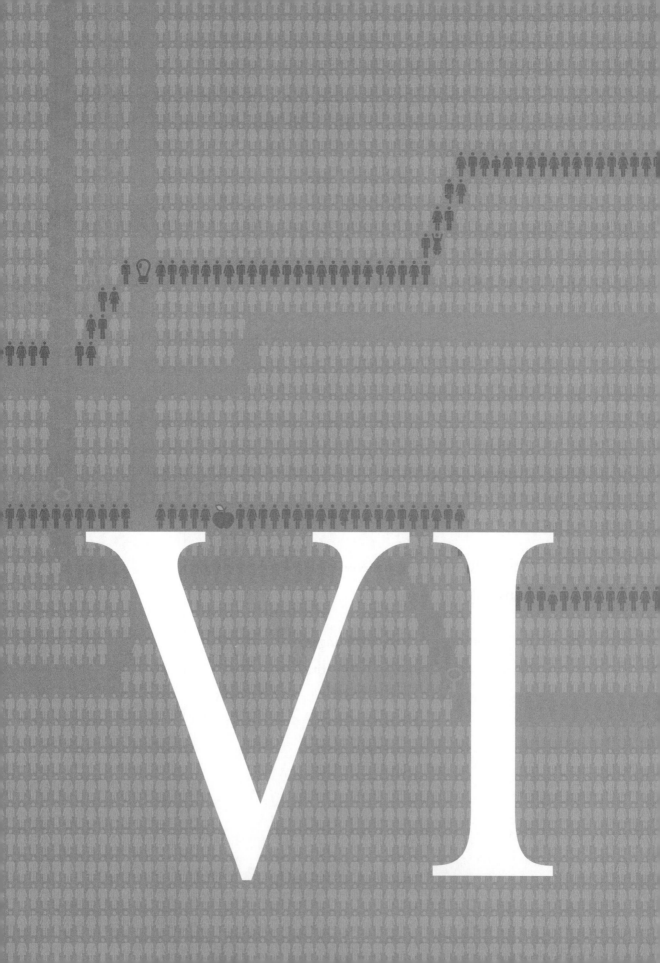

22

Making Sense of Qualitative Data

Pranee Liamputtong and Tanya Serry

CHAPTER OBJECTIVES

In this chapter you will learn:

- [ ] about the fundamental premises and generic concepts of qualitative data
- [ ] about the use of coding strategies
- [ ] how to perform content analysis
- [ ] how to perform thematic analysis

KEY TERMS

Axial coding

Code

Coding

Content analysis

Data analysis

Data display

Data reduction

Descriptive/open coding

Focused coding

Selective coding

Thematic analysis

INTRODUCTION

Data analysis is the process of moving from raw interviews to evidence-based interpretations that are the foundation for published reports. Analysis entails classifying, comparing, weighing and combining material [obtained during data collection] to extract the meaning and implications, to reveal patterns, or to stitch together descriptions of events into a coherent narrative. (Rubin & Rubin 2005, p. 201)

The analysis of qualitative data is a rich experience that requires the researcher to combine creative and reflective thinking alongside systematic and rigorous standards of empirical enquiry. As such, the process of qualitative analysis is data-based and data-driven (Bogdan & Biklen 2007). There are several analytical approaches available to the qualitative researcher in order to be able to turn data, which is often voluminous, into 'a clear, understandable, insightful, trustworthy and even original analysis' (Gibbs 2007, p. 1). In this chapter we will focus on two more commonly used approaches: content analysis and thematic analysis. (For details on other approaches to data analysis, readers are referred to Miles & Huberman 1994; Mason 2002; Ritchie et al. 2003; Liamputtong 2009; Saldaña 2009.)

GENERIC PRINCIPLES REGARDING QUALITATIVE DATA ANALYSIS

Attempting **data analysis** for the novice qualitative researcher can seem daunting. In fact, data analysis in qualitative research is an ongoing, cyclical process that occurs from the very beginning of the research itself (Miles & Huberman 1994; Liamputtong 2009). Researchers need to treat data analysis as an integral component of the research design, the literature review, formation of theory, data collection, the ordering of data, and the writing process (see Northcutt & McCoy 2004; Gibbs 2007; Bryman 2008). In this way, analytic decisions are made from the initial stages of reviewing literature through to data collection, organisation, conclusion drawing and verification. In essence, data analysis continues throughout every step of the research process (Grbich 2007; Liamputtong 2009), such that the process is a 'continuous, iterative enterprise' (Miles & Huberman 1994, p. 12) between the existing data that has been analysed and newly collected data, in order to complete, challenge or resolve issues and queries that arise.

Data analysis: The way that researchers make sense of their data. In qualitative research it involves looking for patterns or themes, whereas in quantitative research numerical data are analysed and statistics are used.

Accordingly, data analysis in qualitative research is not a discrete operation. The interactive and iterative nature of qualitative research also allows data analysis to inform and guide upcoming data collection within the one research project. In turn, data analysis should be an ongoing, lively enterprise that contributes to the energising process of fieldwork. Many other qualitative researchers similarly advise interweaving data collection and analysis from the beginning (see Mason 2002; Gibbs 2007; Bryman 2008; Carpenter & Suto 2008). All these matters will have significant ramifications for how we undertake our data analysis.

Before we discuss traditions and approaches to qualitative data analysis, the concept of data saturation must be mentioned because it is integral to data collection and analysis. A common question of the novice qualitative researcher centres on sample size and 'when to stop' collecting data. Data saturation can address this perplexing question in part. Data saturation occurs when regularities from your analysis emerge such that more information will not offer you new understanding (Liamputtong 2009). At this point, if well-supported conclusions can be drawn via detailed analysis, further data collection is not needed. It is not possible to determine exactly how long this will take before commencing data collection, though the reflective nature of qualitative research does allow further sampling to occur until saturation is reached. See CHAPTERS 1, 5, 7, 8.

Traditions of qualitative data analysis

Carol Grbich (2007, p. 25) outlines a broad, two-step plan for data analysis that provides a useful framework, regardless of the particular analytical approach being used. Phase 1 involves 'preliminary data analysis', which she describes as a means of highlighting emerging issues by keeping track of key information from the data collection process. For example, she suggests that researchers systematically record identifying facts and features from each participant or case using a 'face sheet' (p. 25). This can be followed up by the researcher noting points such as emerging themes, issues of interest and future data collection goals. Phase 2 analysis or 'post data collection' (p. 31) explores data at an increasingly sophisticated or deeper level. In this second phase, the researcher has a number of options for analysing data depending on the nature of the enquiry and the approach used. Researchers typically use a 'block and file' approach in which the data is segmented and categorised into manageable chunks, or 'conceptual mapping' whereby a diagrammatic approach is used to organise data. Frequently, both processes are applied to the data during the analysis phase (Grbich 2007). Techniques used in post-data collection analysis serve to prepare the researcher to draw and verify conclusions that ultimately form the outcomes of your research.

Data analysis in qualitative research is an ongoing, cyclical process that occurs from the very beginning of the research itself.

The cyclical nature of qualitative data analysis

To demonstrate the continuous nature of qualitative data analysis, along with applying Grbich's (2007) two-phase model above, we have used Miles and Huberman's (1994) Components of Data Analysis: Interactive Model as a generic framework for conducting qualitative data analysis. Figure 22.1 displays our version of their model. We describe each component below, with the exception of data collection (see chapters in PART II for discussions about qualitative data collection methods).

Pranee Liamputtong and Tanya Serry

Figure 22.1: Components of data analysis: interactive model

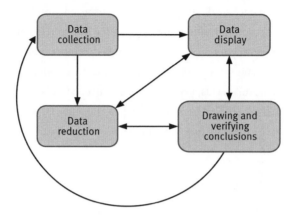

Source: Miles & Huberman 1994, p. 12

Data reduction occurs when raw data is transcribed and transformed into summaries, initial codes and preliminary themes. (We discuss coding and thematic analysis later in this chapter.) Data reduction forms the preliminary phase of analysis. Nevertheless, the process itself requires analytic choices to be made throughout, which form the foundations for deeper levels of analysis. As such, data reduction is a critical component of the entire analytical framework. Yet it is also a fluid process since initial analytic choices are likely to be modified, transformed or collapsed with other themes that emerge. Miles and Huberman (1994) emphasise that data reduction is not a quantitative process. Rather, it is a series of analytic decisions made about the data in which the 'anticipatory' phase should start occurring even before data collection has formally commenced.

> **Data reduction:** The preliminary phase of analysis when raw data is transcribed and transformed into summaries, initial codes and preliminary themes.

Data display is defined by Miles and Huberman (1994, p. 11) as an 'organised, compressed assembly of information that permits conclusion drawing'. For example, data display can take place when rather cumbersome transcripts and observation descriptions are transformed into more accessible forms such as codes, conceptual maps, matrices or even graphs.

> **Data display:** An 'organised, compressed assembly of information that permits conclusion drawing'.

Conclusions are drawn from the data, based on themes and regularities that emerge. Tentative conclusions typically surface as data is collected and analysed, but as Miles and Huberman (1994, p. 11) recommend, 'openness and skepticism' are important qualities that the researcher should maintain until sufficient data is collected and analysed and conclusions can be verified. See also discussions on data analysis processes in CHAPTERS 5, 7, 8.

The reflective practice example below ('Try it yourself') illustrates how this generic framework for data analysis can be applied to a qualitative research project.

TRY IT YOURSELF

FRAMEWORK FOR DATA ANALYSIS

You have started to collect a series of interviews exploring parents' experiences of raising a child who has significant learning difficulty. Each interview was conducted individually and lasted approximately one hour. At this stage you have collected only five interviews although you expect that you will need to collect more. You also decide to summarise your personal reflections of each interview straight after the interview itself. Your summaries act as another form of data and can thus contribute to the overall analysis.

DATA REDUCTION

Your first task is to transcribe your interviews. As a way of further informing your interview protocol as well as conducting some preliminary analyses, you decide to start transcription even though you are only part-way through collecting your interviews. Throughout the transcription of these first few interviews, which is itself a labour-intensive task, you immerse yourself in the content of the interviews. Some initial ideas emerge for you as you transcribe. These ideas included 'parent suspected learning difficulty may occur' and 'parent–school relationship'. You note these ideas in a column in the margin of your transcript. At this point, you are beginning to make analytical choices as you conduct your preliminary data analysis. Furthermore, you decide that there is an important issue raised spontaneously by two of the five parents, which you decide to explore in subsequent interviews. In this way, you are actively engaging in the continuous nature of qualitative research, which means that data analysis can inform ongoing data collection.

DATA DISPLAY

Now that a substantial amount of data has been collected and transcribed and has undergone a preliminary analysis, you decide that the most manageable way to display your data is to code the data into meaningful chunks. (We discuss coding in more depth in the section below.) As part of your coding process, you develop a matrix that has emerged during preliminary analysis. The matrix consists of three broad headings related to the parental experience that you feel will guide deeper analysis for your research:

- impact of the child on parental experience
- impact of the school/institution on parental experience
- impact of family on parental experience
- impact of social networks on parental experience.

CONCLUSIONS

You develop some tentative conclusions based on the data reduction and data display that you have already conducted. But these conclusions will need to be confirmed and verified

Pranee Liamputtong and Tanya Serry

> since you are at an early stage of data analysis in which you have 'stayed close to the data'. To begin the confirmation process of your tentative conclusions, you commence a more detailed process of coding and categorising to make analytic interpretations. It is at this point that you are starting to develop complex and dynamic concepts that sit within your data.

CODING

Coding is central to qualitative research and is typically the starting point for most forms of qualitative analysis. Saldaña (2009, p. 3) defines a **code** as 'a word or short phrase that symbolically assigns a summative, salient essence-capturing and/or evocative attribute for a portion of language-based or visual data'. In essence, coding is the first step that allows researchers to move beyond tangible data to make analytic interpretations (Gibbs 2007; Holton 2007; Corbin & Strauss 2008). According to Charmaz (2006, p. 43), coding is 'the process of defining what the data are about' so that researchers can delve into their data and look for meaning (p. 46). In carrying out coding, researchers name chunks of data with 'a label that simultaneously categorizes, summarizes, and accounts for each piece of data'. These codes ultimately form the foundation for categories and themes that are drawn from the data.

Code: 'A word or short phrase that symbolically assigns a summative, salient essence-capturing and/or evocative attribute for a portion of language-based or visual data.'

Coding: Part of the data analysis process where codes are applied to chunks of data. It is the first step that allows researchers to move beyond tangible data to make analytic interpretations.

The process of coding the data should be dynamic and reflective rather than linear and discrete. This active coding allows the researchers to repeatedly interact with their data and to ask many different questions about it. As a consequence, coding may take the researchers into areas they have not previously considered, such that new or expanded research questions may arise.

While coding, writing marginal notes on the data or transcripts will allow the researchers to maintain their attention to detail (Saldaña 2009). These marginal notes will assist colleagues or other researchers who wish to see how the researchers code their transcripts. Often, later on, marginal notes are used in the coding cycle. As the researchers read through the transcripts again and again, new codes may be added and this can be easily done in the marginal notes. Bryman (2008) points out that the marginal notes the researchers write on the transcripts will gradually be refined into codes.

Some qualitative researchers have provided useful strategies or steps for qualitative researchers to follow (Miles & Huberman 1994; Mason 2002; Charmaz 2006; Liamputtong 2009; Saldaña 2009). Minichiello and colleagues (2008, p. 268) suggest that when experienced researchers develop codes, a strategy often used is to ask the question 'What is this thing (or things) I have before me?' As an example from our own work, we initially set out to explore the perspectives of both parents and teachers regarding children with reading difficulty who were receiving intervention. As our coding progressed, we began to ask further questions of the codes such that we developed a further line of enquiry that explored how parents and teachers differed in their causal attributions for the child's reading difficulty.

Flick (2006, p. 300) suggests the following list of basic questions that qualitative researchers may use as their coding strategies. He also suggests that researchers should examine the text regularly and repeatedly with these questions. With these questions, Flick contends, the researchers will be able to disclose the text.

Table 22.1: Basic questions to use as coding strategies

What?	What is the concern here? Which course of events is mentioned?
Who?	Who are the persons involved? What roles do they have? How do they interact?
How?	Which aspects of the event are mentioned (or omitted)?
When? How long? Where?	Referring to time, course, and location: When does it happen? How long does it take? Where did the incident occur?
How much? How strong?	Referring to intensity: How often is the issue emphasised?
Why?	Which reasons are provided or can be constructed?
What for?	What is the intention here? What is the purpose?
By which?	Referring to means, tactics, and strategies for achieving the aim: What is the main tactic here? How are things accomplished?

The process of coding is a labour-intensive and ongoing task that requires multiple readings of transcripts and other data to complete the progressively more sophisticated levels of coding. It is usual for novice researchers to feel unskilful, clumsy or simply overwhelmed at the beginning of the coding process. More often, the researcher may not feel confident about looking for meanings and naming the codes. However, confidence will gradually increase with their continued efforts with data analysis. Holton (2007, p. 276) points out that 'as coding progresses, patterns begin to emerge. Pattern recognition gives the researchers confidence in the coding process and in their own innate creativity.'

The process of coding the data should be dynamic and reflective rather than linear and discrete.

WHAT CAN BE CODED?

There are several schemes that researchers may use to develop codes from their data. We have found the following suggestions, compiled from Miles and Huberman (1994, p. 61), Bogdan and Biklen (2007, pp. 174–8) and Gibbs (2007, pp. 47–8), to be particularly useful.

☐ Setting and context: general information on surroundings that allows the researchers to place the study in a larger context

- ☐ Definition of the situation: how individuals understand, perceive, or define the setting or the topics on which the study is based
- ☐ Perspectives: ways of thinking about the things that are shared by the participants, such as how things are done here
- ☐ Ways of thinking about people and objects: understandings of each other, of outsiders, of objects in their world, but more detailed than the perspectives
- ☐ Process: sequence of events, flows, transitions, turning points, and changes over time
- ☐ Activities: regularly occurring types of behaviour
- ☐ Actions: what people do or say
- ☐ Events: specific activities, particularly the events that occur infrequently
- ☐ Conditions or constraints: the causes of actions and things that constrain the actions
- ☐ Consequences: types of consequences of the actions or behaviour
- ☐ Strategies: ways of accomplishing things; people's strategies, tactics, methods, techniques for meeting their needs
- ☐ Relationship and social structure: unofficially defined patterns such as cliques, coalitions, romances, friendships, enmities
- ☐ Meanings: the verbal expressions of the participants that 'define and direct action'.

According to Gibbs (2007), those meanings are at the core of most qualitative analysis (see also CHAPTER 1). Meanings include how people see their world and the symbols they use to understand their situation. Meanings direct the actions of the participants. We rely heavily on this schema to code in our own work.

The suggestions we provided above would assist researchers in thinking about categories in which codes will be developed. It is unlikely that all of these aspects will be of relevance in any one study. Researchers will select and focus only on schemes that are relevant to their research (Miles & Huberman 1994), reflecting the importance of the researcher's creativity and reflections. In fact, Creswell (2007, p. 153) recommends that researchers should carefully consider and scrutinise code segments used to represent their data and construct emerging themes rather than adhering solely to the schemes presented above. In turn, the researcher is afforded greater ownership of their analysis with codes that may reveal:

- ☐ data that the researchers may expect to elicit before the study
- ☐ surprising data that the researchers have not expected to discover
- ☐ data that is crucial for the construction of theory, or unusual to the researchers, the readers and even the participants themselves.

STEPS AND STRATEGIES FOR CODING

Our suggestions are paraphrased from Bryman (2008, pp. 550–52) in conjunction with a conceptual framework developed from the work of various qualitative researchers (Miles & Huberman

1994; Strauss & Corbin 1998; Charmaz 2006; Liamputtong 2009). This conceptual framework is discussed below and presented in Figure 22.2. It will lead you through the increasingly deeper and more abstract levels of coding that will allow you to formulate theories and/or key theses arising from your data. See also Chapter 7 for coding in grounded theory research.

Figure 22.2: A conceptual framework for the practice of coding

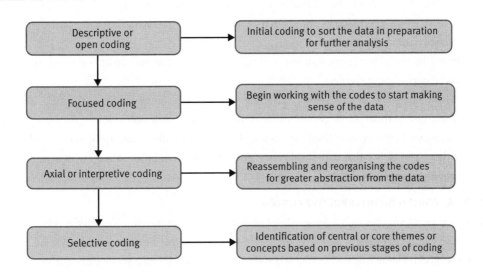

1. DESCRIPTIVE OR OPEN CODING

Coding commences at a **descriptive** (Miles & Huberman 1994) or **open** level (Strauss & Corbin 1998) in which the central aim is to sort and organise the data so that further analysis can take place (Liamputtong 2009). This initial phase of coding stays close to the data itself (Charmaz 2006).

> **Descriptive/open coding**: Often the first step in coding in qualitative data analysis, where the aim is to sort and organise the data so that further analysis can take place.

☐ Commence coding as soon as possible, well before your data collection is complete. As with the practice in grounded theory research, it is wise to start coding while data is still being collected. This will permit you to have a better understanding of the data, to follow up ambiguous data and to help with theoretical sampling. Additionally, it may reduce the feeling of being overwhelmed with too much data, which usually happens when the researchers commence data analysis after all the data is collected.

☐ Read through the initial set of transcripts, field notes or documents without making any notes, or attempting to interpret the data. After reading through the data, you may wish to write down a few notes or keep a reflective journal about what appears to be particularly interesting or significant.

2. FOCUSED CODING

Focused coding (Charmaz 2006) follows descriptive or open coding. This is when you begin working with the codes themselves in order to start making sense of the data. This may involve synthesising the codes and determining relationships between various events or phenomena.

☐ Read through the data again. This time you should start making marginal notes or memos about significant observations or categories that emerge. Make as many of these as possible. This is also coding. Initially, your notes or memos may be very basic. You may use key words expressed by the participants or you may give names to themes in the data. A combination of both is often used.

☐ It may be useful to generate an index of terms or names that may assist you to interpret and theorise about the data.

☐ Review the codes. If you have two or more words or phrases that refer to the same issue, delete one of them. Look closely to see if the developed codes are relevant to concepts and categories in the existing literature. See if there are any connections between the codes or if there is evidence that may suggest one thing that tends to be associated with or caused by something else.

3. AXIAL CODING OR INTERPRETIVE CODING

You are now moving towards a greater level of abstraction from the data. The task at this level of coding will be to evaluate the codes further to determine what needs to be reassembled or reorganised. This may involve processes such as breaking codes into smaller categories or collapsing more than one code into a single category. This interpretation and comparison of coded data is known as the 'Constant Comparison Method' (Flick 2006; Marshall et al. 2007). At this point, coding relies more on inferential analysis in order to make sense of the emerging patterns or themes. **Axial coding** (Strauss & Corbin 1998) essentially refers to drawing data back together once it has been sorted in the initial phase of coding.

4. SELECTIVE CODING

Strauss and Corbin (1998) argue that **selective coding** necessitates a level of analysis beyond axial coding whereby a central or core theme is identified using the previous levels of analysis. At this point, you can begin formulating propositions (Miles & Huberman 1994) by drawing conclusions, making causal connections and developing theoretical constructs. These will need to be verified in order to test their plausibility and conformability (Miles & Huberman 1994). Otherwise, as these authors point out, the researcher runs the risk of writing interesting narrative that may lack scientific rigour.

It is important that you consider more general theoretical understandings in relation to codes and data. By the time you reach this point, you should be able to construct some general theoretical notions or

Focused coding: A step that follows descriptive or open coding, when researchers begin working with the codes themselves in order to start making sense of the data.

Axial coding: The task of further evaluating the codes to determine what needs to be reassembled or reorganised.

Selective coding: A level of analysis where researchers can begin formulating propositions by drawing conclusions, making causal connections and developing theoretical constructs.

concepts about your data. Attempting to outline connections between concepts and categories that you are generating is a good strategy to employ at this time. Also, you should try to see how these tentative concepts and linkages relate to the existing literature.

Further points to consider about coding

☐ In the early stages of your analysis, it is likely that you will generate a large number of codes. You will soon find that some codes will be useful, while others will not. It is important to be inventive and imaginative at the beginning. Things can be tidied up later on.

☐ Recognise that any piece of data can be coded in more than one way or in multiple coding categories.

☐ The process of coding requires the researcher to be rigorous and thorough while maintaining a flexible and receptive approach to the data.

☐ Codes also allow for easy organisation and retrieval of data from a large body of information.

DOING RESEARCH

Examples of codes

To demonstrate some codes we developed into perspectives on identifying and supporting children with reading difficulty, we have provided some examples taken from our analysis of interview data.

When asking educators what factors they thought might influence or be responsible for a child's reading difficulty, one reading specialist said:

'Some kids get really nervous about the whole reading process. You know, it really stresses them. And I have yet to know why. But it really stresses them. And you can't learn effectively if you are highly stressed.'

We coded this text in an umbrella category at the level of focused coding as 'innate factors' and a subcategory or descriptive code that we called 'stress'. From our data, we found that we needed to contrast innate factors with environmental factors such as 'limited exposure to books as a preschooler'.

Similarly, when parents were asked what they thought might have been influential for their child's difficulty learning to read, one of our descriptive codes was 'parent unsure why'. Here are some comments coded accordingly:

'And it's er...I hadn't expected it would happen to us coz I had done all those pre-reading kind of things...'

'I have absolutely no problem with how he was taught. It was really that for some unknown reason, it just didn't seem to be coming together.'

'Honestly, at this point I'm at a loss to see why it's happened. I mean we've read to them and you know, we've spoken to our kids from when they were very young.'

Pranee Liamputtong and Tanya Serry

DOING RESEARCH

Coding

Read the following excerpt from a transcript with a parent about her son, now 10 years old, who has a learning difficulty. Consider the options for coding at a descriptive and focused level.

> 'Jamie's very young for his year. My husband and I were very reluctant whether we should send him to kinder when he turned 3 or hold him back. And a lot of people said to us, because he's a very social child, he should be right. So we put him through. We got to the second year of kinder and the kindergarten teachers were starting to introduce words on cards and simple books for the children to take home. And we found already then that Jamie was struggling. He couldn't do it. And I had already brought up with the kindergarten teacher "should I send Jamie to school?" Coz the way he was interpreting information and that, it just wasn't getting through to him.'

Descriptive codes could include the following:

- ☐ age of child relative to peers
- ☐ shared parenting decision-making
- ☐ reluctance about sending child to kinder
- ☐ social skills of child
- ☐ people said 'he'd be fine'
- ☐ child struggled at kinder
- ☐ child had difficulty interpreting information
- ☐ struggled with reading word cards
- ☐ parent seeking advice from kinder teacher
- ☐ parent worried about child going to school.

Are there any other descriptive codes you might include? Would you consider noting any memos from this excerpt?

Using the codes listed above, focused coding could proceed as follows:

- ☐ parental decision-making processes
- ☐ child attributes used in decision-making regarding kindergarten readiness
- ☐ parental concerns about school readiness.

Are there other focused codes you might draw from the descriptive codes listed above?

TYPES OF DATA ANALYSIS

In the following sections, we describe two different types of qualitative data analysis: content analysis and thematic analysis. Both approaches are widely used, often within the one data set. Content analysis is arguably the most uncomplicated form of qualitative analysis but may not be appropriate for many qualitative research projects. Thematic analysis emphasises the power of words and meaning inherent in those words. There are other kinds of data analysis in qualitative research and we would encourage you to read further (see Liamputtong 2009; CHAPTERS 5, 7, 8).

Content analysis

Content analysis, according to Bryman (2008, p. 275), is an analytic approach that attempts to 'quantify content in terms of predetermined categories and in a systematic and replicable manner'. Although qualitative research does not typically work with numbers or counting, in practice, data analysis sometimes makes use of some underlying counting elements, particularly when judgments about qualities need to be made.

Content analysis:
A form of data analysis used by both qualitative and quantitative researchers in which codes are identified before searching for their occurrence in the data.

> Although qualitative research does not typically work with numbers or counting, in practice, data analysis sometimes makes use of some underlying counting elements, particularly when judgments of qualities need to be made.

An essential goal of qualitative content analysis requires codes to be identified before they are searched for in the data (Morgan 1993; Silverman 2001; Neuendorf 2002; Krippendorf 2004; Flick 2006; Daly 2007). The practice of content analysis, Daly and colleagues (2007) suggest, requires the researchers to know what they want to look for in the text. Accordingly, Morgan and Silverman suggest that content analysis involves developing categories or a consistent set of codes, seeking them out from the data and then systematically recording or counting the number of times the categories occur. In this way, the researcher can get a sense of what is contained within the data.

Furthermore, Grbich (2007) suggests that content analysis is also useful in examining textual data unobtrusively in order to check the patterns and trends of words used, their frequency and relationships. This approach is popularly used for the analysis of published material such as newspapers and magazines, policy documents, visual images, public records, medical records, speeches, and also for interview transcripts (see CHAPTERS 3, 4, 9). We performed a content analysis when looking for theoretical perspectives held by educators involved with supporting young children with reading difficulty. Based on individual interviews that we collected, we searched for particular words that we had identified as critical to our research query. As a result, we were able to propose some novel conclusions from our data (Serry et al. under review). This is an example of content analysis.

We demonstrate content analysis in a study by Shugg and Liamputtong (2002), who examined how the media portray women's health issues in Australian society. Two leading daily newspapers in Melbourne were chosen as sources of articles. A simple statistical analysis was used. They found that the predominant issues in the women's health articles were children/ motherhood and pregnancy. In all, 157 (33.4%) articles related to children/motherhood of 470 women's health articles. The second most frequent subject was pregnancy with 107 articles (22.77%). There was a large gap between these two and the remaining categories, the next being court rulings/damages with 57 articles (12.12%). Table 22.2 presents a selected list of the topic areas.

Table 22.2: Frequency of women's health articles by topics

Categories	Frequency	Percentage
Children/motherhood	157	33.4
Pregnancy	107	22.7
Court rulings/damages	57	12.12
Sexual violence/abuse	34	7.23

DOING RESEARCH

Content analysis

We provide an example from our own research (Serry et al., under review) in which we used content analysis as a small but influential part of our overall data analysis. As part of our investigation exploring how teachers collaborate with their non-teaching colleagues regarding children with learning difficulty, in the individual interviews we noticed differences between the groups in the use of key terminology and jargon. Since we were exploring collaboration, we considered that this variability might be significant enough to explore further. We performed a simple form of content analysis on our interview data where we simply searched for the terminology in question from the texts across all participants. At the outset we did not expect that terminology variability was going to be significant. However, based on our content analysis, we were able to develop a central theme related to the entire study.

Thematic analysis

> [D]iscovering themes is the basis of much social science research. Without thematic categories, investigators have nothing to describe, nothing to compare, and nothing to explain. (Ryan & Bernard 2003, pp. 85–6)

Thematic analysis: The identification of themes through a careful reading and rereading of the data.

Qualitative researchers believe that words are more powerful than numbers (Liamputtong 2009). Hence content analysis may not be appropriate for most qualitative research. A more common type of analysis in qualitative research is **thematic analysis**, sometimes called interpretive thematic analysis (Ryan & Bernard 2003; Braun & Clarke 2006; Liamputtong 2009). Thematic analysis is 'a method for identifying, analysing and reporting patterns (themes) within the data' (Braun & Clarke 2006, p. 79) and is perceived 'as a foundational method for qualitative analysis' (p. 78).

The techniques used for analysing data in thematic analysis and grounded theory are broadly similar (see CHAPTER 7 for data analysis in grounded theory research). In this section, we provide some practical ways of conducting thematic analysis. Much of the discussion about coding presented earlier in this chapter is highly applicable to performing thematic analysis.

There are two main steps. First, you need to read carefully through each transcript. Then, as part of a collective set, you must examine the transcript and make sense of what is being said by the participants as a group (Minichiello et al. 2008). Thematic analysis 'involves searching across a data set—be that a number of interviews or focus groups, or a range of texts—to find repeated patterns of meaning' (Braun & Clarke 2006, p. 86). Coding plays a major part in thematic analysis, whereby the researcher needs to perform the various levels of coding in order to deconstruct data and find links between the various codes. Axial coding is the step that will allow you to connect the different codes that you have identified in the initial coding. It is 'a way of organising the data together by making connections between a major category and its sub-category' (Minichiello et al. 2008, p. 280). This allows the researchers to find themes in the data.

We would like to show the way themes were found in Pranee's recent work on the lived experience of living with HIV/AIDS among women in Central Thailand (see Liamputtong et al. 2009). One woman remarked on her experience:

> People in community tend to see this disease as *rok mua* [promiscuous disease]. As women, we can have only one partner or one husband. But, for those who have HIV/AIDS, people tend to see them as having too many partners and this is not good. They are seen as *pu ying mai dee* [bad women]. And they will be *rang kiat* [discriminated against] more than men who have HIV/AIDS. Men who live with this disease are not seen as bad as the women are. If you are women and have HIV/AIDS, it is worse for you.

From the short transcript of one woman, we may come up with the following codes:

- gender and HIV/AIDS
- HIV/AIDS and discrimination
- HIV/AIDS as promiscuous disease
- HIV/AIDS and bad women
- women and stigma
- gender inequality and HIV/AIDS.

As an illustration, we think the main theme of these codes could be termed 'gender and the stigmatised discourse'. The theme we use here comes from Pranee's own understanding of the story the woman told her. She did not use the word 'stigma' at all, but what she said implied stigma; it is clear from this short transcript that women living with HIV/AIDS are more stigmatised than men living with it. This example is only a simple one based on one short transcript. Once we analyse more transcripts, as Minichiello and colleagues (2008) suggest above, and we find that several other women speak similarly, the theme will become confirmed. However, this theme may change, as there may be other issues emerging from the data. See also CHAPTERS 5, 7, 8.

The following steps proposed by Braun and Clarke (2006, p. 87) are useful for readers to adopt:

☐ Make yourself familiar with your data. This means you should transcribe the data yourself, read and reread the data and write down your initial impressions and ideas.

☐ Start to generate initial codes, as suggested above.

☐ Look for themes by collating codes into tentative themes. At this stage you need to gather all data that is related to each potential theme.

☐ Revise the themes you have developed. Check if the themes work in relation to the codes you have extracted and the entire data set. You may also find it useful to develop a thematic 'map' of the analysis.

☐ Define and name your themes. It is also important to carry out an ongoing analysis to refine the themes so that clear definitions and names for each theme can be generated.

SUMMARY

It's right to say that qualitative data analysis is a craft—one that carries its own disciplines. There are many ways of getting analysis 'right'—precise, trustworthy, compelling, credible—and they cannot be wholly predicted in advance. (Miles & Huberman 1994, p. 309)

In this chapter, we have described the generic principles of qualitative data analysis with particular emphasis on the delicate balance between creative and reflective thinking while maintaining an empirical, data-driven focus. Furthermore, we explored the recursive nature of data analysis as a critical and valuable aspect that highlights the uniqueness of qualitative research overall. We have discussed the centrality of coding as a tool for much qualitative data analysis. In doing so, we outlined steps involved in coding that allow the researcher to work progressively through the data to extract increasingly greater levels of meaning. Finally, we also provided practical suggestions for performing content and thematic analyses. Thematic analysis itself is foundational to qualitative research. There are other approaches that offer different ways of interpreting data but these have not been covered in this chapter.

At the beginning, qualitative researchers are likely to feel overwhelmed with the volume and breadth of the data and ambivalent about the analysis. It is only with exposure and experience that the task becomes not only easier but very rewarding.

TUTORIAL EXERCISES

Here is an extended version of the excerpt from the reflective exercise in the table below. Conduct a data analysis from the transcript sample by doing the following:

1   Conduct initial coding from the transcript portion.

2   From this initial coding, perform a content analysis—what categories have you come up with? How many times does each category appear in the interview?

3   From this initial coding, attempt a thematic analysis—what themes emerge from the text?

4   Look for a missing or hidden agenda within the text—what do you think is not said in the text? And what might be the reason for the missing text?

You need select only one or two of these exercises to practise your analytical skills.

Mother	Jamie's very young for his year. My husband and I were very reluctant whether we should send him to kinder when he turned 3 or hold him back. And a lot of people said to us, because he's a very social child, he should be right. So we put him through. We got to the second year of kinder and the kindergarten was starting to introduce words on cards and simple books for the children to take home. And we found already then that Jamie was struggling. He couldn't do it. And I had already brought up with the kindergarten teacher 'should I send Jamie to school?' Coz the way he was interpreting information and that, it just wasn't getting through to him.
Res.	Mm.
Mother	Even though his social skills were great, his learning skills were very poor. The kindergarten teacher's advice was 'No, he's fine. He's got the social skills, send him to school'. So basically, when you don't know better, you send the child to school. I was very reluctant to send him, but I did. But we found that in prep, he was still struggling, really struggling. But it wasn't just with reading. It was with his motor skills, with writing, with spelling, with basically everything.
Res.	OK.
Mother	We got to grade 1. And even in prep, I was reluctant about sending him to grade 1. But he went into grade 1, and…it would have been probably about March, we got approached by his teacher at the time, and she said 'I would like you to consider keeping Jamie back and repeating grade 1…'.

(Note: 'Res' stands for 'researcher')

FURTHER READING

Bakeman, R. (2000). Behavioral observation and coding. In H.T. Reis & C.M. Judge (eds), *Handbook of research methods in social and personality psychology*. Cambridge: Cambridge University Press, 138–59.

Braun, V. & Clarke, V. (2006). Using thematic analysis in psychology. *Qualitative Research in Psychology*, 3, 77–101.

Bryman, A. (2008). *Social research methods*, 3rd edn. Oxford: Oxford University Press.

Gibbs, G.R. (2007). *Analyzing qualitative data*. London: Sage Publications.

Grbich, C. (2007). *Qualitative data analysis: An introduction*. London: Sage Publications.

Liamputtong, P. (2009). *Qualitative research methods*, 3rd edn. Melbourne: Oxford University Press.

Miles, M.B. & Huberman, A.M. (1994). *Qualitative data analysis*, 2nd edn. Beverley Hills, CA: Sage Publications.

Ryan, G.W. & Bernard, H.R. (2003). Techniques to identify themes. *Field Methods* 15(1), 85–109.

Saldaña, J. (2009). *Coding in qualitative data analysis*. Thousand Oaks, CA: Sage Publications.

Thorne, S. (2000). Data analysis in qualitative research. *Evidence-Based Nursing*, 3, 68–70.

Williamson, T. & Long, A.F. (2005). Qualitative data analysis using data displays. *Nurse Researcher*, 12(3), 7–19.

WEBSITES

www.nova.edu/ssss/QR/QR3-1/carney.html

This website leads you to the paper on a method of categorising, coding and sorting/manipulating qualitative (descriptive) data using the capabilities of a commonly used word processor, WordPerfect®.

www.slais.ubc.ca/RESOURCES/research_methods/qualitat.htm

This website provides the University of British Columbia's directory of online articles on qualitative data analysis.

http://bama.ua.edu/~wevans/content/ppp/ppp_menu.htm

This website provides links to different sites on content analysis.

23

Computer-Assisted Qualitative Data Analysis (CAQDAS)

Tanya Serry and Pranee Liamputtong

CHAPTER OBJECTIVES

In this chapter you will learn:

☐ what computer-assisted qualitative data analysis is and is not

☐ about the functions of CAQDAS

☐ about the benefits and cautions of CAQDAS

☐ how to optimise the use of CAQDAS in qualitative research

KEY TERMS

CAQDAS

Qualitative data analysis

Theory-builders in CAQDAS

INTRODUCTION

In the modern world we are living in, computers have extensively affected our lives, and not surprisingly, this is the case when we do research. For qualitative research, as in other fields of research, the use of computers has gained increasing prominence in both data collection and data analysis.

Computer-assisted qualitative data analysis software (CAQDAS), a term first coined by Lee and Fielding (1991), refers to specifically designed programs (of which there are many) that can take over a substantial amount of the manual labour involved with analysing your data (see CHAPTERS 5, 6, 7, 8, 22). In this chapter we will briefly discuss some of the key functions available via computer-assisted data analysis. We will also describe how we have adopted this software in our own research, along with the circumstances when we have decided not to use it. We do not present a step-by-step approach to using computer programs (see Bryman 2008; Gibbs 2007 for such detail), nor do we promote any one program over another. As Bryman (2008, p. 566) notes, there is 'no industry leader' with regard to computer-assisted qualitative data analysis software options.

> **CAQDAS:** Software specifically designed to offer a highly efficient data management system for storing, coding, organising, sorting and retrieving data.

WHAT IS CAQDAS?

Throughout this chapter we have adopted the acronym CAQDAS since it is widely used. However, you may find the equivalent terms 'Qualitative Data Analysis Software' or QDAS used in certain publications (König 2004). Computer-assisted qualitative data analysis software can take over a substantial amount of the manual labour involved with analysing your data. In this way, it is extremely time-efficient. In particular, it can search, organise, sort and annotate your data. More recently developed CAQDAS programs can store and manage audio and visual data as well as textual data. As such, computer-assisted qualitative data analysis programs can be a valuable asset to your research experience.

As with any software, the program is only as good as the user. Although many of the physical, administrative and clerical tasks involved in qualitative research can be efficiently managed by this software, the rigour of organising, processing and interpreting data remains the province of the researcher (see CHAPTER 1). For example, Bryman (2008, p. 565) suggests that the computer 'takes over the physical task of writing marginal codes, making photocopies of transcripts or field notes, cutting out all chunks of text relating to a code, and pasting them together'. Computer-assisted qualitative data analysis programs can relieve the qualitative researcher from the stereotyped notion that sticky tape, scissors and an empty lounge room floor are all you need for the cutting up and reorganising vast amounts of paper in order to work with your data.

It is important to emphasise that although many researchers limit their use of computer-assisted qualitative data analysis software to data management, a variety of programs can also be used to support theory-building by visualising the various relationships that have been coded in your data. We describe specific functions throughout this chapter.

CAQDAS is a useful tool that can facilitate your qualitative research activity by:

☐ efficiently managing and organising your data

☐ allowing easy retrieval of data such as codes and text content

☐ supporting theory-building (not available in all CAQDAS programs)

☐ acting as a valuable adjunct to the qualitative research process.

What CAQDAS is not

Those who are not overly familiar with qualitative data analysis itself will often say that they 'use' a particular computer-assisted qualitative data analysis software to 'analyse' their data. Such a statement reflects a misinterpretation of how CAQDAS is and is not used. Computer-assisted qualitative data analysis can be a valuable adjunct, assisting researchers to find, categorise and retrieve data or text more quickly than a manual search would. Nevertheless, it cannot analyse data on its own (Gibbs 2007; Bryman 2008; Minichiello et al. 2008). Gibbs (2007, p. 122) reinforces the fact that 'the actual analytic ideas have to be produced by you, the researcher'. As such, we caution against comments such as 'using a CAQDAS to analyse data' because experienced qualitative researchers and reviewers will be alerted to the fact that you lack knowledge about the nature of data analysis in qualitative research (see CHAPTER 22).

> **Qualitative data analysis:**
> Data analysis in qualitative research is an ongoing, cyclical process that occurs from the very beginning of the research itself.

Using computer-assisted qualitative data analysis software can make qualitative analysis easier, more accurate, more reliable and more transparent, but the program will never do the reading and thinking for you. CAQDAS has a range of tools for producing reports and summaries, but the interpretation of these is down to you, the researcher (see Gibbs 2007, p. 106 for a summary of cautions about using CAQDAS).

One of the other risks we have found when using computer-assisted qualitative data analysis is an incorrect assumption that coding equates with analytical reasoning, particularly when the coding is well ordered. We assert that in much qualitative research coding (manually or using computer-assisted qualitative data analysis software) is an early stage step in the analytical process and should be seen as a precursor to the construction of your categories and themes (see CHAPTER 22).

CAQDAS cannot:

☐ analyse your data

☐ generate analytical reports

☐ be a substitute for the reasoning and intellectual rigour required of the researcher.

CAQDAS PROGRAM OPTIONS

There have been several computer packages that qualitative researchers have used (see website references and reflections about various computer-assisted qualitative data analysis programs at the end of this chapter). Before the early 1990s, Ethnograph was the best-known and most widely used software. Since then, other programs have been developed. NUD*IST (Non-numerical Unstructured Data Indexing Searching and Theorizing) became very popular in the 1990s, and later on was developed into QSR NUD*IST Vivo, referred to as NVivo (Bryman 2008). At present, NVivo8 is the most recent version from the QSR team and many qualitative researchers have used the program for their qualitative research. (See Bryman 2008, chapter 23 for detailed step-by-step use of NVivo; see also Gibbs 2002; Bazeley 2007; Gibbs 2007; Lewins & Silver 2007.)

According to Gibbs (2007, p. 107), at present there are three CAQDAS programs that are often used by qualitative researchers: Atlas.ti (now in version 6), MAXqda (the latest version is MAXqda2007) and NVivo8 (this is the latest version). All three have features in common:

- They can transfer text and display it.
- They are able to construct code lists as a hierarchy.
- They permit the researchers to retrieve texts that have been coded.
- They allow the examination of coded texts in the context of the original data.
- They permit the writing of memos that can be linked to codes and data.

Recently, we have also come across a new data analysis package called QDA Miner (v. 3.2) (<www.provalisresearch.com>), which is a software package for coding, annotating, retrieving and analysing documents and images. It claims to provide an easy-to-use model for qualitative data analysis along with having in-built capacity for quantitative analysis as well. NVivo8 also has the facility to work with visual images, documents and media clips.

Tips for choosing the right CAQDAS for your project

- Familiarise yourself with the CAQDAS packages and make your choice based on knowing that the program will be adaptable for what you need it to do. For example, if you are using media clips, your choice of CAQDAS will be restricted.
- Become as familiar as you can with the various functions and features of the program.
- Having said that, sometimes the best way to learn any software package is to simply start using it. In this case it is wise to assume that on your first few attempts at using CAQDAS with your data, you may not be using the program to capacity. You may also find you need to stop and restart. Factor this time into your research schedule. The long-term benefits of optimal use of your CAQDAS should be worth the short-term loss of time.
- Check what support options are available to you for the CAQDAS. Is the HELP function written in a user-friendly manner? Is there access to technical support?
- Find resources in colleagues, friends or even chat rooms that use the CAQDAS you have chosen. We have found sharing and despairing (at times) extremely useful.
- If possible, attend a workshop to help you get started with your CAQDAS.

CAQDAS FUNCTIONS

General features

As a starting point, we have compiled a list of ways that computer-assisted qualitative data analysis software can support your qualitative research. We have compiled this list from Weitzman and Miles (1995), König (2004), Seale (2005) and our own experience. Our list comprises three key sections that depict the general features of CAQDAS. These are storage features, code-and-retrieve features, and assistance with analysis. The first component primarily reflects the clerical aspects of any CAQDAS.

STEPS AND STRATEGIES FOR STORING AND MANAGING YOUR DATA

- entering storing data (including transcripts, journal entries, memos and field notes)
- using CAQDAS to edit and revise your data as needed
- organising storage of all data; typically with back-up function.

CODE-AND-RETRIEVE FEATURES

- coding—such that ideas or concepts are linked to named codes
- recording your memos—in order to support the conceptual leaps made from your raw data (Birks et al. 2008)
- retrieval functions—the ability to locate particular segments of data for closer inspection, including searching for codes, words, combinations of codes and Boolean searches (Weitzman & Miles 1995)
- linking your data to other relevant segments to form categories, clusters, sets, attribute features and themes.

ASSISTING WITH ANALYSIS

- performing content analyses
- displaying data visually, such as a graph, matrix or model
- assistance with theory-building
- assistance with the process of drawing conclusions
- reflecting the transparency of your research.

Code-and-retrieve

Most of the well-known CAQDAS programs are based on the code-and-retrieve theme (Bryman 2008; Minichiello et al. 2008). They enable researchers to code texts while working at the computer and to retrieve the coded text. Bryman (2008, p. 571) tells us that when he used CAQDAS in his work on the Disney Project he carried out the following steps:

1   He read through the interviews both in printed form and in the Document viewer (in the NVivo program).
2   He then developed some codes that were relevant to the documents.
3   He went back into the document and coded them using NVivo.

DOING RESEARCH

Using CAQDAS to code-and-retrieve

We provide an example from our own research experience as new users of CAQDAS. We present the example in diagrammatic form in Figure 23.1 below, as a way of tracking our journey developing familiarity and skill with CAQDAS.

Figure 23.1: Diagrammatic representation of the processes we undertook to 'code-and-retrieve' using CAQDAS

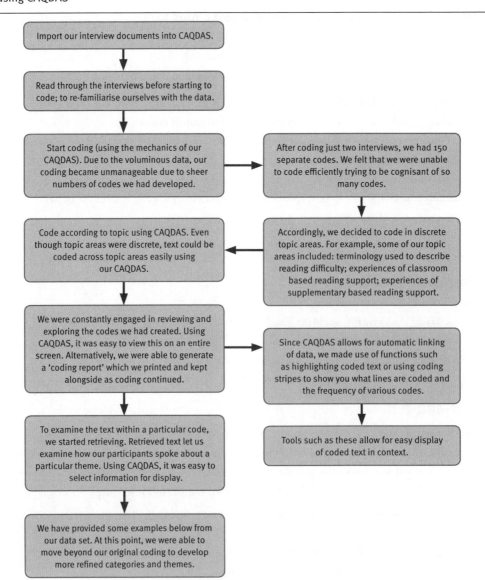

Import our interview documents into CAQDAS.

Read through the interviews before starting to code; to re-familiarise ourselves with the data.

Start coding (using the mechanics of our CAQDAS). Due to the voluminous data, our coding became unmanageable due to sheer numbers of codes we had developed.

After coding just two interviews, we had 150 separate codes. We felt that we were unable to code efficiently trying to be cognisant of so many codes.

Code according to topic using CAQDAS. Even though topic areas were discrete, text could be coded across topic areas easily using our CAQDAS.

Accordingly, we decided to code in discrete topic areas. For example, some of our topic areas included: terminology used to describe reading difficulty; experiences of classroom based reading support; experiences of supplementary based reading support.

We were constantly engaged in reviewing and exploring the codes we had created. Using CAQDAS, it was easy to view this on an entire screen. Alternatively, we were able to generate a 'coding report' which we printed and kept alongside as coding continued.

Since CAQDAS allows for automatic linking of data, we made use of functions such as highlighting coded text or using coding stripes to show you what lines are coded and the frequency of various codes.

To examine the text within a particular code, we started retrieving. Retrieved text let us examine how our participants spoke about a particular theme. Using CAQDAS, it was easy to select information for display.

Tools such as these allow for easy display of coded text in context.

We have provided some examples below from our data set. At this point, we were able to move beyond our original coding to develop more refined categories and themes.

In our work exploring perceptions from parents and educators regarding children with reading difficulty, we undertook a series of steps using CAQDAS. It is important to note that planning the steps shown in Figure 23.1 did not occur at the outset. In many ways, the process of coding and categorising itself was one of trial and error in order to ensure that our data would be optimally managed by our CAQDAS. We argue that this flexibility is well worth it for both the novice and the experienced qualitative researcher.

You will see that despite using CAQDAS, we still had to read and reread transcripts, develop our codes and reflect constantly on our data. Nevertheless, the use of CAQDAS assisted greatly with coding efficiency, visual analysis of data and retrieving coded material in a timely and economical way.

DOING RESEARCH

Retrieved data

As an example from the research mentioned above, we have retrieved items that we coded as 'developmental co-morbidities' under a broad category exploring what educators believed underpinned severe reading difficulty. The steps to retrieve the data are quick and easy. Here are the comments that we coded accordingly. You will note that the CAQDAS we used automatically tells us the percentage of the transcript that each statement made. It also tells us who made each comment as well as providing a hyperlink back to the statement in the original transcript. We have changed the names for the sake of anonymity.

Soula: 0.55% coverage

...little lass that I've got at the moment, she's had a lot of other difficulties. She's got vision difficulties, speech delay. She's very immature.

Jenna: 0.50% coverage

The children that are presenting with severe difficulty have got other learning issues already identified that have already been recognised.

Fiona: 0.43% coverage

...if they've got other issues like it might be sight, hearing, developmental delay, a few things like that...

Although we have not demonstrated it here, we were able to use the retrieval function further to determine whether factors such as years of teaching experience or particular educational role influenced the nature of our participants' responses.

Tanya Serry and Pranee Liamputtong

Assistance with theory-building

Although CAQDAS has been primarily used as a code-and-retrieve tool (Seale 2005), both Gibbs (2007) and Seale (2005) mention that more recent programs have also attempted to provide researchers with analytic procedures that support the generation and testing of theory.

Theory-builders in CAQDAS: This means that the CAQDAS will have various in-built tools that help researchers to make comparisons and develop some theoretical ideas.

These programs offer different facilities such as conceptual mapping to help researchers examine relationships between codes and categories from text. Often these facilities are referred to as '**theory-builders**' (Seale 2005, p. 202). Importantly, this capacity within various programs does not mean that the program itself can build theory on its own. Rather, the CAQDAS will have various in-built tools that help researchers to make comparisons and develop some theoretical ideas.

For example, models that display relationships between codes and memos can assist your conceptual theory-building (Gibbs et al. 2002). Certain CAQDAS programs will create models drawn from the stored data according to your specific instructions. As an example, we have created a model based on our data that maps the views of a particular subset of educators in our cohort regarding issues they raised about a particular treatment to help struggling readers (Figure 23.2). We were attempting to analyse what this subset of educators thought about the treatment beyond the treatment itself. We created models exploring other subsets of educators from our study such that we were able to begin to build theory on factors that influenced various groups of educators' views about the treatment. We found the visual representation of the models using our CAQDAS was powerful in the process of theory-building; acting as a springboard for us to ask further questions of our data.

Figure 23.2: A model we created from our CAQDAS that was used to support our theory-building

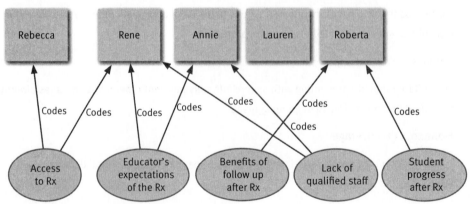

N.B.: Rx is an abbreviation for the treatment program referred to by our participants.

Benefits of CAQDAS

Computer-assisted qualitative data analysis software offers a highly efficient data management system for storing, coding, organising, sorting and retrieving data. As we mentioned above, more recent programs now have the facility to manage data well beyond word-processed documents. Such features widen the scope of many who may find CAQDAS useful to their research. Tanya was recently involved in a training program for new or aspiring users of NVivo8. It was interesting to note the breadth of research fields represented at the workshop. People working in areas such as art history, tourism, advertising and law were all present.

It is essential that users of computer-assisted qualitative data analysis programs have realistic expectations of the program of choice. Although this sounds like an obvious statement for any type of computer software, we want to emphasise this point. The benefits of any program are only as good as the user's analytical thinking, expertise with the program itself, and decision-making. We would encourage anybody who is contemplating using CAQDAS to gain as much familiarity and skill as possible with the program of choice before launching into serious use. For example, Tanya attended a training workshop and sought input from colleagues who are already familiar with the NVivo range before applying computer-assisted qualitative data analysis software to her own data.

Tanya has found the capacity for recent CAQDAS programs to manage documents such as published articles, policy statement and newspaper clips particularly useful. To illustrate an example from her own work, Tanya now imports key published articles (according to the research topic at hand) into NVivo8 and codes these in the same way as she codes interview data. She has found this feature greatly assists the interpretation of her data. Moreover, the efficiency of writing up results is greatly enhanced because everything is stored and accessed in the one location. To reiterate, however, these benefits are only as effective as your analytical processing of your data.

Cautions about CAQDAS

Although many users of computer-assisted qualitative data analysis programs maintain that the computer packages have helped them with data analysis, a number of authors report reservations about the use of CAQDAS. Fielding and Lee (1998) and Gibbs (2007) argue that there is a sense of being distant from the data when using CAQDAS, and that those who use paper-based analysis would feel they are closer to the words of their participants. This may be because many of the early computer-assisted qualitative data analysis programs did not make it easy for researchers to move back and forth between the data to examine the context of coded or retrieved text. Recent programs have allowed this, but many researchers still wish to be closer to their data and hence CAQDAS will limit that closeness.

Tanya Serry and Pranee Liamputtong

As we have pointed out earlier, a computer-assisted qualitative data analysis program does not, and cannot, assist with decisions about coding or the interpretation of findings (Weitzman & Miles 1995; Bryman 2008). We are warned by Minichiello and colleagues (2008, p. 252) that 'the computer does not replace the analytical thinking processes underpinning "interpretive" research'. Computer programs cannot 'develop propositions from the data', or tell the researchers that there are different theories they can apply. Any theoretical framework the researchers will use has to be introduced by the researchers themselves.

Another reservation is that the code-and-retrieve process of CAQDAS may result in a fragmentation of the textual materials (Weaver & Atkinson 1995; Gibbs, 2007). Hence the narrative flow of the data may be lost (Bryman 2008). Context is crucial in qualitative research (Bryman 2008; Liamputtong 2009). Decontexualisation of the data may also occur because of the fragmentation process of coding text into chunks that are then retrieved and grouped into related fragments (Buston 1997; Fielding & Lee 1998). Computer-assisted qualitative data analysis programs then may not be suitable for certain types of qualitative data. From their experience, Catterall and Maclaran (1997) argue that CAQDAS is not appropriate for focus group data because the code-and-retrieve function results in a loss of the communication and interaction process, which is essential in the focus group method (see CHAPTER 4).

For some data analysis, particularly grounded theory (see CHAPTER 7), the use of computer packages for data analysis is a real problem (Glaser 2003). This is because, as Holton (2007, p. 287) makes clear, 'the coding process in classic grounded theory is not a discrete phase but rather an intricate and integral activity woven into and throughout the research process'. Coding in grounded theory requires a much more rigorous method of data analysis than what computer-assisted qualitative data analysis packages such as NVivo8 can offer.

Some qualitative researchers (see Stanley & Temple 1995; La Pelle 2004; Ryan 2004) argue that the coding and retrieval features can be done through powerful word-processing software such as Word for Windows (through the Find function). So researchers may not need to go through a lengthy period of becoming familiar with the operations of CAQDAS. La Pelle (2004, p. 86) tells us she has found that the built-in functions of Microsoft Word 'serve admirably for many qualitative research projects' and they do not require programming skill. Often she prefers to use Word to do many basic data analysis functions.

> I have used Microsoft Word to analyze text from key informant interviews, focus groups, document reviews, and open-ended survey questions, among other sources of data. I use Word functions such as Table, Table Sort, Insert File, Find/Replace, and Insert Comment to do this work. Projects have ranged in size from short simple tasks to complex multiyear research endeavours that involved more than two hundred interviews, more than two thousand pages of transcribed texts, and more than two hundred codes. (La Pelle 2004, p. 86)

CAQDAS: TO USE OR NOT TO USE

Many students and researchers have raised the question of whether they should use computer-assisted qualitative data analysis programs with data analysis. We have suggested several concerns that many qualitative researchers have discussed. However, Bryman (2008, p. 567) has this advice to students and researchers. If you have a small number of cases in your research, it may not be worth the time and trouble learning to master new software. It may also be too expensive for your personal purchase. But if you have a free access or a site licence to the software, you may like to try. If you plan to use it in future research, it may be worthwhile taking the time to learn. Learning new software gives you useful skills that you can make use of in the future. Many of Pranee's postgraduate students take this position.

Our own thoughts on this are that computers can be very useful as adjuncts to qualitative research; CAQDAS can provide efficiencies in data analysis process. But we also argue that computer programs are not always required, nor do they solve many of the central problems of qualitative research. Personally, Pranee remains ambivalent about the role of technology in helping qualitative researchers analyse their data, on the grounds that computer packages cannot do this for us with the thoroughness that we require. Holton (2007, p. 287) says it clearly: 'Experienced classic grounded theorists continue to await a "package" that can replicate the complex capabilities of the human brain for conceptualization of latent patterns of social behaviour.' You can guess then that Pranee does not really use any computer package to do her data analysis. Although she has done CAQDAS training and agrees that it can be useful for many research projects, Pranee works closely with her data by using coloured pens and highlighters, and word-processing to cut and paste the data (see also CHAPTER 22). In contrast, Tanya has used CAQDAS more routinely, but is acutely aware of the importance of the foundational thinking that is required to conduct rigorous and worthy qualitative research.

SUMMARY

In this chapter, we have discussed issues relating to the use of computer-assisted data analysis. We have suggested that CAQDAS can be useful for many qualitative research projects. There are many CAQDAS programs that researchers may wish to use and it is the matter of what you feel most appropriate to your research. Despite the many benefits of CAQDAS, there are some cautions that we must consider. One of the crucial aspects of using CAQDAS is that the software does not do the data analysis for you. It only assists you in doing your data analysis. Hence many qualitative researchers have argued for the non-use of CAQDAS programs. We hope that the discussions in this chapter will help you to decide and consider your own preference in doing qualitative data analysis.

Tanya Serry and Pranee Liamputtong

TUTORIAL EXERCISES

1   In the qualitative studies referenced below, some researchers have chosen to use CAQDAS while others have not. Read one from each group of articles and take careful note of the following issues:
    — How was data storage and management described?
    — How was the code-and-retrieve process managed?

2   Do you think that CAQDAS was beneficial or justified when it was used? Why/Why not?

3   Do you think the use of manual coding and retrieving was justified? Why/Why not?

4   Would you have done anything differently if you were one of the authors? Justify your responses.

PAPERS USING CAQDAS

Marshall, J., Goldbart, J. & Phillips, J. (2007). Parents' and speech and language therapists' explanatory models of language development, language delay and intervention. *International Journal of Language & Communication Disorders*, 42(5), 533–55.

Williamson, P., Koro-Ljungberg, M. E. & Bussing, R. (2009). Analysis of critical incidents and shifting perspectives: Transitions in illness careers among adolescents with ADHD. *Qualitative Health Research*, 19, 352–65.

PAPERS NOT USING CAQDAS

Lasser, J. & Corley, K. (2008). Constructing normalcy: A qualitative study of parenting children with Asperger's Disorder. *Educational Psychology in Practice*, 24(4), 335–46.

Bailey, R.L, Stoner, J. B., Angell, M. E. & Fetzer, A. (2008). School-based speech-language pathologists' perspectives on dysphagia management in the schools. *Language, Speech & Hearing Services in Schools*, 39(4), 441–450.

SOFTWARE OPTIONS

The versions documented in the websites were the latest releases at the time of publication of this book. It is likely that there will be updates as programs are revised, refined and enhanced. We have listed the CAQDAS programs alphabetically because we do not advocate the use of any specific CAQDAS.

‹www.quarc.de/software_overview_table.pdf›

Provides a useful table comparing the functionality of six CAQDAS packages. This may help you decide which program or programs will be appropriate for your research.

AnnoTape: ‹www.quarc.de/software_overview_table.pdf›

Atlas.ti: ‹www.atlasti.com/de›

Ethnograph 6.0: ‹www.qualisresearch.com›

HyperResearch 2.8: ‹www.researchware.com/hr›

MAXQDA: ‹www.maxqda.com›

NVivo8: ‹www.qsrinternational.com›

NVivo8 superseded NUD*IST 6.

QDA Miner 3.2 ‹www.provalisresearch.com/QDAMiner/QDAMinerDesc.html›

This CAQDAS is specifically designed to incorporate mixed methods

FURTHER READING

Bazeley, P. (2007). *Qualitative data analysis with NVivo*, 3rd edn. London: Sage Publications.

Bryman, A. (2008). *Social research methods*, 3rd edn. Oxford: Oxford University Press.

Gibbs, G. R. (2007). *Analyzing qualitative data*. London: Sage Publications.

Kelle, U., Prein, G. & Bird, K. (1995). *Computer-aided qualitative data analysis: Theory, methods and practice*. Thousand Oaks, CA: Sage Publications.

La Pelle, N. (2004). Simplifying qualitative data analysis using general purposes software tools. *Field Methods*, 16(1), 85–108.

Marshall, H. (2002) Horses for courses: Facilitating postgraduate students' choice of Computer assisted Qualitative data analysis Systems (CAQDAS), *Contemporary Nurse*, 13(1), 29–37. Available online at < www.contemporarynurse.com/13.1/13-1p29.htm>.

Richards, L. & Morse, J. (2007). *Read me first for a user's guide to qualitative methods*, 2nd edn. Thousand Oaks, CA: Sage Publications.

WEBSITES

www.lynrichards.org

> *This website allows you to download a copy of* Up and Running in NVivo. *The author described this handbook to be useful 'If you need further help in moving from learning software to getting going in your own project…' See the following three websites.*

www.uk.sagepub.com/richards

http://caqdas.soc.surrey.ac.uk

http://sophia.smith.edu/~jdrisko/Qualitative.PDF

www.soc.surrey.ac.uk/caqdas

> *This site is the CAQDAS Networking Project at Surrey University.*

www.qualisresearch.com

> *Qualis Research Associates for the Ethnograph.*

www.scolari.co.uk

> *This is a Scolari: Sage Publications Software for CAQDAS programs.*

www.provalisresearch.com

> *A new data analysis package called QDA Miner (v. 3.2).*

24

Data Analysis in Quantitative Research

Jane Pierson

CHAPTER OBJECTIVES

In this chapter you will learn:

☐ about the purpose of data analysis in health research

☐ about considerations in selecting data analysis procedures

☐ about the use of procedures to examine differences between two or more measures of central tendency

☐ about the use of procedures to examine relationships between two or more sets of measures

KEY TERMS

ANOVA

Chi-square test

Correlation coefficient

Degrees of freedom

Descriptive statistics

Inferential statistics

Interval data

MANOVA

Multiple regression analysis

Nominal data

Ordinal data

Ratio data

t-test

STATISTICS IN HEALTH RESEARCH

Descriptive statistics include measures of central tendency such as means, median (50th percentile) or mode (most frequently occurring score), and measures of dispersion (e.g. the standard deviation and the range).

Inferential statistics include various procedures commonly referred to as statistical tests.

Statistical significance: Whether or not an outcome is statistically significant is established by using a statistical test to decide whether the outcome is likely to be due to chance, or to be real.

Quantitative health research involves the measurement of health phenomena (see chapters in PART III). The resulting data are commonly summarised and analysed using statistics. Descriptive statistics are used to summarise data, and inferential statistics to analyse data. **Descriptive statistics** include measures of central tendency (e.g. the mean and the median), and measures of dispersion (e.g. the standard deviation and the range). **Inferential statistics** include a variety of procedures that are commonly referred to as statistical tests. While these tests differ from each other in terms of their specific characteristics, they all have essentially the same purpose, which is to determine whether or not a particular outcome of a research study is statistically significant (see also CHAPTER 25).

Statistical significance

Establishing whether or not an outcome has **statistical significance** is accomplished by using a statistical test to decide whether the outcome is likely to be due to chance or to be real. To appreciate what is meant by chance in this context, consider the (hypothetical) study summarised in Table 24.1. This study was a randomised controlled trial (see CHAPTER 15) that examined the effectiveness of a new drug in lowering blood pressure (BP), in those who suffer from hypertension (high blood pressure).

Table 24.1: Mean diastolic blood pressure (BP) and standard deviation (in brackets), pre and post treatment

Group	Treatment	Control (placebo)
Pre-treatment BP (mmHg)	100.25 (8.76)	98.04 (8.94)
Post-treatment BP (mmHg)	86.25 (7.97)	96.17 (9.09)

In this study, participants were randomly assigned to one of two groups: treatment or control, with 24 participants per group. Before the commencement of the treatment phase of the trial, each participant's BP was measured and the mean diastolic BP was calculated for each group. While it could be expected that the means would be similar before the treatment phase began, it would not be expected that these means would be exactly the same (or at least this would not happen very often). This is because individuals differ from each other and there are different individuals in the groups. However, random assignment to groups means that they should be effectively equivalent to each other, so any difference between them before treatment comes about just by chance. While the means for the two groups at the conclusion of the treatment phase are, again, not the same as each other, the difference between them now reflects both chance and any action of the drug. See also CHAPTER 15.

A statistical test allows the determination of the probability of obtaining an effect (which in this case can be thought of as the difference between the group's means after treatment), by chance. If the probability of obtaining the effect by chance is relatively high, it is concluded that the effect is due to chance. If, however, the probability of obtaining the effect by chance is low, it is concluded that the effect is real, that is, it is statistically significant. (In this example a real effect is one that is due to the drug being effective in lowering diastolic BP.) The probability of getting an effect by chance is considered to be low if it is equal to or less than a criterion probability value. While this value (the alpha level) may be one of a range of values, it is conventionally set at .05 (which corresponds to a probability of occurrence by chance of 5 times in 100). So if a statistical test determines that the probability of getting an effect by chance is equal to or less than .05, it can be concluded that the effect is statistically significant (i.e. real). If the probability of getting the effect by chance is greater than .05, it is concluded that the effect is not statistically significant (i.e. due to chance).

Conducting a statistical test involves calculating the value(s) of a statistic, which can be thought of as standing for the effect(s). The probability of obtaining the calculated value of the statistic by chance is then determined. If this probability is equal to or less than the alpha level, the effect is deemed to be statistically significant. If the probability is higher than the alpha level, the effect is deemed not to be statistically significant. See also CHAPTER 25, which deals with reading statistical data.

CHOOSING STATISTICAL TESTS

As noted above, there is a large variety of statistical tests that can be employed in the analysis of quantitative data. Thus deciding which statistical test is appropriate is often viewed as being somewhat complex. In practice, however, there are just two key criteria that need to be considered when choosing a statistical test: the characteristics of the study design, and the characteristics of the data that are collected during the study.

Study design characteristics

The first study design characteristic that needs to be considered when choosing a statistical test is whether it is experimental, quasi-experimental or correlational. Broadly speaking, experimental and quasi-experimental designs look for differences between sets of measures (for two or more groups or two or more conditions), while correlational designs look for relationships between two or more sets of measures. Experimental designs involve random assignment to groups, while in quasi-experimental designs the groups are naturally occurring or are formed on the basis of pre-existing characteristics of the participants. Designs where the same participants are observed under two or more conditions, or at two or more time-points (within subjects or repeated measures designs), can be considered as special cases of experimental designs, where each participant serves as their own control.

For both experimental and quasi-experimental designs, the study design characteristics that need to be considered when choosing a statistical test are the number of independent variables, the number of levels of each independent variable, whether measures are repeated or not across the levels of each independent variable, and the number of dependent variables. In practice, all this comes down to deciding how many groups or conditions are to be compared with each other, whether the measures (or scores) that are to be compared come from the same participants (or from matched pairs), or from different participants, and how many characteristics were measured (for each group or for each condition). For correlational designs, the study design characteristic that needs to be considered when selecting statistical procedures is the number of variables (i.e. the number of sets of measures). See chapters in PART III.

Data characteristics

For both experimental/quasi-experimental designs and correlational designs, the characteristic of the data that is important in the choice of statistical test is related to the level of measurement (i.e. to the properties of the measurement scale) that is used for data collection. There are four types of measurement scales, and therefore four levels of measurement: nominal, ordinal, interval and ratio (see also CHAPTERS 11, 13). The points on a nominal scale correspond to categories that are different from each other, but cannot be ordered with respect to each other (e.g. the response categories yes, no, don't know). The points on an ordinal scale can be put in order with respect to each other, but the intervals between each of the points are not necessarily equal to each other (e.g. a rating scale with the points strongly disagree, disagree, neutral, agree, strongly agree). On an interval scale the intervals between each of the points are all equal to each other but the scale does not have a fixed zero point that corresponds to the absence of what is measured (e.g. the Celsius and Fahrenheit temperature scales). A ratio scale has both equality of intervals and a fixed zero point that corresponds to the absence of what is measured (e.g. scales for measuring weight).

For interval and ratio data, another characteristic, which is related to the degree of normality of the data, needs to be considered when deciding on the appropriate statistical test. Normality is assessed in terms of the extent to which the distribution of the scores (i.e. the distribution of the study data) approximates that of the normal distribution (for further discussion of the normal distribution and related concepts see, for example, Grove 2007).

The study that is summarised in Table 24.1 can serve as an example of the use of the criteria (outlined above) for choosing statistical tests. This study used an experimental design. There are two groups to be compared with each other and, as participants were randomly assigned to one or other of the two groups, the scores that are to be compared come from different participants. One characteristic (diastolic blood pressure) has been measured for each member of the two groups. Thus there is one independent variable (Group), which has two levels (treatment and control) and, as there are different participants in the two groups, measures are not repeated across the levels of the independent variable. There is one dependent variable (diastolic blood pressure). The level of measurement is ratio (as blood pressure is measured using a ratio scale), and the distribution of the scores approximates that of the normal distribution. The specifics of the study design, together with the data characteristics, indicate that an independent t-test is the appropriate statistical test for analysing the study's data. The conduct of t-tests is discussed in the next section.

CONDUCTING STATISTICAL TESTS

Experimental and quasi-experimental designs

There are a number of statistical tests that we can use with these designs. These include the t-test, analysis of variance (and of covariance), and multivariate analysis of variance (and of covariance).

THE T-TEST

The **t-test** is used to compare two means with each other, to establish if there is a statistically significant difference between them. There are several versions of the t-test. These include the one-sample t-test, used to compare a mean for a single set of scores with another mean, and the two-sample t-test, used when there are two sets of scores, the means of which are to be compared with each other. As the latter are the most commonly encountered t-tests in health research, the following discussion will be limited to them. Two-sample t-tests are appropriate when there is one independent variable with two levels, and one dependent variable, when the level of measurement is interval or ratio, and the data are approximately normally distributed. When the two sets of scores come from different participants (i.e. measures are not repeated across the levels of the independent variable), the independent t-test (unpaired t-test) is used. When the two sets of scores come from the same participants or from matched pairs (i.e. measures are repeated across the levels of the independent variable) the related t-test (paired-samples t-test) is used.

> A **t-test** is used to compare two means with each other, to establish if there is a statistically significant difference between them.

A two-sample t-test is conducted by calculating a value of the t statistic that stands for the effect, which can be thought of as the mean difference (i.e. the difference between the means for the two groups or the difference between the means for the two conditions). The probability of obtaining the calculated value of t (and therefore the effect) by chance, with the applicable **degrees of freedom** (df)[1] is then determined. If this probability is equal to or less than the alpha level set for the test, then the t value (and therefore the effect) is deemed to be (statistically) significant. If the probability is greater than the alpha level, then the t value (and therefore the effect) is deemed to be not significant. As the conduct of the two types of two sample t-tests is essentially the same, only the use of the independent t-test is described in what follows.

> **Degrees of freedom:** Value(s) that represent the number of scores that are free to vary associated with a test statistic. Used to calculate the statistical significance of a test statistic.

As discussed above, the study summarised in Table 24.1 has one independent variable with two levels, and one dependent variable. The level of measurement is ratio and the data are approximately normally distributed. The two sets of scores come from different participants. An independent t-test is therefore applicable. For the post-treatment data summarised in Table 24.1, the calculated value of t is 4.02. With 46 degrees of freedom, the probability of getting this t value by chance is .0002. As this value is lower than the alpha level (.05) set for the test, this t value, and therefore the effect (the mean difference), is significant.

Strictly speaking, the distribution of the data should be approximately normal for t-tests to be used. This is because the value of t (which is calculated using the data) will be distorted if the distribution of scores is non-normal. However, so-called parametric tests, including the t-test, and the various types of analysis of variance (see below), are regarded as being robust to violations of the assumption of normality, and therefore the calculated value of the statistic is little affected, unless the deviation from normality is extreme (Maxwell & Delaney 2003; Elliot & Woodward 2006). Therefore t-tests can be used for most interval and ratio data.

When the data's non-normality is such that t-tests would be inappropriate, a non-parametric equivalent can be used. Non-parametric statistics are sometimes called distribution-free statistics, because they do not have assumptions about the characteristics of the distribution of the scores. There are two non-parametric statistical tests that are equivalent to (two sample) t-tests. The Mann-Whitney U-test is used when different participants provide the two sets of scores, and the Wilcoxon signed-rank test is used when the two sets of scores come from the same participants (or from matched pairs). The conduct of these tests is essentially equivalent to that of the corresponding parametric t-tests. These non-parametric statistical tests are also used when the level of measurement is ordinal, and two medians are to be compared with each other. While detailed discussion of these and other non-parametric statistics is beyond the scope of this chapter, there are a number of texts that provide such discussion (see Siegel & Castellan 1988; Gibbons 1993).

ANALYSIS OF VARIANCE

Analysis of variance (ANOVA) is one of the most commonly used data analysis procedures. An ANOVA is used to compare the means of three or more sets of scores to determine if there are statistically significant differences between them. An ANOVA can be used when the level of measurement is interval or ratio, and the data are reasonably normally distributed. As there are a number of types of ANOVA, the decision about which one is appropriate depends on consideration of the study design. When there is one independent variable (factor) with three or more levels, and one dependent variable (measure), a one-way ANOVA is appropriate. When the three or more sets of scores come from different participants (i.e. measures are not repeated across the levels of the independent variable) the independent variable is termed

An **ANOVA** is used to compare the means of three or more sets of scores to determine if there are statistically significant differences between them.

a between-subjects factor, and the one-way ANOVA for independent groups is used. When the three or more sets of scores come from the same participants, the independent variable is termed a within-subjects factor and the design is referred to as a within-subjects (repeated-measures) design. For such designs, a one-way ANOVA for repeated measures is used.

A one-way ANOVA is conducted by calculating a value of the *F* statistic that stands for the effect, which can be thought of as the set of differences between the means (for the three or more groups, or the three or more conditions). Thus a single ANOVA simultaneously compares all of the means with each other. The probability of obtaining the calculated value of *F* (and therefore the effect) by chance, with the applicable degrees of freedom[2] is then determined. If this probability is equal to or less than the alpha level set for the test, then the value of *F* (and therefore the effect) is (statistically) significant. If the probability is greater than the alpha level, then the value of *F* (and therefore the effect) is not significant. Therefore a significant value of *F* indicates that there is at least one statistically significant difference between the means. However, the test does not allow for a decision to be made as to which of the mean differences are significant. To determine which of the differences are likely to be significant, follow-up tests, referred to as post-hoc tests, are required (see Grove 2007).

As the processes involved in the conduct of the two types of one-way ANOVA are essentially the same, only an example of the application of the one-way ANOVA for independent groups is given in what follows. The (hypothetical) study summarised in Table 24.2 compared three different diet plans, each of which aimed to produce weight loss, in those who are overweight. There were 30 participants in each group. The data shown in Table 24.2 relate to the amount of weight lost by participants, over a 2-month period.

Table 24.2: Mean amount of weight loss and standard deviation (in brackets) for Plan A, Plan B, and Plan C participants

Group	Plan A	Plan B	Plan C
Weight loss (kg)	8.12 (2.38)	6.75 (1.97)	6.87 (2.01)

This study has one independent variable (one between-subjects factor): Group, which has three levels: plan A, plan B, and plan C, and one dependent variable: Weight loss. The level of measurement is ratio and the data are approximately normally distributed. The sets of scores come from different participants. A one-way ANOVA for independent groups is therefore appropriate. For the data summarised in Table 24.2, the calculated value of *F* is 3.81. With (2, 87) degrees of freedom, the probability of getting this value of *F* by chance is .026. As this probability is lower than the alpha level (.05) set for the test, this value of *F* (and therefore the effect) is significant. It can be seen from Table 24.2 that the mean for Plan A was significantly higher than the means for Plans B and C, which were similar to each other. It is therefore likely that the mean for Plan A is significantly different from those for both Plan B and C. However, a post-hoc procedure would be needed to confirm this.

As discussed above (in the context of the t-test), the distortion of the value of *F*, due to non-normality of the data, is only of consequence when the departure from normality is very marked. It is also relatively robust to another assumption about the data, that is, homogeneity of variance (Maxwell & Delaney 2003). Therefore the ANOVA can be used for most interval or ratio data. When the data's non-normality is such that an ANOVA would be inappropriate, a non-parametric equivalent can be used. The Kruskal-Wallis test is used when different participants provide the three or more sets of scores. The Friedman test is used when the three or more sets of scores come from the same participants. These non-parametric statistics are also used when the level of measurement is ordinal, and three or more medians are to be compared with each other. Detailed discussion of these non-parametric tests is provided in Siegel and Castellan (1988) and Gibbons (1993).

When there are two or more independent variables (factors), and one dependent variable (measure), the level of measurement is interval/ratio, and the data are reasonably normally distributed, a factorial ANOVA is used. Each factor can have two or more levels. Measures on each factor can be non-repeated or repeated and therefore designs can be fully independent, fully within subjects, or mixed (repeated measures on one or more factors and non-repeated measures on one or more factors).

The (hypothetical) study summarised in Table 24.3 investigated the effectiveness of a new therapy in reducing asthma symptomology for people diagnosed with allergic asthma and people diagnosed with idiopathic asthma. The therapy was administered at two times of day, 8 a.m. and 8 p.m. Thus there are two factors: Type of asthma, which has two levels, allergic and idiopathic, and Time of day, which also has two levels, a.m. and p.m. Forty-eight asthmatic participants were divided into two groups on the basis of whether their asthma was allergic or idiopathic. Members of each group were then randomly assigned to one of the two administration times, with 12 participants in each of the resulting four groups. After one month of therapy, peak flow volumes were measured for each participant. (Note that higher peak flow represents a lower degree of asthma symptomology.) As there are two independent variables (factors), the level of measurement is ratio, the data are approximately normally distributed, and there are different participants in each of the groups, a factorial ANOVA (for independent groups) is applicable.

Table 24.3: Mean peak flow volume (L/min) and standard deviation (in brackets)

Type of asthma	Allergic	Idiopathic
a.m. administration	468.33 (63.94)	424.17 (44.81)
p.m. administration	426.67 (44.99)	478.33 (56.22)

A factorial ANOVA yields a number of values of F (and the probability of obtaining each of these by chance, with the corresponding degrees of freedom). These values of F correspond to the main effect for each factor and to the interaction(s) between factors. In the context of the study summarised in 24.3, the main effect for Type of asthma corresponds to the difference between the overall means for allergic and idiopathic, and the main effect for Time of day corresponds to the difference between the overall means for a.m. and p.m. Thus the overall mean for allergic asthma is 447.50 and the overall mean for idiopathic asthma is 451.25, and the overall mean for a.m is 446.25 and the overall mean for p.m. is 452.50. The means that correspond to the interaction effect are those shown in Table 24.3. In this study, neither of the main effects was significant (i.e. there was no statistically significant difference between the overall means for Type of asthma or for Time of day). There was, however, a significant interaction between Type of asthma and Time of day. Thus for allergic asthma, a.m. administration was more effective than was p.m. administration; while for idiopathic asthma, p.m. administration was more effective than was a.m. administration. Note that interactions can take on a number of forms, according to which means differ from each other.

A modified version of ANOVA, namely analysis of covariance (ANCOVA), is used when a (continuous) extraneous variable is systematically confounded with the levels of the independent variable(s). A confounding variable of this kind is referred to as a covariate. (Such a situation is not uncommon when quasi-experimental designs are used.) To appreciate the nature of this situation, consider the following (hypothetical) study. This study aims to compare the level of strain (as measured by the carer-strain index) experienced by people who are acting as a carer for a person with one of three different medical conditions: severely disabling osteoarthritis, cancer, or dementia. Thus the independent variable of interest is the care-recipient's condition. The confounding variable is the carer's health status (as measured by the MOS SF 36). Hence there are apparent differences in the health status of participants in the three groups. Those caring for a person with cancer have, on average, poorer health status than do those caring for a person with osteoarthritis, and those caring for a person with dementia, have, on average, the poorest health status. As it has been established through previous research that level of carer strain (irrespective of the health condition(s) experienced by the care-recipient) increases with declines in the health status of the carer, any differences in this study may be due only to the differences in health status of the three carer groups, or due to both differences in health status and differences in the nature of the care-recipient's condition. In order to allow the means for carer strain to be compared, to look for differences that are attributable to the differences in the nature of the care-recipient's condition, an ANCOVA is needed.

In simple terms, an ANCOVA identifies, and puts to one side, differences between the groups that are due to the covariate. It therefore adjusts for any influence of the covariate, and allows for the examination of differences between the groups that are due to the variable of interest. In the example study described above, the variable of interest is the care-recipient's condition. The ANOVA removes the effects of the covariant, which for this example is the carer's health status, and allows the groups to be compared to look for differences that are due to the differences in the health condition of the care-recipient.

MULTIVARIATE ANALYSIS OF VARIANCE

Multivariate analysis of variance (MANOVA) is used when there are two or more dependent variables (measures), each of which is measured on an interval or ratio scale, and where the set of scores for each is reasonably

A **MANOVA** is used when there are two or more dependent variables, each of which is measured on an interval or ratio scale.

normally distributed. A MANOVA can be applied to designs where there are one or more independent variables, each with two or more levels.

A MANOVA determines if there is a significant difference(s) between the groups, in terms of scores on a 'new' dependent variable, which can be thought of as an amalgam of the scores (for each participant) on the two or more dependent variables. If the groups are shown to differ significantly by the MANOVA, separate ANOVAs, one for each dependent variable, are then used. These tests are used to determine if the groups are significantly different for only one of the dependent variables, or for some or all of the dependent variables. When there are two or more dependent variables and one or more covariates (as described above) a multivariate analysis of covariance (MANCOVA) is usually used. Further consideration of MANOVA and MANCOVA is beyond the scope of this chapter. Likewise, profile analysis, which is recommended as an alternative to MANOVA when there are two or more dependent variables and repeated measures on one or more of the independent variables, will not be covered here. Further discussion of these procedures can be found in a number of texts (e.g. Tabachnick & Fidell 2006).

DOING RESEARCH

A research student's dilemma

For her thesis project, Elaine Tsang examined self-perceived quality of life among older Chinese people living in Melbourne. She recruited older Chinese people who were living in the general community, and older Chinese people who were living in a Chinese-specific aged care facility. The study used a mixed-methods approach. Participants were interviewed, and measures were made of a number of characteristics that are likely to be associated with quality of life. These measures included the MOS SF 36, the Geriatric Depression Scale, and a life satisfaction index. Each participant also completed a questionnaire that collected basic demographic information, including age (in years). Elaine had intended to compare the measures for the two groups, but when she examined the demographic data, she realised that such comparison would be problematic. This was because the people living in the aged care facility were older, on average, than were the people who were living in the community. She knew that previous research had shown that quality of life declines with advancing age, and realised that this meant that any difference between the groups could be due to the difference in age, rather than to differences in measures of self-perceived quality of life. Elaine was concerned about this problem, until she consulted several statistics texts. She learnt from them that she could use analysis of covariance (specifically multivariate analysis of covariance) to analyse her data. This analysis would adjust for the age difference between the two groups, and allow her to compare the two groups on the measures that related to quality of life. For more discussion of the methods used in this study, see Tsang et al. (2003).

Correlational designs

For correlational designs, there are a number of statistical procedures that researchers can use. These include chi-square tests, correlation coefficients, and multiple regression.

CHI-SQUARE TESTS

There are two types of **chi-square test**, which are used when the level of measurement is nominal and the data therefore consist of frequency counts for categories. These are the one-way chi-square test, which is sometimes called the goodness of fit test, and the two-way chi-square test. While the one-way chi-square test has some applications in health research, it will not be considered further here. The two-way chi-square test is commonly encountered in health research. It is used when there are two variables and it determines if the relationship (association) between the two variables is statistically significant. The data are arranged in a contingency table, which shows the frequency counts (the observed frequencies) for a number of categories. Such a contingency table is shown in Table 24.4.

> A **chi-square test** is used when the level of measurement is nominal and the data therefore consist of frequency counts for categories with different names.

Table 24.4: Number of female and male participants in each response category

	Yes	No
Females	55	45
Males	38	62

The table summarises participants' responses to two of a number of questions on a (hypothetical) survey. The first question asked participants to specify their gender. Responses were measured on a nominal scale, which had two points: male and female. The second question asked participants whether or not they had visited a GP in the preceding 6 months. Again responses were measured on a nominal scale with the points yes and no. On the basis of their responses, participants were classified into one of four categories. It can be seen from the table that there does appear to be some degree of association between the variable Gender, and the variable GP visits. Thus more females say yes than no, while more males say no than yes. In other words, more females than males report having visited a GP. As there are two variables and the level of measurement is nominal, a two-way chi-square test is appropriate.

The two-way chi-square test compares the observed frequencies for the categories, with the expected (on the basis of chance) frequencies for these categories. It is conducted by calculating a value of the chi-square statistic, which stands for the effect (the association between the two variables). The probability of obtaining the calculated value of chi-square (and therefore the effect) by chance, with the applicable degrees of freedom[3] is then determined. If this probability is equal to or less than the alpha level set for the test, then the chi square value (and therefore the effect) is (statistically) significant. If the probability is greater than the alpha level, then the chi-square value (and therefore the effect) is not significant.

For the data summarised in Table 24.4, the calculated value of chi-square is 5.81. With 1 df, the probability of getting this chi-square value by chance is .016. As this probability is lower than the alpha level (.05) set for the test, this chi-square value, and therefore the effect (the association between Gender and GP visits), is deemed to be significant. Thus it can be concluded that significantly more females than males reported having visited a GP in the preceding 6 months.

For designs where the two-way chi-square test is applicable, it is possible for each variable to have any number of levels (i.e. points of the scale, or categories). Hence a contingency table can have an unlimited number of both rows and columns. In practice, however, there are limits on these numbers. This is partly because a prerequisite for the use of the chi-square test is that no more than 50 per cent of the expected frequencies can be less than 5. As the expected frequencies are based on the observed frequencies, this essentially limits the number of categories. A multivariate analysis (based on chi-square) can be used to examine associations between three or more variables, all of which are measured using a nominal scale. This procedure, namely multi-way frequency analysis, is yet to come into common use in health research. Discussion of this analysis is provided by Tabachnick and Fidell (2006).

CORRELATION COEFFICIENTS

Correlation coefficients summarise the degree of relationship (correlation) between variables. In the case of bivariate correlation, these variables correspond to two sets of measures (or scores) for one group of participants. The value of a correlation coefficient ranges from +1 (a perfect positive correlation), through 0 (no correlation), to −1 (a perfect negative correlation). There are a number of correlation coefficients, two of which are commonly encountered in health research. These are the Pearson correlation coefficient and the Spearman correlation coefficient. The former is used when the level of measurement (for both variables) is interval or ratio. The latter is a non-parametric statistic that is used when the level of measurement is ordinal or where one variable is measured using an ordinal scale and one is measured using an interval or ratio scale (in which case the higher scale is reduced to an ordinal scale). While these correlation coefficients are descriptive statistics, they can also function as inferential statistics (i.e. as statistical tests, effectively), as it is possible to establish the probability of obtaining the value of the coefficient by chance. It is therefore possible to decide if the effect that the coefficient summarises (i.e. the correlation between the two variables) is statistically significant (i.e. real) or due to chance. As the use of the two coefficients for this purpose is essentially the same, only one example, using the Spearman coefficient, is given here.

The data shown in Table 24.5 is (hypothetical) data from a study that assessed basic life support (BLS) knowledge, and BLS performance, for a group of 12 health care professionals

Correlation coefficients are used to summarise the degree of relationship (correlation) between variables.

who had recently completed BLS training. Both knowledge and performance were measured on a 5-point scale, where 1 equated to very poor and 5 equated to very good. As there are two variables and the level of measurement is best characterised as ordinal, a Spearman correlation coefficient is the appropriate statistic. It can be seen from the table that there appears to be some degree of positive correlation between the two sets of scores. The calculated value of the Spearman correlation coefficient for these data is .45. When the number of participants, and therefore the number of pairs of scores (N) is 12, the probability of getting this value by chance is .13. As this probability is higher than the applicable alpha level (.05), this value of the correlation coefficient, and therefore the effect (the correlation), is deemed to be not significant.

Table 24.5 Ratings of BLS knowledge and performance

BLS knowledge	5, 4, 3, 4, 2, 3, 4, 2, 3, 3, 4, 3
BLS performance	4, 3, 3, 3, 1, 2, 2, 4, 3, 2, 4, 2

MULTIPLE REGRESSION

A **multiple regression analysis** is a multivariate procedure that can be used when there are three or more variables and the level of measurement is interval or ratio. It assesses the degree to which scores for a subset of these variables predict scores for another variable in the set. The degree of predictability is related to the degree of correlation between the predicted variable and its predictor variables. For example, measures could be made, for a group of participants, of blood cholesterol level, blood sugar level and level of physical activity, and the degree to which scores on these variables predict scores on a measure of body mass index could be assessed using a multiple regression analysis.

> **Multiple regression analysis:** A multivariate procedure that assesses the degree to which scores for a subset of variables predict scores for another variable in the set.

Multiple regression and associated procedures, such as logistic regression (where the predicted variable is nominal), are being used increasingly in health research. While these procedures are beyond the scope of this chapter, discussion is provided in a number of texts (see e.g. Tabachnick & Fidell 2006; Grove 2007).

SUMMARY

In this chapter, I have outlined the nature and the purpose of inferential statistics (i.e. statistical tests). I have explained that the purpose of these tests is to determine if the outcome of a research study (an effect) is statistically significant (real) or due to chance. Two broad classes of effects (mean differences, and correlation) have been distinguished. The meaning of statistical significance has been explained. The study design and data characteristics that need to be considered when selecting statistical tests have been outlined. I have also provided details of the use of a number of statistical procedures to analyse quantitative data. These procedures include t-tests, ANOVA (and its variants), chi-square tests, and correlation coefficients. Non-parametric statistics have been briefly discussed, as have some multivariate procedures. These discussions, I hope, have provided readers with better understandings about data analysis in quantitative research.

TUTORIAL EXERCISES

1   The (hypothetical) study summarised in Table 24.6 examined the effect of alcohol consumption on video-game playing performance. Each of the participants played the video-game under two conditions: sober, and under the influence.
    —   Describe the design of this study.
    —   What was measured in this study and what level of measurement was used?
    —   Which statistical test could be used to analyse these data?

Table 24.6: Mean number of points scored on the video-game and standard deviation (in brackets) when participants were sober and when they were under the influence of alcohol

State	Sober	Under the influence
Number of points	932.50 (18.32)	921.92 (15.13)

2   The (hypothetical) study summarised in Table 24.7 examined the relationship between degree of overweight and cholesterol level.
    —   Describe the design of this study.
    —   What was measured in this study and what level of measurement was used?
    —   What statistic could be used in the analysis of this data?

Table 24.7: Body mass index (BMI) and blood cholesterol level

BMI	30, 28, 25, 26, 32, 31, 29, 26, 27, 28, 29, 30
Cholesterol level (mmol/L)	7.5, 6.5, 6.0, 6.5, 8.5, 7.5, 5.5, 5.5, 6.0, 7.0, 8.5

3   Locate a journal paper online, which reports a study in which ANOVA was used for data analysis.
    —   Describe the design of this study.
    —   What was measured in this study and what level of measurement was used?
    —   For one of the ANOVAs, what was/were the value, or values of F? What were the associated degrees of freedom? What was/were the probability or probabilities of obtaining the result by chance?

NOTES

1   For an independent groups t-test, the degrees of freedom are equal to (the number of participants in the first group plus the number of participants in the second group) minus 2. For a related t-test, the degrees of freedom are equal to the number of participants minus 1.

2   There are two types of degrees of freedom associated with a value of F. The first is equal to the number of levels minus 1, and the second is equal to the total number of participants minus the number of levels (for an independent groups ANOVA).

3   For the two-way chi-square, the number of degrees of freedom is equal to (the number of rows multiplied by the number of columns) minus 1.

FURTHER READING

Elliot, A.C. & Woodward, W.A. (2006). *Statistical analysis quick reference and guide book with SPSS examples*. Thousand Oaks, CA: Sage Publications.

Grove, S.K. (2007). *Statistics for health care research: A practical workbook*. Edinburgh: Elsevier Saunders.

Maxwell, S.E. & Delany, H.D. (2003). *Designing experiments and analysing data: A model comparison perspective*. Mahwah, NJ: Lawrence Erlbaum Associates.

Tabachnick, B.G. & Fidell, L.S. (2006). Usi*ng multivariate statistics*, 5th edn. Boston, MA: Pearson/Allyn & Bacon.

WEBSITES

There are a number of websites that provide calculators that can be used to conduct statistical tests, as well as providing information about these tests. Such websites can be found by typing the name of the test (along with the word 'calculator') into an internet search engine (e.g. t-test calculator; chi-square calculator).

25

How to Read and Make Sense of Statistical Data

Paul O'Halloran

CHAPTER OBJECTIVES

In this chapter you will learn:

☐ to identify key issues when interpreting descriptive and inferential statistics

☐ to describe the differences between statistical and clinical significance

☐ to describe how clinical significance can be determined

☐ how to calculate effect size

☐ how to read results sections of quantitative research papers or mixed methods papers with confidence

KEY TERMS

ANOVA

Clinical significance

Confidence intervals

Degrees of freedom

Descriptive statistics

Effect size

Inferential statistics

p value

Statistical significance

Type I & II statistical error

INTRODUCTION

I have been teaching research methods at undergraduate and postgraduate levels for some 10 years now. One of the biggest challenges students report when reading research papers is interpreting the results sections of quantitative research papers. Indeed, many students will comment that they just bypass the results section entirely and go straight to the discussion section of a research paper. While you can often get the gist of the results in the opening paragraphs of the discussion, the problem with this approach is that the consumer (student, practitioner or other researcher) of the research article must assume that the researcher has interpreted the results without bias and correctly. Unfortunately, this is not always the case. As readers will discover in this chapter, even researchers can occasionally make errors when interpreting their results. The ability to interpret quantitative results is important even if you choose not to do any of your own research. As a practitioner, you will need to be able to read research papers for information regarding the latest techniques and so on, and be able to make some preliminary distinctions between good and poor research papers.

The main purpose of this chapter is to provide foundation knowledge and skills for you to be able to read and interpret statistical data, whether it be your own that you obtained in a small research project or more typically what you are reading in refereed research articles.

Where to begin

Students often comment that when reading a results section of a research article they become overwhelmed by the mass of figures, whether these are in a table, in text, or in a graph or some other pictorial representation of the data. One of the first questions students ask is 'Where do I begin?' One of the best places to begin when reading quantitative data is with the summary or **descriptive statistics**.

Descriptive statistics include measures of central tendency such as means, median (50th percentile) or mode (most frequently occurring score), and measures of dispersion (e.g. the standard deviation and the range).

READING AND INTERPRETING DESCRIPTIVE STATISTICS

Descriptive statistics include measures of central tendency such as means, median (50th percentile) or mode (most frequently occurring score) (see CHAPTER 24). However, these figures are difficult to interpret unless we also have some measure of dispersion, such as variance, standard deviation or semi inter-quartile range. These measures of dispersion give the reader an indication of how much variation there is in scores. In other words, they provide an indicator of how representative or reliable the mean or median is. Let's illustrate this with a data set from my own study, which examined the effect of a walking program on mood in persons with type 2 diabetes (O'Halloran 2007).

Paul O'Halloran

Interpreting descriptive statistics: illustrative example

TYPE 2 DIABETES AND MOOD STUDY

Background to the study: Physical activity plays an important role in the management of type 2 diabetes. Yet people with type 2 diabetes are less active than the general population (Dunstan et al. 2002). One of the challenges when working with people with type 2 diabetes is to have people make long-term changes to their physical activity patterns. It has been suggested that how individuals feel immediately after a bout of physical activity can affect the likelihood of maintaining involvement in the activity (e.g. Biddle et al. 2000). Thus my study determined if sessions of walking led to improvements in mood in persons with type 2 diabetes. Specifically, using the Subjective Exercise Experience Scale (SEES: McAuley & Courneya 1994), the mood of 24 previously sedentary people with type 2 diabetes was measured before and after 20- and 40-minute bouts of group walking. The data that relate to the Positive Well-Being scale of the SEES are presented in the table below.

Table 25.1 Pre- and post-exercise Positive Well-Being scores: Means, standard deviations, and effect sizes

SEES subscale	Pre-exercise		Post-exercise		
	M	SD	M	SD	d#
Positive Well-Being					
20-minute walk	17.7	5.2	21.8	5.1	.79
40-minute walk	18.4	5.8	22.1	5.4	.67

 # Effect sizes were calculated by subtracting mean scores at the post-exercise assessment from the pre-exercise mean and then dividing this by the pooled standard deviation.

As you can see in the table, there are a number of figures in columns under the symbol headings M, SD, and d. Often one of the first things that students become confused by is the symbols that are used by researchers. I have included some commonly used statistical symbols in Table 25.2.

Table 25.2: Statistical symbols

Name	Symbol (examples)	Definition
Mean	M	The arithmetic mean
Median	MD	The point that cuts the distribution in half
Mode	Mode	The most common value
Variance	s^2	Squared average amount of variability around the mean
Standard deviation	sd, s, SD	Average amount of variability around the mean

Effect size	ES, d, r, q, g, w, f, f^2	A measure of change or association that is independent of sample size
Correlation coefficients	r	Measures the degree of relationship between 2 variables
Confidence interval	CI	An expected range in which the population value will be found at a given level of probability
t-test	t	Compares differences between 2 means
ANOVA	F	Compares differences between 3 or more means
Regression	R^2	The prediction of the relationship between 2 or more variables
Chi-square	x^2	Measure of association when categorical data are used

M is one of the symbols that is used for mean. *SD* is used to represent standard deviation and *d* for Cohen's (1992) effect size. We will be referring to effect size a little later when we discuss key considerations when interpreting inferential statistics.

From Table 25.1 we can ascertain that the mean for Positive Well-Being was *M* = 17.7 before the 20-minute walk and *M* = 21.8 after the walk. In order to obtain a sense of the meaning of these figures, it is important to have some understanding of the scale on which they were measured. From the measures section of this paper (O'Halloran 2007), we would be able to see that people rated their moods on the SEES on a 7-point scale (from 1 = not at all to 7 = very much so), and since each mood subscale has four items, the minimum score must be 4 and the maximum 28. Thus higher scores are indicative of a more positive mood. A score of around 18 on the Positive Well-Being scale before exercise would suggest that people were feeling relatively positive before exercise. That people scored 21.8 after exercise indicated that they were feeling even better after exercise. However, we cannot confidently reach conclusions about data on the basis of descriptive statistics only. This requires reference to inferential statistics, which will be discussed shortly. Once these steps have been followed, the next thing to examine is the standard deviation or average amount of variation around the mean.

As can be seen in Table 25.1, the standard deviation for the 20-minute walk on the Positive Well-Being scale was *sd* = 5.2 before exercise and *sd* = 5.1 after exercise. This suggests that scores varied on average about 5 from the means. Given this value relative to the means of 17.7 and 21.8, the standard deviation suggests a relatively small amount of variation between scores and that the mean may be representative of scores at each assessment. Had the standard deviation being around the 15–20 mark rather than 5, these conclusions would have been less certain. Students often ask, 'When should I worry about the size of the standard deviation?' There is no definitive answer here, but common sense is often a useful guide (e.g. how large is it relative to the mean and what does this degree of variation indicate given the scale used to measure the variable of interest?).

Confidence intervals

A further important indicator of the representativeness of the mean, particularly with respect to a population, is that of **confidence intervals**. Whenever a mean is calculated using a sample, there is always going to be a degree of error. One way of ascertaining the amount of error is to calculate the confidence interval of the mean. While confidence intervals are actually an **inferential statistic**, I will discuss them here because they provide one of the best indicators of the representativeness of the mean. A common practice for researchers is to calculate the 95 or 99 per cent confidence intervals for reported means (Edwards 2008). The 95 per cent confidence interval, for example, enables us to be able to conclude that we are 95 per cent certain that the true population mean lies between two values.

Confidence interval:
An important indicator of the representativeness of the mean, particularly with respect to a population.

Inferential statistics
includes a variety of procedures that are commonly referred to as statistical tests.

Returning to the type 2 diabetes and mood study (O'Halloran 2007), if the 95 per cent confidence intervals for the Positive Well-Being scale means for the 20 minutes of walking were calculated, it would appear in text as follows: for the Pre-exercise mean (M= 17.7, 95% CI 15.6–19.9) and for the Post-exercise mean (M= 21.8, 95% CI 19.6–23.9). The way that this would be interpreted is that we are 95 per cent certain that the true population mean of the Positive Well-Being scale before exercise for people with type 2 diabetes lies somewhere between 15.6 and 19.9 and after exercise it lies somewhere between 19.6 and 23.9.

The narrower the range in these values, the more representative the mean. Conversely, a wide range in these values suggests that the sample mean does not give a useful guide to the population value. The relatively small range of values reported above suggests that the mean values of 17.7 before exercise and 21.8 after exercise are fairly good representations of the true population value. If you would like to read more about confidence intervals and how to calculate and interpret them, please consult Polgar and Thomas (2007) or Edwards (2008).

Where does that leave us? Making sense of descriptive statistics in the type 2 diabetes and mood study

For illustrative purposes, we examined descriptive statistics relating to a measure of Positive Well-Being in persons with type 2 diabetes before and after a 20-minute session of group walking. Reference to the mean values and standard deviations in the summary table (Table 25.1) in conjunction with an understanding of what scores represent, suggested that people scored fairly high on Positive Well-Being before exercise and even higher after exercise (although we could not yet determine if this was statistically significant). Further, we were able to conclude that variation among the mean scores was small to moderate at both assessment points, and the calculation of confidence intervals enabled us to determine that these mean scores were a reasonable indicator of population values. Our next key question is, are the differences between these mean scores before and after exercise 'real' or did they occur by chance? This determination requires inferential statistics.

Steps for reading/making sense of descriptive statistics

1 Go to summary table or figure.

2 Examine measures of central tendency (e.g. means, medians).

3 Examine method section for a description of the measure/questionnaire etc. to understand what scores represent.

4 Examine measures of dispersion (e.g. variance, standard deviation).

5 Look for confidence intervals.

READING AND INTERPRETING INFERENTIAL STATISTICS

While descriptive statistics provide a useful starting point for reading and interpreting quantitative statistics, they only tell part of the story. They provide a preliminary overview of what was found in a particular study and might give some clues about the effect of a treatment or intervention or the relevance of associations between factors in health settings. But descriptive statistics alone are not sufficient for reaching valid conclusions about what seem to be meaningful associations or treatment effects. This is because whenever you are using a sample to make inferences about what is happening in a population (generally the essence of quantitative research), there is going to be some error involved with issues such as sampling and the measurement of the variable of interest. For example, in the type 2 diabetes and mood study discussed above, although the mean mood scores were based on 24 people with type 2 diabetes, we are hoping to make inferences about what is happening in the wider population of previously sedentary persons with type 2 diabetes. In other words, we aim to generalise our findings to the wider population of persons with type 2 diabetes. However, there would have been a degree of error involved in activities in the study such as the measurement of mood. Thus there are two major potential interpretations for the increase in Positive Well-Being scores from before the 20-minute walk (M =17.1) to after the walk (M = 21.8). One interpretation is that the walk seemed to have some positive influence on mood in these people and the other is that the means differed due to chance. Inferential statistics enable us to determine which one of these explanations is more probable or likely to be correct (see Chapter 24).

Interpreting outcomes from inferential tests

As discussed in CHAPTER 24, there are a host of *inferential tests* such as t-tests, chi-square, ANOVA and so on that can be used to determine the probability of an outcome being due to chance. The appropriateness of these tests will be determined by questions such as the number of groups, type of data, and the studies of particular research question(s) (Polgar & Thomas 2007). However, all inferential tests produce a common value that is crucial in the interpretation of findings. That particular value is the **p value**. This *p* value is the first thing to examine when reading inferential statistics, because it represents the probability of the 'null hypothesis' being true. That is, the probability of no treatment effect (i.e. no effect of exercise on mood in persons with type 2 diabetes) or no association between two variables (such as the consumption of green leafy vegetables and colon cancer). The way that this hypothesis-testing works is that if the probability of there being no treatment effect or no association is low enough this suggests that there must indeed be a treatment effect or association. While this sounds a little convoluted, mathematically you can only assess the probability of a null effect (e.g. no difference between means or treatment effects), not the probability of a treatment effect being true. If this *p* value is equal to or below a predetermined value (i.e. the alpha level, α) set by researchers before the study, we say that the finding is **statistically significant**. If on the other hand the *p* value exceeds this predetermined value set by researchers, we say that the finding is not statistically significant. This predetermined alpha level is most typically set at .05 or .01 (Cowles & Davis 1982). If an alpha level of $\alpha = .05$ is set, it means that in order for something to be considered statistically significant the probability of it being due to chance must be equal to or below 5 in 100. If an alpha level of $\alpha = .01$ is set, it means that in order for something to be considered statistically significant the probability of it being due to chance must be equal to or below 1 in 100.

p **value:** All inferential tests produce a common value, the *p* value, which is crucial in the interpretation of findings. It is one thing to examine when reading inferential statistics.

Statistical significance is established by using a statistical test to decide whether the outcome is likely to be due to chance or to be real.

Interpreting inferential statistics: type 2 diabetes and mood study

Let's examine this in relation to data from the type 2 diabetes and mood study (O'Halloran 2007). In order to examine if walking had an effect on mood in these people, a form of **ANOVA** (see CHAPTER 24) was calculated that enabled the researcher to compare two different levels of a variable or factor (in this case duration of the walks) across time. This two-way repeated Measures ANOVA is able to examine if there are differences over time (i.e. from the pre-exercise assessment of mood to that following exercise), duration (i.e. do average means during the 20-minute walk differ form those in the 40-minute walk?), or between walks of different durations (i.e. the interaction effect that examines if the pattern of change in mood differs between the 20- and 40-minute walks). This analysis produced a single significant finding in relation to Positive Well-Being. Specifically, there was a significant time effect for Positive Well-Being. If you look at the Positive Well-Being means in Table 25.1, average scores were higher at the post-exercise assessments than they were prior to exercise for both the 20-and 40-minute walks. This was reported as follows ($F(1,23) = 25.61, p = .000$). There are several important pieces of information contained in these brackets, which are discussed below.

ANOVA: One of the most common analyses in quantitative data analysis procedures, used to compare the means of three or more sets of scores to determine if there are statistically significant differences.

How to make sense of reported inferential statistics: a step-by-step approach

The following example relates to a form of ANOVA, but the same principles hold true regardless of whether you are reading statistical output from a t-test, correlation coefficient, chi-square, or multiple regression (see CHAPTER 24). There will always be at least three sets of values: a test statistic (in this case $F = 25.61$), some figures in parentheses known as degrees of freedom (in this case (1,23)) and a p value, which is the probability of the null hypothesis being true (in this case $p = .000$). The meaning of each of these values and how to interpret them further is outlined in the two steps below.

STEP 1: LOOK AT THE p VALUE

The thing that most people will examine first is the p value. Remember, this indicates the probability of the null hypothesis being true. While the p was $= .000$ in the type 2 diabetes study, it does not indicate that we can be 100 per cent certain that the null hypothesis is false. This can never be the case in inferential statistics. There is always going to be some probability of the null hypothesis being true. What it does suggest is that the probability of the null hypothesis being true in this example was less than 1 in 1000. It is convention to report to two or three decimal places, so it may have been $p = .00001$ and then rounded to $p = .000$. Therefore in this case, the p value indicates that there was a very low probability of there being no difference between means at the pre-exercise assessment and those at the post-exercise assessment (i.e. the 'null hypothesis' being true). In other words, the probability was so low, well below the predetermined level set by the researcher ($\alpha = .05$), that the finding would be deemed statistically significant. We would therefore conclude that there must be a difference in means between these time-points. It is worth noting that since most statistical tests are calculated using computer programs, exact probabilities are typically reported. But in some research articles, instead of the statistic been reported as ($F(1,23) = 25.61, p = .000$), you may see ($F(1,23) = 25.61, p < .05$) or ($F(1,23) = 25.61, p < .01$). In all cases, this clearly indicates that the result was statistically significant

What if instead of being ($F(1,23) = 25.61, p = .000$), it was ($F(1,23) = 2.61, p = .08$)? This would suggest that the probability of there being no difference between means is now 8 in 100. This is higher than most alpha levels set by researchers, and had this been the case we would have concluded that there was no difference between Positive Well-being means before and after exercise. The finding would have been considered not statistically significant.

STEP 2: EXAMINE TEST VALUES AND DEGREES OF FREEDOM

In addition to examining the p value, it is also important to look at the specific value produced by the test such as $F = 25.61$ in the example above or $t = 8.91$ in the case of a t-test or $r = .7$ in the case of a correlation coefficient. These values refer to different things in different tests, and it is important to have an understanding of what the test is actually calculating (see

CHAPTER 24). At a basic level, typically the larger the value the stronger the effect, whether that be a treatment effect as reflected by differences in means or an association or correlation between variables such as number of physiotherapy sessions attended and flexibility in a knee joint during rehabilitation. In the example reported above in the diabetes study, an F of 25.61 is large. This can be determined by looking at an F table in most books on quantitative statistics (see Schwartz & Polgar 2003).

Degrees of freedom are the values reported in the parentheses or brackets before the test value. In the above example, these degrees of freedom were (1,23). The precise meaning of degrees of freedom will vary across different tests. As well, for some tests such as Pearsons correlation coefficient there will be only one value in these brackets (e.g. r (41) = .7) and for others, such as an ANOVA, there will be two. In all cases, these degrees of freedom refer in some way to the number of scores in a sample that are free to vary. Larger degrees of freedom are typically reflective of larger sample sizes.[1]

Degrees of freedom: Value(s) that represent the number of scores that are free to vary associated with a test statistic. Used to calculate the statistical significance of a test statistic.

The larger the test statistic and degrees of freedom (typically), the more likely you are to have a significant p value.

HOW TO INTERPRET FINDINGS THAT ARE STATISTICALLY SIGNIFICANT

So far we have looked at an illustrative example of how to read and interpret inferential statistics as they relate to whether a finding is statistically significant or not. But it does not end there. There can be a number of potential explanations for results that are statistically significant. These are outlined below.

The finding was *not* due to chance, and it was meaningful

In most cases this is the ideal scenario for researchers and this type of finding is clearly interpretable. Not only is the finding unlikely to be due to chance but it also has some 'real' meaning. This begs the question of how we determine if a finding has some real meaning. There are several indicators of determining whether a finding may be meaningful as well as statistically significant. One is to examine the effect size of a statistic, if reported. **Effect size**, which can be measured in various ways and depends on the particular statistical test that was undertaken (Cohen 1992), is a measure of the strength of a finding (whether that is difference between means or relationships between factors) that is independent of sample size. You might ask why such a measure is important. The reason is that the size of a sample plays a substantial role in determining whether a finding is statistically significant or not. For instance, if you have hundreds or thousands of people

Effect size is a measure of the strength of a finding that is independent of sample size.

in a sample, the study has so much power to detect findings that even very minor differences or relationships can be deemed statistically significant.

Let's illustrate this with an example from a study that asked a sample of more than 350 students whether they thought it was okay for a therapist to tell a client's partner that the client was HIV-positive, even if it meant going against a client's wishes (Collins & Knowles 1995). The researchers asked female (n = 164) and male students (n = 203) to rate this on a 5-point scale from 1 (strongly agree/always) to 5 (strongly disagree/never). Results showed a significant difference ($F(1) = 17.51, p<.001$) between the mean for females ($M = 2.71$) and that for males ($M = 2.11$). However, since it seems that both females and males were undecided on this issue and that scores only differed by .6 on a 5-point scale, it would be difficult to argue that the results were meaningful. The researchers in this study would have been well advised to calculate an effect size, or measure of the differences between these means that did not take sample size into account. The appropriate effect size statistic for comparing two means is Cohen's (1992)

$$d = \frac{M_A - M_B}{\sigma}$$

With this measure of effect size, one mean is subtracted from the other, divided by the standard deviation (the standard of the comparison group is often used or the average standard deviation of the two groups). You will notice that sample size is not included in this calculation. Once this has been calculated, this value can be compared to some criteria that Cohen (1992) developed for interpreting the magnitude of an effect or finding. According to Cohen (1992), a small effect is defined as $d = .20$, a medium effect as $d = .50$, and a large effect as $d = .80$. Examination of the data in Table 25.1 shows that the effects for differences between pre- and post-exercise Positive Well-Being means in the 20-minute ($d = .79$) and 40-minute ($d = .67$) walks were in the medium to large range. Thus this would be one indicator that as well as being statistically significant, these results are also likely to be meaningful.

Another very useful indicator of whether statistical findings are meaningful is **clinical significance**. Clinical significance refers to the practical or applied value of a finding or sets of findings (Kazdin 2003). As such, there are no precise calculations for determining if something is clinically significant. Rather, according to Kazdin (2003), clinical significance can be gauged by factors such as:

Clinical significance:
The practical or applied value of a finding or sets of findings.

1   *Amount of change* as a result of an intervention (can be determined by effect size, or if clients or patients are no longer experiencing problems or symptoms).

2   *Subjective evaluations* from a client or patient regarding the effects of a factor or intervention. That is, do participants from a study report noticeable differences in how they are feeling or functioning, and are these differences noticed by significant others in the person's life?

3   *Social impact*. That is, can the information from the study or a new treatment or intervention have a measurable impact on things such as rates of an illness, days missed at work, or days of hospitalisation?

4   *Comparison*. Here the client or patient is compared with the performance of others such as a normative sample or a patient group. For example, if a physiotherapist developed a new intervention for assisting patients to rehabilitate following a hip replacement, it would be useful to examine not only if there has been a significant improvement in this group's quality of life or some measure of disability but also how these people compare with normative samples on these measures.

The finding was *not* due to chance but it was *not* meaningful

As noted above, findings can occasionally be statistically significant without necessarily being meaningful. That is, the findings are unlikely to be due to chance but they also have little practical significance or meaning. This can occur when you have particularly large sample sizes.[2] This was illustrated above in the study by Collins & Knowles (1995), where relatively minute mean differences in the responses of males and females were found to be statistically significant. There are also cases where a correlation coefficient can be as low as $r = .2$ yet still be significant if the sample size is large enough. The key, as suggested above, is to give an indicator of the meaningfulness of a result such as effect size or clinical significance. When reading statistical findings, it is therefore useful to ask yourself 'has the investigator or investigators provided a measure of effect size or an indicator of clinical significance?' Even if they have not, by referring to the factors that are indicators of clinical significance (Kazdin 2003) you can often get a sense of this yourself. For example, applying these clinical significance criteria to findings in Collins and Knowles's study, it would be fair to conclude that while this gender difference in opinions about disclosing information on HIV status was indeed significant there is little practical or applied value in a difference so small.

The finding was in fact due to chance—an error was made

By its nature, statistical testing is probabilistic. As such, there is always going to be some probability that a mistake has been made. We can, for example, mistakenly conclude that something was statistically significant when this was not the case. This is termed a **Type I error**. The maximum probability of making such an error is equal to the alpha level in the study. If

---

Type I statistical errors occur when researchers mistakenly conclude that a finding was statistically significant when it may be a result of chance rather than being a real difference.

the researcher selected an alpha level of .05, the researcher will mistakenly conclude that a finding is significant a maximum of 5 times in 100. This is why some researchers will adopt a more conservative alpha level such as .01. This means that the probability of a researcher mistakenly concluding that a result is significant will be 1 in 100. You might wonder why researchers do not always go with a more conservative alpha level such as .01.

The reason is that the lower the alpha level, the greater the chance of incorrectly concluding a result to be non-significant. This is termed a **Type II error** and will be discussed below (see also CHAPTER 15).

Therefore, we can summarise this by saying there are two key steps in interpreting findings that are statistically significant.

Type II statistical errors occur when researchers mistakenly conclude that there was no difference, no association and so on when in fact there was.

Steps for interpreting findings that are statistically significant

Step 1. Ask 'how likely is it that the result was due to chance?' In other words, what is the probability that we have made a mistake (i.e. Type I error)? This can be determined by examining the *p* value. Look for confidence intervals.

Step 2. Determine if the finding was meaningful. This can be determined in several ways. This can include examining factors such as the effect size (Cohen 1992), if reported and certainly by looking at indicators of clinical significance.

HOW TO INTERPRET FINDINGS THAT ARE *NOT* STATISTICALLY SIGNIFICANT

Just as there are several explanations for findings that are statistically significant, there is more than one explanation for findings that are not deemed statistically significant. These are outlined below.

The finding was due to chance and was *not* meaningful

This type of finding is generally clearly interpretable. Let's illustrate this by referring to the type 2 diabetes and mood study (O'Halloran 2007) discussed above. In this study, as well as examining the effect of walking on positive mood (i.e. Positive Well-Being), Psychological Distress was also measured before and after the 20- and 40-minute walks. This information is presented in Table 25.3 below.

Table 25.3 Pre- and post-exercise Psychological Distress scores: Means, standard deviations, and effect sizes

SEES subscale	Preexercise		Post-exercise		
	M	**SD**	**M**	**SD**	**d#**
Psychological Distress					
20-minute walk	7.0	4.4	6.1	3.7	−.22
40-minute walk	7.1	3.7	7.0	4.0	−.01

 # Effect sizes were calculated by subtracting mean scores at the post-exercise assessment from the pre-exercise mean and then dividing this by the pooled standard deviation.

Paul O'Halloran

As can be seen in Table 25.3, there is very little difference between pre-exercise and post-exercise means for both the 20- and 40-minute walks. In contrast to the findings regarding Positive Well-Being, there was no significant effect for time for Psychological Distress ($F(1,23)$ = .89, p = .355). Reference to the table shows that the effect size was d =−.22 for the 20-minute walk and d = −.01 for the 40-minute walk. Reference to the criteria supplied by Cohen (1992) suggests the differences between pre- and post-exercise Psychological Distress means were small to very small. Thus by considering these results you could clearly conclude that walking did not seem to influence Psychological Distress in this study.

The finding was due to chance but possibly meaningful

Let's suppose for a minute that the effect sizes for Psychological Distress had been around d=.5 to d=.8 and above. This finding would have been more difficult to interpret as these effect sizes would be indicators of medium to large differences (Cohen 1992). Had this been the case, the correct interpretation would have been that this finding, while seemingly due to chance, is nevertheless potentially meaningful. This can occur quite often, particularly when sample sizes are relatively small, which reduces the probability of being able to detect a true difference (i.e. the test has low power). Therefore it is always worth considering the possibility that non-significant findings could potentially be meaningful. In order to rule this possibility out, it is sensible to examine information such as the effect size for the result and other potential indicators of clinical significance such as whether participants with a physical condition are no longer troubled by symptoms after a treatment or whether their scores on a measure following a treatment place them within a 'normal range'. Another example where you need to be careful in interpreting a non-significant result is where a correlation appears moderate to large (e.g. r = .5 or more) yet not significant. This can also occur when the sample size is low. Once you have examined these indicators of clinical significance, you are able to make an interpretation with some confidence one way or another.

The finding was not due to chance—an error was made

As with findings that are statistically significant, it is also possible to make an error when a non-significant result is produced in a study. This is a Type II error, where the researcher or researchers mistakenly concludes that there was no difference, no association and so on. This is more likely to occur when sample sizes are low and/or a stringent alpha level has been adopted in the study (α < .01). For instance, in some studies alpha levels of .008 or less can be adopted, particularly when researchers are trying to account for multiple comparisons in their study. Such situations reduce the power of the study, therefore making it more difficult to correctly identify a true difference or relationship. As well, a further useful indicator of whether a Type II error has occurred is if the effect size of the statistic is in the medium to high range (Cohen 1992).

Therefore we can summarise this by saying there are two key steps in interpreting findings that are *not* statistically significant.

> Steps for interpreting findings that are *not* statistically significant
>
> **Step 1.** Determine if the finding was meaningful. This can be determined by examining factors such as the effect size (Cohen 1992) and certainly by looking at indicators of clinical significance (Kazdin 2003).
>
> **Step 2.** Determine if a Type II error may have occurred. Examine the sample size in the study and see if the alpha level set by the researchers was low.

WHAT IT ALL MEANS: SOME SIMPLE DECISION RULES FOR MAKING SENSE OF INFERENTIAL STATISTICS

Before the last 20 years or so, interpreting statistical tests was as simple as examining the probability levels and ensuring that a Type I error had not occurred (Schmidt 1996). If a finding was statistically significant, it was interpreted as meaningful, and if not significant, the assumption was made that no effect was present. However, as can be ascertained in the discussion above, there has been a shift to recognising that interpretation of quantitative data cannot rely on the outcome of inferential statistics in isolation (Cohen 1996; Schmidt 1996; Kazdin 2003). Indeed, there are multiple considerations that need to be taken into account when interpreting the outcome of inferential statistics. These include the size of the effect, potential errors in statistical decision-making, the influence of sample size and alpha levels on the power to detect differences, and indicators of clinical significance. These considerations can lead a consumer of quantitative data to feel somewhat confused about how this can all fit together, particularly how statistical and clinical significance influences our interpretations of data. One way of simplifying this is to create some simple decision rules for combining statistical and clinical significance to reach an overall conclusion regarding a result. These are given in Table 25.4.

Table 25.4 Simple decision rules for interpreting inferential statistics

<table>
<tr><td colspan="2"></td><th colspan="2">Statistical significance</th></tr>
<tr><td colspan="2"></td><th>YES</th><th>NO</th></tr>
<tr><th rowspan="2">Clinical Significance</th><th>YES</th><td>**Clear**
Strong evidence for a treatment effect or finding</td><td>**Inconclusive**
Suspend judgment
There is a need for further research (e.g. with larger samples)</td></tr>
<tr><th>NO</th><td>**Inconclusive**
Suspend judgment
Suggests findings may not be meaningful—need for further research</td><td>**Clear**
Strong evidence for lack of a treatment effect or lack of relationship between factors</td></tr>
</table>

Paul O'Halloran

Using the information in this table, we would conclude that the findings regarding the effect of Positive Well-Being and Psychological Distress in the type 2 diabetes and mood study could both be interpreted clearly. For Positive Well-Being, both the 20- and 40-minute walks resulted in significant improvements on this measure and the size of the effects suggested that these improvements could also be clinically significant. Further, there was consistency between statistical and clinical significance in relation to the effect of walking on Psychological Distress. In both cases, neither seemed to be significant (i.e. p was $>$ .05 and the effect sizes were small). On the other hand, in the Colin and Knowles (1995) study, where the difference between males and females with respect to their views on confidentiality of information about HIV status was statistically significant yet seemingly minor in magnitude (i.e. unlikely to be clinically significant), we would conclude that results are inconclusive. The recommendation using these decision rules in Table 25.4 would be to suspend judgment about this finding until confirmation with further research.

SUMMARY

The primary purpose of this chapter was to provide information to help you read and interpret statistical data. I have suggested that the best place to start is with the studies summary or descriptive statistics. With descriptive statistics, it was recommended that as a minimum, it is important to examine the measures of central tendency, such as the mean or median, in conjunction with measures of dispersal such as the standard deviation and confidence intervals if available. This examination will leave you with an indicator of how representative the mean or median is of what is happening in the sample and/or population. As well, these descriptive statistics often provide an overall indicator of how data relate to a study's aims or research questions. For example, the descriptive statistics in the investigation of the effect of walking on mood in persons with type 2 diabetes revealed that walking for either 20 or 40 minutes may have led to an improvement in Positive Well-Being. But before we could make such conclusions with any confidence, I suggested that inferential statistics had to be examined to determine the probability that such findings were not due to chance. Through inspection of the p values from the statistical test that was used to examine the effect of walking on mood, we were able to conclude that is was very unlikely that these improvements in Positive Well-being were in fact due to chance. However, it was emphasised that statistical significance alone is not adequate to interpret results from statistical tests. It is crucial to consider whether findings have any practical or applied value. That is, the potential clinical significance of the finding(s) must be examined. I have argued that it is only by examining statistical and clinical significance in conjunction that we can reach meaningful conclusions from statistical tests. This discussion concluded with a set of simple decision rules that combine statistical and clinical significance.

TUTORIAL EXERCISES

1   When interpreting descriptive statistics, why is it important to examine measures of dispersal as well as the means or medians?

2   Why is it important to examine inferential statistics?

3   What does it mean when a researcher concludes that their findings were statistically significant?

4   What are some of the limitations of relying of statistical significance alone when interpreting statistical data?

5   What conclusions would you reach in interpreting the following sets of results:
   — A researcher found that the difference between a new and old treatment for rehabilitation from a hip replacement was significant. As well, the patients that received the new treatment returned to their usual work and leisure activities substantially earlier than the group receiving the old treatment.
   — A researcher found that the correlation between sessions of treatment in a health setting and recovery time in 1200 patients was significant (r (1199) = .2, p = .021).
   — Researchers found that differences in two treatments for stuttering were not significant in a sample of 18 people who experience stuttering. They calculated an effect size on the number of times that people in each treatment group stuttered and they found that d =.72.

NOTES

1   This is true of statistical tests such as t-tests, correlation coefficients, and outputs from an ANOVA such as interaction effects, where participant numbers feature in the calculations of the degrees of freedom etc. However, with some statistical tests such as chi-square, sample sizes are not used to compute the degrees of freedom (see Edwards 2008).

2   This is not to suggest that large sample sizes are a negative. On the contrary, the larger the sample size the better in terms of power and often in terms of generalisability.

FURTHER READING

Edwards, T. (2008). Research design and statistics: A bio-behavioural approach. Boston, MA: McGraw-Hill.

Kazdin, A.E. (ed.) (2003). *Methodological issues and strategies in clinical research*, 3rd edn. Washington, DC: American Psychological Association.

Phillips, J.L. (2001). *How to think about statistics*, 6th edn. New York: W.H. Freeman & Co.

Paul O'Halloran

Websites

www.statsoft.com/textbook/esc.html#What_is_"statistical_significance"_(p-level)

For further explanation of significance testing.

www.sportsci.org/resource/stats/generalize.html#effect

For discussion of confidence intervals.

www.indiana.edu/~stigtsts/quotsagn.html

For discussion of limitations of significance testing.

www.musc.edu/dc/icrebm/statisticalsignificance.html

For clear definitions of key terms and concepts such as Confidence intervals and type I and type II errors.

26

Presentation of Research Findings: Writing a Qualitative and Quantitative Research Report

Pranee Liamputtong and Nora Shields

CHAPTER OBJECTIVES

In this chapter you will learn:

☐ how to provide discussions on writing up research papers

☐ about commonalities and differences in writing qualitative and quantitative papers

☐ to suggest structures for writing a research paper

☐ about examples from both qualitative and quantitative approaches in writing research papers

INTRODUCTION

Once we have conducted a good piece of research, what shall we do with our interesting and important findings? We need to put our information down on paper. We need to write about it so that our research findings can be disseminated and other people can read and make use of them, whether for improving current health and welfare practices or using them as the basis for developing new research projects. We also have an obligation to our participants to make sure their contributions to our work reach as wide a target audience as possible.

THE NATURE OF QUALITATIVE RESEARCH WRITING

> Writing is an ongoing and socially embedded practice. It is about 'textwork'…or the practice, art, and craft of writing. (Marvasti 2008, p. 613)

Qualitative writing is different from quantitative writing. A quantitative report consists of a concise presentation of the methods and results of the study. Qualitative writing, on the other hand, 'must be a convincing argument systematically presenting data to support the researcher's case and to refute alternative explanations' (Morse 1994b, p. 231; see also Silverman 2000; Oermann 2001; Belgrave et al. 2002; Hansen 2006; Marvasti 2008; Wolcott 2009). Richardson (2003, p. 501) argues that unlike quantitative work, which relies heavily on tables and summaries, 'qualitative work depends upon people reading it. Just as a piece of literature is not equivalent to its "plot summary", qualitative research is not contained in its abstracts. Qualitative research has to be read, not scanned; its meaning is in the reading.'

For this reason, writing that is based on qualitative research, be it a report, article or book, tends to be long. The written report must contain enough detail to tell readers about the research and its findings. So qualitative papers tend to be longer than quantitative writing. There are several reasons for this (Neuman 2006; Liamputtong 2009):

1   Qualitative data are more difficult to condense. Qualitative data contain words, not numbers, and include many quotes and extended case examples.

2   In a qualitative report, detailed descriptions of the research sites and the population under study need to be provided so that readers will have a better understanding of the research setting.

3   Qualitative researchers employ less standardised data collection methods, ways of developing analytic categories, and modes of organising evidence. The methods chosen depend on the conditions of the research site and the researchers' preferences. Hence qualitative researchers need to explain what they did, and why, at greater length.

4   The goals of qualitative studies are to explore new settings and construct new theories. Detailed descriptions of the development of new concepts, their relationships, and the interpretations of evidence need to be provided. This adds to the length of the report.

5   The nature of qualitative data gives the writer freedom to use literary devices to keep the reader's interest and accurately translate a meaning system for the reader. This, again, lengthens the paper.

There are other distinctive characteristics of qualitative writing. This is particularly so in the presentation of research findings. There are three ways that we can write to present the results of our research (Liamputtong 2009). First, the findings are given without comments or interpretations; interpretations can be discussed later on in the discussion section. Second, interpretations can be added up to a point in order to make some connections between lines of evidence; further detail is again provided in the discussion section. Last, the results and discussion of each point may need to go together if an in-depth discussion is required to give meaning to the findings. However, because of the nature of qualitative research, which needs some interpretations to make the findings more meaningful, qualitative writing tends to include discussion throughout (as opposed to the specific 'Discussion' section in quantitative reports). This makes the report's organisational structure more critical for ensuring clarity. Writing a qualitative report therefore requires careful attention to structure and meaning. Writers need to make a special effort to achieve coherence and conciseness (Belgrave et al. 2002; Neuman 2006; Liamputtong 2009; Wolcott 2009).

In qualitative reports, the language is not as objective or formal as in quantitative papers. A writer usually uses the first person (I, we) in describing the research processes and in discussing the findings (Neuman 2006; Liamputtong 2009; Wolcott 2009). Wolcott argues that since the researcher's role is an integral part of qualitative study, descriptive accounts need to be made in the first person. This is what Pranee tends to use in her qualitative research reports, whether these are a journal paper, report or book.

Like quantitative reports, qualitative reports also make use of graphic representations, such as figures, pictures and illustrations. Very often tables are used to describe the major background characteristics of the people under study, but the tables and graphics are used to supplement the discussion, not to replace it (Liamputtong 2009).

One important point we wish to make is that in reporting qualitative findings it is not essential to state the number of people who discuss a particular issue. For example, when you write about the perceptions of infant feeding among Australian mothers, you will not say that four women believe breastfeeding is the best option for newborn infants. You will explain in detail about how these mothers, whatever the number, see breastfeeding. You need to present how the women perceive breastfeeding, and there can be a range of perceptions, but not how many of them perceive each of the perceptions. Some researchers who do not have a good understanding of the nature of qualitative research may demand that you do so. But we suggest that you should adhere to the practice of qualitative research when writing up a qualitative research piece.

Pranee Liamputtong and Nora Shields

THE NATURE OF QUANTITATIVE RESEARCH WRITING

Quantitative research writing often reflects the type of research it is describing: it is quite a standardised affair. Here you are more likely to include tables of numerical data to describe participant characteristics, or to display your overall findings in graphic form. Quantitative research writing is usually written in the third person, although many health-related journals are now encouraging authors to write in the first person, particularly when describing what methods they used and how they were applied. This is similar to how authors of qualitative research write their reports. Although there is a basic framework for presenting the results from any quantitative study, the fundamental point to remember is that you are telling a story to your reader. In this regard, quantitative research writing is similar to qualitative research writing.

One of the major problems with many published reports on quantitative research (particularly clinical research reports) is that the methods used and the results found are often inadequately described. This has implications for the readers. For example, if a report of a clinical trial does not tell you that the person employed to recruit the participants did not know which group the participants were allocated to, you might not believe the results to the same extent as when the authors explicitly state this information. The reason you may not believe the outcomes is that an assessor who is not blind to group allocation is a potential source of bias to the results. So it is very important that you describe your research methods, providing as much detail as possible.

In a positive move to address poor reporting of clinical trials, various groups have taken the initiative of developings guidelines on how to write about this type of research. For example, the CONSORT statement (see CHAPTER 15) is an evidence-based set of recommendations for reporting randomised controlled trials and offers a standard way for authors to prepare the reports of their research findings (Altman et al. 2001). Although the statement focuses on randomised controlled trials, many of its recommendations are relevant and applicable to all types of quantitative clinical research. CONSORT have also recently published a statement for clinical trials of non-pharmological treatments (Boutron et al. 2008).

It is also important when writing a quantitative research report for publication in a health journal to keep in mind who is likely to read your article. Health professionals generally read research reports because they want to be effective clinicians and offer their patients the most up-to-date treatment approaches and management strategies. Most clinicians read journal articles as part of their continued professional development and are 'research consumers'. It can be easy for them to get lost in the technical jargon and statistical analysis of a research report. Writing about your research in a clear and transparent way helps those who read your research to interpret it with greater ease.

You also need to think about why people might read your article. What most readers are interested in is how your work might endorse their approaches to practice or how it suggests ways for them to change their practice. So it is important when writing a quantitative research report that you discuss the implications of your statistical analysis for everyday clinical practice.

If you want clinicians and health professionals to change their practice as a result of your research, you need to tell them in a simple and straightforward way how your analysis applies to them (see CHAPTER 25).

THE STRUCTURE OF RESEARCH WRITING: COMMONALITY AND DIVERGENCE

There are common structures that make the presentation of the findings clear and easy to follow:

- ☐ title
- ☐ abstract or summary
- ☐ introduction
- ☐ research design and method
- ☐ findings or results
- ☐ discussion and conclusion
- ☐ acknowledgments
- ☐ references

Title

It is best to have a title that captures the essence of your text. So you need to provide one that reflects what you write. Sometimes researchers may use a very interesting title to catch the attention of the audiences. Some journals also like the title to include the research design of the study because this can help readers locate literature more quickly and easily.

Abstract or summary

This section needs to be brief but to contain essential information about your paper. When readers read this section, they can immediately see what the paper is about, how you carried out the research and what are the main findings of the study. Structured abstracts are best for quantitative research. A structured abstract includes a series of subheadings (such as research design, participants, method, results, discussion and keywords), and generally the information included under each heading is standardised (Haynes et al. 1990). Writing your abstract using a structured format helps readers find the information they need more easily (Hartley et al. 1996). In qualitative research, you will include essential parts such as we have presented above, but they do not need to be separated by subheadings, though subheadings may be required by particular journals that publish qualitative papers. You need to follow the guidelines of a journal if you wish to write your work for publication.

Introduction

The introduction explains the reasons why you did your research. It indicates the nature, importance and urgency of the research. The emphasis here is typically on relevant previous research. It also emphasises the situation and factors that prompt the proposed project. Evidence from a literature review or a systematic review should be used to explain the exact nature and extent of the health issue that has led to the development of your research. This section is important since it demonstrates how much you understand and how familiar you are with the literature. It also allows you justify the need for your research in a strong and compelling way (see the CONSORT website).

Additionally, many researchers also include in this section the theoretical framework they are using. This is to give readers enough detail about the theory or framework that they use to explain their findings. It must be noted that this theoretical framework may not be referred to by all researchers, and is more common among papers that make use of the qualitative approach.

At the end of your introduction you should list the specific aims and objectives of your research. These are the questions you want to answer in your study. For qualitative research, you need to provide your research questions or suppositions (see Liamputtong 2009). For quantitative research, you should also include your hypotheses. These are more specific than your objectives and can be tested using statistical methods (see the CONSORT website). Often your objectives and hypotheses will be very similar.

Research design and method

This section discusses the design of the research and the method you employ. It generally contains six subheadings: participants, method, intervention, outcome measures, procedure, data analysis. For a qualitative piece, you will not have the intervention and outcome measures, but you will have to explain the need for the qualitative approach and give a discussion on rigour (see also CHAPTER 1). Often too, you may need to discuss some ontological and epistemological positions of your research (see CHAPTER 1).

Every research study addresses an issue relevant to a particular population or people with a particular health issue, concern or condition. The participants section includes some descriptions of the research participants, for example who they were and how they were selected. A description of the participants usually includes some of their socio-demographic characteristics such as age, sex, gender, education level, employment and diagnosis. These 'eligibility criteria' or 'inclusion and exclusion criteria' are particularly important in clinical research because they help the reader know who the information will be relevant to or how generalisable the research findings are. How the participants were recruited should also be described (e.g. by referral or self-selection through advertising). In qualitative research you also include some socio-demographic characteristics of the participants as indicated above.

The method section must outline the method used in the study and give some explanation of it. We cannot assume that readers will know what the method is about without some explanation. For example, if you use a focus group method for data collection, you must explain what a focus group is, what the method can offer you, and how it is usually conducted (see

CHAPTER 4). Similarly, if you use a survey method, you will have to provide some discussion on what the method can offer and how it is generally used (see CHAPTER 13)

Some quantitative research studies investigate the effect of a particular intervention or treatment. If your study does, then you should describe fully the intervention that was implemented. Relevant details might include what the intervention is, what it does, the dose applied (intensity, frequency and duration), who administered it (what personnel, were they trained or untrained?), any specific equipment used and where it took place (contextual factors). It is also important to give details about any control or placebo interventions. For example, if your control group was a usual care group, you need to describe what usual care is.

One of the key features of quantitative research study is the outcome measures used; they are what determine whether an intervention was effective; or in a comparative study, if there is a difference between groups of participants (see CHAPTER 11). A full description of the outcome measures would include information on the psychometric properties of the outcome measure (such as validity and reliability) relevant to the study participants; details of how the outcomes were measured; and steps taken to improve reliability (e.g. were multiple measures taken and the average calculated, or were the assessors trained to perform the assessments in a standard way?). Most research studies employ several outcome measures, but the most important outcome is the primary outcome measure. All other outcome measures are secondary outcome measures. The sample size calculation is usually based on data relating to the primary outcome measure. It is important to document if the participant and assessor are blind to group allocation since this removes a potential source of bias. In health research, while it is often possible to employ an assessor who is blinded, it is not always possible to blind the participant to the intervention.

In the procedure section you describe what happened during the study in time sequence. In qualitative research, you describe the process of data collection and how you went about doing your research. For example, say you select a focus group method as your data collection tool, you need to explain in detail about how you actually used it in your research. In quantitative research, you describe when the outcome measures were assessed, particularly if they were assessed on more than one occasion. Other important aspects to mention about the research design are randomisation and concealment of group allocation.

The final part of your methods section is the data analysis. In qualitative research, you need to explain what data analysis method you employ, for example thematic or content analysis (see CHAPTER 22). An important thing to remember is that it is not enough for you to say that the data analysis is carried out using thematic data analysis. The readers may not know what this method is about. You must explain the nature of the method and how you used it in your study. Even though you may use computer programs to help you to analyse the data (see CHAPTER 23), you still have to give some explanation of what the package can do and the way you used it.

In quantitative research, this is where you describe the statistical methods used to complete your analysis, and state why you chose those particular methods. You might start

Pranee Liamputtong and Nora Shields

by saying how you analysed the participant's demographic data (e.g. calculating means and standard deviations). When comparing groups, you might calculate an estimate of how large the treatment effect was (an effect size) and the associated 95 per cent confidence interval. This analysis helps the reader interpret the difference in outcome between the groups and the range of uncertainty around the true treatment effect. Many people report the statistical significance of their findings using p-values; these values are the probability that your findings could have occurred by chance. It is always best to report the actual p value (e.g. $p = 0.023$) rather than stating the threshold ($p < 0.05$) (see CHAPTERS 24, 25).

Findings

The results of your research are presented in this section. In qualitative research, the findings are separated into different themes, and verbatim quotations are used to elaborate your explanation of the findings. In quantitative research, the results are often presented as tables and figures.

Discussion and conclusion

What you have found in your research is discussed at great length in this section. An important aspect that you should remember is that you need to link your findings with the literature and theory you have provided in the introduction. Readers would like to see how your study can confirm or contribute to new knowledge in the area or discipline. In the conclusion, often researchers make some recommendations for further research or implications for health care practices. This will allow readers to see that your research findings can be used in real life and/ or others can duplicate or extend your research in the field.

Acknowledgment

It is customary to acknowledge the assistance of others in this section. In particular, you express your sincere gratitude to your research participants, who have given you valuable knowledge so that you could undertake your research. You should also acknowledge funding agencies who have given you money to carry out the research.

References

This section lists all the references you have cited in the text. You need to ensure that they are complete and that the format is consistent throughout.

DOING RESEARCH

Qualitative writing

Here is an example from Pranee's qualitative research. The research is based on the work of one of her doctoral students and was published in *Sexual Health* (see Rawson & Liamputtong 2009).[1] For reasons of length, we only present certain sections of the paper and exclude all references cited. You may wish to read this paper from the journal directly (see detail in the References).

Title

'The Influence of Traditional Vietnamese Culture on the Utilisation of Mainstream Health Services for Sexual Health Issues by Second Generation Vietnamese Australian Young Women.'

Abstract

This paper discusses the impact traditional Vietnamese culture has on the uptake of mainstream health services for sexual health matters by Vietnamese Australian young women. It is part of a wider qualitative study which explored the factors that shaped the sexual behaviour of Vietnamese Australian young women living in Australia. A grounded theory methodology was employed, involving in-depth interviews with 15 Vietnamese Australian young women aged 18–25 years who reside in Victoria. The findings demonstrated that the ethnicity of the general practitioner had a clear impact on the women utilising the health service. They perceived that a Vietnamese doctor would hold the traditional view of sex held by their parents' generation. They reasoned that due to cultural mores, optimum sexual health care could only be achieved with a non-Vietnamese health professional. It is evidenced from the present study that cultural influences can impact on the sexual health of young people from culturally diverse backgrounds and in Australia's multicultural society, provision of sexual health services must acknowledge the specific needs of ethnically diverse young people.

Introduction

The sexual and reproductive development and health of young people are important global health concerns, and while its importance is widely acknowledged in contemporary research, research centres primarily on young people's sexual activity, unsafe sexual practices and the potential outcomes of risk-taking behaviour (such as sexually transmitted infections and teenage pregnancies), and sex education. A biomedical perspective underpins this body of work to the exclusion of the relevance of prevailing social factors and processes, thus effectively denying the importance of socially informed enquiry. It has been argued that a comprehensive sexual health strategy, involving medical, social, cultural, gendered and age-specific aspects, is needed to ensure that the global population receives and maintains optimum sexual and reproductive health. As part of a wider study, we sought to help fill this void by exploring the factors which influence the sexual behaviour of young women in Australia with a specific cultural heritage.

In this paper, we discuss how the parental Vietnamese culture influences the way these young women utilised mainstream health services for sexual health matters.

Pranee Liamputtong and Nora Shields

Specifically, we examine how the parental Vietnamese culture influenced the young women's choice of general practitioner (GP).

Method

This research adopted a qualitative methodology as this enabled us to examine and learn from the experiences of the young women who are living them. In addition, the exploratory nature of this research into the complex interplay of sexuality, second generation and gender issues is well suited to a qualitative research design. Grounded theory allowed us to uncover the young women's thoughts, perceptions and feelings, and so ensure that behaviour is understood through the meanings and interpretations they attach to it. Data were gathered by in-depth interviews with 15 second-generation Vietnamese young women living in Melbourne, Australia. An 'interview guide' was utilised and consisted of a list of topics deemed pivotal to the research question. The inclusion criterion for participation in the study were (1) be a second-generation immigrant; that is, be born or live in Australia, in accordance with national census data; (2) be Vietnamese Australian; that is, have lived in Australia from a young age with one or both parents being born in Vietnam; (3) be aged 18 to 25 years; and (4) be fluent in English.

The 15 interviews were audiotaped, allowing for an uninterrupted flow of discussion, and the tapes transcribed by the first author and analysed. In keeping with grounded theory method, the tapes were transcribed and analysed at the completion of each interview. Data analysis was informed by grounded theory and involved assessment and interpretation of the commonalities, contradictions and differences of the young women's lived experiences using open, axial and selective coding. To ensure anonymity, the young women are referred to by pseudonyms.

Findings

The analysis process for the wider study resulted in the development of four main categories as shaping the sexual behaviour of Vietnamese Australian young women. The results presented in this section relate to the category 'The Impact of Sexual and Reproductive Health Services on Sexual Behaviour', specifically the subcategory we have termed 'Choice of General Practitioner', and how accessing health care for sexual health purposes is influenced and impacted by the parental Vietnamese culture. This subcategory consisted of two key elements: 'Parental influence over choice of General Practitioner' and 'Ethnicity of General Practitioner'. Analysis of the interview data produced significant insights into the young women's preferences regarding optimum sexual health care and factors which would hinder their access to such care.

Parental influence over choice of general practitioner

The young women who lived with their parents viewed them as controlling their choice of GP. They had the same GP as their parents and expressed concern about this situation, feeling that it could create problems if they wanted, or needed, to see the GP about sexual health matters. This concern was generated, and fuelled, by fear and resulted in participants 'changing' their GP for consultations about sex-related issues.

The young women viewed having access to adequate and appropriate health care as important in relation to sexual and reproductive health. While they stated that they 'occasionally' needed to visit their family GP, or other family health practitioners, they indicated their reluctance to so. This reluctance was based on two concerns: first, having the 'same GP as parents' and second, the ethnicity of the GP. Participants voiced the need for 'trust' when talking about sexual health issues. They had a 'fear of being found out'. They used phrases such as 'concerned about people finding out', 'parents might find out' and 'Vietnamese people gossip'. Their preferred site for 'treatment' was a family health clinic, which they viewed as offering the possibility of a confidential and anonymous service.

The generation of fear

The young women's concern about having the same GP as their parents arose from the fear that their parents, or other members of the Vietnamese community, may learn that a visit concerned sexual health matters. Nga indicated her concern:

> It's a bit scary. I'd feel 'Are they [the doctors] going to say something and it gets back to my parents?'

Changing general practitioner for sexual health issues

To avoid the possibility of being 'exposed', the young women indicated that they would change their GP. Those who no longer lived in the parental home stated that they *had* changed their GP from the one they shared with their parents:

> When I lived at home we all had the same doctor as my parents and that's awkward for certain things. Now I have my own doctor, nothing to do with my family. (Lan)

Discussion and conclusion

In the traditional Vietnamese culture the prescribed conduct of women is rooted in Confucian tenets which enjoin female submission and premarital female chastity. Young women are deemed to be guardians of the 'traditional moral values', and immense importance is placed on female virginity before marriage and on family honour. Thus, the young women perceived that a Vietnamese GP would be upholding this traditional moral code. Their expressions of fear, embarrassment and judgment stemmed from this perception of sexuality within the Vietnamese community. In most Asian cultures, open discussion about sexuality is unusual, even among close friends, since sex is considered a very sensitive and taboo subject and is generally not discussed. During their interviews the young women stressed that within the traditional culture, discussion of sexual issues would be perceived as indicative of engagement in sexual activities. They were only too aware of the cultural expectations and the notion that any premarital sexual expression could compromise their, and their family's, moral reputation within the community. They later discussed the consequences of shame and dishonour for non-adherence to traditional sexual mores. (This will be addressed in a later paper.) For these young women, trust was the underlying component in gaining optimum sexual health care. They believed this to be unachievable with a Vietnamese GP.

The findings indicate that the factors which impact on the sexual behaviour of Vietnamese Australian young women have significant implications for the provision of sexual health services. Cultural taboos can limit young people's access to sexual and reproductive services and information. Thus there is a clear need for health care providers working within a multicultural society such as Australia to acknowledge that cultural context and social environment constitute multifaceted aspects of human behaviour. If the overall morbidity of young Australians is to be addressed through the development and implementation of appropriate strategies then, in addition to having culturally based and appropriate sex education information, the sexual health care services provided must be culturally sensitive.

DOING RESEARCH

Quantitative writing

Here we provide an example from Nora's quantitative research. The research was published in *Archives of Physical Medicine and Rehabilitation* in 2008.[2] Again, we present only certain sections of the paper and exclude all references. You may wish to read this paper from the journal directly (see Shields et al. 2008).

Title

'Effects of a Community-Based Progressive Resistance Training Program on Muscle Performance and Physical Function in Adults with Down Syndrome: A Randomised Controlled Trial.'

Structured abstract

Objective Does progressive resistance training improve muscle strength, muscle endurance, and physical function in adults with Down syndrome? *Design* Single-blind randomised controlled trial. *Participants* Adults (N = 20) with Down syndrome (13 men, 7 women; mean age, 26.8±7.8y) were randomly assigned to either an intervention group (n = 9) or a control group (n = 11). *Intervention* The intervention was a supervised, group progressive resistance training program, using weight machines performed twice a week for 10 weeks. Participants completed 2–3 sets of 10–12 repetitions of each exercise until they reached fatigue. The control group continued with their usual activities.

Main Outcome Measures The outcomes measured by blinded assessors were muscle strength (1-RM), muscle endurance (number of repetitions at 50% of 1-RM) for chest press, and the grocery shelving task. *Results* The intervention group demonstrated significant improvement in upper-limb muscle endurance compared to the control group (mean difference 16.7 reps, 95% confidence interval, [CI] 7.1–26.2); and a trend towards an improvement in upper-limb muscle strength (mean difference 8.6kg, 95% CI, −1.3–18.5kg) and in upper-limb function (mean difference −20.3s, 95% CI, −45.7–5.2s). *Conclusions* Progressive resistance training is a safe and feasible fitness option that can improve upper-limb muscle endurance in adults with Down syndrome.

Introduction

People with Down syndrome (DS) have reduced muscle strength and muscular endurance compared to their peers without disability. Muscle weakness can impact the ability of people with DS to perform everyday activities. Only three trials have investigated the effects of progressive resistance training in people with DS. Each of these trials found improved muscle strength with training, but none of the trials reported the effects of the programs on muscle endurance or functional activities. These trials were also limited as none employed blinded assessors to collect the data and two studies did not include a control group in their design. As no randomised controlled trial (RCT) has been conducted, it is not known to what extent the reported effects of progressive resistance training in people with DS are due to the strength training intervention rather than due to series effects. The aim of this trial was to determine if a progressive resistance training program for adults with DS can lead to increased muscle strength and endurance, and to improved physical function in this population.

Methods

We conducted an RCT. The trial received ethics approval from the university ethics committee, and all participants and their carers gave written informed consent to take part.

Participants

Adults with DS were included if they were aged 18 years or more, had the ability to follow simple verbal instructions in English, and were well enough to participate in a progressive resistance training program. The exclusion criterion was participation in a strength training program in the six months prior to the start of the study. Adults with DS were randomised using a concealed allocation, block randomisation method to either an intervention group or a control group.

Intervention

Participants in the intervention group completed a 10-week, twice a week progressive resistance training program at a community gymnasium. The program included three exercises for the upper limbs using weight machines (shoulder press, seated chest press, seated row). Participants completed 2–3 sets of 10–12 repetitions of each exercise until they reached fatigue. A 2-minute rest period was given between each set, and the resistance was increased when two sets of 12 repetitions of an exercise could be completed. Participants completed the program as a group, supervised by two accredited fitness trainers. Participants in the control group continued with their typical daily activities.

Outcome measurements

All participants were assessed at baseline and immediately after the intervention period. The outcome measurements were taken by assessors who were blind to group allocation. Maximal muscle force generation was tested by establishing the amount of weight each participant could lift in a single seated chest press (1-RM). Muscle endurance was measured by counting the number of repetitions that could be completed when the weight on the seated chest press was lowered to 50% of 1-RM. Physical function was measured using the grocery shelving task. Participants were asked to carry two grocery bags each containing 10 x 410 g items to a bench 2 m away. The participants then stacked the items onto a shelf at shoulder height. Participants completed the task as quickly as possible and the time taken was measured.

Data analysis

Data were analysed using SPSS statistical software to determine if there were any significant baseline demographic differences between the groups. Outcomes were analysed using analysis of covariance on the change scores with the baseline measure of that variable used as the covariate. The mean difference within each group and the mean difference between the groups and the 95% CIs of the mean differences were also calculated. Effect sizes and 95% CIs were also calculated for the change scores.

Results

Twenty adults (13 men, 7 women) with DS took part (see Table 26.1). Participants in the intervention group attended 92.8% of scheduled training sessions. No sessions were missed due to injury. The intervention group had a statistically significant improvement in upper-limb muscle endurance compared to the control group (mean difference in repetitions of the chest press at 50% of 1-RM, 16.7; 95% CI, 7.1–26.2; P<.01). There were also trends towards improvement in upper-limb muscle strength (mean difference 1-RM, 8.6kg; 95% CI −1.3 to 18.5kg; P=.08) and upper-limb function (mean difference in grocery shelving task, −20.3s; 95% CI, −45.7 to 5.2s; P=.11) that favoured the intervention group (Table 26.2).

Table 26.1: Demographic data for intervention and control groups

Characteristic	Intervention (n = 9)	Control (n = 11)
Mean age ± SD (y)	25.8±5.4	27.6±9.5
Sex (male/female)	7/2	6/5
Height (cm)	158.8 (7.12)	152.0 (10.0)
Weight (kg)	78.4 (13.5)	61.2 (6.7)
Level of perceived ID		
Mild	2	2
Moderate or severe	7	9

Table 26.2: Mean (SD) score and mean (95%CI) difference between groups for upper-limb outcomes for the intervention group and the control group

Outcome	Score				Difference between groups		
	Baseline (week 0)		Post-intervention (week 10)		Week 10–Week 0[†] (95 % CI)	p-value	Effect size (95 % CI)
	Int	Con	Int	Con	Int-Con		
Chest press 1RM (kg)	35.9 (15.4)	28.0 (10.2)	44.9 (15.2)	31.6 (13.3)	8.6 (-1.3 to 18.5)	0.08	0.63 (-0.20 to 1.59)
Chest press endurance (no. of repetitions)	15.0 (4.7)	19.0 (8.1)	25.9 (8.3)	17.5 (9.5)	16.7 (7.1 to 26.2)	0.00	1.51 (0.46 to 2.44)
Grocery Shelving Task (sec)	85.1 (49.1)	122.8 (84.0)	67.5 (33.4)	110.7 (66.4)	-20.3 (-45.7 to 5.2)	0.11	0.22 (-0.68 to 1.09)

Note: [†] = derived from ANCOVA with dependent variable on admission and baseline weight as covariates
Con, control group; Int, intervention group

Discussion and Conclusion

The main finding was that upper-limb muscle performance improved in adults with DS after a 10-week progressive resistance exercise program. There was a significant increase in chest press endurance and also a trend toward an increase in upper-limb strength as measured by a 1-RM chest press and upper-limb functional activity as measured by a grocery shelving task. The effect sizes observed were moderate to large (.76–.90) and the changes in upper-limb strength carried over to trends to changes in upper-limb physical function tasks suggests that these results may be clinically significant. The change in upper-limb endurance may be relevant in these adults, whose employment involves manual work of the upper limbs.

The progressive resistance exercise program implemented for this study was feasible for adults with DS. It might be expected that adults with DS have difficulty taking part in or being motivated to continue with a progressive resistance exercise program. The participants were all capable of taking part in the program and experienced benefits from doing so despite their intellectual disability. Compliance with the program was excellent, and there were also no withdrawals from the study, indicating that a strength training program was an acceptable form of exercise to the participants. Another positive finding was that the training program appeared to be a safe intervention for people with DS. No major adverse events were reported during the program. This finding is consistent with conclusions that strength training appears to be a relatively safe intervention for people with a broad range of health conditions.

The main strength of this trial was that it was an RCT. It adds to an area of research where to date only three previous studies have investigated if strength training programs are beneficial for adults with DS. This trial was limited by the relatively small sample size of 20 participants, which required the effects of the intervention to be large in order to detect any changes as a result of the strength training program.

SUMMARY

We strongly believe that writing up our research findings is an essential component of the research process if we wish to complete it. Writing about our findings helps to communicate the important issues arising from our research to wider audiences, be they academics, health and welfare professionals or policy-makers. More importantly, what we find in conducting any piece of research may prove useful in improving the health and well-being of many individuals and in the provision of health and welfare services for many people in the society. Our research findings can be used as 'evidence' in health and social care. So it is our moral obligation to write after we have completed our research. How will anyone find this information if we do not write about it? Research dissemination through writing is therefore an important part of the research process. Precisely for this reason, van Manen (2006, p. 715) writes that:

> It is in the act of…writing that insights emerge. The [writing] involves textual material that possesses…interpretive significance. It is precisely in the process of writing that the data of the research are gained as well as interpreted and that the fundamental nature of the research question is perceived.

TUTORIAL EXERCISES

1   Obtain four articles on any issue relevant to your study from journals. Two papers
must be based on qualitative methods and the other two on quantitative methods.
You need to read through each paper and critically examine the format that each
paper has adopted. Do you see any commonality or differences between these four
papers? Please discuss the commonalities and differences between them.

2   You have done a piece of research using one of the methods that we have covered in
this book. You have just finished your data analysis. Now it is time for you to write up
your research findings. Please start composing your paper using the structures we
have provided in this chapter.

NOTES

1   This paper is used with permission from CSIRO Publishing. The link to this issue of *Sexual Health* is
<www.publish.csiro.au/nid/166/issue/5048.htm>.

2   This paper is used here with permission from Elsevier Science.

FURTHER READING

Belgrave, L.L., Zablotsky, D. & Guadagno, M.A. (2002). How do we talk to each other?
Writing qualitative research for quantitative readers. *Qualitative Health Research*, 12(10),
1427–39.

Berg, K. & Latin, R. (2008). *Essentials of research methods in health, physical education, exercise science,
and recreation*, 3rd edn. Baltimore, MA: Lippincott Williams & Williams.

Goodall, H.L. (2008). *Writing qualitative inquiry: Self, stories, and academic life*. Walnut Creek, CA:
Left Coast Press.

Johnstone, M-J. (2004). *Effective writing for health professionals: A practical guide to getting published*.
Sydney: Allen & Unwin.

Liamputtong, P. (2009). *Qualitative research methods*, 3rd edn. Melbourne: Oxford University
Press.

Moore, N. (2006). *How to do research: A practical guide to designing and managing research projects*,
3rd edn. London: Facet.

Richardson, L. (1990). *Writing strategies: Reaching diverse audiences*. Newbury Park, CA:
Sage Publications.

Pranee Liamputtong and Nora Shields

Rugg, G. & Petre, M. (2004). *The unwritten rules of PhD research.* Maidenhead, UK: Open University Press.

Wolcott, H.F. (2009). *Writing up qualitative research*, 3rd edn. Thousand Oaks, CA: Sage Publications.

WEBSITES

www.consort-statement.org

The CONSORT website.

http://donotstopwriting.wordpress.com/2007/07/12/how-to-write-a-qualitative-study

This website provides some tips for writing qualitative paper and there is a section where readers can see comments from users and make their comments.

www.crisanet.org/docs/conference_08/Writing_Publishing_Workshop/How_Write_Paper_Qualitative_Data.pdf

This website provides a set of slides that discuss how to write up qualitative papers.

http://cnx.org/content/m14576/latest

The webpage contains vivid discussions on writing up qualitative theses. It gives some ideas about what the author calls the haziness of writing a qualitative dissertation that readers may find useful.

Glossary

Allocation bias: A type of selection bias that occurs when the process of allocating participants to groups leads to differences in the baseline characteristics of those groups.

Allocation concealment refers to where the randomised allocation sequence is concealed from investigators who are involved in recruiting participants.

Alternating treatment design: Two or three treatments of interest are provided in rapid succession and in an alternating format, within a session, in a session-by-session format or in a day-by-day format. The results are graphed together to show clearly the difference in rate and stability of learning in each treatment condition.

Analysis of narratives: The type of data analysis where themes are derived across the stories to demonstrate commonalities and dissimilar experiences.

Analytical cross-sectional study: A study that involves taking a 'snapshot' or cross-section of the population at a particular point in time. It aims to address questions about associations between exposures and outcomes.

Analytical epidemiological studies are designed to test hypotheses about associations between an exposure of interest and a particular health outcome. Thus they aim to identify or describe cause-and-effect relationships or associations between exposure and outcome factors.

Anonymity refers to a person being unknown to the researcher and hence to anyone else. Furthermore, where the person took part in any health research their confidentiality is maintained.

ANOVA (Analysis of variance): One of the most commonly used analyses in quantitative data analysis procedures. An ANOVA is used to compare the means of three or more sets of scores to determine if there are statistically significant differences between them.

Ascertainment bias occurs when the results or conclusions of the trial are distorted by the knowledge of which intervention each participant is receiving.

Assessment: It is referred to as an evaluation that is used to describe the process of gathering quantitative data in general.

Assessment bias occurs if an investigator's assessment of a participant lacks objectivity. Subjective outcome measures are prone to exaggerate the effect of the intervention.

Axial coding: The step in coding that requires moving towards a greater level of abstraction from the data. The task at this level of coding will be to further evaluate the codes to determine what needs to be reassembled or reorganised. This may involve processes such as breaking codes into smaller categories or collapsing more than one code into a single category. A phase of the Straussian mode of grounded theory in which categories and subcategories are systematically related to one another.

Bias: A concept used in randomised controlled trials and other positivist research designs. Researchers may unknowingly influence or bias the outcome of a study. Such bias can distort the results or conclusions away from the truth, the result being a poor-quality trial that underestimates, or more likely overestimates the benefits of an intervention. They are five main types of bias: selection, allocation, assessment, ascertainment and stopping rule biases.

Blinding: A technique used in randomised controlled trials to prevent assessors, participants or data analysis staff knowing which group the participant is in after s/he has been allocated.

Bracketing or **epoche**: The fundamental concept underpinning phenomenological reduction. The aim is to suspend all judgments and prior ideas about the phenomenon 'in order to enter the unique world of the individual whose experience is the focus of the research' (Carpenter & Suto 2008, p. 67). The concept of bracketing is characteristic of descriptive phenomenology.

CAQDAS (computer-assisted qualitative data analysis software): A term first coined by Lee and Fielding (1991), it refers to a specifically designed program (of which there are many versions) that can take over a substantial amount of the manual labour involved with analysing the data. Computer-assisted qualitative data analysis software offers a highly efficient data management system for storing, coding, organising, sorting and retrieving data.

Case-control study: A study that compares a group of people who have the outcome factor of interest (cases) with a group of people who do not (controls). Investigators then look back through time to identify exposures in the two groups. The two groups are then compared using measures of association, most commonly the odds ratio.

Case study in qualitative research: The study of a particular issue that is examined through one or more cases within a 'bounded system' (such as a setting *or* context).

Chi-square test: A test of statistical significance, used when the level of measurement is nominal and the data therefore consist of frequency counts for categories. These are the one-way chi-square test, which is sometimes called the goodness of fit test, and the two-way chi-square test. The latter, which is commonly encountered in health research, is used when there are two variables and determines if the relationship (association) between the two variables is statistically significant.

Citation bias occurs where articles that have statistically significant findings are cited more often than others.

Clinical audit: A process that provides a systematic framework for establishing care standards based on best evidence. It is a practical way to compare day-to-day practice with best evidence care standards and it can identify areas of care that require improvement.

Clinical data-mining provides practice-based evidence, i.e. evidence or information derived from practice. Such evidence underscores the importance of experiential knowledge in clinical decision-making and its contribution to establishing broad-based best practice models.

Clinical observation: Data that the the professional has identified from direct observation of empirical aspects of the practice field, either from their immediate perceptions or by means of instrumentation.

Clinical practice guidelines: 'Systematically developed statements which assist the health professional and the patient to make decisions about what is the appropriate health care in specific circumstances' (Field & Lohr 1990, p. 38).

Clinical significance: The practical or applied value of a finding or set of findings. Clinical significance can be gauged by factors such as amount of change as a result of an intervention, subjective evaluations from a client or patient regarding the effects of a factor or intervention, and social impact of the intervention.

Clinical trial: A trial that is conducted to determine if an intervention is effective; that is, whether it is beneficial to patients. A clinical trial can be used to investigate the efficacy of interventions.

Code: 'A word or short phrase that symbolically assigns a summative, salient essence-capturing and/or evocative attribute for a portion of language-based or visual data' (Saldaña 2009, p. 3).

Coding: Part of the data analysis process where codes are applied to segments, or chunks, of data. It is central to qualitative research and is typically the starting point for most forms of qualitative analysis. Coding is the first step that allows researchers to move beyond tangible data to make analytic interpretations.

Cohort study: It follows a group (or cohort) of people over time who have been exposed to a possible risk factor for a health outcome and another group who have not been exposed. The incidence of the outcome in the exposed group is then compared to the incidence of the outcome in the group that is not exposed. This enables the relationship between the exposure and outcome to be assessed.

Collaborative participatory research: A term that highlights the importance of collaboration and participation. This model recognises that the researcher has certain technical expertise, and that community leaders and community members have knowledge of their community needs and perspectives. The approach involves a transfer of knowledge, including knowledge of how to undertake research with community organisations.

Community can refer to a geographic community or a community of 'interest' or 'identity'.

Concurrent design: With this design, the questions that the researchers ask would tend to be framed from the start and they could consider using multiple reference points where intact, but separate data sets are collected concurrently.

Confidence interval: An important indicator of the representativeness of the mean, particularly with respect to a population. One way of ascertaining the amount of error in statistical analysis is to calculate the confidence interval of the mean. The narrower the range in these values, the more representative the mean.

Confidentiality aims to conceal the true identity of people who participate in the research. Revealing their true identities could lead to danger and other negative consequences for these people. It is extremely important with some vulnerable groups, particularly those who are marginalised and stigmatised in the society.

Consolidated Standards of Reporting Trials (CONSORT) Statement: This statement aims to ensure accurate and complete reporting of the design, conduct, analysis and generalisability of trials, thus ensuring the highest possible standards are met when clinical trials are published.

Constant comparison allows the researchers to see patterns in the data, and in the initial stages of analysis, the researcher simply groups like 'incidents' together and applies a name to the group, and this group is called a category. By comparing each incident within that category to one another, the properties of that category begin to emerge.

Constructivism: An epistemology that dominates the qualitative approach, also referred to as interpretivism. It suggests that 'reality' is socially constructed. Constructivist researchers reject the ideal of a single truth. They believe that there are multiple truths, which are individually constructed.

Reality is seen as being shaped by social factors such as class, gender, race, ethnicity, culture and age. To constructivist researchers, reality is not firmly rooted in nature, but is a product of our own making.

Content analysis: A form of data analysis used by both qualitative and quantitative researchers that involves the identification of codes before searching for their occurrence in the data. It is a deductive method, in contrast to the inductive method of thematic analysis.

Convenience sampling: This technique allows researchers to find individuals who are conveniently available and willing to participate in a study. Convenience sampling is crucial when it is difficult to find individuals who meet some specified criteria such as age, gender, ethnicity or social class. It is a form of a non-probability sampling technique.

Correlation coefficient: It is used to summarise the degree of relationship (correlation) between variables. In the case of bivariate correlation, these variables correspond to two sets of measures (or scores) for one group of participants.

Cross-sectional study: A study that involves the measurement of exposure and outcome simultaneously within the population of interest. Cross-sectional studies are often described as providing a snapshot of the frequency and characteristics of a disease in a population at a particular point in time. Cross-sectional studies are also referred to as prevalence studies.

Cross-sectional survey: It is used where the primary purpose is descriptive. A cross-sectional survey provides a profile of the sample at one point in time. It cannot make inferences about past or future and relies largely on descriptive and correlational analyses. A cross-sectional survey can tell us what proportion of a sample or population reports certain symptoms, diseases or characteristics, and whether these are more prevalent among certain sections of the population.

Culture: The knowledge people use to generate and interpret social behaviour.

Data analysis: The way that researchers make sense of their data. Data analysis in qualitative research differs from that of the quantitative approach. In qualitative research, data analysis looks for patterns (themes), whereas in quantitative research numerical data are analysed and statistics are used.

Data display: An 'organised, compressed assembly of information that permits conclusion drawing' (Miles & Huberman 1994, p. 11).

Data-mining: The process of extracting and analysing data to uncover hidden patterns and useful information. It is used commonly in retail, marketing and fraud detection. In social work research and practice, it is a form of research most often done by practitioners themselves, rather than by external researchers.

Data reduction occurs when raw data is transcribed and transformed into summaries, initial codes and preliminary themes. Data reduction forms the preliminary phase of analysis.

Data saturation: A concept associated with grounded theory, used by qualitative researchers as a way of justifying the number of research participants, and established during the data collection process. Saturation is considered to occur when little or no new data is being generated and new data fits into the categories already developed.

Degrees of freedom: Value(s) that represent the number of scores that are free to vary associated with a test statistic. Degrees of freedom are used to calculate the statistical significance of a test statistic.

Deontological ethics is an approach to ethics that holds that acts are inherently good or evil, regardless of their consequences.

Descriptive or **open coding:** Often the first level or step in coding in qualitative data analysis, in which the central aim is to sort and organise the data so that further analysis can take place. In grounded theory, this is referred to as open coding. This initial phase of coding stays close to the data itself.

Descriptive epidemiology focuses on describing health states and events and their distribution. It describes morbidity and mortality within the population using person, place and time variables. Descriptive studies are often carried out using pre-existing population health data. There are two common types of descriptive epidemiological studies: cross-sectional studies and longitudinal studies.

Descriptive phenomenology: Phenomenology as an approach to studying 'things as they appear' in order to arrive at a rigorous and unbiased understanding of the essential human consciousness and experience. Descriptive phenomenology develops detailed concrete descriptions of experience.

Descriptive statistics include measures of central tendency such as the mean (average), median (50th percentile) or mode (most frequently occurring score), and measures of dispersion (e.g. the standard deviation and the range).

Descriptive test: It describes the difference between individuals within a group.

Discourses provide 'historically variable ways of specifying knowledge and truth—what is possible to speak of at any given moment' (Ramazanoğlu 1993, p. 19). In other words, discourses are not simply systems of signs, but systems of practices, and these systems or discourses bring objects into existence as they are spoken.

Discriminative test: It distinguishes between individuals with and without a characteristic or trait.

Ecological study: An epidemiological study in which the unit of analysis is groups or aggregates rather than individuals. For instance, an ecological study may look at the association between rates of smoking and lung mortality in different countries. A limitation of ecological studies is that one cannot infer that associations observed at the aggregate level exist at the individual level—this is known as the ecological fallacy.

Effect size, which can be measured in various ways and depends on the particular statistical test that was undertaken, is a measure of the strength of a finding (whether that is difference between means or relationships between factors) that is independent of sample size.

Emic: An insider's perspective. It is a perspective conducted in one's own culture, such as an intensive care nurse conducting research within an intensive care ward.

Epidemiology is concerned with the study of the distribution and determinants of health states in populations. Epidemiology can provide the answers to questions asked in the health sector such as: How much disease is there? Who gets it? Where are most people affected? When did they have it? What happens over time?

Epistemology is concerned with the nature and scope (limitations) of the nature of knowledge. It addresses the questions: What is knowledge? How is knowledge acquired? What do people know? How do we know what we know? Why do we know what we know?

Ethical principles: There are four principles that researchers must adhere to in their research: *respecting autonomy*—the person making an informed decision about being involved; *beneficence*—the obligation to provide benefits, not to the participant necessarily, but certainly to the 'public good'; *non-maleficence*—avoiding bad intention or the causation of harm or discomfort disproportionate to the benefits of the research; and *justice*—the concept that benefits, risks and costs are equitably distributed.

Ethnography: A research method that focuses on the scientific study of the lived culture of groups of people, used to discover and describe individual social and cultural groups. Crucial features include the use of participant observation with other qualitative methods in the fieldwork, including in-depth interviewing, focus groups and unobtrusive methods.

Ethno-nursing: The use of ethnography as a method for research in nursing allows nursing to be studied within the natural setting and viewed within the context in which it occurs as well as studying areas that have not been previously explored. It can be used to document, describe and explain nursing phenomena in relation to care, health, illness prevention and illness or injury recovery by nurses, clients and nursing or health institutions. It can provide in-depth data and detailed accounts of nursing phenomena or experiences, and a holistic view, not otherwise gained through other research methods.

Etic: An outsider's perspective. In ethnographic studies conducted from the etic perspective, the researcher has no knowledge or experience in the culture s/he is studying.

Evaluative tests: are designed to measure change over time and are often called outcome measures. To accurately measure the amount of change, evaluative tools need to collect data at interval or ratio levels.

Evidence: 'Information' which can be used to support and guide practices, programs and policies in health and social care in order to enhance the health and well-being of individuals, families and communities.

Evidence in the context of evidence-based practice: is what results from a systematic review and appraisal of all available literature relevant to a carefully designed question and protocol. It is information that can be used to support and guide practices, programs and policies in health and social care in order to enhance the health and well-being of individuals, families and communities.

Evidence-based practice in health care: A process that requires the practitioner to find empirical evidence about the effectiveness or efficacy of different treatment options and then determine the relevance of the evidence to a particular client's situation. The information is carefully considered in light of the available resources and the clinician's expertise in order to determine the selected treatment plan for the client. EBP emphasises the importance of practice being based on, and supported by, sound empirical research, with the preferred 'gold standard' to such research being the conduct of randomised controlled trials.

Explanatory trial: A trial that is highly controlled and hence reduces the number of variables that can affect the final outcome. It has more ability to explain what variable caused the result detected. However, because of the tight controls placed on the trial, the results of an explanatory trial may not necessarily be able to be generalised to everyday practice.

Exposure: Exposure refers to a potential risk or protective factor for a health state. The exposure may represent an actual exposure (e.g. environmental pollution), a behaviour (e.g. physical inactivity, cigarette smoking) or an individual attribute (e.g. age) (Oleckno 2002). Exposure is also often referred to as a study factor or independent variable.

Fieldwork: A period of data collection commonly employed in the ethnographic method. Fieldwork may take a year or longer. The researcher usually stays in the community being studied throughout the period.

Focused coding: A step that follows descriptive or open coding. This is when researchers begin working with the codes themselves in order to start making sense of the data. This may involve synthesising the codes and determining relationships between various events or phenomena.

Focused ethnography concentrates on a single problem in a particular setting. Rather than attempting to portray an entire cultural system, focused ethnography draws on the cultural ethos of a microcosm to study selected aspects of everyday life. It gives emphasis to particular behaviours in specific settings and allows researchers to work within time and scope limitations by narrowing the focus and providing objectives that are more manageable. Focused ethnography is also known as specific, particularistic, or mini-ethnography.

The focus group method: A data collection method based on group discussion. Typically, there is a moderator who acts as leader of the group and a notetaker who records field notes of the discussion. The participants (usually between eight and ten) express their views by interacting in a group discussion of the issues.

Funnel format survey: In this model, the questions move from a broad focus to more specific content, from non-sensitive questions to more sensitive questions, and from more impersonal to more personal. In an **inverted funnel format survey**, questions move from more specific to more general, from more sensitive to less sensitive, and from personal to impersonal.

Grounded theory: A qualitative research approach that aims to generate theory from the data. Theories are grounded in the empirical data and built up inductively through a process of careful analysis and comparison.

Hermeneutics: A theory of the process of interpretation. Hermeneutics is used in qualitative research to examine the way people develop interpretations of their life in relation to their life experiences.

Human Research Ethics Committee: It includes researchers, health and social care professionals, a lawyer, lay members, and someone with a pastoral role in the community. They also indicate the need to have a balance of men and women as well as people who are regularly present or are co-opted for specialist expertise.

Incidence: The number of new cases of a health state in a particular population at a specific point in time. There are two types of incidence: cumulative incidence and incidence rate. The *incidence rate* is a measure of the rate at which new cases of the health state occur in the population during a specified time. *Cumulative incidence* measures the risk of a person developing the health state in a defined time-period.

In-depth interviewing: A method of qualitative data collection. The interview does not use fixed questions, though it can be guided by a set of broad questions. It aims to engage interviewees in conversation to elicit their understandings and interpretations. Within this method, it is assumed that people have particular and essential knowledge about the social world that is obtainable through verbal messages.

Indigenous people: The original inhabitants of a country. They are usually a minority group and have often been exploited and oppressed through processes of colonisation. Indigenous peoples are widely recognised to be disadvantaged across a range of social, political and health indicators.

Inferential statistics include a variety of procedures that are commonly referred to as statistical tests.

Informed consent: A process that precedes the data collection. The people to be involved in the research process are informed of the aims and methods of the research and then asked for their consent to participation in the research project. It is suggested that people from whom data was collected understood the research and agreed to participate based on this understanding.

Institutional ethnography: A qualitative mode of social inquiry that was developed with the aim of discovering or exposing the chains of coordination and control in a social system or among settings of everyday life. Institutional ethnography in not empirically focused on 'experience' or 'culture', but rather on social organisation, and is concerned with exploring and describing social and institutional forces that shape, limit and otherwise organise people's everyday worlds.

Intentionality: The assumption that the life-world 'is not an objective environment or a subjective consciousness or a set of beliefs; rather, [it] is what we perceive and experience it to be' (Finlay 1999, p. 302).

Intention-to-treat analysis: A concept used in randomised controlled trials. It should be conducted as the primary analysis. With this type of analysis, outcome measures are obtained regardless of compliance with the trial protocol, and data from all participants are analysed according to allocation, even if the participants had adverse events or unexpected outcomes.

Interpretive or **hermeneutic phenomenology** focuses on describing the meanings attributed by individuals' 'being in the world and how these meanings influence the choices that they make' (Lopez & Willis 2004, p. 729). Researchers working in this tradition would encourage participants to describe interactions, relations with others, physical experiences and so on in order to place the lived experience in the context of daily life.

Interval data have the property of a rank order, and in addition, distances or intervals between the units of measurement are equal. Interval data meet the criteria for measurement because it is possible to define the distance between values and therefore identify *how much* one individual or group differs from another.

Interview transcript: The written record of an interview that has been transcribed from the verbal conversation. It is used for in-depth data analysis in qualitative research.

Inverted funnel format survey: see **Funnel format survey.**

Key informant: An individual who is able to provide in-depth information to an ethnographer in ethnographic research. It is a concept that is used more often in ethnographic research than other qualitative methods.

Knowledge: 'An accepted body of facts or ideas that is acquired through the use of the senses or reasons' (Grinnell et al. 2008, p. 9). However, it is recognised that knowledge can also be acquired through research methods.

Knowledge acquisition: It takes the position that the most efficient way of 'knowing something' is through research findings, which have been gathered through the use of research methods.

Life-world: 'The world of experience as it lived' (Finlay 1999, p. 301), 'our sense of lived life' (Rapport 2005, p. 131).

Likert scale: It is used to measure subjective variables such as attitudes. The researcher generates a number of statements (e.g. attitudes) and wishes to measure the extent to which participants agree or disagree with the statements.

Longitudinal cohort survey: A type of survey in which the primary purpose is to track changes over time. Longitudinal surveys administer the same set of questions to individuals on repeated occasions and seek to understand how individuals or groups change over time. They could be undertaken simply to monitor changes in health or some other variable over time, or they may be undertaken to measure outcomes of certain interventions or treatments.

Longitudinal studies are useful to identify new cases (incidence) of a health state in a defined population and time-period. They follow a group of people over time to identify new cases (incidence) of a health state in a defined population and period.

Measurement: This term is used in a number of different contexts, including where the instrument or tool meets the requirements for being a measure—that is, it is capable of measuring the magnitude of the attribute under evaluation using a calibrated scale. Measurement involves the process of description and quantification. It involves recording physical or behavioural characteristics by assigning a value to aspects such as the quality, quantity, frequency or degree of these attributes.

Measurement errors occur when researchers do not measure accurately or when they measure a different variable from the one intended. Measurement errors can either be systematic or random depending on whether or not they have a constant pattern.

Measures of association determine strengths of associations or relationships between exposures and outcomes. The measure of association used depends on the study design. Relative risks are a common measure of association and are primarily used for the analysis of associations in cohort studies. The odds ratio is mainly used in case-control studies and is the 'odds' of exposure among the cases compared to the 'odds' among the controls.

Memos in grounded theory: An important part of the coding process in grounded theory. It is a note to self that researchers write as they analyse the data and continue data collection. Memos help the researcher to look more deeply into the developing categories and properties, and to come up with 'grounded' hypotheses (based on the data) about what is going on.

Meta-analysis: A statistical technique that combines the results of similar studies into a single result that provides an estimate of the overall effect.

Metaphor is used in narrative enquiry to enhance the meaning of stories by making an analogy with something familiar, or emphasising the meaning of experience that might be difficult to understand or convey in any other way.

Method: The actual strategies and techniques that researchers use to acquire knowledge and collect data.

Methodology: 'A specific philosophical and ethical approach to developing knowledge; a theory of how research should, or ought, to proceed given the nature of the issue it seeks to address' (Hammell 2006, p. 167).

Mixed format survey: This is particularly relevant for longer surveys covering a number of domains. Here the questions are organised in sections or domains and particular formats are applied within domains.

Mixed methods: A research design that combines research methods from qualitative and quantitative research approaches within a single research study.

Moderator: A key person in focus groups method, who may or may not be the researcher. A moderator leads and controls group discussions; in some contexts a facilitator is a preferred term.

Morbidity: The state of a person's health, that is, illness, disability, chronic disease and so forth.

Mortality: Death.

Multiple baseline design: When it is unlikely that treated behaviours will return to baseline levels after withdrawal of the treatment, multiple baseline designs are frequently the design of choice. In this design, the effects of treatment are replicated across several participants or across different target behaviours. The design also allows for replication across different treatment conditions within a single participant so that the relative effectiveness of one treatment over another can be investigated.

Multiple probe design: In some situations the multiple probe design offers a cost-effective alternative to the multiple baseline design. Not all probes are taken in every session but rather some are taken at a predetermined and less frequent schedule or once a requisite skill is obtained.

Multiple realities: The idea of multiple realities relates to the concept of intentionality, that the same objects or situations can mean different things to different people, and that people and the worlds they occupy are inextricably intertwined (Carpenter & Suto 2008, p. 66).

Multiple regression analysis is a multivariate procedure that can be used when there are three or more variables and the level of measurement is interval or ratio. It assesses the degree to which scores for a subset of these variables predict scores for another variable in the set.

Multivariate analysis of variance (MANOVA) is used when there are two or more dependent variables (measures), each of which is measured on an interval or ratio scale, and where the set of scores for each is reasonably normally distributed. A MANOVA can be applied to designs where there are one or more independent variables, each with two or more levels.

Narrative analysis: An approach to the analysis of data generated mainly from a narrative enquiry approach, which can also used to analyse other qualitative data. Within this method, a story is created by imposing order on narrative data.

Narrative enquiry: A research method that focuses on the structure and nature of the narratives, or stories, produced.

Narrative review: It aims to provide 'a critical interpretation of the literature that it covers' (Bryman 2008, p. 696). It is now seen as contrasting to, and less focused than, a systematic review.

Nominal data occur where objects or people are assigned to named categories according to some criterion, for example male/female.

Non-probability sampling: In this method, the probability of a potential research participant being selected is not known in advance. This sampling method does not provide 'representative samples' for the populations from which they are drawn, so the findings cannot be generalised to a larger group of people. However, these methods are useful for research questions that do not need to involve large populations, and particularly for qualitative research projects.

Observation: The process of collecting data by looking rather than listening.

Observational epidemiological study: This type of study does not seek to intervene or change people's exposure status. Rather, the aim is to collect information about people's exposure and health outcomes as these naturally occur within the population. Observational studies can be considered as either descriptive or analytical.

Observationally based research: It refers to research that is based on observation. The work of Jean Piaget is often cited as an example of this approach. From his observations of his young children within the family home, Piaget envisaged his theory that the infant's cognitive development proceeded by way of particular stages.

Ontology: the study of the nature of being, existence or reality in general. It is concerned with understanding the kinds of things that construct the world. It asks whether or not there is a single objective reality in this world.

Open coding: see **Descriptive coding**.

Ordinal data result when observations are rank-ordered and values are assigned sequentially to reflect the logical ordering of categories. Common examples are Likert scales, which rank responses from low to high.

Outcome: The health state that is under investigation and of interest. The outcome of interest is also often referred to as the dependent variable. Other authors use the term 'disease'. In epidemiology, however, not all outcomes are diseases and in fact some outcomes may be desirable or favourable health states. As such, it would be unfortunate and inappropriate to label these outcomes as disease.

Outcome measure: A term used in reference to the evaluative test used to measure the effect of the intervention (see **Evaluative tests**). Outcome measures should be both valid and reliable.

p **value:** All inferential tests produce a common value, the *p* value, that is critical in the interpretation of findings. This *p* value is one thing to examine when reading inferential statistics. That is because this value represents the probability of the 'null hypothesis' being true.

Participant observation: A data collection method used in ethnography and behavioural studies. The researcher is more or less embedded with the group being studied so as to observe activities first hand.

Participatory action research: A method in which research and action are joined in order to plan, implement and monitor change. The informants become co-researchers and hence have their voices heard in all aspects of the research. The researcher becomes a participant in the initiatives and uses his/her research knowledge and expertise to assist the informants in self-research.

Patient-reported outcome: The outcome where the patient, rather than the clinician, reports on the impact of a disease or intervention on the status of their health. When evaluating the effect of an intervention on a patient, the patient's perspective on whether that intervention is effective or not is most important.

Phenomenological reduction: The goal is to search for all possible meanings, to describe rather than explain, to gain rich, 'thick' information that represents the essential nature of the individuals' experiences and that 'communicates the sense and logic of the phenomenon to others' (Todres 2005, p. 110) in a new way.

Phenomenology: A methodological approach that has a strong and dynamic philosophical and epistemological foundation that seeks to understand, describe and interpret human behaviour and the meaning individuals make of their experiences. Phenomenologists study people's understandings and interpretations of their experiences in their own terms, emphasising these as explanations for their actions.

Photovoice: This method rejects traditional paradigms of power and the production of knowledge within the research relationship. It allows people to record and reflect the concerns and needs of their community by taking photographs. It also promotes critical discussion about important issues through dialogue about the photographs. Using a camera to record their concerns and needs allows individuals who rarely have contact with those who make decisions over their lives to make their voices heard.

Physiotherapy Evidence Database (PEDro): For the profession of physiotherapy, a relatively large body of relevant research evidence is available and has been collected, appraised and made available.

PICO concept or logic grid: A useful process to start off a systematic review. PICO stands for: **P**opulation, **I**ntervention or indicator, **C**omparator or control, and **O**utcome.

Plot: A forestructure of narrative indicating how people think in recounting stories and revealing the meaning and significance of various story elements. Plot also indicates how people extract understanding from past events to make sense of present circumstances.

Population: In statistical research, the group, or cases, from which the sample in a research project is selected. The term is used in epidemiology to refer to all the people who live in a defined area or country.

Population-based health data: 'Ongoing systems that collect and register all cases of a particular disease or class of diseases as they develop in a defined population' (Oleckno 2002, p. 349). Common sources of population health data that are routinely collected include census data and disease registries (such as births, deaths, cancer and infectious diseases). The collection of registry data is a national responsibility and often this data is provided to both the United Nations and the World Health Organization. Other sources of data include regular surveys such as the National Health Survey and hospital records.

Population health data: There are a number of sources of population health data that are freely available both internationally and nationally. Common sources of population health data that are routinely collected include census data and disease registries (such as births, deaths, cancer and infectious diseases). The collection of registry data is a national responsibility and often this data is provided to both the United Nations and the World Health Organization. Other sources of data include regular surveys such as the National Health Survey and hospital records.

Positionality is related to the 'position' from which one 'chooses' to speak. The research question or aim is developed from this 'position' and to some extent it lends credibility and authority to the study. In addressing issues of positionality researchers need to make a full explanation of their experience and knowledge of the research topic and their relationship with the participants.

Positivism: An approach to research that believes social science research methods should be scientific in the same way as the physical sciences such as physics or chemistry. Qualitative researchers reject the arguments of positivism, pointing out that meanings and interpretations cannot be measured like physical objects. Positivism views reality as being independent of our experiences of it, and being accessible through careful thinking, and observing and recording of our experiences.

Postmodern ethnography: Postmodern ethnography still requires a traditional methodological commitment in realist ethnography to observation and the use of key informants as the basis for detailed description and structural analysis of the social world, and the use of cases, particularly conflicts where individual interests seem opposed to social forces. But it also requires an embedded sense of what it is like to live in the social world so described, and here the approaches used most commonly are life history. Ethnographers use these techniques in combination with each other to provide greater ethnographic richness, as well as to improve the reliability of both data and interpretation.

Practice-based research has the following essential attributes: it is inductive (concepts derived from practice wisdom); it makes use of non-experimental or quasi-experimental designs; it seeks descriptive or correlational knowledge; it may be either retrospective or prospective; it may be quantitative or qualitative, but tends to rely on instruments tailored to the needs of social practice rather than external standardised research instruments; it is collaborative in nature; and practice requirements tend to outweigh research considerations.

Pragmatic trial: One in which the investigators attempt to mimic common practice, thereby endeavouring as much as possible to make the results generalisable to everyday practice. Pragmatic trials have become more common over the past decade or so in an effort to make clinical trials more meaningful to clinicians and the public.

Pragmatism: A paradigm that has been promoted as an attractive philosophy within 'methodological pluralism'. It argues that reality does not exist only as natural and physical realities, but also as psychological and social realities, which include subjective experience and thought, language, and culture. Knowledge is both constructed and based on the reality of the world in which we live and which we experience. Therefore researchers should employ a combination of methods that work best for answering their research questions.

Predictive test: It aims to assess individuals in terms of their likely future outcomes, e.g., hospital admission scores on the Functional Independence Measure were used to predict length of stay and discharge scores.

Prevalence: The frequency of existing cases of a health state in a particular population at a specific point in time or time period.

Prevalence rate ratio: The ratio of the prevalence in the exposed to the prevalence in the unexposed. The ratio is calculated as:

$$P \; = \; \frac{\text{Prevalence in the exposed}}{\text{Prevalence in the unexposed}}$$

Prevalence study: see **Cross-sectional study**.

Probability sampling method: The method that requires that the probability of an element being selected is known in advance. This method is important in quantitative research where, in most cases, the intent is to generalise the findings for the sample to the population from which the sample was taken. The four most common methods for drawing random samples include simple random sampling, systematic random sampling, stratified random sampling, and cluster random sampling.

Project agreement or **memorandum of understanding:** It is drawn up to clarify the roles, responsibilities and expectations of the researcher and the community partners around particular issues such as ownership of data, outcomes and publications. While MOUs are seldom legally binding, this process is important for the collaborating partners to develop an understanding of each other's values and expectations.

Publication bias occurs when a trial is published or not published because of the direction of its findings. Studies that have a positive result are more likely to be published and trials finding no difference between groups are, on average, less likely, or will take longer to be published.

Purposive sampling: Purposive sampling looks for cases that will be able to provide rich or in-depth information about the issue being examined in the research. It does not look for cases that will provide a representative sample, as in random sampling techniques in quantitative research.

Q^2 or Q squared: The combination of quantitative and qualitative approaches in a research study. It is the concept used in mixed methods research design.

Qualitative research: A research strategy that has its emphasis on words rather than numbers in the process of data collection and analysis. The focus of qualitative research is on the generation of theories.

Qualitative data analysis: Data analysis in qualitative research is an ongoing, cyclical process that occurs from the very beginning of the research itself.

Quality assessment: An integral part of the systematic review process. The quality assessment process can guide the interpretation of the review findings and help determine the strength of inferences we can make from the results.

Quantitative research: Research strategies that place their emphasis on numbers in the process of data collection and analysis. The focus of the quantitative approach is on the testing of theories.

Questionnaire: A specific type of written survey made up of a structured series of questions. Questionnaires usually have highly standardised response options so that data can be easily analysed and compared across individuals or groups.

Randomisation: A mechanism where participants are randomly allocated an intervention (e.g. the active test intervention versus a placebo or a sham intervention). It is a powerful tool that ensures the study groups are as similar as possible except for the intervention being studied.

Randomised controlled trial: A clinical trial where participants are randomly assigned to groups in order to receive different interventions. This randomisation removes many of the effects that may bias the true result. It is currently considered the 'gold standard' for evaluating the efficacy of an intervention as it removes many of the effects that may bias the true result. Randomised controlled trials can either be explanatory or pragmatic.

Ratio data have the same properties as interval data, and in addition, have an empirical rather than an arbitrary zero. This is the highest level of measurement and data from ratio scales have the greatest statistical utility because of their mathematical properties.

Reflexivity: An essential strategy that makes explicit the deep-seated views and judgments that affect the research topic, including a full assessment of the influence of the researcher's background, assumptions, perceptions, values, beliefs and interests on the research process.

Reliability: The extent to which a measurement instrument is dependable, stable and consistent when repeated under identical conditions. Reliability refers to the ability of the scale to provide consistent, stable information across time and across respondents. For instance, if someone completes the scale today and again in two days' time, do you get essentially the same responses?

Research-based practice has the following characteristics: it is deductive (concepts derived from theory); it seeks causal knowledge therefore it gives priority to experimental, randomised control group designs; it is prospective; and it relies on standardised, quantitative research instruments. While it is collaborative, research requirements tend in the main to outweigh practice considerations.

Research ethics: Contemporary research ethics is understood as finding the balance between the risks associated with a research project and its benefits. Risks relating to issues such as confidentiality, anonymity, discomfort from the procedures and so forth are set against the benefits not just to the pariticpants but to the public at large. Decisions about research proposals are usually made by ethics committees. See **Human Research Ethics Committee**.

Research participant: A person who agrees to take part in the study on equal terms.

Rigour: Rigorous qualitative research is trustworthy and can be relied upon by other researchers. 'Rigour' is preferred to the terms 'validity' and 'reliability', used by quantitative researchers, because 'rigour' indicates the different methodology involved in research that focuses on meanings and interpretations.

Sample size: In a randomised controlled trial this must be determined before the start of the trial, and should be large enough to be able to detect if the intervention being evaluated leads to a clinically worthwhile effect.

Secondary data analysis: An analysis of data collected for purposes other than for a specific piece of research. Often the data are taken from existing research results that other researchers have undertaken.

Selection bias arises if the investigators systematically manipulate enrolment into the trial.

Selective coding: A level of analysis beyond axial coding whereby a central or core theme is identified using the previous levels of analysis. At this point, researchers can begin formulating propositions by drawing conclusions, making causal connections and developing theoretical constructs.

Semi-structured interview: A technique that is often referred to as an in-depth interview but more accurately refers to an interview where the researchers have prepared some pre-interview questions (theme lists) and used them to elicit information, but at the same time allow the participants to elaborate on their responses.

Sensitive topics may include research that involves the private sphere of an individual. Sensitive research includes studies that are 'intimate, discreditable or incriminating' and may cause emotional upset or pose some physical and emotional risk to the participants.

Sequential design: A research design when one data set follows another and extends or explores the findings from the first set. For example, a qualitative study is undertaken to explore a particular issue or phenomenon and researchers could create hypotheses from these results that they could test using a survey or experimental design.

Single-subject experimental design: An experimental research method that focuses on a single individual and their response to treatment(s) across time. Several terms have been used interchangeably for SSEDs. These include: Single-case designs or single-case experimental designs; Single-subject designs; Interrupted time series designs; N of 1; Small N designs.

Snowball sampling: Sampling that relies on existing participants to identify acquaintances who fit the inclusion criteria of a study in order to increase the size of the sample, particularly when a population is difficult to locate.

Standardised scale: It provides a scientific form of health assessment that is particularly useful for measuring subjective constructs such as pain, mood and level of symptoms. Standardised scales are made up of a series of self-report questions, ratings or items that measure a specific concept, and where the response categories are in the same format and can be summed or aggregated in some weighted form.

Statistical significance: Establishing whether or not an outcome is statistically significant is accomplished by using a statistical test to decide whether the outcome is likely to be due to chance, or to be real. If the probability of obtaining the effect by chance is low, then it is concluded that the effect is real, that is, it is statistically significant.

Steering committee or **advisory group:** Researchers using CPR often establish a steering committee or advisory group to provide advice and guidance on all matters pertaining to the community with whom and for whom the research is being conducted.

Stopping rule bias: A concept relevant to randomised controlled trials. It can occur if a trial is stopped inappropriately.

Survey: A descriptive research method where respondents are asked a series of questions in a standard manner so that responses can be easily quantified and analysed statistically. This enables the researcher to describe the characteristics of the sample being studied and to make generalisations to the larger population of interest.

Survey to test intervention effects: A survey in which the primary question is whether a particular intervention or experiment produces change in outcomes. It takes measures before and after a treatment or intervention to determine whether the intervention is associated with hypothesised improvement.

Symbolic interactionsim: An American tradition that typically uses qualitative research methods to study the way people make sense of their experiences through common symbols and symbolic processes.

Systematic review: A comprehensive identification and synthesis of the available literature on a specified topic. Systematic reviews are different from narrative reviews in that they provide an objective or scientific summary of the literature rather than a subjective opinion-based summary. In a systematic review, literature is treated as data.

Thematic analysis: The identification of themes through a careful reading and rereading of the data. The method is inductive, building up concepts and theories from the data, compared with the deductive method of content analysis.

Theme: A grouping of data emerging from the research and to which the researcher gives a name.

Theoretical assumptions are hypothetical statements that explain, or are used to predict, certain phenomena. Theoretical models are diagrammatic explanations of hypothetical relationships. They are used to guide what is to be measured. If the intention is to improve participation, then participation must be carefully defined and measured. If the intention is to investigate relationships between constructs within the model, for example the relationship between impairments of body function and participation, then both elements must be evaluated. Careful consideration of the theoretical assumptions under investigation (in practice and research) is an essential component of all test selection.

Theoretical sampling: A technique in grounded theory whereby sampling (of people, events or other data) is guided by the developing theory and not based on statistical or other predetermined grounds. New units are selected to be part of the sample on the basis of the need to fill out particular concepts or theoretical points.

Theory-builders in CAQDAS: CAQDAS programs offer different facilities such as conceptual mapping to help researchers examine relationships between codes and categories from text. Often these facilities are referred to as 'theory-builders'. Importantly, this capacity within various programs does not mean that the program itself can build theory on its own. Rather, the CAQDAS will have various in-built tools that help researchers to make comparisons and develop some theoretical ideas.

Theory in grounded theory: A set of categories, related to one another to form a framework that explains the main concern of the participants and shows how this concern is resolved or managed. When a grounded theory is developed, it is never a 'final product'; it is dynamic, ongoing, and 'under development'. A grounded theory is able to explain and relate concepts that are important and relevant in the area studied. Because the theory defines a set of concepts, and does not just provide a description about 'what happened' in the data, it is applicable in different situations.

Thick description: Descriptions based on qualitative research, typically ethnography, where ample detail and background information are provided so that people's actions can be understood in the context of the experiences and patterns of meaning that influence them.

Triangulation: The use of multiple methods, researchers, data sources, or theories in a research project. It recognises the value of different methods of data collection and/or different methods of analysis in teasing out answers to complex questions regarding health-related behaviours.

t-test: It is used to compare two means with each other, to establish if there is a statistically significant difference between them. There are several versions of the t-test. These include the one-sample t-test, which is used to compare a mean for a single set of scores with another mean, and two-sample t-tests, which are used when there are two sets of scores, the means of which are to be compared with each other.

Type I statistical error: It occurs when the researchers mistakenly conclude that a finding was statistically significant when it may be a result of chance rather than being a real difference. Testing multiple non-prespecified hypotheses inflates the Type I statistical error rate, resulting in spurious and often implausible findings.

Type II statistical error: It occurs when the investigators conclude that there is no significant difference between the groups (i.e. that the intervention being studied is not effective); there may have been a clinically important effect but the trial did not have a sufficiently large sample size to detect it statistically. This is more likely to occur when sample sizes are low.

Unobtrusive method: A method that does not require direct contact with the informants. It makes use of data that have been published or are available in libraries, the press, or other media. Indirect and unobtrusive observation, where the informants have no knowledge about the research, is also employed.

Utilitarian: An ethical issue based on the assumption that it is possible to predict the likely consequences of an action (in this case research) and the likely benefit it will have for the greatest number of people.

Validity: The extent to which an instrument measures what it is intended to measure. Validity refers to the degree to which the scale measures what it is supposed to measure (content and construct validity). For instance, does it have a good correlation with another 'gold standard' measure?

Verbal rating scale: It is commonly used where a question is asked and a range of verbal response categories provided for the participant to circle the response that most closely represents their view.

Virtue ethics: A situation where judgments are made about a person (*qua* researcher) by their demonstrated moral character.

Visual analogue scale: One that provides the opportunity for respondents to rate items on a continuous line between two end points. Typically, participants are asked to mark a position on the line that goes from 0 to 10 or from 0 to 100.

Vulnerable people: Individuals who are marginalised and discriminated against in society because of their social positions, based on class, ethnicity, gender, age, illness, disability or sexual preferences. Often they are difficult to reach and require special considerations when they are involved in research. The term is also used to refer to people who are difficult to access in societies.

References

Aamodt, A. (1982). Examining ethnography for nurse researchers. *Western Journal of Nursing Research*, 4(2), 209–21.

ABS (Australian Bureau of Statistics) & AIHW (Australian Institute of Health and Welfare) (2008). *The health and welfare of Australia's Aboriginal and Torres Strait Islander peoples*. ABS Cat. No. 4704.0. AIHW Cat. No. AIHW 21. Canberra: ABS & AIHW.

ABS (2006a). *National health survey: Summary of results, Australia 2004–05*. Cat. No. 4364.0. Canberra: ABS. <www.ausstats.abs.gov.au/ausstats/subscriber.nsf/0/3B1917236618A042CA25711F00185526/$File/43640_2004-05.pdf>, accessed 5 April 2009.

ABS (2006b). *2004–05 National Health Survey: User's guide—electronic publication*. Cat. No. 4363.0.55.001. Canberra: ABS.

ABS (2006c). *A picture of the nation*. Canberra: ABS.

ABS (2009). Births. <www.abs.gov.au/AUSSTATS/abs@.nsf/DSSbyCollectionid/C25FB9875049D14ACA256BD000281108?opendocument>, accessed 23 March 2009.

Ahern, K.J. (1999). Ten tips for reflexive bracketing. *Qualitative Health Research*, 9, 407–11.

AIHW (Australian Institute of Health and Welfare) (2008). *Aboriginal and Torres Strait Islander health performance framework, 2008 report: Detailed analyses*. Cat. no. IHW 22. Canberra: AIHW.

AIHW (2008). GRIM (General Record of Incidence of Mortality) books. <www.aihw.gov.au/hospitals/nhm_database.cfm>, accessed 23 March 2009.

AIHW (2009). National hospital morbidity data collection. <www.aihw.gov.au/hospitals/nhm_database.cfm>, accessed 19 January 2009.

AIHW (n.d.). Data Online 2009. /<www.aihw.gov.au/dataonline.cfm>, accessed 19 January 2009.

Albrechtsen, J. (2006). Muslim world requires a dose of girl power. <www.theaustralian.news.com.au/story/0,20867,20975680-32522,00.html>, accessed 24 March 2008.

Alexopoulos, G.S., Abrams, R.C., Young, R.C. & Shamoian, C.A. (1988). Cornell scale for depression in dementia. *Biological Psychiatry*, 23, 271–84.

Altman, D.G. (1980). Statistics and ethics in research: III How large a sample? *British Medical Journal*, 281, 1336–38.

Altman, D.G. (1996). Better reporting of randomised controlled trials: The CONSORT statement. *British Medical Journal*, 313, 570–71.

Altman, D.G., Schulz, K.F., Moher, D., Egger, M., Davidoff, F., Elbourne, D., et al. (2001). The revised CONSORT statement for reporting randomized trials: Explanation and elaboration. *Annals of Internal Medicine*, 134(8), 663–94.

American Association for the Advancement of Science, & Mead, M. (1968). *Science and the concept of race*. New York: Columbia University Press.

American Educational Research Association, A.P.A., National Council on Measurement in Education (1999). *Standards for educational and psychological testing*. Washington, DC: American Educational Research Association.

Anastas, J. (2005). Observation. In R. Grinnell & Y. Unrau (eds), *Social work research and evaluation: Quantitative and qualitative approaches*. New York: Oxford University Press, 213–30.

Angen, M.J. (2000). Evaluating interpretive inquiry: Reviewing the validity debate and opening the dialogue. *Qualitative Health Research*, 10(3), 378–95.

Annells, M. (1996). Grounded theory method: Philosophical perspectives, paradigm of inquiry, and postmodernism. *Qualitative Health Research*, 6(3), 379–93.

Annells, M. (1997a). Grounded theory method, part I: Within the five moments of qualitative research. *Nursing Inquiry*, 4, 120–29.

Annells, M. (1997b). Grounded theory method, part II: Options for users of the method. *Nursing Inquiry*, 4, 176–80.

Annells, M. (2005). A qualitative quandary: Alternative representation and meta-synthesis. *Journal of Clinical Nursing*, 14, 535–6.

Aoun, S.M. & Kristjanson, L.J. (2005). Evidence in palliative care research: How should it be gathered? *Medical Journal of Australia*, 183(5), 264–6.

Argyris, C. & Schon, D. (1974). Theory and practice: Increasing professional effectiveness. Jossey-Bass: San Francisco.

Arminio, J.L. & Hultgren, F.H. (2002). Breaking out from the shadow: The question of criteria in qualitative research. *Journal of College Student Development*, 43(4), 446–56.

Arndt, M., Murchie, F., Schembri, A. & Davidson, P. (2009). 'Others had similar problems and you were not alone': Evaluation of an open group mutual aid model in cardiac rehabilitation. *Journal of Cardiovascular Nursing*, 24(4), 328–35.

Arroll, B., Robb, G. & Sutich, E. (2003). *The diagnosis and management of soft tissue knee injuries: Internal derangements. Best practice evidence-based guideline.* New Zealand Guidelines Group.

Audet, J. & d'Amboise, G. (2001). The multi-site study: An innovative research methodology. *The Qualitative Report*, (2). <www.nova.edu/ssss/QR/QR6-2/index.html>, accessed 1 January 2009.

Auslander, G., Dobrof, J. & Epstein, I. (2001). Comparing social work's role in renal dialysis in Israel and the United States: A practice-based research potential of available clinical information. *Social Work in Health Care*, 33(3/4), 129–51.

Austin, P.C., Mamdani, M.M., Juurlink, D.N. & Hux, J.E. (2006). Testing multiple statistical hypotheses resulted in spurious associations: A study of astrological signs and health. *Journal of Clinical Epidemiology*, 59(9), 964–9.

Australian Council on Healthcare Standards (2004). ACHS News, 12, 4.

Avis, M. (2003). Do we need methodological theory to do qualitative research. *Qualitative Health Research*, 13(7), 995–1004.

Bailey, A. (2008). Let's tell you a story: Use of vignettes in focus group discussions on HIV/AIDS among migrant and mobile men in Goa, India. In P. Liamputtong (ed.), *Doing cross-cultural research: Ethical and methodological perspectives.* Dordrecht, The Netherlands: Springer, 253–64.

Baillie, L. (1995). Ethnography and nursing research: A critical appraisal. *Nurse Researcher*, 3(2), 5–21.

Baluch, B. & Davis, P. (2008). Poverty dynamics and life trajectories in rural Bangladesh. *International Journal of Multiple Research Approaches*, 2(2), 176–90.

Bamberg, M. (2007). *Narrative: State of the Art.* Amsterdam: John Benjamins.

Barbour, R. (2008). *Introducing qualitative research: A student's guide to the craft of doing qualitative research.* London: Sage Publications.

Barratt, R. (1991). *Culture and conduct: An excursion in anthropology*, 2nd edn. Belmont, CA: Wadsworth Publishing Company.

Barter-Godfrey, S.H. & Taket, A.R. (2007). Understanding women's breast screening behaviour: A study carried out in South East London, with women aged 50–64 years. *Health Education Journal* 66(4), 335–46.

Bateson, G. (1973). *Steps towards an ecology of mind*. London: Paladin.

Bateson, G. & Mead, M. (1942). *Balinese character: A photographic analysis*. New York: New York Academy of Sciences.

Baum, F. (2008). *The new public health*, 3rd edn. Melbourne: Oxford University Press.

Bauman, Z. (2005). Afterthought: On writing: On writing sociology, In N.K. Denzin & Y.S. Lincoln (eds), *The SAGE handbook of qualitative research*. Thousand Oaks, CA: Sage Publications, 1089–98.

Bazeley, P. (2007). *Qualitative data analysis with NVivo*, 3rd edn. London: Sage Publications.

Beadle-Brown, J., Mansell, J. & Kozma, A. (2007). De-institutionalization in intellectual disabilities. *Current Opinion in Psychiatry* 20, 437–42.

Beauchamp, T.L. & Childress, J.F. (2001). *Principles of biomedical ethics*, 5th edn. Oxford: Oxford University Press.

Beaudin, C.L. & Pelletier, L.R. (1996). Consumer-based research: Using focus groups as a method of evaluating quality of care. *Journal of Nursing Care Quality*, 10, 28–33.

Beaver, K. & Luker, K.A. (2005). Follow-up in breast cancer clinics: Reassuring for patients rather than detecting recurrence. *Psycho-Oncology*, 14(2), 94–101.

Becker, P. (1993). Common pitfalls of published grounded theory research. *Qualitative Health Research*, 3(2), 254–60.

Beckerman, H., Roebroeck, M.E., Lankhorst, G.J., Becher, J.G., Bezemer, P.D. & Verbeek, A.L.M. (2001). Smallest real difference, a link between reproducibility and responsiveness. *Quality of Life Research*, 10, 571–78.

Begg, C., Cho, M., Eastwood, S., Horton, R., Moher, D., Olkin, I., et al. (1996). Improving the quality of reporting of randomized controlled trials: The CONSORT statement. *Journal of the American Medical Association*, 276, 637–39.

Beilby, J., Wutzke, S.E., Bowman, J., Mackson, J.M. & Weekes, L.M. (2006). Evaluation of a national quality use of medicines service in Australia: An evolving model. *Journal of Evaluation in Clinical Practice*, 12(2), 202–17.

Belgrave, L.L., Zablotsky, D. & Guadagno, M.A. (2002). How do we talk to each other? Writing qualitative research for quantitative readers. *Qualitative Health Research*, 12(10), 1427–39.

Benjaminse, A., Gokeler, A. & van der Schans, C.P. (2006). Clinical diagnosis of an anterior cruciate ligament rupture: A meta-analysis. *Journal of Orthopaedic & Sports Physical Therapy*, 36(5), 267–88.

Beretvas, S. & Chung, H. (2008). A review of meta-analyses of single-subject experimental designs: Methodological issues and practice. *Evidence-based Communication Assessment and Intervention*, 2(3), 129–41.

Bettelheim, B. (1943). Individual and mass behavior in extreme situations. *Journal of Abnormal and Social Psychology*, 38, 417–52.

Bhangwanjee, S., Muchar, D.J.J., Jeena, P.M. & Moddley, P. (1997a). Does HIV status influence the outcome of patients admitted to a surgical intensive care unit? A prospective double blind study. *British Medical Journal*, 314, 1077–81.

Bhangwanjee, S., Muchar, D.J.J., Jeena, P.M. & Moddley, P. (1997b). Letter: Why we did not seek informed consent before testing patients for HIV. *British Medical Journal*, 314, 1081–84.

Biddle, S.J.H., Fox, K.R., Boutcher, S.H. & Faulkner, G.E. (2000). The way forward for physical activity and the promotion of psychological well-being. In *Physical activity and psychological well-being*. New York: Routledge, 154–68.

Bingham, S.A., Day, N.E., Luben, R. et al. (2003). Dietary fibre in food and protection against colorectal cancer in the European Prospective Investigation into Cancer and Nutrition (EPIC): An observational study. *Lancet*, 361, 1496–501.

Birks, M., Chapman, Y. & Francis, K. (2008). Memoing in qualitative research: Probing data and processes *Journal of Research in Nursing*, 13(1), 68–75.

Bland, J.M. & Altman, D.G. (1986). Statistical methods for assessing agreement between two methods of clinical measurement. *The Lancet*, 1(8476), 307–10.

Blumer, H. (1969/1986). *Symbolic interactionism: Perspective and method*. Berkeley, CA: University of California Press.

Bogdan, R.C. & Biklen, S.K. (2007). *Qualitative research for education: An introduction to theory and methods*, 5th edn. Boston, MA: Pearson.

Bond, T.G. & Fox, C. (2007). *Applying the Rasch model: Fundamental measurement in the human sciences*, 2nd edn. New Jersey: Lawrence Erlbaum Associates, Inc.

Booth, T. (1999). Doing research with lonely people. *British Journal of Learning Disabilities*, 26(1), 132–4.

Boutron, I., Guittet, L., Estellat, C., Moher, D., Hróbjartsson, A. & Ravaud, P. (2007). Reporting methods of blinding in randomized trials assessing nonpharmacological treatments. *PLoS Medicine*, 4(2), e61.

Boutron, I., Moher, D., Altman, D., Schulz, K. & Ravaud, P. (2008). Methods and processes of the CONSORT Group: Example of an extension for trials assessing nonpharmacologic treatments. *Annals of Internal Medicine*, 148, W60–W66.

Bourgois, P.I. (1995). *In search of respect: Selling crack in El Barrio*. Cambridge: Cambridge University Press.

Bourgois, P.I. & Schonberg, J. (2009). *Righteous dopefiend*. Berkeley, CA: University of California Press.

Bowling, A. (1995). *Measuring disease*. Buckingham, UK: Open University Press.

Bowling, A. (2002). *Research methods in health: Investigating health and health services*. 2nd edn. Buckingham, UK: Open University Press.

Bowling, A. (2005). *Measuring health: A review of quality of life measurement scales*, 3rd edn. Maidenhead, UK: Open University Press.

Boychuk-Duchscher, J.E. & Morgan, D. (2004). Grounded theory: Reflections on the emergence vs. forcing debate. *Journal of Advanced Nursing, 48*, 605–12.

Bragge, P., Bialocerkowski, A. & McMeeken, J. (2006). A systematic review of prevalence and risk factors associated with playing-related musculoskeletal disorders in pianists. *Occupational Medicine*, 56, 28–38.

Braun, V. & Clarke, V. (2006). Using thematic analysis in psychology. *Qualitative Research in Psychology*, 3, 77–101.

Bray, J., Lee, L., Smith, S. & Yorks, L. (eds) (2000). *Collaborative inquiry in practice: Action, reflection and making meaning.* Thousand Oaks, CA: Sage.

Britten, N. (2000). Qualitative interviews in health care research. In C. Pope & N. Mays (eds), *Qualitative research in health care*, 2nd edn. London: BMJ Books, 11–29.

Broom, A. & Willis, E. (2007). Competing paradigms and health research. In M. Saks & J. Allsop (eds), *Researching health: Qualitative, quantitative and mixed methods.* London: Sage Publications, 16–31.

Bruce, C., Parker, A. & Renfrew, L. (2006). 'Helping or something': Perceptions of students with aphasia and tutors in further education. *International Journal of Language & Communication Disorders*, 41(2), 137–54.

Bryman, A. (2007). Barriers to integrating qualitative and quantitative research. *Journal of Mixed Methods Research*, 1(1), 8–22.

Bryman, A. (2008). *Social research methods*, 3rd edn. Oxford: Oxford University Press.

Bulmer, M. (ed.) (1982). *Social research ethics.* London: Macmillan.

Buston, K. (1997). NUD*IST in action: Its use and its usefulness in a study of chronic illness in young people, *Sociological Research Online*, 2(3). <www.socresonline.org.uk/socresonline/2/3/6.html>, accessed 8 September 2008.

Butera-Prinzi, F. & Perlesz, A. (2004). Children's experience of living with a parent with a head injury. *Brain Injury*, 18(1), 83–101.

Byham-Gray, L.D., Gilbride, J.A., Dixon, B. & Stage, F.K. (2005). Evidence-based practice: What are dieticians' perceptions, attitudes, and knowledge? *Journal of the American Dietetic Association*, October, 1574–81.

Byrne, M. (2001). Ethnography as a qualitative research method. *AORN Journal*, 74(1), 82–4.

Cadman, D., Gafni, A. & McNamee, J. (1984). Newborn circumcision: An economic perspective. *Canadian Medical Association Journal*, 131, 1353–5.

Caplan B. & Reidy, K. (1996). Staff–patient–family conflicts in rehabilitation: Sources and solutions. *Topics in Spinal Cord Injury Rehabilitation*, 2, 21–33.

Carding, P. & Hillman, R. (2001). More randomised controlled studies in speech and language therapy. *British Medical Journal*, 323, 645–6.

Carpenter, C. (1994). The experience of spinal cord injury: The individual's perspective: implications for rehabilitation practice. *Physical Therapy*, 74(7), 614–29.

Carpenter, C. & Hammell, K. (2000). Evaluating qualitative research. In K. Walley Hammell, C. Carpenter & I. Dyck (eds), *Using qualitative research: A practical introduction for occupational and physical therapists.* Edinburgh: Churchill Livingstone, 107–19.

Carpenter, C. & Suto, M. (2008). *Qualitative research for occupational and physical therapists: A practical guide.* Oxford: Wiley-Blackwell.

Carr, W. & Kemmis, S. (1986). *Becoming critical: Education, knowledge, and action research.* Philadelphia, PA: Falmer Press.

Catterall, M. & Maclaran, P. (1997). Focus group data and qualitative analysis programs: Coding the moving picture as well as snapshots. *Sociological Research Online*, 2(1). <www.socresonline.org.uk/2/1/6.html>, accessed 6 April 2009.

Centre for Evidence-Based Medicine (2009). *Levels of evidence.* <www.cebm.net/levels_of_evidence.asp>, accessed 30 March 2009.

Centre for Reviews and Dissemination (2001). Report No 4: Undertaking systematic reviews of research on effectiveness. University of York <www.york.ac.uk/inst/crd/index.htm>, accessed 30 March 2009.

Cesario, S., Morin, K. & Santa-Donator, A. (2002). Evaluating the level of evidence of qualitative research. *Journal of Gynaecology and Neonatal Nursing*, 31(6), 708–14.

Chalmers, T.C., Celano, P., Sacks, H.S. & Smith, H., Jr. (1983). Bias in treatment assignment in controlled clinical trials. *New England Journal of Medicine*, 309(22), 1358–61.

Chan, A.-W., Hrobjartsson, A., Haahr, M.T., Gotzsche, P.C. & Altman, D.G. (2004). Empirical evidence for selective reporting of outcomes in randomized trials: Comparison of protocols to published articles. *Journal of the American Medical Association*, 291(20), 2457–65.

Charles, P., Giraudeau, B., Dechartres, A., Baron, G. & Ravaud, P. (2009). Reporting of sample size calculation in randomised controlled trials: Review. *British Medical Journal*, 338, b1732, doi: 10.1136/bmj.b1732.

Charmaz, K. (2000). Grounded theory: Objectivist and constructivist methods. In N.K. Denzin & Y.S. Lincoln (eds), *Handbook of qualitative research,* 2nd edn. Thousand Oaks, CA: Sage, 509–35.

Charmaz, K. (2002). Stories and silences: Disclosures and self in chronic illness. *Qualitative Inquiry*, 8(3), 302–328.

Charmaz, K. (2006). *Constructing Grounded Theory*. London: Sage Publications.

Cheek, J., Onslow, M. & Cream, A. (2004). Beyond the divide: Comparing and contrasting aspects of qualitative and quantitative research approaches. *Advances in Speech-Language Pathology*, 63, 147–52.

Chester, R., Costa, M.L., Shepstone, L., Cooper, A. & Donell, S.T. (2008). Eccentric calf muscle training compared with therapeutic ultrasound for chronic Achilles tendon pain: A pilot study. *Manual Therapy*, 13(6), 484–91.

Christiansen, O.B., Mathiesen, O. & Lauritsen, J.G. (1992). Study of the birthweight of parents experiencing unexplained recurrent miscarriages. *British journal of Obstetrics and Gynaecology*, 99(5), 408–11.

Chronister, J.A., Lynch, R.T., Chan, F. Rosenthal, D. & da Silva Cardoso, E. (2008). The evidence-based practice movement in healthcare: Implications for rehabilitation. *Journal of Rehabilitation*, 74(2), 6–15.

Clandinin, J.D. (ed.) (2007). *Handbook of narrative inquiry: Mapping the methodology.* Thousand Oaks, CA: Sage Publications.

Clayton, A.M. & Thorne, T. (2000). Diary data enhancing rigour: Analysis framework and verification tool. *Journal of Advanced Nursing*, 32(6), 1514–21.

Closs, S.J. & Lewin, B.J.P (1998). Education and research. Perceived barriers to research utilization: A survey of four therapies. *British Journal of Therapy & Rehabilitation*, 5(3), 151–5.

Coates, V. (2004). Qualitative research: A source of evidence to inform nursing practice? *Journal of Diabetes Nursing*, 8(9), 329–34.

Cochrane, A.L. (1979). 1931–1971: A critical review, with particular reference to the medical profession. In *Medicines for the year 2000*. London: Office of Health Economics, 1–11.

Coffin, J., Drysdale, M., Hermeston, W., Sherwood, J. & Edwards, T. (2008). Ways forward in Indigenous health. In S-T. Liaw & S. Kilpatrick (eds), *A textbook of Australian rural health*. Canberra: Australian Rural Health Education Network, 141–52.

Cohen, J. (1977). *Statistical power analysis for the behavioural sciences*. New York: Academic Press.

Cohen, J. (1992). A power primer. *Psychological Bulletin*, 112, 155–9.

Colaizzi, P.F. (1978). Psychological research as the phenomenologist views it. In R.S. Valle & M. King (eds), *Existential phenomenological alternatives for psychology*. New York: Oxford University Press, 48–71.

Collins, J. & Fauser, B. (2005). Balancing the strengths of systematic and narrative reviews. *Human Reproduction Update*, 11, 103–04.

Collins, K., Onwuegbuzie, T. & Jaio, Q. (2007). A mixed-methods investigation of mixed methods in sampling designs in social and health science research. *Journal of Mixed Methods Research*, 1(3), 267–94.

Collins, N. & Knowles, A.D. (1995). Adolescents' attitudes towards confidentiality between the school counsellor and the adolescent client. *Australian Psychologist*, 30(3), 179–82.

Concato, J. (2004). Observational versus experimental studies: What's the evidence for a hierarchy? *Journal of the American Society for Experimental Neuro-therapeutics*, 1, 341–7.

Cook, D., Mulrow, C. & Haynes, R.B. (1997). Systematic Reviews: Synthesis of Best Evidence for Clinical Decisions. *Annals of Internal Medicine*, 126, 376–80.

Cooper, A.F., Jackson, G., Weinman, J. & Horne, J. (2005). A qualitative study investigating patients' beliefs about cardiac rehabilitation. *Clinical Rehabilitation*, 19, 87–96.

Cooper, K., Smith, B.H. & Hancock, E. (2009). Patients' perceptions of self-management of chronic low back pain: Evidence for enhancing patient education and support. *Physiotherapy*, 95, 43–50.

Corbin, J. & Strauss, A. (2008). *Basics of qualitative research: Techniques and procedures for developing grounded theory*, 3rd edn. Thousand Oaks, CA: Sage Publications.

Corti, L. & Thompson, P. (2004). Secondary analysis of archived data. In C. Seale, G. Gobo, J.F. Gubrium & D. Silverman (eds), *Qualitative research practice*. London: Sage Publications, 327–43.

Cott, C. (2007). Client-centred rehabilitation: Client perspectives. *Disability and Rehabilitation*, 26(24), 1411–22.

Council for Aboriginal Reconciliation (1994). *Addressing disadvantage: A greater awareness of the causes of Indigenous Australians' disadvantage*. Canberra: Australian Government Publishing Service.

Coupland, H., Ritchie, J. & Maher, L. (2004). *Within reach: A participatory needs assessment of young injecting drug users in South Western Sydney*. Sydney: UNSW Publishing and Printing Service.

Covey, S.R. (2004). The 8th habit: From effectiveness to greatness. New York: Free Press.

Cowles, M. & Davis, D. (1982). On the origins of the .05 level of statistical significance. *American Psychologist*, 37, 553–8.

Cox, K. (2003). Assessing the quality of life of patients in phase I and II anti-cancer drug trials: Interviews versus questionnaires. *Social Science & Medicine*, 56, 921–34.

Coyne, I.T. (1997). Sampling in qualitative research. Purposeful and theoretical sampling: Merging or clear boundaries? *Journal of Advanced Nursing*, 26, 623–30.

Crapanzano, V. (1980). *Tuhami, portrait of a Moroccan*. Chicago: University of Chicago Press.

Creswell, J.W. (1998). *Qualitative inquiry and research design: Choosing among five traditions*. Thousand Oaks, CA: Sage Publications.

Creswell, J.W. (2007). *Qualitative inquiry & research design: Choosing among five approaches*, 2nd edn. Thousand Oaks, CA: Sage Publications.

Creswell, J.W. & Plano Clark, V.L. (2007). *Designing and conducting mixed methods research*. Thousand Oaks, CA: Sage Publications.

Crowther, M. & Cook, D. (2007). Trials and tribulations of systematic reviews and meta-analyses. *Hematology*, 2007, 493–7.

Cumming, S., Fitzpatrick, E., McAuliffe, D., McKain, S., Martin, C. & Tonge, A. (2007). Raising the Titanic: Rescuing social work documentation from the sea of ethical risk. *Australian Social Work*, 60(2), 239–57.

Cusick, A., Vasquez, M., Knowles, L. & Wallen, M. (2005). Effect of rater training on reliability of Melbourne Assessment of Unilateral Upper Limb Function scores. *Development Medicine & Child Neurology*, 47(1), 39–45.

Cutcliffe, J.R. (2000). Methodological issues in grounded theory. *Journal of Advanced Nursing*, 31(6), 1476–84.

Cutcliffe, J. & Ramcharan, P. (2002). Leveling the playing field? Exploring the merits of the ethics-as-process approach for judging qualitative research proposals. *Qualitative Health Research*, 12, 1000–10.

Dahm, P., Poolman, R.W., Bhandari, M., Fesperman, S.F., Baum, J., Kosiak, B., et al. (2009). Perceptions and competence in evidence-based medicine: A survey of the American Urological Association Membership. *Journal of Urology*, 181(2), 767–77.

Dalley J. & Sim J. (2001). Nurses' perceptions of physiotherapists as rehabilitation team members. *Clinical Rehabilitation*, 15, 380–89.

Daly, J., Willis, K., Small, R., Green, J., Welch, N., Kealy, M. & Hughes, E. (2007). A hierarchy of evidence for assessing qualitative health research. *Journal of Clinical Epidemiology*, 60, 43–9.

Daly, K.J. (2007). *Qualitative methods for family studies and human development*. Thousand Oaks, CA: Sage Publications.

D'Arcy Hart, P. (1999). A change in scientific approach: From alternation to randomised allocation in clinical trials in the 1940s. *British Medical Journal*, 319, 572–3.

Dattilio, F. (2006). Case-based research in family therapy. *Australian and New Zealand Journal of Family Therapy*, 27(4), 208–13.

David, R. & Whitehouse, J. (1998). Modelling the consultation process in a secondary referral unit for children. *International Journal of Language & Communication Disorders*, 33(Suppl), 532–7.

Davidson, M. (2002). The interpretation of diagnostic tests: A primer for physiotherapists. *Australian Journal of Physiotherapy*, 48(3), 227–32.

Davidson, P.M., Daly, J., Hancock, K., Chang, E., Moser, D., K. & Cockburn, J. (2003). Perceptions and experiences of heart disease: A literature review and identification of a research agenda in older women. *European Journal of Cardiovascular Nursing*, 2(4), 255–64.

Davies, D. & Dodd, J. (2002). Qualitative research and the question of rigor. *Qualitative Health Research*, 12(2), 279–89.

Davison, C., Davey-Smith, G. & Frankel, S. (1991). Lay epidemiology and the prevention paradox: The implication of coronary candidacy for health education. *Sociology of Health and Illness*, 13(1), 1–19.

Davison, C., Davey-Smith, G. & Frankel, S. (1992). The limits of lifestyle: Re-assessing 'fatalism' in the popular culture of illness prevention. *Social Science & Medicine*, 34, 675–85.

Day, S.J. & Altman, D.G. (2000). Statistics notes: Blinding in clinical trials and other studies. *British Medical Journal*, 321, 504.

De Bie, R. (2001). Critical appraisal of prognostic studies: An introduction. *Physiotherapy Theory & Practice*, 17, 161–71.

de Koning, K. & Martin, M. (1996). *Participatory research in health: Issues and experiences*. London: Zed Books.

De Laine, M. (2000). *Fieldwork, participation and practice: Ethics and dilemmas in qualitative research*. London: Sage Publications.

de Vaus, D.A. (2007). *Social surveys 2: Survey instruments and data sources*, vol. 2. London: Sage.

De Vries, R., DeBruin, D.A. & Goodgame, A. (2004). Ethics review of social, behavioural and economic research: Where should we go from here? *Ethics and Behavior*, 14(4), 351–68.

Del Mar, C., Glasziou, P. & Mayer, D. (2004). Teaching evidence based medicine. *British Medical Journal*, 329, 989–90.

Denzin, N.K. (1982). On the ethics of disguised observation: An exchange between Norman K. Denzin and Kai T. Erikson. In M. Bulmer (ed.), *Social research ethics*. London: Macmillan, 139–51.

Denzin, N.K. (2008). The new paradigm dialogs and qualitative inquiry. *International Journal of Qualitative Studies in Education*, 21(4), 315–25.

Denzin, N.K. (2009). The elephant in the living room: Or extending the conversation about the politics of evidence. *Qualitative Research*, 9(2), 139–60.

Denzin, N.K. & Lincoln, Y.S. (2005). Methods of collecting and analysing empirical materials. In N.K. Denzin & Y.S. Lincoln (eds), *The Sage handbook of qualitative research*. Thousand Oaks, CA: Sage Publications, 641–9.

Denzin, N.K. & Lincoln, Y.S. (2008). Introduction: The discipline and practice of qualitative research. In N.K. Denzin & Y.S. Lincoln (eds), *Strategies of qualitative inquiry*, 3rd edn. Thousand Oaks, CA: Sage Publications, 1–43.

Department of Health (1994). *Standards for local research ethics committees: A framework for ethical review*. London: Department of Health.

Department of Health (2001). *The expert patient: A new approach to chronic disease management in the twenty-first century*. London: Department of Health.

Department of Health (2005a). Research governance framework for health and social care. London: Department of Health. <www.dh.gov.uk/en/Publicationsandstatistics/Publications/PublicationsPolicyAndGuidance/DH_4008777>, accessed 6 April 2009.

Department of Health (2005b). *Creating a patient-led NHS: Delivering the NHS Improvement Plan*. London: Author.

Department of Veterans' Affairs (2007). Constipation: A quality of life issue for veteran patients. *Therapeutic brief*, <www.va.gov/oig/54/reports/VAOIG-06-03145-23.pdf> and <www.va.gov/oig/54/reports/VAOIG-06-03145-23.pdf>, accessed 4 February 2009.

DeVault, M. & McCoy, L. (2002). Institutional ethnography: Using interviews to investigate ruling relations. In J. Gubrium & J. Holstein (eds), *Handbook of interview research: Context and method*. Thousand Oaks, CA: Sage Publications.

de Visser, R.O., Smith, A.M.A., Rissel, C., Richters, J. & Grulich, A.E. (2003). Sex in Australia: Safer sex and condom use among a representative sample of adults. [The Australian Study of Health and Relationships, a survey of 19 307 people aged 16–59 years which had a broad focus across many aspects of sexual and reproductive health]. *Australian and New Zealand Journal of Public Health*, 27(2), 223–9.

Dew, K. (2007). A health researcher's guide to qualitative methodologies. *Australian and New Zealand Journal of Public Health*, 31(5), 433–7.

Dickson-Swift, V., James, E. & Liamputtong, P. (2008). *Undertaking sensitive research in the health and social sciences: Managing boundaries, emotions and risks.* Cambridge: Cambridge University Press.

Dillman, D.A., Smyth, J.D. & Christian, L.M. (2008). *Internet, mail, and mixed-mode surveys: The tailored design method*, 3rd edn. Hoboken, NJ: John Wiley.

Dixon-Woods, M., Shaw, R.L., Agarwal, S. & Smith, J.A. (2004). The problem of appraising qualitative research. *Quality and Safety in Health Care*, 13, 223–5.

Dobrof, J., Dolinko, A., Lichtiger, E., Uribarri, J. & Epstein, I. (2001). Dialysis patient characteristics and outcomes: The complexity of social work practice with the end stage renal disease population. *Social Work in Health Care*, 33(3/4), 105–28.

Dobrof, J., Ebenstein, H., Dodd, S-J. & Epstein, I. (2006). Caregivers and professionals partnership caregiver resource center: Assessing a hospital support program for family caregivers. *Journal of Palliative Medicine*, 9(1), 196–205.

Dodd, K. & Shields, N. (2005). A systematic review on the outcomes of cardiovascular exercise programs for people with Down syndrome. *Archives of Physical Medicine and Rehabilitation*, 86, 2051–58.

Doll, R. (1998). Controlled trials: The 1948 watershed. *British Medical Journal*, 317, 1217–20.

Doll, R., Peto, R., Boreham, J. & Sutherland, I. (2005). Mortality from cancer in relation to smoking: 50 years observations on British doctors. *British Journal of Cancer*, 92(3), 426–9.

Dominelli, L. & Holloway, M. (2008). Ethics and governance in social work research in the UK. *British Journal of Social Work*, 38(5), 1009–28.

Donovan, J., Mills, N., Smith, M., Brindle, L., Jacoby, A., Peters, T., Frankel, S., Neal, D. & Hamdy, F. (2002). Improving design and conduct of randomised trials by embedding them in qualitative research: ProtecT (prostate testing for cancer and treatment) study. *British Medical Journal*, 325, 766–70.

Douglas, J.D. (1976). *Investigative social research*. Beverley Hills, CA: Sage Publications.

Dowling, M. (2007). From Husserl to van Manen: A review of different phenomenological approaches. *International Journal of Nursing Studies*, 44(1), 131–42.

Duley, L. & Farrell, B. (2002). *Clinical trials*. London: BMJ Books.

Duncan, S. & Edwards, R. (1997). Lone mothers and paid work: Rational economic man or gendered moral rationalities? *Feminist Economics*, 3(2), 29–61.

Dunning, H., Williams, A., Abonyi, S. & Crooks, V. (2008). A mixed method approach to quality of life research: A case study approach. *Social Indicators Research*, 85, 145–58.

Dunstan, D.W., Zimmet, P.Z., Welborn, T.A., de Courten, M.P., Cameron, A.J., Sicret, R.A. et al. (2002). The rising prevalence of diabetes mellitus and impaired glucose tolerance: The Australian Diabetes, Obesity and Lifestyle study. *Diabetes Care*, 25, 829–34.

Dysart, A.M. & Tomlin, G.S. (2002). Factors related to evidence-based practice among US occupational therapy clinicians. *American Journal of Occupational Therapy*, 56(3), 275–84.

Edmonds, V.M. (2005). The nutritional patterns of recently immigrated Honduran women. *Journal of Transcultural Nursing*, 16(3), 226–36.

Edwards, S.J.L., Ashcroft, R. & Kirchin, S.T. (2004). Research ethics committees: Differences and moral judgements. *Bioethics*, 18(5), 407–27.

Edwards, T. (2008). *Research design and statistics: A bio-behavioural approach*. Boston, MA: McGraw-Hill.

Egger, M., Jüni, P., Bartlett, C., Holenstein, F. & Sterne, J. (2003). How important are comprehensive literature searches and the assessment of trial quality in systematic reviews? Empirical study. *Health Technology Assessment*, 7, 1.

Ellen, R.F. (1984). *Ethnographic research: A guide to general conduct*. London: Academic Press.

Elliot, A.C. & Woodward, W.A. (2006). *Statistical analysis quick reference and guide book with SPSS examples*. Thousand Oaks, CA: Sage Publications.

Embretson, S.E. & Hershberger, S.L. (1999). *The new rules of measurement: What every psychologist and educator should know*. Mahwah, NJ: Lawrence Erlbaum Associates.

Epstein, I. (2001). Using available clinical information in practice-based research: Mining for silver while dreaming of gold. *Social Work in Health Care*, 33(3/4), 15–32.

Epstein, I. & Auslander, G. (2001). Clinical data-mining in practice-based research: A workshop on using available clinical information. Workshop presented at the Third International Conference on Social Work in Health and Mental Health, Tampere, Finland, 1–5 July.

Epstein, I., Zilberfein, F. & Snyder, S. (1997). Using available information in practice-based outcomes research: A case study of psycho-social risk factors and liver transplant outcomes. In E.J. Mullen & J.L. Magnabosco (eds), *Outcomes in the human services: Cross-cutting issues and methods*. Washington, DC: NASW Press, 224–33.

Erikson, K.T. (1967). A comment on disguised observation in sociology. *Social Problems*, 14, 366–73.

Esterberg, K.G. (2002). *Qualitative methods in social research*. Boston, MA: McGraw Hill.

Evans, D. (2003). Hierarchy of evidence: A framework for ranking evidence evaluating healthcare interventions. *Journal of Clinical Nursing*, 12, 77–84.

Evans-Pritchard, E.E. (1937). *Witchcraft, oracles, and magic among the Azande*. Oxford: Clarendon Press.

Evans-Pritchard, E.E. (1951). *Social anthropology*. London: Cohen & West.

Fawcett, A.J.L. (2007). Principles of assessment and outcome measurement for occupational therapists and physiotherapists: Theory, skills and application. <http://library.latrobe.edu.au/record=b2264691~S5>, accessed February 2009.

Feldman, S. & Howie, L. (2009). Looking back, looking forward: Reflections on using a life history review tool with older people. *Journal of Applied Gerontology*, 28(5), 621–37.

Fergusson, D., Aaron, S.D., Guyatt, G. & Hebert, P. (2002). Post-randomisation exclusions: The intention to treat principle and excluding patients from analysis. *British Medical Journal*, 325, 652–4.

Ferguson, F.C., Brownless, M. & Webster, V. (2008). A Delphi study investigating consensus among expert physiotherapists in relation to the management of low back pain. *Musculoskeletal Care*, 6(4), 197–210.

Field, M.J. & Lohr, K.N. (1990). Clinical practice guidelines: Directions for a new program. Institute of Medicine, Washington, DC: National Academy Press.

Fielding, N. & Lee, R.M. (1998). *Computer analysis and qualitative research*. London: Sage Publications.

Figert, A. & Kuehnert, P. (1997). Reframing knowledge about the AIDS epidemic: Academic and community-based interventions. In P. Nyden, A. Figert, M. Shibley & D. Burrows (eds), *Building community: Social science in action*. Thousand Oaks, CA: Pine Forge Press, 154–60.

Finfgeld, D.L. (2003). Metasynthesis: The state of the art—so far. *Qualitative Health Research*, 13(7), 893–904.

Finlay, L. (1999). Applying phenomenology in research: Problems, principles and practice. *British Journal of Occupational Therapy*, 62(7), 299–306.

Finlay, L. & Ballinger, C. (2006). *Qualitative research for allied health professionals: Challenging choices*. West Sussex: John Wiley & Sons.

Fisher, A.G. & Fisher, A.G. (1993). The assessment of IADL motor skills: An application of many-faceted Rasch analysis. *American Journal of Occupational Therapy*, 47(4), 319–29.

Fleck, C. & Muller, A. (1997). Bruno Bettelheim and the concentration camps. *Journal of the History of Behavioural Sciences*, 33(1), 1–37.

Flemming, K. (1998). EBN notebook: Asking answerable questions. *Evidence Based Nursing*, 1(2), 36–7.

Flick, U. (2006). *An introduction to qualitative research*, 3rd edn. Newbury Park, CA: Sage Publications.

Floersch, J. (2000). Reading the case record: The oral and written narratives of social workers. *Social Service Review*, 74(2), 169–91.

Floersch, J. (2004). A method for investigating practitioner use of theory in practice. *Qualitative Social Work*, 3(2), 161–77.

Fontana, A. & Prokos, A.H. (2007). *The Interview: From Formal to Postmodern*. Walnut Creek, CA: Left Coast Press.

Fook, J. (ed.) (1996). *The reflective researcher: Social workers' theories of practice research*. Sydney: Allen & Unwin.

Fook, J. & Gardner, F. (2007). *Practising critical reflection: A resource book*. Maidenhead, UK: Open University Press.

Fossey, E., Harvey, C., Mcdermott, F. & Davidson, L. (2002). Understanding and evaluating qualitative research. *Australian and New Zealand Journal of Psychiatry*, 36(6), 717–32.

Foucault, M. (1971). Orders of discourse. *Social Science Information* 1971(10), 7. Available at <http://ssi.sagepub.com>, accessed 1 April 2009.

Foucault, M. (2009) <www.eng.fju.edu.tw/crit.97/Foucault/Foucault.htm#power>, accessed 24 March 2009.

Franklin, R., Allison, D. & Gorman, B. (eds) (1996). Design and analysis of single-case research. New Jersey: Lawrence Erlbaum Associates.

Freire, P. (1972). *Pedagogy of the oppressed*. London: Sheed & Ward.

Freud, S. (1974). *The standard edition of the complete psychological works of Sigmund Freud*. <http://freud.org.uk/furfaq.htm>, accessed 19 April 2009.

Freudenthal, S., Ahlberg, B.M., Mtweve, S., Nyindo, P., Poggensee, G. & Krantz, I. (2006). School-based prevention of schistosomiasis: Initiating a participatory action research project in northern Tanzania. *Acta Tropica*, 100, 79–87.

Friedman, L.M., Furberg, C.D. & DeMets, D.L. (1998). *Fundamentals of clinical trials*. New York: Springer.

Fritz, J.M. & Wainner, R.S. (2001). Examining diagnostic tests: An evidence-based prespective. *Physical Therapy*, 81(9), 1546–64.

Furlong, M. (1998). Cases and clinicians. *Psychotherapy in Australia*, 4(3), 48–52.

Gamberini, L. & Spagnolli, A. (2003). Display techniques and methods for cross-medial data analysis. *PsycNology Journal* 1 (2), 131–40. <www.psychology.org/File/PSYCHNOLOGY_JOURNAL_1_2_GAMBERINI.pdf >, accessed 1 January 2009.

Gearing, R.E. (2004). Bracketing in research: A typology. *Qualitative Health Research*, 14(10), 1429–52.

Geertz, C. (1973). *The Interpretation of Cultures: Selected Essays*. New York: Basic Books.

Geertz, C. (1995). *After the Fact*. Cambridge, MA: Harvard University Press.

Genat, W. (2006). *Aboriginal Health Workers: Primary Health Care at the Margins*. Perth: University of Western Australia Press.

Gergen, K.J. & Gergen, M. (1988). Narrative and the self as relationship. In L. Berkowitz (ed). *Advances in Experimental Social Psychology*. San Diego: Academic Press.

Gergen, M.M. & Gergen, K.J. (2006). Narratives in Action. *Narrative Inquiry*, 16, 112–21.

Gholizadeh, L. (2009). The discrepancy between perceived and estimated absolute risks of coronary heart disease in Middle Eastern women: Implications for cardiac rehabilitation. Unpublished PhD thesis, University of Western Sydney, Sydney.

Gibbons, J.D. (1993). *Nonparametric statistics: An introduction*. Newbury Park, CA.: Sage Publications.

Gibbs, A. (1997). Focus groups. <www.soc.surrey.ac.uk/sru/SRU19.html>, accessed 12 December 2006.

Gibbs, G.R. (2007). *Analyzing qualitative data*. London: Sage Publications.

Gibbs, L. & Gambrill, E. (2002). Evidence-based practice: Counterarguments to objections. *Research on Social Work Practice*, 12(3), 452–76.

Gibson, B.E. & Martin, D.K. (2003). Qualitative research and evidence-based physiotherapy practice. *Physiotherapy*, 89, 350–58.

Gibson, B.E. & Martin, D.K. (2003). Qualitative research and evidence-based physiotherapy practice. *Physiotherapy*, 89(6), 350–58.

Gilles, M.T., Dickinson, J.E., Cain, A., Turner, K.A., McGuckin, R., Loh, R., et al. (2007). Perinatal HIV transmission and pregnancy outcomes in indigenous women in Western Australia. *Australian and New Zealand Journal of Obstetrics and Gynaecology*, 47, 362–7.

Giorgi, A.P. & Giorgi, B.M. (2003). The descriptive phenomenological psychological method. In P.M. Camic, J.E. Rhodes & L. Yardley (eds), *Qualitative research in psychology: Expanding perspectives in methodology and design*. Washington, DC: American Psychological Association, 243–71.

Glaser, B.G. & Strauss, A. (1967). The *discovery of grounded theory: Strategies for qualitative research*. New York: Aldine.

Glaser, B.G. (1978). *Theoretical sensitivity: Advances in the methodology of grounded theory*. Mill Valley, CA: Sociology Press.

Glaser, B.G. (1992). *Emergence vs forcing: Basics of grounded theory analysis*. Mill Valley, CA: Sociology Press.

Glaser, B.G. (ed.) (1996). *Gerund grounded theory: The basic social process dissertation*. Mill Valley, CA: Sociology Press.

Glaser, B.G. (1998). *Doing grounded theory: Issues and discussions*. Mill Valley, CA: Sociology Press.

Glaser, B.G. (2001). *The grounded theory perspective: Conceptualization contrasted with description*. Mill Valley, CA: Sociology Press.

Glaser, B.G. (2002a). Conceptualisation: On theory and theorizing using grounded theory [electronic version]. *International Journal of Qualitative Methods*, 1, 1–31. <www.ualberta.ca/~iiqm/backissues/1_2Final/pdf/glaser.pdf>, accessed 10 March 2009.

Glaser, B.G. (2002b). Constructivist grounded theory? [electronic version]. *Forum: Qualitative Social Research*, 3. <http://nbn-resolving.de/urn:nbn:de:0114-fqs0203125>, accessed 14 January 2009.

Glaser, B.G. (2003). *The grounded theory perspective II: Description's remodelling of grounded theory*. Mill Valley, CA: Sociology Press.

Glaser, B.G. (2004). Naturalistic inquiry and grounded theory [electronic version]. *Forum: Qualitative Social Research*, 5. <http://nbn-resolving.de/urn:nbn:de:0114-fqs040170>, accessed 10 March 2009.

Glaser, B.G. & Holton, J. (2004). Remodeling grounded theory [electronic version]. *Forum: Qualitative Social Research*, 5. <www.qualitative-research.net/fqs-texte/2-04/2-04glaser-e.pdf>, accessed 12 March 2009.

Goffman, I. (1969). *Where the action is: Three essays*. London: Allen Lane.

Golafshani, N. (2003). Understanding reliability and validity in qualitative research. *The Qualitative Report*, 8(4), 597–607.

Goleman, D. (2006). *Social intelligence: The new science of human relationships*. New York: Bantam Books.

Gomm, R. (2004). *Social research methodology: A critical introduction*. London: Palgrave Macmillan.

Goodfellow, J. (1997). Narrative inquiry: Musings, methodology and merits. In J. Higgs (ed.), *Qualitative research: Discourse on methodologies*. Sydney: Hampden Press, 61–74.

Gordis, L. (2009). *Epidemiology*, 4th edn. Saunders: Elsevier.

Goulding, C. (2002). *Grounded theory: A practical guide for management, business and market researchers*. London: Sage Publications.

Grady, C. (2001). Money for research participation: Does it jeopardize informed consent? *American Journal of Bioethics*, 1(2), 40–44.

Grant, S., Aitchison, T., Henderson, E., Christie, J., Zare, S., McMurray, J. & Dargie, H. (1999). A comparison of the reproducibility and the sensitivity to change of visual analogue scales, Borg scales, and Likert scales in normal subjects during submaximal exercise. *Chest*, 116, 1208–17.

Graves, J. (2007). Factors influencing indirect speech and language therapy interventions for adults with learning disabilities: The perceptions of carers and therapists. *International Journal of Language and Communication Disorders*, 42(suppl 1), 103–21.

Grazian, D. (2003). Blue *Chicago: The search for authenticity in urban blues clubs*. Chicago: Chicago University Press.

Grbich, C. (2007). *Qualitative data analysis: An introduction*. London: Sage Publications.

Green, J. & Britten, N. (1998). Qualitative research and evidence based medicine. *British Medical Journal*, 316, 1230–32.

Green, J. & Thorogood, N. (2009). *Qualitative methods for health research*, 2nd edn. London: Sage Publications.

Greene, J.C. (2007). *Mixed methods in social inquiry*. San Francisco: Wiley.

Greenfield, B.H. (2006). The meaning of caring in five experienced physical therapists. *Physiotherapy Theory and Practice*, 22, 175–87.

Greenfield, B.H., Anderson, A., Cox, B. & Tanner, M.C. (2008). Meaning of caring to 7 novice physical therapists during their first year of clinical practice. *Physical Therapy*, 88(10), 1154–66.

Greenhalgh, T. (1997). How to read a paper: Papers that summarise other papers (systematic reviews and meta-analyses). *British Medical Journal*, 315, 672–5.

Greenhalgh, T. (2001). *How to read a paper: The basics of evidence based medicine*. London: BMJ books.

Greenhalgh, T. (2006). *How to read a paper: The basics of evidenced based medicine*, 2nd edn. Malden, MA: Blackwell Publishing/BMJ Books.

Greenhalgh, T. & Peacock, R. (2005). Effectiveness and efficiency of search methods in systematic reviews of complex evidence: Audit of primary sources. *British Medical Journal*, 331, 1064–65.

Grinnell, R.M. & Unrau, Y.A. (eds) (2005). *Social work research and evaluation: Quantitative and qualitative approaches*. New York: Oxford University Press.

Grinnell Jr, R.M., Unrau, Y.A. & Williams, M. (2008). Introduction. In R.M. Grinnell & Y.A. Unrau (eds), *Social work research and evaluation: Foundations of evidence-based practice*, 8th edn. New York: Oxford University Press, 4–27.

Grove, S.K. (2007). *Statistics for health care research: A practical workbook*. Edinburgh: Elsevier Saunders.

Grypdonck, M.H.F. (2006). Qualitative health research in the era of evidenced-based practice. *Qualitative Health Research*, 16(10), 1371–85.

Guba, E.G. & Lincoln, Y.S. (1981). *Effective evaluation: Improving usefulness of evaluation results through responsive and naturalistic approach*. San Francisco: Jossey-Bass.

Guba, E.G. & Lincoln, Y.S. (1989). *Fourth generation evaluation*. Newbury Park, CA: Sage Publications.

Guba, E.G. & Lincoln, Y.S. (1994). Competing paradigms in qualitative research. In N.K. Denzin & Y.S. Lincoln (eds), *Handbook of qualitative research*. Thousand Oaks, CA: Sage Publications, 105–17.

Guba, E.G. & Lincoln, Y.S. (2005). Paradigmatic controversies, contradictions and emerging confluences. In N.K. Denzin & Y.S. Lincoln (eds), *The Sage handbook of qualitative research*. Thousand Oaks, CA: Sage Publications, 191–215.

Guba, E.G. & Lincoln, Y.S. (2008). Paradigmatic controversies, contradictions, and emerging confluences. In N.K. Denzin & Y.S. Lincoln (eds), *The landscape of qualitative research*, 3rd edn. Thousand Oaks, CA: Sage Publications, 255–86.

Gubrium, J.F. & Holstein, J.A. (2002). *Handbook of interview research: Context and method*. Thousand Oaks, CA: Sage Publications.

Guest, G., Bunce, A. & Johnson, L. (2006). How many interviews are enough? An experiment with data saturation and variability. *Field Methods*, 18(1), 59–82.

Guillemin, M. & Gillam, L. (2004). Ethics, reflexivity and 'ethically important moments' in research. *Qualitative Inquiry*, 10(2), 261–81.

Guyatt, G.H., Haynes, R.B., Jaeschke, R.Z., Cook, D.J., Green, L., Naylor, C.D., et al. (2000). Evidence-based medicine: Principles for applying the users' guides to patient care. *Journal of the American Medical Association*, 284(10), 1290–96.

Haahr, M.T. & Hrobjartsson, A. (2006). Who is blinded in randomized clinical trials? A study of 200 trials and a survey of authors. *Clinical Trials*, 3(4), 360–65.

Hagey, R.S. (1997). The use and abuse of participatory action research [editorial]. *Chronic Diseases in Canada*, 18(1), 1–4.

Hajiro, T. & Nishimura, K. (2002). Minimal clinically significant difference in health status: The thorny path of health status measures? *European Respiratory Journal*, 19, 390–91.

Halcomb, E.J., Gholizadeh, L., Phillips, J. & Davidson, P. (2007). Literature review: Considerations in undertaking focus group research with culturally and linguistically diverse groups. *Journal of Clinical Nursing*, 16(6), 1000–11.

Hall, W.A. & Callery, P. (2001). Enhancing the rigor of grounded theory: Incorporating the reflexivity and relationality. *Qualitative Health Research*, 11(2), 257–72.

Hammell, K.W. (2006). *Perspectives on disability and rehabilitation: Contesting assumptions; challenging practice.* Edinburgh: Churchill Livingstone/Elsevier.

Hammell, K.W. & Carpenter, C. (2000). Introduction to qualitative research in occupational therapy and physical therapy. In K.W. Hammell, C. Carpenter & I. Dyck (eds), *Using qualitative research: A practical introduction for occupational and physical therapists.* Edinburgh: Churchill Livingstone, 1–12.

Hammell, K.W. & Carpenter, C. (2004). *Qualitative research in evidence-based rehabilitation.* Edinburgh: Churchill Livingstone.

Hammersley, M. (1996). The relationship between qualitative and quantitative research: Paradigm loyalty versus methodological eclecticism. In J.T.E. Richardson (ed.), *Handbook of research methods for psychology and the social sciences.* Leicester: BPS Books, 159–74.

Hammersley, M. (2005). Close encounters of a political kind: The threat from the evidence-based policy-making and practice movement. *Qualitative Researcher,* 1, 2–4.

Hammersley, M. (2008). The issue of quality in qualitative research. *International Journal of Research & Method in Education,* 30(3), 287–305.

Hammersley M. & Atkinson P. (1995). *Ethnography: Principles in practice,* 2nd edn. London: Routledge & Kegan Paul.

Hammersley, M. & Atkinson, P. (2007). *Ethnography: Principles in practice,* 3rd edn. Milton Park, Abingdon, UK: Routledge.

Hanna, S., Russell, D., Bartlett, D., Kertoy, M., Rosenbaum, P. & Swinton, M. (2005). *Clinical Measurement Guidelines for Service Providers.* <http://canchild.icreate3.esolutionsgroup.ca/en/canchildresources/resources/ClinicalMeasurement.pdf>, accessed 15 March 2009.

Hansen, E.C. (2006). *Successful qualitative health research: A practical introduction.* Sydney: Allen & Unwin.

Hart, E. & Bond, M. (1995). *Action research for health and social care: A guide to practice.* Buckingham, UK: Open University Press.

Hartley, J., Sydes, M. & Blurton, A. (1996). Obtaining information accurately and quickly: Are structured abstracts more efficient? *Journal of Information Science,* 22, 349–56.

Hartsock, N. (1987). The feminist standpoint: Developing the ground for a specifically feminist historical materialism. In S. Harding (ed.), *Feminism and methodology.* Bloomington, IN: Indiana University Press, 157–80.

Hawker, S., Payne, S., Kerr, C., Hardey, M. & Powell, J. (2002). Appraising the evidence: Reviewing disparate data systematically. *Qualitative Health Research,* 12(9), 1284–99.

Hay, D.P., Franson, K.L., Hay, L. & Grossberg, G.T. (1998). Depression. In E.H. Duthie & P.R. Katz (eds), *Practice of geriatrics,* 3rd edn. Philadelphia, PA: W.B. Saunders Company, 286–94.

Haynes, R.B., Mulrow, C.D., Huth, E.J., Altman, D.G. & Gardner, M.J. (1990). More informative abstracts revisited. *Annals of Intern Medicine,* 113, 69–76.

Heinemann, A.W., Linacre, J.M., Wright, B.D. & Hamilton, B.B. (1994). Prediction of rehabilitation outcomes with disability measures. *Archives of Physical Medicine and* Rehabilitation, 75, 133–43.

Hennink, M.M. (2007). *International focus group research: A handbook for the health and social sciences.* Cambridge: Cambridge University Press.

Henry, J., Dunbar, T., Arnott, A., Scrimgeour, M., Matthews, S., Murakami-Gold, L., et al. (2002a). *Indigenous research reform agenda: Changing institutions,* vol. 3. Casuarina, NT: Cooperative Research Centre for Aboriginal and Tropical Health.

Henry, J., Dunbar, T., Arnott, A., Scrimgeour, M., Matthews, S., Murakami-Gold, L., et al. (2002b). *Indigenous research reform agenda: Rethinking methodologies*. Casuarina, NT: Cooperative Research Centre for Aboriginal and Tropical Health.

Herbert, R., Jamtvedt, G., Mead, J. & Birger Hagen, K. (2005). *Practical evidence-based physiotherapy*. Edinburgh: Elsevier/Butterworth/Heinemann.

Hersh, D. (2003). 'Weaning' clients from aphasia therapy: Speech pathologists' strategies for discharge. *Aphasiology*, 17(11), 1007–29.

Hesse-Biber, S.N. & Leavy, L.P. (2005). *The practice of qualitative research*. Thousand Oaks, CA: Sage Publications.

Hewitt, C., Hahn, S., Torgerson, D.J., Watson, J. & Bland, J.M. (2005). Adequacy and reporting of allocation concealment: Review of recent trials published in four general medical journals. *British Medical Journal*, 330, 1057–58.

Higgins, J.P.T. & Green, S. (2008). Cochrane Handbook for Systematic Reviews of Interventions 5.0.1 [updated September 2008]. <www.cochrane-handbook.org/>.

Hill, E., Graham, M. & Shelley, J. (2007). *A comparison of hysterectomy trends in Australian*. Melbourne: Deakin University.

Hirschi, T. (1969). *Causes of delinquency*. Berkeley, CA: University of California Press.

Hochschild, A. (1990). *The second shift: Working parents and the revolution of the home*. New York: Viking.

Hochschild, A. (2003). *The commercialization of intimate life: Notes from home and work*. Berkeley, CA: University of California Press.

Hollis, S. & Campbell, F. (1999). What is meant by intention to treat analysis? Survey of published randomised controlled trials. *British Medical Journal*, 319, 670–74.

Holloway, I. (2005). *Qualitative research in health care*. Maidenhead, UK: Open University Press.

Holloway, I. & Wheeler, S. (2002). *Qualitative research in nursing*, 2nd edn. Oxford: Blackwell Science.

Holmefur, M. (2009). The Assisting Hand Assessment: Continued development, psychometrics and longitudinal use. Doctoral dissertation, Karolinska Institutet, Stockholm.

Holroyd, E., Twinn, S. & Adab, P. (2004). Socio-cultural influences on Chinese women's attendance for cervical screening. *Journal of Advanced Nursing*, 46(1), 42–52.

Holton, J. (2007). The coding process and its challenges. In A. Bryant & K. Charmaz (eds), *The Sage handbook of grounded theory*. London: Sage Publications, 265–89.

Holton, J.A. (2007). The coding process and its challenges. In A. Bryant & K. Charmaz (eds), *The Sage handbook of grounded theory*. London: Sage Publications, 265–89.

Horner, R.D. & Baer, D.M. (1978). Multiple-probe technique: A variation of the multiple baseline. *Journal of Applied Behavior Analysis*, 11(1), 189–96.

Howard, D., Best, W. & Nickels, L. (submitted). Optimising the design of intervention studies: Critiques and ways forward. *Journal of Speech Language and Hearing Research*.

Howie, L., Coulter, M. & Feldman, S. (2004). Crafting the self: Narratives of occupational identity. *American Journal of Occupational Therapy*, 58(4), 446–54.

Hrobjartsson, A., Gotzsche, P. & Gluud, C. (1998). The controlled clinical trial turns 100 years: Fibiger's trial of serum treatment of diptheria. *British Medical Journal*, 317, 1243–45.

Hughes, C. (1992). 'Ethnography': What's in a word—process? product? promise? *Qualitative Health Research*, 2(4), 439–50.

Humphery, K. (2001). Dirty questions: Indigenous health and 'Western research'. *Australian and New Zealand Journal of Public Health*, 25(3), 197–202.

Humphreys, L. (1975). *Tearoom trade: Impersonal sex in public places*. New York: Aldine.

Iacono. T. (2006). Ethical challenges and complexities of including people with intellectual disability as participants in research. *Journal of Intellectual and Developmental Disability*, 31(3), 173–9.

Iles, R. & Davidson, M. (2006). Evidence based practice: A survey of physiotherapists' current practice. *Physiotherapy Research International*, 11(2), 93–103.

International Committee of Medical Journal Editors (2009). *Uniform requirements for manuscripts submitted to biomedical journals: Writing and editing for biomedical publication. III. J. Obligation to Register Clinical Trials.* <www.icmje.org/#clin_trials>.

Ioannidis, J.P.A. (1998). Effect of the statistical significance of results on the time to completion and publication of randomized efficacy trial. *Journal of the American Medical Association*, 279(4), 281–86.

Israel, B.A., Eng, E., Schulz, A.J. & Parker, E.A. (2005). *Methods in community-based participatory research for health*. San Francisco: Jossey-Bass.

Ittenback, R. & Lawhead, W. (1996). Historical and philosophical foundation of single-case research. In R. Franklin, D. Allison & B. Gorman (eds), *Design and analysis of single-case research*. New Jersey: Lawrence Erlbaum Associates, 13–39.

Jackson, J.L., O'Malley, P.G. & Kroenke, K. (2003). Evaluation of acute knee pain in primary care. *Annals of Internal Medicine*, 139(7), 575–88.

Jadad, A. (1998). *Randomised controlled trials*. London: BMJ Books.

Jadad, A.R., Moore, R.A., Carroll, D., Jenkinson, C., Reynolds, D.J.M., Gavaghan, D.J., et al. (1996). Assessing the quality of reports of randomized clinical trials: Is blinding necessary? *Controlled Clinical Trials*, 17, 1–12.

Jamtvedt, G., Young. J.M., Krisotffersen, D.T., O'Brien, M.A. & Oxman, A.D. (2006). Audit and feedback: Effects on professional practice and health care outcomes. *Cochrane Database of Systematic Reviews. Issue 2.* <www.cochrane.org/reviews/en/ab000259.html>.

Jenkinson, C. & McGee, H. (1998). *Health status measurement: A brief but critical introduction*. Oxford: Radcliffe Medical Press.

Jette, D.U., Bacon, K., Batty, C., Carlson, M., Ferland, A., Hemingway, R.D., et al. (2003). Evidence-based practice: Beliefs, attitudes, knowledge, and behaviors of physical therapists. *Physical Therapy*, 83(9), 786–805.

Joanna Briggs Institute (2000). Best practice information sheet: *Identification and management of dysphagia in adults with neurological impairment*, 4(2), Adelaide: Joanna Briggs Institute.

Joanna Briggs Institute (2008). Best practice information sheet: *Management of constipation in older adults*, 12(7). Adelaide: Joanna Briggs Institute.

Johnson, B. (2008). Editorial: Living with tensions: The dialectic approach. *Journal of Mixed Methods Research*, 2(3), 203–07.

Johnson, J.M. (2002). In-depth interviewing. In J.F. Gubrium & J.A. Holstein (eds), *Handbook of interview research: Context and method*. Thousand Oaks, CA: Sage Publications, 103–19.

Johnson, L.M., Randall, M., Reddihough, D., Oke, L.E., Byrt, T.A. & Bach, T.M. (1994). Development of a clinical assessment of quality of movement for unilateral upper limb function. *Developmental Medicine & Child Neurology*, 36, 965–73.

Johnson, R. & Onwuegbuzie, T. (2006). Mixed methods research: A research paradigm whose time has come. *Educational Researcher*, 33(7), 14–26.

Johnson, R. & Waterfield, J. (2004). Making words count: The value of qualitative research. *Physiotherapy Research International*, 9(3), 121–31.

Johnson, R.B., Onwuegbuzie, A.J. & Turner, L.A. (2007). Toward a definition of mixed methods research. *Journal of Mixed Methods Research*, 1(2), 112–33.

Jones, P. (1987). The untreatable family. *Child Abuse and Neglect*, 11, 409–20.

Jorgensen, D. L. (1989). *Participant observation: A methodology for human studies*. Newbury Park, CA: Sage Publications.

Josselson, R. (2006). Narrative research and the challenge of accumulating knowledge. *Narrative Inquiry*, 16, 4–10.

Josselson, R. (2007). The ethical attitude in narrative research: Principles and practicalities. In J.D. Clandinin (ed.), *Handbook of narrative inquiry: Mapping the methodology*. Thousand Oaks, CA: Sage Publications, 537–66.

Jüni, P., Altman, D. & Egger, M. (2001). Assessing the quality of controlled clinical trials. *British Medical Journal*, 323, 42–6.

Jüni, P., Altman, D.G. & Egger, M. (2001). Systematic reviews in health care: Assessing the quality of controlled clinical trials. *British Medical Journal*, 323, 42–6.

Jüni, P., Witschi, A., Bloch, R. & Egger, M. (1999). The hazards of scoring the quality of clinical trials for meta-analysis. *Journal of the American Medical Association*, 282(11), 1054–60.

Kaida, A., Gray, G., Bastos, F.I., Andia, I., Maier, M., McIntyre, J., et al. (2008). The relationship between HAART use and sexual activity among HIV-positive women of reproductive age in Brazil, South Africa and Uganda. *AIDS Care*, 20(1), 21–5.

Kale, R. (1997). Letter: Failing to seek patients' consent to research is always wrong. *British Medical Journal*, 314, 1081–84.

Kazdin, A.E. (2003). Clinical significance: Measuring whether interventions make a difference. In A.E. Kazdin (ed.), *Methodological issues and strategies in clinical research*, 3rd edn. Washington, DC: American Psychological Association, 547–68.

Kearney, M. (2001). Levels and applications of qualitative research evidence. *Research in Nursing & Health*, 24, 145–53.

Keech, A., Gebski, V. & Pike, R. (eds) (2007). *Interpreting and reporting clinical trials: A guide to the CONSORT statement and the principles of randomised controlled trials*. Sydney: MJA Books.

Keene, J. (2001). *Clients with complex needs: Inter-professional practice*. Oxford: Blackwell Science.

Kellehear, A. (1993). *The unobtrusive researcher: A guide to methods*. Sydney: Allen & Unwin.

Keller, C., Fleury, J., Perez, A., Ainsworth, B. & Vaughan, L. (2008). Using visual methods to uncover context. *Qualitative Health Research*, 18(3), 428–36.

Kelly, T. & Howie, L. (2007). Working with stories in nursing research: Procedures used in narrative analysis. *International Journal of Mental Health Nursing*, 16, 136–44.

Kent, G. (1996). Shared understandings for informed consent: The relevance of psychological research on the provision of information. *Social Science and Medicine*, 43(10), 1517–23.

Khanlou, N. & Peter, E. (2004). Participatory action research: Considerations for ethical review, *Social Science and Medicine*, 60(10), 2333–40.

Kielhofner, G. (2008). *Model of Human Occupation: Theory and Application*, 4th edn. Baltimore, MA: Lippincott Williams & Wilkins.

Kielhofner, G., Borrell, L., Holzmueller, R., Jonsson, H., Josephson, S., Keonen, R. et al. (2008). Crafting occupational life. In G. Kielhofner (ed.). *Model of human occupation: Theory and application*, 4th edn. Baltimore. MA: Lippincott Williams & Wilkins, 110–25.

Kingma, J.J., de Knikker, R., Wittink, H.M. & Takken, T. (2007). Eccentric overload training in patients with chronic Achilles tendinopathy: A systematic review. *British Journal of Sports Medicine*, 41(6), e3.

Kirkham, S. (2003). The politics of belonging and intercultural health care. *Western Journal of Nursing Research*, 25(7), 762–80.

Kitson, A., Harvey, G. & McCormack, B. (1998). Enabling the implementation of evidence-based practice: A conceptual framework. *Quality in Health Care*, 7, 149–58.

Kline, T.J.B. (2005). *Psychological testing: A practical approach to design and application*. Thousand Oaks, CA: Sage Publications.

Klingels, K., De Cock, P., Desloovere, K., Huenaerts, C., Molenaers, G., Van Nuland, I., et al. (2008). Comparison of the Melbourne Assessment of Unilateral Upper Limb Function and the Quality of Upper Extremity Skills Test in hemiplegic CP. *Development Medicine & Child Neurology*, 50(12), 904–09.

Koch, T. & Kralik, D. (2001). Chronic illness: Reflections on a community-based action research programme. *Journal of Advanced Nursing*, 36(1), 23–31.

Koch, T., Selim, P. & Kralik, D. (2002). Enhancing lives through the development of a community-based participatory action research programme. *Journal of Clinical Nursing*, 11, 109–17.

Koehn, M.L. & Lehman, K. (2008). Nurses' perceptions of evidence-based nursing practice. *Journal of Advanced Nursing*, 62(2), 209–15.

König, T. (2004). *CAQDAS—A primer*. <www.lboro.ac.uk/research/mmethods/research/software/ caqdas_primer.html#what>, accessed 30 March 2009.

Kovacs, M., Feinberg, T.L., Paulaskas, S., Finkelstein, R., Pollock, M. & Crouse-Novak, M. (1985). Initial coping responses and psychosocial characteristics of children with insulin-dependent diabetes mellitus. *Journal of Pediatrics*, 106, 827–34.

Krippendorff, K. (2004). *Content analysis: An introduction to its methodology*, 2nd edn. Thousand Oaks, CA: Sage Publications.

Krueger, R.A. (1998). *Focus group kit: Analyzing & reporting focus group results*, 6th edn. Thousand Oaks, CA: Sage Publications.

Krueger, R.A. & Casey, M.A. (2009). *Focus groups: A practical guide for applied research*, 4th edn. Thousand Oaks, CA: Sage Publications.

Krumlinde-Sundholm, L. & Eliasson, A. (2003). Development of the Assisting Hand Assessment: A Rasch-built measure intended for children with unilateral upper limb impairments. *Scandinavian Journal of Occupational Therapy*, 10(1), 16–26.

Kummerer, S.E., Lopez-Reyna, N.A. & Hughes, M.T. (2007). Mexican immigrant mothers' perceptions of their children's communication disabilities, emergent literacy development, and speech-language therapy program. *American Journal of Speech-Language Pathology*, 16(3), 271–82.

Kvale, S. (2007). *Doing interviews*. London: Sage Publications.

Kvale, S. & Brinkmann, S. (2008). *InterViews: Learning the craft of qualitative research interviewing*. London: Sage Publications.

La Pelle, N. (2004). Simplifying qualitative data analysis using general purposes software tools. *Field Methods*, 16(1), 85–108.

Lacey, E.A. (1998). Social and medical research: Is there a difference? *Social Sciences in Health*, 4(4), 211–17.

Lai Fong Chiu (2002). *Straight talking: Communicating breast screening information in primary care*. Leeds, UK: Nuffield Institute for Health.

Laine, C., Horton, R., DeAngelis, C.D., Drazen, J.M., Frizelle, F.A., Godlee, F., et al. (2007). Clinical trial registration: Looking back and moving ahead. *New England Journal of Medicine*, 356(26), 2734–6.

Laine, M.D. (1997). *Ethnography: Theory and applications in health research*. Sydney: MacLennan & Petty.

Landorf, K.B. & Burns, J. (2009). Health outcome assessment. In B. Yates (ed.), *Merriman's assessment of the lower limb*. Edinburgh: Elsevier/Churchill Livingstone, 35–51.

Landorf, K.B., Radford, J.A., Keenan, A-M. & Redmond, A.C. (2005). Effectiveness of low-dye taping for the short-term management of plantar fasciitis. *Journal of the American Podiatric Medical Association*, 95(6), 525–30.

Lang, T.A. & Secic, M. (1997). *How to report medical statistics in medicine*. Philadelphia, PA: American College of Physicians.

Last, J.M., Abramson, J.H., Friedman, G.D., Porta, M., Spasoff, R.A. & Thuriaux, M. (eds), (1995). *A dictionary of epidemiology*, 3rd edn. New York: Oxford University Press.

Laugharne, C. (1995). Ethnography: Research method or philosophy? *Nurse Researcher*, 3(2), 45–54.

Law, M. (2004). Outcome measures rating form guidelines. <www.canchild.ca/Default.aspx?tabid=192>, accessed 12 March 2009.

Lee, P. (2005). The process of gatekeeping in health care research. *Nursing Times*, 101(32), 36–8.

Lee, C. & Gramotnev, H. (2006). Predictors and outcomes of early motherhood in the Australian longitudinal study on women's health. *Pyschology, Health and Medicine*, 11(1), 29–47.

Lee, R. & Fielding, N.G. (1991). Computing for qualitative research: Options, problems and potential. In N.G. Fielding & R.M. Lee (eds), *Using computers in qualitative research*. London: Sage Publications, 1–13.

Lee, R.M. & Renzetti, C.M. (1993). The problems of researching sensitive topics: Introduction. In C.M. Renzetti & R.M. Lee (eds), *Researching sensitive topics*. London: Sage Publications, 3–13.

Leininger, M.M. (1979). *Transcultural nursing*. New York: MASSON International Nursing Publications.

Leininger, M.M. (1985). *Qualitative research methods in nursing*. Orlando, FL: Grune & Stratton.

Leininger, M.M. (1994). *Nursing and anthropology: Two worlds to blend*. Columbus, OH: Greyden Press.

Letts, L., Wilkins, S., Law, M., Stewart, D., Bosch, J. & Westmorland, M. (2007a). Critical review form: Qualitative studies. Occupational Therapy Evidence-Based Research Group, McMaster University. Available at: <www.srs-mcmaster.ca/Default.aspx?tabid=630>, accessed 20 July 2009.

Letts, L. et al. (2007b). Guidelines for critical review form: Qualitative studies (version 2.0). Occupational Therapy Evidence-Based Research Group, McMaster University. Available at: <www.srs-mcmaster.ca/Default.aspx?tabid=630>, accessed 20 July 2009.

Levy, R.I. (1988). *Tahitians: Mind and experience in the society islands* (Midway reprint edn). Chicago: University of Chicago Press.

Lewin, K. (1946/1988). Action research and minority problems. In Deakin University (ed.), *The action research reader*. Melbourne: Deakin University. Originally published in 1946, 41–6.

Lewins, A. & Silver, C. (2007). *Using software in qualitative research: A step-by-step guide*. Los Angeles: Sage Publications.

Liamputtong, P. (2007). Researching the vulnerable: A guide to sensitive research methods. London: Sage Publications.

Liamputtong, P. (2009). *Qualitative research methods*, 3rd edn. Melbourne: Oxford University Press.

Liamputtong, P. (2010). *Performing qualitative cross-cultural research*. Cambridge: Cambridge University Press.

Liamputtong, P. (in press). *Focus group methodology: Principles and practices*. London: Sage Publications.

Liamputtong, P., Haritavorn, N. & Kiatying-Angsulee, N. (2009). HIV and AIDS, stigma and AIDS support groups: Perspectives from women living with HIV and AIDS in central Thailand. *Social Science and Medicine*, special issue on Women, Mothers and HIV Care in Resource Poor Settings, 69(6), 862–8.

Lincoln, Y.S. & Guba, E.G. (1985). *Naturalistic inquiry*. Beverly Hills, CA: Sage Publications.

Lincoln, Y.S. & Guba, E.G. (1989). *Fourth generation evaluation*. Newbury Park, CA: Sage Publications.

Logemann, J.A. (2004). Evidence-based practice. *Advances in Speech-Language Pathology*, 6(2), 134–5.

Long, C.L. & Hollin, C.R. (1997). The scientist-practitioner model in clinical psychology: A critique. *Clinical Psychology and Psychotherapy*, 4(2), 75–83.

Lopez, K.A. & Willis, D.G. (2004). Descriptive versus interpretive phenomenology: The contributions to nursing knowledge. *Qualitative Health Research*, 14(5), 726–35.

Low, J. (2007). Unstructured interviews and health research. In M. Saks and J. Allsop (eds), *Health research: Qualitative, quantitative and mixed methods*. London: Sage Publications, 74–91.

Lynoe, N., Sandlund, M. & Jacobsson, L. (1999). Research ethics committees: A comparative study of assessment of ethical dilemmas. *Scandinavian Journal of Psychiatry*, 2, 152–9.

MacKenzie, A. (1992). Learning from experience in the community: An ethnographic study of district nurse students. *Journal of Advanced Nursing*, 17, 682–91.

Madriz, E. (2000). Focus groups in feminist research. In P. Labella (ed.), *Handbook of qualitative research*. London: Sage Publications, 835–9.

Maher, L., Tran, T., Sargent, P., Tran, M.G. & Musson, R. (2002). Participatory action research with PLWHA in Vietnam. In *Proceedings of the XIV international AIDS conference*, Barcelona, 7–12 July 2002, 14.

Malanga, G.A., Andrus, S., Nadler, S.F. & McLean, J. (2003). Physical examination of the knee: A review of the original test description and scientific validity of common orthopedic tests. *Archives of Physical Medicine & Rehabilitation*, 84(4), 592–603.

Malinowski, B. (1922/1961). *Argonauts of the western Pacific: An account of native enterprise and adventure in the archipelagoes of Melanesian New Guinea*. New York: E. P. Dutton.

Malinowski, B. (1932). *The sexual life of savages in north-western Melanesia: An ethnographic account of courtship, marriage and family life among the natives of the Trobriand islands, British New Guinea*, 3rd edn. London: Routledge & Kegan Paul.

Mansell, J. & Beadle-Brown, J. (2004). Person-centred planning or person-centred action? A response to the commentators. *Journal of Applied Research in Intellectual Disabilities* 17, 31–5.

Manuel, J., Fang, L., Bellamy, J.L. & Bledsoe, S.E. (2008). Evaluating evidence. In R.M. Grinnell & Y.A. Unrau (eds), *Social work research and evaluation: Foundations of evidence-based practice*, 8th edn. New York: Oxford University Press, 482–95.

Marcus, G.E. & Fischer, M.M.J. (1999). *Anthropology as cultural critique: An experimental moment in the human sciences*, 2nd edn. Chicago: University of Chicago Press.

Markham, C. & Dean, T. (2006). Parents' and professionals' perceptions of quality of life in children with speech and language difficulty. *International Journal of Language & Communication Disorders*, 41(2), 189–212.

Marshall, J., Goldbart, J. & Phillips, J. (2007). Parents' and speech and language therapists' explanatory models of language development, language delay and intervention. *International Journal of Language & Communication Disorders*, 42(5), 533–55.

Martone, M. (2001). Decisionmaking issues in the rehabilitation process. *Hastings Center Report*, 31, 36–41.

Marvasti, A. (2008). Writing and presenting social research. In P. Alasuutari, L. Bickman & J. Brannen (eds), *The Sage handbook of social research methods*. London: Sage Publications, 602–16.

Marvasti, A.B. (2004). *Qualitative research in sociology*. London: Sage Publications.

Mason, J. (2002). *Qualitative researching*, 2nd edn. London: Sage Publications.

Matthews, J.N.S. (2006). *An introduction to randomized controlled clinical trials*. Boca Raton, FL: Chapman & Hall/CRC.

Matyas, T.A. & Greenwood, K.M. (1990). Visual analysis of single-case time series: Effects of variability, serial dependence, and magnitude of intervention effects. *Journal of Applied Behavioral Analysis*, 23, 333–9.

Maxwell, S.E. & Delany, H.D. (2003). *Designing experiments and analysing data: A model comparison perspective*. Mahwah, NJ: Lawrence Erlbaum Associates.

Mayo, K., Tsey, K. & the Empowerment Research Team (2009). *Research dancing: Reflections on the relationships between university-based researchers and community-based researchers at Gurriny Yealamucka Health Services Aboriginal Corporation, Yarabah*. Casuarina, NT: Cooperative Research Centre for Aboriginal Health.

McAuley, E. & Courneya, K. S. (1994). The subjective exercise experiences scale (SEES): Development and preliminary validation. *Journal of Sport and Exercise Psychology*, 16, 163–77.

McCann, T.V. & Clark, E. (2003a). Grounded theory in nursing research, Part 1: Methodology. *Nurse Researcher*, 11(2), 7–18.

McCann, T.V. & Clark, E. (2003b). Grounded theory in nursing research, Part 2: Critique. *Nurse Researcher*, 11(2), 19–28.

McCurdy, D.W., Spradley, J.P. & Shandy, D.J. (2005). *The cultural experience: Ethnography in complex society*, 2nd edn. Long Grove, IL.: Waveland Press.

McDonald, K. (1999). *Struggles for subjectivity*. Cambridge: Cambridge University Press.

McDonald, M., Townsend, A., Cox, S.M., Paterson, N.D. & Lafreniere, D. (2008). Trust in health research relationships: accounts of human subjects. *Journal of Empirical Research on Human Research Ethics*, 3(4), 35–47

McDowell, I. (2006). *Measuring health: A guide to rating scales and questionnaires*. New York: Oxford University Press.

McDowell, I. & Newell, C. (1996). *Measuring health: A guide to rating scales and questionnaires*. New York: Oxford University Press.

McLauchlan, G. & Handoll, H.H.G. (2001). Interventions for treating acute and chronic Achilles tendinitis. (Vol. Art. No.: CD000232. DOI: 10.1002/14651858.CD000232.): *Cochrane Database of Systematic Reviews*.

McPherson, K., Herbert, A., Judge, A., Clarke, A., Bridgman, S., Maresh, M., et al. (2005). Psychosexual health 5 years after hysterectomy: Population-based comparison with endometrial ablation for dysfunctional uterine bleeding. *Health Expectations*, 8, 234–43.

McReynolds, L. & Kearns, K. (1984). *Single-subject experimental designs in communicative disorders*. Baltimore. MA: University Park Press.

Mead, M. (1942). *Growing up in New Guinea: A study of adolescence and sex in primitive societies*. Harmondsworth: Penguin.

Mead, M. (1944). *The American character*. Harmondsworth: Penguin.

Mead, M. (1949). *Male and female, A study of the sexes in a changing world*. New York: W. Morrow.

Mead, M. (1951). *The school in American culture*. Cambridge, MA: Harvard University Press.

Mead, M. (1956). *New lives for old: Cultural transformation—Manus, 1928–1953*. London: Gollancz.

Mead, M. (1961). *Coming of age in Samoa: A psychological study of primitive youth for Western civilization*. New York: W. Morrow.

Mead, M. (1965). *And keep your powder dry: An anthropologist looks at America (A new expanded edn)*. New York: Morrow.

Mead, M. (1968). *The mountain Arapesh*. Garden City, NY: Natural History Press.

Mead, M. (1977). *Sex and temperament in three primitive societies*. London: Routledge & Kegan Paul.

Mead, M. & American Museum of Natural History (1970). *Culture and commitment: A study of the generation gap*. London and Sydney: Bodley Head.

Mead, M. & Baldwin, J. (1971). *A rap on race*. Philadelphia, PA: Lippincott.

Mead, M. & Heyman, K. (1965). *Family*. New York: Macmillan.

Mead, M. & Macgregor, F.M.C. (1951). *Growth and culture: A photographic study of Balinese childhood*. New York: Putnam.

Mead, M. & Wolfenstein, M. (1955). *Childhood in contemporary cultures*. Chicago: University of Chicago Press.

Meltzer, P.J., Abbott, P. & Spradling, P. (2002). Teaching gerontology using the Self-Discovery Tapestry: An innovative instrument. *Gerontology & Geriatrics Education*, 23(2), 49–63.

Merighi, J., Ryan, M., Renouf, N. & Healy, B. (2005). Reassessing a theory of professional expertise: A cross-national investigation of expert mental health social workers. *British Journal of Social Work*, 35, 709–25.

Miles, M.B. & Huberman, A.M. (1994). *Qualitative data analysis*, 2nd edn. Beverley Hills, CA: Sage Publications.

Milgram, S. (1974). *Obedience and authority: An experimental view*. New York: Harper Collins

Miller W.L. & Crabtree, B.F. (2005). Clinical research. In N.K. Denzin & Y.S. Lincoln (eds), *The Sage handbook of qualitative research*, 2nd edn. Thousand Oaks, CA: Sage Publications, 605–39.

Minichiello, V., Aroni, R. & Hays, T. (2008). *In-depth interviewing*, 3rd edn. Sydney: Pearson Prentice Hall.

Minkler, M. & Wallestein, N. (2008). *Community-based participatory research for health: From process to outcomes*, 2nd edn. San Francisco: Jossey-Bass.

Mirabito, D. (2001). Mining treatment termination data in an adolescent mental health service: A quantitative study. *Social Work in Health Care*, 33(3/4), 71–90.

Mirkovic, M., Green, R., Taylor, N. & Perrott, M. (2005). Accuracy of clinical tests to diagnose superior labral anterior and posterior (SLAP) lesions. *Physical Therapy Reviews*, 10, 5–14.

Mishler, E.G. (1999). *Storylines: Craftartists' narratives of identity*. Cambridge, MA: Harvard University Press.

Moffatt, S., White, M., Mackintosh, J. & Howel, D. (2006). Using quantitative and qualitative data in health services research: What happens when mixed method findings conflict? *BMC Health Services Research*, 6.

Moher, D. & Tricco, A. (2008). Issues related to the conduct of systematic reviews: A focus on the nutrition field. *American Journal of Clinical Nutrition*, 88, 1191–9.

Moher, D., Dulberg, C.S. & Wells, G.A. (1994). Statistical power, sample size, and their reporting in randomized controlled trials. *Journal of the American Medical Association*, 272(2), 121–4.

Moher, D., Cook, D., Eastwood, S., Olkin, I., Rennie, D. & Stroup, D. (1999). Improving the quality of reports of meta-analyses of randomised controlled trials. *The Lancet*, 354, 1896–900.

Moher, D., Schulz, K.F., Altman, D.G. for the CONSORT Group (2001a). The CONSORT statement: Revised recommendations for improving the quality of reports of parallel-group randomised trials. *The Lancet*, 357, 1191–4.

Moher, D., Schulz, K.F., Altman, D.G. for the CONSORT Group (2001b). The CONSORT dtatement: Revised tecommendations for improving the quality of reports of parallel-group randomized trials. *BMC Medical Research Methodology*, 1, 2.

Moher, D., Schulz, K.F., Altman, D.G. for the CONSORT Group (2009). *The CONSORT statement: Revised recommendations for improving the quality of reports of parallel-group randomized trials*. <www.consort-statement.org/>.

Moran, G., Fongay, P., Kurtz, A., Bolton, A. & Brook, C. (1991). A controlled study of the psychoanalytic treatment of brittle diabetes. *Journal of the American Academy of Child and Adolescent Psychiatry*, 30(6), 926–35.

Morgan, D. (2007). Paradigms lost and pragmatism regained: Methodological implications of combining qualitative and quantitative methods. *Journal of Mixed Methods Research*, 1(January), 48–76.

Morgan, D.L. (1993). Qualitative content analysis: A guide to paths not taken. *Qualitative Health Research*, 3, 112–21.

Morgan, D.L. (1998). *Focus group kit*, vol. 1: *Focus group guidebook*. Thousand Oaks, CA: Sage Publications.

Morgan, D. & Morgan, R. (2009). *Single-case research methods for the behavioural and health sciences*. Los Angeles: Sage Publications.

Morrell, C. & Harvey, G. (2003). *The clinical audit handbook*. London: Elsevier Science.

Morse, J.M. (1994a). Designing funded qualitative research. In N.K. Denzin & Y.S. Lincoln (eds), *Handbook of qualitative research*. Thousand Oaks, CA: Sage Publications, 220–35.

Morse, J.M. (1994b). *Critical issues in qualitative research methods*. Thousand Oaks, CA: Sage Publications.

Morse, J.M. (1998). What's wrong with random selection. *Qualitative Health Research*, 8(6), 733–5.

Morse, J.M. (2005). Beyond the clinical trail: Expanding criteria for evidence. *Qualitative Health Research*, 15(1), 3–4.

Morse, J.M. (2007). Strategies of intraproject sampling. In P.L. Munhall (ed.), *Nursing research: A qualitative perspective*, 4th edn. Sudbury, MA: Jones & Bartlett, 529–39.

Morse, J.M., Barrett, M., Mayan, M., Olson, K. & Spiers, J. (2002). Verification strategies for establishing reliability and validity in qualitative research. *International Journal of Qualitative Methods*, 1(2), Article 2. <www.ualberta.ca/~iiqm/backissues/1_2Final/pdf/morseetal.pdf>, accessed 29 July 2008.

Morse, J.M. & Richards, L. (2002). *Read me first for a user's guide to qualitative methods*. Thousand Oaks, CA: Sage Publications.

Moses, J.W. & Knutsen, T.L. (2007). *Ways of knowing: Competing methodologies in social and political research*. Basingstoke: Palgrave Macmillan.

Moustakas, C. (1994). *Phenomenological research methods*. Thousand Oaks, CA: Sage Publications.

Muecke, M. (1994). On the evaluation of ethnographies. In J. Morse (ed.), *Critical issues in qualitative research methods*. Thousand Oaks, CA: Sage Publications, 187–209.

Muir Gray, J. (1997). *Evidence-based healthcare*. London: Churchill Livingstone.

Muldoon, M.F., Barger, S.D., Flory, J.D. & Manuck, S.B. (1998). What are quality of life measurements measuring? *British Medical Journal*, 316, 542–5.

Mullen, E.J., Bellamy, J.L. & Bledsoe, S.E. (2008). Evidence-based practice. In R.M. Grinnell & Y.A. Unrau (eds), *Social work research and evaluation: Foundations of evidence-based practice*, 8th edn. New York: Oxford University Press, 508–24.

Munhall, P.L. (2007). The landscape of qualitative research in nursing. In P.L. Munhall (ed.), *Nursing research: A qualitative perspective*, 4th edn. Sudbury, MA: Jones & Bartlett, 3–36.

Murphy, A. & McDonald, J. (2004). Power, status and marginalisation: Rural social workers and evidence-based practice in multidisciplinary teams. *Australian Social Work*, 57(2), 127–36.

Mykhalovskiy, E. & McCoy, L. (2002). Troubling ruling discourses of health: Using institutional ethnography in community-based research. *Critical Public Health*, 12(1), 17–37.

Nathan, P. & Gorman, J. (eds) (2002). *A guide to treatments that work*, 2nd edn. Oxford: Oxford University Press.

Nathan, P., Gorman, J. & Salkind, N. (1999). *Treating mental health disorders: A guide to what works*. New York: Oxford University Press.

National Aboriginal and Torres Strait Islander Health Council (2003). National strategic framework for Aboriginal and Torres Strait Islander health 2003–2013: Framework for Action by Governments. Canberra: NATSIHC.

National Aboriginal Health Strategy Working Party (1989). *A national Aboriginal health strategy*. Canberra: Australian Government Publishing Service.

Nay, R. (1993). Benevolent oppression: Lived experiences of nursing home life. Unpublished PhD thesis, University of New South Wales, Sydney.

Nay, R. & Fetherstonhaugh, D. (2007). Evidence-based practice: Limitations and successful implementation. *Annals of the New York Academy of Science*, 1114, 456–63.

Nettleton, J. & Reilly, O. (1998). Facilitating effective learning during clinical placement. *International Journal of Language & Communication Disorders*, 33(Suppl.), 250–4.

Neuendorf, K.A. (2002). *The content analysis guidebook.* Thousand Oaks, CA: Sage Publications.

Neuman, W.L. (2006). *Social research methods: Qualitative and quantitative approaches*, 6th edn. Boston, MA: Pearson/Allyn & Bacon.

Newell, D.J. (1992). Intention-to-treat analysis: Implications for quantitative and qualitative research. *International Journal of Epidemiology*, 21, 837–41.

NHMRC (National Health and Medical Research Council) (1999a). *A guide to the development, implementation and evaluation of clinical practice guidelines.* Canberra: Commonwealth of Australia.

NHMRC (1999b). *National statement on research involving humans.* Canberra: Commonwealth of Australia.

NHMRC (2003). *Values and ethics: Guidelines for ethical conduct in Aboriginal and Torres Strait Islander health research.* Canberra: NHMRC.

NHMRC (2005). *Keeping research on track: A guide for Aboriginal and Torres Strait Islander peoples about health research ethics.* Canberra: Australian Government Publishing Service.

NHMRC (2007). *National statement on ethical conduct in human research.* Canberra: NHMRC and AVCC.

NHMRC (2008a). *NHMRC additional levels of evidence and grades for recommendations for developers of guidelines* Stage 2 Consultation early 2008 to end June 2009: Canberra: Australian Government.

NHMRC (2008b). *NHMRC evidence hierarchy.* <www.nhmrc.gov.au/guidelines/_files/Stage%202%20 Consultation%20Levels%20and%20Grades.pdf>, accessed 20 April 2009.

Nieminen, P., Rucker, G., Miettunen, J., Carpenter, J. & Schumacher, M. (2007). Statistically significant papers in psychiatry were cited more often than others. *Journal of Clinical Epidemiology*, 60(9), 939–46.

Nilsson, D. (2001). Psycho-social problems faced by 'frequent flyers' in a paediatric diabetes unit. *Social Work in Health Care*, 33(3/4), 53–69.

NOP World (2005). International survey on breast cancer. Offprint of study tables provided on request. The survey is reported on <http://info.cancerresearchuk.org/news/archive/pressreleases/2005/ june/75016?a=5441>.

Northam, E., Anderson, P., Werther, G., Adler, R. & Andrewes, D. (1995). Neuropsychological complications of insulin dependent diabetes in children. *Child Neuropsychology*, 1(1), 74–87.

Northam, E., Anderson, P., Adler, R., Werther, G. & Warne, G. (1996). Psychosocial and family functioning in children with insulin-dependent diabetes at diagnosis and one year later. *Journal of Pediatric Psychology*, 21(5), 699–717.

Northcutt, N. & McCoy, D. (2004). *Interactive qualitative analysis: A systems method for qualitative research.* London: Sage Publications.

Nyden, P. & Wiewel, W. (1992). Collaborative research: Harnessing the tensions between researcher and practitioner. *American Sociologist*, 23(4), 43–55.

Oakley, A. (2009). Interviewing women: A contradiction in terms. In N. Fielding (ed.), *Interviewing II*, vol. 1. London: Routledge, 93–115.

O'Cathain, A., Murphy, E. & Nicholl, J. (2007). Why, and how, mixed methods research is undertaken in health services research in England, A mixed methods study. *BMC Health Services Research*, 7.

Oermann, M.H. (2001). *Writing for publication in nursing*. Philadelphia, PA: Lippincott Williams & Wilkins.

O'Halloran, P.D. (2007). Mood Changes in weeks 2 and 6 of a graduated group walking program in previously sedentary persons with type 2 diabetes. *Australian Journal of Primary Health*, 13, 68–73.

Oleckno, W.A. (2002). *Essential epidemiology: Principles and applications*. Long Grove, IL: Waveland Press.

Orbach, S. (1984). *Fat is a feminist issue*. London: Hamlyn.

Orbach, S. (2009). *Bodies*. London: Picador.

Osterlind, S.J. (2006). *Modern measurement: Theory, principles, and applications of mental appraisal*. New Jersey: Pearson Education/Merrill Prentice Hall.

Padgett, D.K. (2008). *Qualitative methods in social work research*, 2nd edn. Los Angeles: Sage Publications.

Palisano, R.J., Rosenbaum, P.L., Bartlett, D. & Livingston, M.H. (2008). Content validity of the expanded and revised gross motor function classification system *Developmental Medicine & Child Neurology*, 50, 744–50.

Patton, M. (1990). *Qualitative evaluation and research methods*. Thousand Oaks, CA: Sage Publications.

Patton, M. (2002). *Qualitative research and evaluation methods*, 3rd edn. Thousand Oaks, CA: Sage Publications.

Peat, J.K. (2001). *Health science research: A handbook of quantitative methods*. Sydney: Allen & Unwin.

PEDro (2009). *PEDro rating scale*. Sydney: Centre for Evidence-based Physiotherapy. <www.pedro.org.au/>.

Pellatt, G.C. (2007). Patients, doctors, and therapists perceptions of professional roles in spinal cord injury rehabilitation: Do they agree? *Journal of Interprofessional Care*, 21(2), 165–77.

Pelto, P.J. & Pelto, G.H. (1978). *Anthropological research: The structure of inquiry*, 2nd edn. Cambridge: Cambridge University Press.

Perlesz, A., Furlong, M. & the 'D' Family (1996). A systemic therapy unravelled: In through the out door. In C. Flaskas & A. Perlesz (eds), *The therapeutic relationship in systemic therapy*. London: Karnac Books, 142–57.

Perlesz, A., Furlong, M. & McLachlan, D. (1992). Family work and Acquired Brain Injury. *Australian and New Zealand Journal of Family Therapy*, 13(3), 145–53.

Perlesz, A., Kinsella, G.J. & Crowe, S. (2000). Psychological distress and family satisfaction following Traumatic Brain Injury: Injured individuals and their primary, secondary and tertiary carers. *Journal of Head Trauma Rehabilitation*, 15(3), 909–29.

Pfeffer, N. (2004). Screening for breast cancer: Candidacy and compliance. *Social Science and Medicine*, 58, 151–60.

Phillips, D. (1973). *Abandoning method*. San Francisco: Jossey-Bass.

Phillips, J. & Davidson, P. (2009). Action Research as a mixed method design. In E.J. Halcomb & S. Andrew (eds), *Mixed methods in health research*. Sydney: John Wiley & Sons, 195–216.

Piantadosi, S. (2005). *Clinical trials: A methodologic perspective*. New York: Wiley Interscience.

Pilling, S. & Slattery, J. (2004). Management competencies: Intrinsic or acquired? What competencies are required to move into speech pathology management and beyond? *Australian Health Review*, 27(1), 84–92.

Pilote, L. & Hlatky, M. (1995). Attitudes of women toward hormone therapy and prevention of heart disease. *American Heart Journal*, 129, 1237–38.

Pinnegar, S. & Daynes, G.J. (2007). Locating narrative inquiry historically: Thematics in the turn to narrative. In J.D. Clandinin (ed.), *Handbook of narrative inquiry: Mapping the methodology*. Thousand Oaks, CA: Sage Publications, 3–34.

Piper, M.C. & Darrah, J. (1994). *Motor assessment of the developing infant*. Philadelphia, PA: W.B. Saunders.

Plath, D. (2006). Evidence based practice: Current issues and future directions. *Australian Social Work*, 59(1), 56–72.

Pocock, S.J. (ed.) (1983). *Clinical trials: A practical approach*. Chichester: John Wiley & Sons.

Polgar, S. & Thomas, S.A. (2007). *Introduction to research in health sciences*, 5th edn. Edinburgh: Churchill Livingstone.

Polkinghorne, D.E. (2005). Narrative configuration in qualitative analysis. In A.J. Hatch & R. Wisniewski (eds), *Life history and narrative: Qualitative study series 1*. London: RoutledgeFalmer, 5–24.

Poolman, R.W., Sierevelt, I.N., Farrokhyar, F., Mazel, J.A., Blankevoort, L. & Bhandari, M. (2007). Perceptions and competence in evidence-based medicine: Are surgeons getting better? A questionnaire survey of members of the Dutch Orthopaedic Association. *Journal of Bone & Joint Surgery—American Volume*, 89(1), 206–15.

Popay, J., Rogers, A. & Williams, G. (1998). Rationale and standards for the systematic review of qualitative literature in health services research. *Qualitative Health Research*, 8, 341–51.

Portney, L.G. & Watkins, M.P. (2000). *Foundations of clinical research: Applications to practice*, 2nd edn. Upper Saddle River, NJ: Prentice Hall Health.

Portney, L. & Watkins, M. (2009). *Foundations of clinical research: Applications to practice*, 3rd edn. New Jersey: Prentice Hall Health.

Prasad, K.R.S. & Reddy, K.T.V. (2004). Auditing the audit cycle: An open-ended evaluation. *Clinical Governance: An International Journal*, 9(2), 110–14.

Pravikoff, D.S., Tanner, A.B. & Pierce, S.T. (2005). Readiness of U.S. nurses for evidence-based practice. *American Journal of Nursing*, 105(9), 40–51; quiz 52.

Priest, N., Mackean, T., Waters, E., Davis, E. & Riggs, E. (2009). Indigenous child health research: A critical analysis of Australian studies. *Australian and New Zealand Journal of Public Health*, 33(1), 55–63.

Procter, R., Carmichael, R. & Laterza, V. (2008). Co-interpretation of usage data: A mixed methods approach to evaluation of online environments. *International Journal of Multiple Research Approaches*, 2(1), 44–56.

Proschan, M.A. & Waclawiw, M.A. (2000). Practical guidelines for multiplicity adjustment in clinical trials. *Controlled Clinical Trials*, 21, 527–39.

Pyett, P. & VicHealth Koori Health Research and Community Development Unit. (2002). Towards reconciliation in Indigenous health research: The responsibilities of the non-Indigenous researcher. *Contemporary Nurse*, 14(1), 56–65.

Pyett, P., Waples-Crowe, P. & van der Sterren, A. (2008). Challenging our own practices in Indigenous health promotion and research. *Health Promotion Journal of Australia*, 19(3), 179–83.

Pyett, P., Waples-Crowe, P. & van der Sterren, A. (2009). Engaging with Aboriginal communities in an urban context: Some practical suggestions for public health researchers. *Australian and New Zealand Journal of Public Health*, 33(1), 51–4.

Quimby, E. (2006). Ethnography's role in assisting mental health research and clinical practice. *Journal of Clinical Psychology*, 62(7), 859–79.

Radcliffe-Brown, A.R. (1922/1964). *The Andaman Islanders*. New York: Free Press of Glencoe.

Radcliffe-Brown, A.R. (1931). *The social organization of Australian tribes*. Melbourne: Macmillan.

Radford, J.A., Landorf, K.B., Buchbinder, R. & Cook, C. (2006). Effectiveness of low-dye taping for the short-term treatment of plantar heel pain: A randomised trial. *BMC Musculoskeletal Disorders*, 7, 64.

Raines, J.C. (2008). Evaluating qualitative research studies. In R.M. Grinnell & Y.A. Unrau (eds), *Social work research and evaluation: Foundations of evidence-based practice*, 8th edn. New York: Oxford University Press, 446–1.

Ramazanoğlu, C. (ed.) (1993). *Up against Foucault: Explorations of some tensions between Foucault and feminism*. London: Routledge.

Ramcharan, P. (2006). Ethical challenges and complexities of including vulnerable people in research: some pre-theoretical considerations. *Journal of Intellectual and Developmental Disability*, 31(3), 183–5.

Ramcharan, P. & Cutcliffe, J. (2001). Judging the ethics of qualitative research: Considering the ethics as process model. *Journal of Health and Social Care in the Community*, 9(6), 358–66.

Ramsden, I. (1990). Cultural safety. *New Zealand Nursing Journal*, 83(11), 18–19.

Randall, M. (2009). Modification and psychometric evaluation of the Melbourne assessment of unilateral upper limb function. Unpublished PhD thesis, La Trobe University, Melbourne.

Randall, M., Imms, C. & Carey, L. (2008). Establishing validity of a modified Melbourne assessment for children aged 2–4 years. *American Journal of Occupational Therapy*, 62(4), 373–84.

Randall, M., Johnson, L. & Reddihough, D. (1999). *The Melbourne Assessment of unilateral upper limb function: Test administration manual*. Melbourne: Royal Children's Hospital.

Rapley, T. (2004). Interviews. In C. Seale, G. Gobo, J.F. Gubrium & D. Silverman (eds), *Qualitative research practice*. London: Sage Publications, 15–33.

Rapley, T. (2007). *Doing conversation, discourse and document analysis*. London: Sage Publications.

Rapport, F. (2005). Hermeneutic phenomenology: The science of interpretation of texts. In I. Holloway (ed.), *Qualitative research in health care*. Oxford: Blackwell, 125–46.

Rapport, N. & Overing, J. (2000). *Social and cultural anthropology: The key concepts*. Routledge: London.

Rauscher, L. & Greenfield, B.H. (2009). Advancements in contemporary physical therapy research: Use of mixed methods designs. *Physical Therapy*, 89(1), 91–100.

Rawson, H. & Liamputtong, P. (2009). Influence of traditional Vietnamese culture on the utilisation of mainstream health services for sexual health issues by second-generation Vietnamese Australian young women. *Sexual Health*, 6, 75–81.

Read, C. & Bateson, D. (2009). Marrying research, clinical practice and cervical screening in Australian Aboriginal women in western New South Wales, Australia. *Rural and Remote Health*, 9(1117). <www.rrh.org.au>, accessed 20 May 2009.

Registered Nurses Association of Ontario (2005). *Prevention of constipation in the older adult population*. Ontario: RNAO.

Reid, W.J. (1994). *Qualitative research in social work*. New York: Columbia University Press.

Reilly, S. (2004). The move to evidence-based practice in speech pathology. In S. Reilly, J. Douglas & J. Oates (eds), *Evidence-based practice in speech pathology*. London: Whurr, 3–17.

Reissman, C.K. (2008). *Narrative methods for the human sciences*. Los Angeles: Sage Publications.

Richardson, L. (2003). Writing: A method of inquiry. In N.K. Denzin & Y.S. Lincoln (eds), *Collecting and interpreting qualitative materials research*, 2nd edn. Thousand Oaks, CA: Sage Publications, 499–501.

Richters, J., Grulich, A.E., De Visser, R.O., Smith, A.M.A. & Rissel, C. (2003). Sex in Australia: Contraceptive practices among a representative sample of women. [The Australian Study of Health and Relationships, a survey of 19 307 people aged 16–59 years which had a broad focus across many aspects of sexual and reproductive health.]. *Australian and New Zealand Journal of Public Health*, 27(2), 210–16.

Ritchie, J. & Lewis, J.E. (2005). *Qualitative research practice*. London: Sage Publications.

Ritchie, J., Spencer, L. & O'Connor, W. (2003). Carrying out qualitative analysis. In J. Ritchie & J. Lewis (eds), *Qualitative Research Practice: A Guide for Social Science Students* London: Sage.

Robertson, M. & Boyle, J. (1984). Ethnography: Contributions to nursing research. *Journal of Advanced Nursing*, 9(1), 43–9.

Rogers, G. & Bouey, E. (2005). Participant observation. In R. Grinnell & Y. Unrau (eds), *Social work research and evaluation: Quantitative and qualitative approaches*. New York: Oxford University Press, 232–44.

Roland, M. & Torgerson, D. (1998a). Understanding controlled trials: What outcomes should be measured? *British Medical Journal*, 317, 1075–80.

Roland, M. & Torgerson, D. (1998b). Understanding controlled trials: What are pragmatic trials? *British Medical Journal*, 316, 285.

Rolfe, G. (2006). Validity, trustworthiness and rigour: Quality and the idea of qualitative research. *Journal of Advanced Nursing*, 53(3), 304–10.

Rolls, L. & Relf, M. (2006). Bracketing interviews: Addressing methodological challenges in qualitative interviewing in bereavement and palliative care. *Mortality,* 11(3), 286–305.

Romanello, M. & Knight-Abowitz, K. (2000). The 'ethic of care' in physical therapy practice and education: Challenges and opportunities. *Journal of Physical Therapy Education*, 14(5), 20–25.

Rorty, R. (1989). *Contingency, irony and solidarity*. Cambridge: Cambridge University Press.

Rosaldo, M. (1980). Knowledge and passion: Ilongot notions of self and social life. Cambridge: Cambridge University Press.

Rose, M. (2009). Single-subject experimental designs. In A. Perry, M. Morris & S. Cotton (eds), *Menzies Foundation: Handbook for allied health* researchers. Melbourne: Menzies Foundation, ch. 2.4.

Rose, M. Douglas, J. & Matyas, T. (2002). The comparative effectiveness of gesture and verbal treatments for a specific phonologic naming impairment. *Aphasiology*, 15(10/11), 977–90.

Rose, M. & Douglas, J. (2006). A comparison of verbal and gesture treatments for a word production deficit resulting from acquired apraxia of speech. *Aphasiology*, 20(12), 1186–209.

Rose, M. & Sussmilch, G. (2008). The effects of semantic and gesture treatments on verb retrieval and verb use in aphasia. *Aphasiology*, 22(7), 691–706.

Rosenberger, W.F. & Lachin, J.M. (2002). *Randomization in clinical trials: Theory and practice*. New York: Wiley Interscience.

Rossman, G.B. & Rallis, S.F. (2003). *Learning in the field: An introduction to qualitative research*, 2nd edn. Thousand Oaks, CA: Sage Publications.

Royal College of Nursing Research Society (2005).*Informed consent in health and social care: RCN Guidance for Nurses.* London: RCN.

Rubin, A. & Parrish, D. (2007). Views of evidence-based practice among faculty in Master of Social Work programs: A national survey. *Research on Social Work Practice*, 17(1), 110–22.

Rubin, H.J. & Rubin, I.S. (2005). *Qualitative interviewing: The art of hearing data*, 2nd edn. Thousand Oaks, CA: Sage Publications.

Ryan, G.W. (2004). Using a word processor to tag and retrieve blocks of text. *Field Methods*, 16(1), 109–30.

Ryan, G.W. & Bernard, H.R. (2003). Techniques to identify themes. *Field Methods*, 15(1), 85–109.

Ryan, M. & Sheehan, R. (in press). Research articles in 'Australian Social Work' from 1998–2007: A content analysis. *Australian Social Work.*

Sackett, D.L., Rosenburg, W.M., Gray Muir, J.A., Haynes, R.B. & Richardson, W.S. (1996). Evidence based medicine: What it is and what it isn't. *British Medical Journal*, 312, 71–2.

Sackett, D.L., Richardson, W.S., Rosenberg, W. & Haynes, R.B. (1997). *Evidence-based medicine: How to practice and teach EBM.* London: Churchill Livingstone.

Sackett, D., Straus, S., Richardson, W., Rosenberg, W. & Haynes, R. (2000). *Evidence-based medicine: How to practice and teach EBM*, 2nd edn. Edinburgh: Churchill Livingstone.

Sajatovic, M. & Ramirez, L.F. (2003). *Rating scales in mental health,* 2nd edn. Hudson, OH: Lexi-Comp.

Saks, M. & Allsop, J. (2007). *Researching health: Qualitative, quantitative and mixed methods.* London: Sage Publications.

Salbach, N.M., Jaglal, S.B., Korner-Bitensky, N., Rappolt, S. & Davis, D. (2007). Practitioner and organizational barriers to evidence-based practice of physical therapists for people with stroke. *Physical Therapy*, 87(10), 1284–303.

Saldaña, J. (2009). *Coding in qualitative data analysis.* Thousand Oaks, CA: Sage Publications.

Sale, J.E.M., Lohfeld, L.H. & Brazil, K. (2002). Revisiting the quantitative-qualitative debate: Implications for mixed-methods research. *Quality & Quantity*, 36(1), 43–53.

Sandelowski, M. (2004). Using qualitative research. *Qualitative Health Research*, 14(10), 1366–86.

Sarantakos, S. (2005). *Social research*, 3rd edn. New York: Palgrave Macmillan.

Satyendra, L. & Byl, N. (2006). Effectiveness of physical therapy for Achilles tendinopathy: An evidence based review of eccentric exercises. *Isokinetics and Exercise Science*, 14(1), 71–80.

Savage, J. (2000). Ethnography and health care. *British Medical Journal*, 321, 1400–02.

Savage, J. (2006). Ethnographic evidence. *Journal of Research in Nursing*, 11(5), 383–93.

Scally G. & Donaldson L.J. (1998). The NHS's 50th anniversary. Clinical governance and the drive for quality improvement in the new NHS in England. *British Medical Journal*, 317, 61–5.

Schachter, C., Stalker, C. & Teram, E. (1999). Toward sensitive practice: Issues for physical therapists working with survivors of childhood abuse. *Physical Therapy,* 79(3), 248–61.

Schade, D.S., Drumm, D.A., Duckworth, W.C. & Eaton, R.P. (1985). The etiology of incapacitating Brittle Diabetes. *Diabetes Care*, 1, 12–20.

Schmidt, F.L. (1996). Statistical significance testing and cumulative knowledge in psychology: Implications for the training of researchers. *Psychological Methods*, 1, 115–29.

Scholten, R.J.P.M., Opstelten, W., van der Plas, C.G., Bijl, D., Deville, W.L.J.M. & Bouter, L.M. (2003). Accuracy of physical diagnostic tests for assessing ruptures of the anterior cruciate ligament: A meta-analysis. *Journal of Family Practice*, 52(9), 689–94.

Schon, D. (1983). *The reflective practitioner*. Basic Books: New York.

Schulz, K.F. (1995). Subverting randomization in controlled trials. *Journal of the American Medical Association*, 274(18), 1456–58.

Schulz, K.F. (1996). Randomised trials, human nature, and reporting guidelines. *The Lancet*, 348, 596–8.

Schulz, K.F., Chalmers, I., Hayes, R.J. & Altman, D.G. (1995). Empirical evidence of bias: Dimensions of methodological quality associated with estimates of treatment effects in controlled trials. *Journal of the American Medical Association*, 273(5), 408–12.

Schulz, K.F. & Grimes, D.A. (2002a). Allocation concealment in randomised trials: Defending against deciphering. *The Lancet*, 359, 614–18.

Schulz, K.F. & Grimes, D.A. (2002b). Blinding in randomised trials: Hiding who got what. *The Lancet*, 359, 696–700.

Schulz, K.F. & Grimes, D.A. (2002c). Sample size slippages in randomized trials: Exclusions and the lost and wayward. *The Lancet*, 359, 781–5.

Schutt, R.K. (2008). Sampling. In R.M. Grinnell & Y.A. Unrau (eds), *Social work research and evaluation: Foundations of evidence-based practice*, 8th edn. New York: Oxford University Press, 136–56.

Schwandt, T. (1997). *Qualitative inquiry: A dictionary of terms*. Thousand Oaks, CA: Sage Publications

Schwartz, H. & Jacobs, J. (1979). *Qualitative sociology*. New York: Free Press.

Schwartz, D. & Lellouch, J. (2009). Explanatory and pragmatic attitudes in therapeutical trials. *Journal of Clinical Epidemiology*, 62(5), 499–505.

Schwartz, M. & Polgar, S. (2003). *Statistics for evidence based health care*. Melbourne: Tertiary Press.

Scott, K. & McSherry, R. (2008). Evidence-based nursing: Clarifying the concepts for nursing in practice. *Journal of Clinical Nursing*, 18, 1085–95.

Seale, C.F. (2005). Using computers to analyse qualitative data. In D. Silverman (ed.), *Doing qualitative research: A practical handbook*, 2nd edn. London: Sage Publications, 188–208.

Seeley, J., Biraro, S., Shafer, L.A., Nasirumbi, P., Foster, S., Whitworth, J. & Grosskurth, H. (2008). Using in-depth qualitative data to enhance our understanding of quantitative results regarding the impact of HIV and AIDS on households in rural Uganda. *Social Science and Medicine*, 67(10), 1434–46.

Serry, T., Liamputtong, P. & Rose, M. (under review). Perspectives about the role of oral language as a function of learning to read: Views from primary school educators. *Language, Speech and Hearing Services in Schools*.

Shagi, S., Vallely, A., Kasindi, S., Chiduo, B., Desmond, N., Soteli, S., et al. (2008). A model for community representation and participation in HIV prevention trials among women who engage in transactional sex in Africa. *AIDS Care*, 20(9), 1039–49.

Shapiro, D. (2002). Renewing the scientist-practitioner model. *The Psychologist*, 15, 232–4.

Shaw, I. & Gould, N. (2001). *Qualitative research in social work*. London: Sage Publications.

Shields, N., Murdoch, A., Loy, Y., Dodd, K. & Taylor, N. (2006). A systematic review of the self concept of children with cerebral palsy compared with children without disability. *Developmental Medicine and Child Neurology*, 48, 151–57.

Shields, N., Taylor, N. & Dodd, K.J. (2008). Effects of a community-based progressive resistance strength training program on muscle performance and physical function in adults with Down syndrome: A randomized controlled trial. *Archives of Physical Medicine and Rehabilitation*, 89, 1215–20.

Shore, B. (1982). *Sala'ilua, a Samoan mystery*. New York: Columbia University Press.

Shostak, M. (1983). *Nisa: The life and words of a !Kung woman* (1st Vintage Books edn). New York: Vintage Books.

Shugg, J. & Liamputtong, P. (2002). Being female: The portrayal of women's health in print media. *Health Care for Women International*, 23(6–7), 715–28.

Siegel, S. & Castellan, N.J. (1988). *Nonparametric statistics for the behavioural sciences*, 2nd edn. New York: McGraw-Hill.

Sillitoe, P., Dixon, P. & Barr, J. (2005). Indigenous knowledge inquiries: A methodologies manual for development. Rugby: ITDG Publishing.

Silverman, D. (2000). *Doing qualitative research: A practical handbook*. London: Sage Publications.

Silverman, D. (2001). *Doing qualitative research*, 2nd edn. London: Sage Publications.

Simonds, J.F. (1977). Psychiatric status of diabetic youth matched with a control group. *Diabetes*, 26(10), 921–25.

Sinha, S., Curtis, K., Jayakody, A., Viner, R. & Roberts, H. (2007). 'People make assumptions about our communities': Sexual health amongst teenagers from black and minority ethnic backgrounds in East London. *Ethnicity & Health*, 12(5), 423–41.

Skeat, J. & Perry, A. (2008). Exploring the implementation and use of outcome measurement in practice: A qualitative study. *International Journal of Language & Communication Disorders*, 43(2), 110–25.

Slingsby, B.T. (2006). Professional approaches to stroke treatment in Japan: A relationship-centred model. *Journal of Evaluation in Clinical Practice*, 12(2), 218–26.

Smith, A.M.A., Rissel, C., Richters, J., Grulich, A.E. & De Visser, R.O. (2003). Sex in Australia: The rationale and methods of the Australian Study of Health and Relationships. [A survey of 19 307 people aged 16–59 years which had a broad focus across many aspects of sexual and reproductive health.]. *Australian and New Zealand Journal of Public Health*, 27(2), 106–17.

Smith, B. (2007). The state of the art in narrative inquiry. *Narrative Inquiry*, 17, 391–8.

Smith, D.E. (1987). *The everyday world as problematic: A feminist sociology*. Boston, MA: Northeastern University Press.

Smith, E. (2008). *Using secondary data in educational and social research*. Maidenhead, UK: McGraw-Hill/Open University Press.

Smith, J., Osman, C. & Goding, M. (1994). Reclaiming the emotional aspects of the therapist–Family system. *Australian and New Zealand Journal of Family Therapy*, 11(3), 139–46.

Smith, J.A. (1995). Semi-structured and qualitative analysis. In J.A. Smith, R. Harre & L. Van Langenhove (eds), *Rethinking methods in psychology*. London: Sage Publications, 9–25.

Smith, L.K., Draper, E.S., Manktelow, B.N., Dorling, J.S. & Field, D.J. (2007). Socioeconomic inequalities in very preterm birth rates. *Archives of Disease in Childhood—Fetal and Neonatal Edition*, 92, F11–14.

Smith, L.T. (1999). *Decolonizing methodologies: Research and Indigenous peoples*. Dunedin, NZ: University of Otago Press.

Solomon, D.H., Simel, D.L., Bates, D.W., Katz, J.N. & Schaffer, J.L. (2001). The rational clinical examination. Does this patient have a torn meniscus or ligament of the knee? Value of the physical examination. *Journal of the American Medical Association*, 286(13), 1610–20.

Stacey, J. (1988). Can there be a feminist ethnography? *Women's Studies Forum*, 11(1), 21–7.

Stalker, K. (1998). Some ethical and methodological issues in research with people with learning disabilities. *Disability and Society*, 13(1), 5–19.

Stanley, L. & Temple, B. (1995). Doing the business? Evaluating software packages to aid the analysis of qualitative data sets. *Studies in Qualitative Methodology*, 5, 169–97.

Stanley, M. & Cheek, J. (2003). Grounded theory: Exploiting the potential for occupational therapy. *British Journal of Occupational Therapy*, 66(4), 143–50.

Stapleton, E. (2008). The occupation of caring in later life for an adult child with a mental illness: A narrative study. Unpublished honours thesis. La Trobe University, Melbourne.

Stern, P. N. (1994). Eroding grounded theory. In J. Morse (ed.), *Critical issues in qualitative research methods*. Thousand Oaks, CA: Sage, 212–23.

Strathern, M. (ed.) (2000). Audit cultures: Anthropological studies in accountability, ethics and the academy. London: Routledge.

Straus, S.E., Richardson, W.S., Glasziou, P. & Haynes, R.B. (2005). *Evidence-based medicine: How to practice and teach EBM*. Edinburgh: Churchill Livingstone.

Strauss, A. (1987). *Qualitative analysis for social scientists*. Cambridge: Cambridge University Press.

Strauss, A. & Corbin, J. (1990). *Basics of qualitative research: Grounded theory procedures and techniques*. Newbury Park, CA: Sage.

Strauss, A. & Corbin, J. (1998). *Basics of qualitative research: Grounded theory procedures and techniques*, 2nd edn. Newbury Park, CA: Sage Publications.

Streiner, D.L. & Norman, G.R. (2003). *Health measurement scales: A practical guide to their development and use*, 3rd edn. Oxford: Oxford University Press.

Stringer, E.T. (1999). *Action research*, 2nd edn. Thousand Oaks, CA: Sage Publications.

Stringer, E. & Genat, W. (2004). *Action research in health*. New Jersey: Pearson.

Strolla, L.O., Gans, K.M. & Risica, P.M. (2006). Using qualitative and quantitative formative research to develop tailored nutrition intervention materials for a diverse low-income audience. *Health Education Research*, 21(4), 465–76.

Suddick, K.M. & De Souza, L. (2006). Therapists' experiences and perceptions of teamwork New York in neurological rehabilitation: Reasoning behind the team approach, structure and composition of the team and teamworking process. *Physiotherapy Research International,* 11(2), 72–83.

Sumsion, T. & Law, M. (2006). A review of evidence on the conceptual elements informing client-centred practice. *Canadian Journal of Occupational Therapy*, 73(3), 153–62.

Szklo, M. & Nieto, F.J. (2007). *Epidemiology: Beyond the basics*, 2nd edn. Boston, MA: Jones & Bartlett.

Tabachnick, B.G. & Fidell, L.S. (2006). *Using multivariate statistics*, 5th edn. Boston, MA: Pearson/Allyn & Bacon.

Takeuchi, R., O'Brien, M.M., Ormond, K.B., Brown, S.D.J. & Maly, M.R. (2008). 'Moving forward': Success from a physiotherapist's point of view. *Physiotherapy Canada*, 60, 19–29.

Tashakkori, A. & Teddlie, C. (2003). A general typology of research designs featuring mixed methods. *Research in the Schools*, 13(1), 12–28.

Tashakkori, A. & Teddlie, C. (2003). *Handbook of mixed methods in social & behavioral research*. Thousand Oaks, CA: Sage Publications.

Tashakkori, A. & Teddlie, C. (2003). Issues and dilemmas in teaching research methods courses in social and behavioural sciences: US perspective *International Journal of Social Research Methodology*, 6(1), 61–77.

Tattersall, R.B. (1985). Brittle diabetes. *British Medical Journal*, 291, 555–6.

Taylor, M.C. (2005). Interviewing. In I. Holloway (ed.), *Qualitative research in health care*. Maidenhead, UK: Open University Press, 39–55.

Teddlie, C. & Yu, F. (2007). Mixed method sampling: A typology with examples. *Journal of Mixed Methods Research*, 1(1), 77–100.

Teddlie, C. & Tashakkori, A. (2009). *Foundations of mixed methods research: Integrating quantitative and qualitative approaches in the social and behavioral sciences*. Thousand Oaks, CA: Sage Publications.

Tedlock, B. (2005). The observation of participation and the emergence of public ethnography. In N.K. Denzin & Y.S. Lincoln (eds), *The Sage handbook of qualitative research*. Thousand Oaks, CA: Sage Publications, 467–78.

Terwee, C.B., Bot, A.D.M., de Boer, M.R., van der Windt, D.A.W.M., Knol, D.L., Dekker, J., et al. (2007). Quality criteria were proposed for measurement properties of health status questionnaires. *Journal of Clinical Epidemiology*, 60, 34–42.

Thompson, C. & Learmonth, M. (2002). How can we develop an evidence based culture? In J. Craig & R. Smyth (eds), *The evidence-based practice manual for nurses*. Edinburgh: Churchill Livingstone, 211–36.

Thorne, S. (2000). Data analysis in qualitative research. *Evidence Based Nursing*, 3(3), 68–70.

Thurston, W., Cove, L. & Meadows, L. (2008). Methodological congruence in complex and collaborative mixed method studies. *International Journal of Multiple Research Approaches*, 2(1), 2–14.

Tobin, G.A. & Begley, C.M. (2004). Methodological rigour within a qualitative framework. *Journal of Advanced Nursing*, 48(4), 388–96.

Todres, I. (2005). Clarifying the life-world: Descriptive phenomenology. In I. Holloway (ed.), *Qualitative research in health care*. Oxford: Blackwell, 104–24.

Torgerson, D.J. & Roberts, C. (1999). Understanding controlled trials: Randomisation methods: concealment. *British Medical Journal*, 319, 375–6.

Torgerson, D.J. & Torgerson, C.J. (2008). *Designing randomised trials in health education and the social sciences: An introduction*. Basingstoke, UK: Palgrave Macmillan.

Torrance, H. (2008). Building confidence in qualitative research: Engaging the demands of policy. *Qualitative Inquiry*, 14(4), 507–27.

Travers, K. (1996). The social organization of nutritional inequities. *Social Science and Medicine*, 43, 543–53.

Trulsson, U. & Klingberg, G. (2003). Living with a child with a severe orofacial handicap: Experience from the perspectives of parents. *European Journal of Oral Science*, 111(1), 19–25.

Tsang, E.Y.L., Liamputtong, P. & Pierson, J. (2003). The views of older Chinese people in Melbourne about their quality of life. *Ageing and Society*, 24, 51–74.

Turner, V.W. (1968). *Schism and continuity in an African society: A study of Ndembu village life*. Manchester: Published on behalf of the Institute for Social Research, University of Zambia, by Manchester University Press.

Ukrainetz, T.A. & Frequez, E.F. (2003). 'What isn't language?': A qualitative study of the role of the school speech-language pathologist. *Language, Speech, and Hearing Services in Schools*, 34(4), 284–98.

Unrau, Y.A., Grinnell, R.M. & Williams, M. (2008). The quantitative research approach. In R.M. Grinnell & Y.A. Unrau (eds), *Social work research and evaluation: Foundations of evidence-based practice*, 8th edn. New York: Oxford University Press, 62–81.

Vallely, A., Shagi, C., Kasindi, S., Desmond, N., Lees, S., Chiduo, B., et al. (2007). The benefits of participatory methodologies to develop effective community dialogue in the context of a microbicide trial feasibility study in Mwanza, Tanzania. *BMC Public Health*, 7, 133.

van Manen, M. (1997). From meaning to method. *Qualitative Health Research*, 7(3), 345–69.

van Manen, M. (2006). Writing qualitatively, or the demands of writing. *Qualitative Health Research*, 16(5), 713–22.

van Tulder, M., Assendelft, W., Koes, B., Bouter, L. & the Editorial Board of the Cochrane Collaboration Back Review Group. Method guidelines for systematic reviews in the Cochrane Collaboration Back Review Group for Spinal Disorders. *Spine*, 22, 2323–30.

van Usen, C. & Pumberger, B. (2007). Effectiveness of eccentric exercises in the management of chronic Achilles tendinosis. *Internet Journal of Allied Health Sciences and Practice*, 5(2), 1–14.

Velicer, W.F., Prochaska, J.O., Fava, J.L., Norman, G.J. & Redding, C.A. (1998). Smoking cessation and stress management: Applications of the transtheoretical model of behavior change. *Homeostasis*, 38, 216–33.

Victorian Department of Human Services (2009). Victorian Health Information Surveillance System. <www.health.vic.gov.au/healthstatus/vhiss/index.htm>, accessed 23 March 2009.

Vlayen, J., Aertgeerts, B., Hannes, K., Sermeus, W. & Ramaekers, D. (2005). A systematic review of appraisal tools for clinical practice guidelines: Multiple similarities and one common deficit. *International Journal for Quality in Health Care*, 17(3), 235–42.

Vogt, D.S., King, D.W. & King, L.A. (2004). Focus groups in psychological assessment: Enhancing content validity by consulting members of the target population. *Psychological Assessment*, 16(3), 231–43.

Wacjman, J. & Martin, B. (2002). Narratives of identity in modern management: The corrosion of gender difference? *Sociology* 36(4), 985–1002. <http://soc.sagepub.com/cgi/content/abstract/36/4/985>, accessed 1 January 2009.

Walsh, D. & Downe, S. (2005). Meta-synthesis method for qualitative research: A literature review. *Journal of Advanced Nursing*, 94, 661–4.

Wand, A. & Eades, S. (2008). Navigating the process of developing a health research project in Aboriginal health. *Medical Journal of Australia*, 188(10), 584–6.

Wang, D. & Bakhai, A. (2006). *Clinical trials: A practical guide to design, analysis, and reporting*. London: Remedica.

Wang, R., Lagakos, S.W., Ware, J.H., Hunter, D.J. & Drazen, J.M. (2007). Statistics in medicine: Reporting of subgroup analyses in clinical trials. *New England Journal of Medicine*, 357(21), 2189–94.

Waples-Crowe, P. & Pyett, P. (2005). *The making of a great relationship: A review of a healthy partnership between mainstream and Indigenous organisations*. Melbourne: Victorian Aboriginal Community Controlled Health Organisation.

Ware, J.E., Kosinski, M. & Keller, S.D. (1994). *SF-36 Physical and Mental Health Summary Scales: A user's manual*. Boston, MA: The Health Institute, New England Medical Center.

Warr, D. & Pyett, P. (1999). Difficult relations: Sex work, love and intimacy. *Sociology of Health & Illness*, 21(3), 290–309.

Waterman, H. (1998). Embracing ambiguities and valuing ourselves: Issues of validity in action research. *Journal of Advanced Nursing*, 28(1), 101–05.

Waters, M. (Writer) (2004). *Mean girls*. In L. Michaels, T. Shimkin, L. Rosner, J.S. Messick & J. Guinier (Producer). USA: Paramount Pictures.

Weaver, A. & Atkinson, P. (1995). *Microcomputing and qualitative data analysis*. Aldershot: Avebury.

Weitzman, E.A. & Miles, M.B. (1995). Choosing software for qualitative data analysis: An overview. *Field Methods*, 7, 1–5.

Westhues, A., Ochocka, J., Jacobson, N., Simich, L., Maiter, S., Janzen, R. & Fleras, A. (2008). Developing theory from complexity: Reflections on a collaborative mixed method participatory action research study. *Qualitative Health Research*, 18(5), 701–17.

White, S. (2001). Auto-ethnography as reflexive inquiry: The research act as self-surveillance. In I. Shaw & N. Gould (eds), *Qualitative research in social work*. Newbury Park, CA: Sage Publications, 100–15.

Whiting, P., Rutjes, A., Reitsma, J., Bossuyt, P. & Kleijnen, J. (2003). The development of QUADAS: a tool for the quality assessment of studies of diagnostic accuracy included in systematic reviews. *BMC Medical Research Methodology*, 3, 25.

WHO (World Health Organization), Health and Welfare Canada & Canadian Public Health Association. (1986). *Ottawa charter for health promotion*. Ottawa: World Health Organization.

WHO (2001). *International classification of functioning, disability and health: Short version*. Geneva: World Health Organisation.

WHO (2006). *Reproductive Health Indicators. Guidelines for their generation, interpretation and analysis for global monitoring*. Geneva: World Health Organization.

WHO (2008). *Indicator definitions and metadata, 2008*. <www.who.int/whosis/indicators/compendium/2008/en/>, accessed 13 February 2009.

WHO (2009). *International Clinical Trials Registry Platform (ICTRP)*: World Health Organization. <www.who.int/ictrp/en/>.

Wiles, R., Heath, S. & Crow, G. (2005). Methods briefing 2: Informed consent and the research process (ESRC Research Methods Programme). Available at <www.esrc.ac.uk/methods/>.

Wilkinson, S. (1998). Focus groups in health research: Exploring the meanings of health and illness. *Journal of Health Psychology*, 3(3), 329–48.

Williams, M., Unrau, Y.A. & Grinnell, R.M. (2008). The qualitative research approach. In R.M. Grinnell & Y.A. Unrau (eds), *Social work research and evaluation: Foundations of evidence-based practice*, 8th edn. New York: Oxford University Press, 84–101.

Williamson, K. (2008). Where information is paramount: A mixed methods, multidisciplinary investigation of Australian on-line investor. *iRinformationresearch* 13(4). <http://informationr.net/ir/13-4/paper365.html>, accessed 1 January 2009.

Willke, R.J., Burke, L.B. & Erickson, P. (2004). Measuring treatment impact: A review of patient-reported outcomes and other efficacy endpoints in approved product labels. *Controlled Clinical Trials*, 25(6), 535–52.

Willis, J.W. (2007). *Foundations of qualitative research: Interpretive and critical approaches*. Thousand Oaks, CA: Sage Publications.

Willis, J. & Saunders, M. (2007). Research in a post-colonial world. In M. Pitts & A. Smith (eds), *Researching the margins: Strategies for ethical and rigorous research with marginalised communities*. Basingstoke, UK: Palgrave Macmillan, 96–113.

Willis, K., Green, J., Daly, J., Williamson, L. & Bandyopadhyay, M. (2009). Perils and possibilities: Achieving best evidence from focus groups in public health research. *Australian and New Zealand Journal of Public Health*, 33(2), 131–6.

Wilson, H.S. & Hutchinson, S.A. (1996). Methodological mistakes in grounded theory. *Nursing Research*, 45(2), 122–4.

Wilson, M.G., Goetzel, R.Z., Ozminkowski, R.J., Dejoy, D.M., Della, L., Roemer, E.C., Schneider, J., Tully, K.J., White, J.M. & Baase, C.M. (2007). Using formative research to develop environmental and ecological interventions to address overweight and obesity. *Obesity*, 15, 37S–47S.

Winbolt, M., Nay, R. & Fetherstonhaugh, D. (in press). Taking a TEAM (Translating Evidence into Aged care Methods) approach to practice change. In R. Nay & S. Garrett (eds), *Older people: Issues and innovations in care*. Sydney: Elsevier Australia, 442–55.

Winkelman, W. & Halifax, N. (2007). Power is only skin deep: An institutional ethnography of nurse-driven outpatient psoriasis treatment in the era of clinic web sites. *Journal of Medical Systems*, 31(2), 131–39.

Wolcott, H. (1990). Making a study 'more ethnographic'. *Journal of Contemporary Ethnography*, 19(1), 44–72.

Wolcott, H.F. (2009). *Writing up qualitative research*, 3rd edn. Thousand Oaks, CA: Sage Publications.

Wood, L., Egger, M., Gluud, L.L., Schulz, K.F., Jüni, P., Altman, D.G., et al. (2008). Empirical evidence of bias in treatment effect estimates in controlled trials with different interventions and outcomes: Meta-epidemiological study. *British Medical Journal*, 336, 601–05.

Woodley, B.L., Newsham-West, R.J. & Baxter, G.D. (2007). Chronic tendinopathy: effectiveness of eccentric exercise. *British Journal of Sports Medicine,* 41(4), 188–98; discussion 199.

World Medical Association (2008). World Medical Association Declaration of Helsinki: *Ethical principles for medical research involving human subjects*. <www.wma.net/e/policy/b3.htm>.

World Medical Organisation (2008). *The World Medical Association Declaration of Helsinki: Ethical principles for medical research involving human subjects*. Seoul: Department of Health.

Wright-Mills, C. (1967). *The sociological imagination*. London: Oxford University Press.

Zwarenstein, M. & Treweek, S. (2009). What kind of randomized trials do we need? *Journal of Clinical Epidemiology*, 62(5), 461–3.

Index